Resources for Instructor Success—

Instructor's Resource Manual
ISBN 0-13-113732-8
This manual contains a wealth of material to help faculty plan and manage their LPN/LVN nursing courses. It includes detailed learning outcomes, lecture outlines, teaching suggestions for the classroom and clinical settings, and more for each chapter. This supplement is available to faculty upon adoption of the textbook as an online download.

Instructor's Resource CD-ROM
ISBN: 0-13-113733-6
This comprehensive resource CD-ROM is available to faculty upon adoption of the textbook and provides:

- Instructor's Resource Manual. This manual contains a wealth of material to help faculty plan and manage their LPN/LVN nursing courses. It includes detailed learning outcomes, lecture outlines, teaching suggestions for the classroom and clinical settings and more for each chapter.
- Animations and video library
- Image Library
- Test Generator
- PowerPoint Lecture Slides

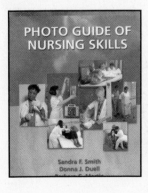

Photo Guide of Nursing Skills
Provides a full-color atlas of all basic and intermediate skills. Its unique, easy-to-use format presents each procedure in logical steps—complete with appropriate illustrations, descriptions, and rationales. A critical thinking section focuses on unexpected outcomes.
ISBN: 0-8385-8174-9
Smith, Duell & Martin

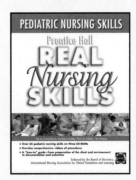

Prentice Hall Real Nursing Skills
The volumes in this series consist of CD-ROMs with comprehensive procedures and rationales demonstrated in hundreds of realistic video clips, animations, illustrations, and photographs. This is the only skills series designed to help students and practicing nurses visualize how to perform clinical nursing skills and understand the concepts and rationales for each skill.
Pediatric Nursing Skills
ISBN: 0-13-191524-X

Brief Table of Contents

Pediatric

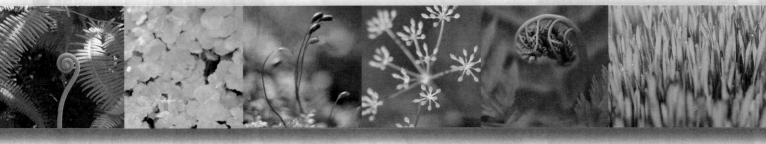

Nursing Care

Pediatric

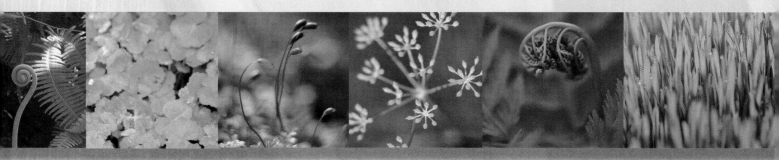

Nursing Care

Ellise D. Adams, CNM, MSN, CD (DONA), ICCE
Clinical Assistant Professor
University of Alabama Huntsville
Huntsville, Alabama

Mary Ann Towle, RN, MEd, MSN
Faculty
Boise State University
Boise, Idaho

PEARSON

Prentice
Hall

Upper Saddle River, New Jersey 07458

Library of Congress Cataloging-in-Publication Data

Adams, Ellise D.
   Pediatric nursing care / Ellise D. Adams, Mary Ann Towle.
      p. ; cm.
   Includes bibliographical references and index.
   ISBN-13: 978-0-13-237986-1
   ISBN-10: 0-13-237986-4
   1. Pediatric nursing. I. Towle, Mary Ann. II. Title.
   [DNLM: 1. Pediatric Nursing—methods. 2. Community
   Health Nursing—methods. 3. Nursing, Practical—methods.
   WY 159 A193p 2009]
   RJ245.A315 2009
   618.92'00231—dc22   2007042125

Publisher: Julie Levin Alexander
Assistant to Publisher: Regina Bruno
Editor-in-Chief: Maura Connor
Senior Acquisitions Editor: Kelly Trakalo
Development Editor: Rachel Bedard
Editorial Assistant: JulieAnn Oliveros
Media Product Manager: John Jordan
Director of Marketing: Karen Allman
Senior Marketing Manager: Francisco Del Castillo
Marketing Coordinator: Michael Sirinides
Managing Editor, Production: Patrick Walsh
Production Liaison: Yagnesh Jani
Production Editor: Carol Singer, GGS Book Services
Media Project Manager: Stephen Hartner
Manufacturing Manager/Buyer: Ilene Sanford
Composition: GGS Book Services
Printer/Binder: R.R. Donnelley
Senior Design Coordinator: Maria Guglielmo-Walsh
Cover Designer: Mary Siener
Cover Illustration: Ti Leaves Background and Image, Dana Edmunds/Pacific Stock; Fern Bud, Eyewire/Getty Images, Inc.; Plant Buds, Photodisc/Getty Images, Inc.; Fiddlehead, Mary Siener; Sprouting Plants, Creatas Images/Jupiter Images; Flower buds (close-up), Michael Banks/Getty Images Inc.; Greenery, Creatas Images/Jupiter Images.
Pearson Education LTD.
Pearson Education Australia PTY, Limited
Pearson Education Singapore, Pte. Ltd
Pearson Education North Asia Ltd
Pearson Education Canada, Ltd.
Pearson Educación de Mexico, S.A. de C.V.
Pearson Education—Japan
Pearson Education Malaysia, Pte. Ltd
Pearson Education, Upper Saddle River, New Jersey

Notice: Care has been taken to confirm the accuracy of information presented in this book. The authors, editors, and the publisher, however, cannot accept any responsibility for errors or omissions or for consequences from application of the information in this book and make no warranty, express or implied, with respect to its contents.

The authors and publisher have exerted every effort to ensure that drug selections and dosages set forth in this text are in accord with current recommendations and practice at time of publication. However, in view of ongoing research, changes in government regulations, and the constant flow of information relating to drug therapy and reactions, the reader is urged to check the package inserts of all drugs for any change in indications or dosage and for added warning and precautions. This is particularly important when the recommended agent is a new and/or infrequently employed drug.

10 9 8 7 6 5 4 3 2 1
ISBN-13: 978-0-13-237986-1
ISBN-10: 0-13-237986-4

Student Success is built-in from the start...

Practical and vocational nurses from around the country told us that they needed two things to succeed as students in order to achieve their LPN/LVN licenses. First, they needed books that explain what the LPN/LVN needs to know and do. Second, they needed a variety of excellent review materials to reinforce their learning. ***Pediatric Nursing Care*** contains power-packed, built-in support to ensure your success throughout your LPN/LVN education.

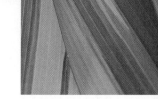

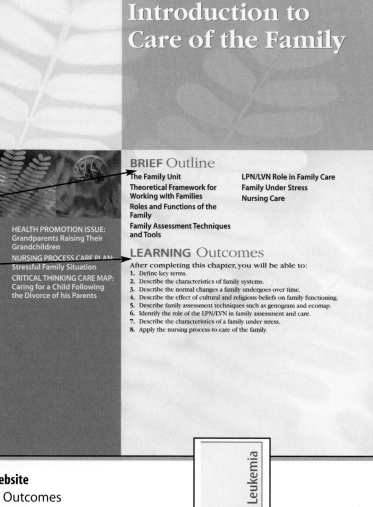

Chapter 4

Introduction to Care of the Family

HEALTH PROMOTION ISSUE: Grandparents Raising Their Grandchildren

NURSING PROCESS CARE PLAN: Stressful Family Situation

CRITICAL THINKING CARE MAP: Caring for a Child Following the Divorce of his Parents

BRIEF Outline

The Family Unit
Theoretical Framework for Working with Families
Roles and Functions of the Family
Family Assessment Techniques and Tools
LPN/LVN Role in Family Care
Family Under Stress
Nursing Care

LEARNING Outcomes

After completing this chapter, you will be able to:
1. Define key terms.
2. Describe the characteristics of family systems.
3. Describe the normal changes a family undergoes over time.
4. Describe the effect of cultural and religious beliefs on family functioning.
5. Describe family assessment techniques such as genogram and ecomap.
6. Identify the role of the LPN/LVN in family assessment and care.
7. Describe the characteristics of a family under stress.
8. Apply the nursing process to care of the family.

As you start each chapter—

Brief Outlines preview what the chapter will cover for quick access and review.

Learning Outcomes identify what you can expect to learn from each chapter and help you focus your reading.

MediaLinks call your attention to the additional learning tools that are available on the CD-ROM and Companion Website that accompany your textbook, including:

Prentice Hall Nursing MediaLink CD-ROM
- Learning Outcomes
- Audio Glossary—key terms, definitions, and pronunciations
- NCLEX-PN® Review Questions
- Animations & Videos—difficult concepts brought to life

Companion Website
- Learning Outcomes
- Chapter Outlines
- Audio Glossary
- NCLEX-PN® Review Questions
- Key Term Review—matching questions and crossword puzzles to help with new terminology and definitions.
- Case Studies—scenarios and critical-thinking questions
- Challenge Your Knowledge—visual critical thinking questions
- WebLinks—content-related hyperlinks
- Nursing Tools—handy reference materials

MediaLink Tabs MediaLink Tabs prompt you to explore videos, animations, and activities on the Student CD-ROM and Companion Website.

Makes need-to-know information easy to find and use!

Pediatric Nursing Care contains color-coded boxes and tables with important information for you to remember.

BOX 11-4 CLIENT TEACHING

Toilet Training

Determining Readiness

Although readiness is individualized, the child must have achieved the following developmental skills:

- Stand and walk
- Pull pants up and down
- Recognize need to "go"
- Can wait to reach bathroom

Helpful Hints

- If child is afraid of toilet, use small chair or small toilet seat insert.
- If using toilet, place sturdy stool in front of toilet for child to stand on to reach the seat.
- Place child on seat upon rising in the morning, before and after naps, before bath, before bed, and at regular intervals through the day.
- Teach hand washing after toileting.
- Praise success. Do not punish accidents.
- If child does not cooperate, wait a few weeks and try again.

Client Teaching and Nutrition Therapy boxes help you prepare for your role as educators in health care settings.

BOX 25-3 NUTRITION THERAPY

Foods for a Low-Salt, Low-Protein Diet

Low-Salt Diet

- The health care professional will order the amount of restriction (e.g., a 2-g Na diet). Most foods do contain some sodium, so foods that are lowest in sodium should be selected.
- The nurse reinforces the following guidelines to help the client (or parents) maintain a low-salt diet:
  - Check labels for Na (sodium).
  - Add no salt to foods.
  - Avoid salty snacks (chips, salty popcorn, pretzels with salt).
  - Avoid processed, prepared foods because they tend to contain higher levels of sodium.

Low-Protein Diet

- The health care professional will order the amount of restriction (e.g., a 40-g protein diet)
- The nurse reinforces the following guidelines to help the client (or parents) maintain a low-protein diet:
  - All meats and milk are high in protein (about 3 oz meat = 8 g protein).
  - Cereal/bread and vegetables are moderate to low in protein.
    - ½ cup cereal or 1 slice bread = 2 g protein
    - ½ cup vegetables = 1 g protein
  - Avoid seafood.
  - Limit meat to half of a serving.
  - Use bread and vegetables for foo

Life Span Considerations boxes and **Communicating Across the Lifespan** provide perspective on adapting nursing interventions to different developmental levels.

---

clinical ALERT

Because of the life-threatening nature of epiglottitis, infants and toddlers who cannot ask for help must not be left alone during the acute phase of epiglottitis.

Clinical Alerts call the student's attention to clinical roles and responsibilities for heightened awareness, monitoring, and/or reporting

---

BOX 18-9 LIFE SPAN CONSIDERATIONS

Vaccine Against Human Papillomavirus

Parents have a new immunization decision to make with the recent recommendation from the FDA and the CDC regarding Gardasil, the vaccine against HPV. The nurse can assist parents in understanding how HPV is transmitted, how it relates to cervical cancer, and how it can be prevented. Parents should be taught that the vaccine is most effective when given prior to the initiation of sexual activity. Parents may have concerns that vaccinating their daughters is an acknowledgment that they will become sexually active. The nurse can help parents explore these feelings and compare risks and benefits related to the vaccine. The nurse can help parents understand that even if their daughters abstain from sexual activity until they are in a monogamous relationship, there is no guarantee that their partner has been abstinent. Therefore it is possible that he carries the virus. This is an appropriate time for the nurse to assist parents in health promotion teaching regarding sexual activity.

TABLE 14-4

Pharmacology: Drugs Used for Conscious Sedation

DRUG	USUAL ROUTE/DOSE	CLASSIFICATION	SELECTED SIDE EFFECTS	DON'T GIVE IF
Diazepam (Valium)	IM/IV # 5 years 0.2–0.5 mg slowly every 2–5 minutes up to 5 mg $ 5 years 1 mg every 5 minutes up to 10 mg	Anxiolytic, anticonvulsant	Drowsiness, dizziness, hypotension, respiratory distress	Other drugs are being administered; (do not mix)
Midazolam (Versed)	IM 0.08 mg/kg IV 0.15 mg/kg followed by 0.05 mg/kg every 2 minutes × one to three doses	Short-acting benzodiazepine anxiolytic, sedative hypnotic	Retrograde amnesia, respiratory distress, hypotension	Severe organic heart disease; caution with renal or hepatic impairment
Lorazepam (Ativan)	PO, IV, IM 0.05 mg/kg	Benzodiazepine anxiolytic, sedative hypnotic	Drowsiness, sedation, respiratory distress	Child is younger than 12 years

Pharmacology tables reinforce selected common medications nurses will encounter in practice. Additional boxes and tables offer information on key topics.

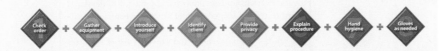

PROCEDURE 13-26 Administering Oxygen to Children

Purpose
- To provide the prescribed concentration of oxygen to the child

Equipment
- Oxygen supply, including a flowmeter
- Device to humidify the oxygen
- Nasal cannula, face masks, or oxygen tent
- Oxygen tubing

Check order + Gather equipment + Introduce yourself + Identify client + Provide privacy + Explain procedure + Hand hygiene + Gloves as needed

Interventions
- Perform preparatory steps (see icon bar).
- Set up oxygen delivery method, including humidification.
- Turn on oxygen to prescribed flow rate.
- Place the face mask over the bridge of the child's nose to the cleft of the chin (see Figure 13-33). OR
- Place the nasal cannula into the anterior nares and put an elastic band around the child's head. OR
- Surround the child in the hospital bed with the oxygen tent. Secure the edges of the tent to deliver prescribed oxygen dosage and prevent escape of oxygen.

SAMPLE DOCUMENTATION

(date) 0700 (Note: Oxygenation portion only. This is a focused part of a complete documentation entry.) O₂ per nasal cannula at 2 L/minute applied. Band secured around head.

_____ K. Coffey, LPN

Procedures Procedures give step-by-step instructions and rationales for nursing actions. Special icons in the procedures reinforce essential preliminary steps in client care. "Live" documentation at the end of each procedure demonstrates samples of good record-keeping.

HEALTH PROMOTION ISSUE

DEVELOPING A THERAPEUTIC RELATIONSHIP WITH A PEDIATRIC CLIENT

The LPN/LVN working in a pediatrician's office is approached by a recently hired LPN/LVN. Her past nursing experience has been with adult clients in an acute-care setting. She states that she has never worked with children before and is having some difficulty relating to them. She is most distressed that the children seem afraid of her. The children will not open up to her and talk to her about issues related to their health care. She is concerned that these factors will affect the type of nursing care she is able to give and ultimately affect the child's health care. She wants some assistance in performing her nursing tasks without scaring the children.

DISCUSSION

For the nurse to assist the child to become healthy, a positive nurse–client relationship must be established. This relationship develops over time, demonstrates respect and confidentiality, is client focused and not nurse focused, and has respect and mutual trust as its basis.

For the relationship between a child and a nurse to be therapeutic, the nurse must display caring behaviors mixed with a professional attitude that conveys competence. Trust develops when children believe that the nurse cares about them and is capable of helping them through a situation. Trust develops as the nurse:

- Listens attentively to what the child says, even if the child is talking about cartoons or toys.
- Displays empathy. Empathy includes recognizing the child's needs, acknowledging the child as real, and showing the child that the nurse is working diligently to meet expressed needs.
- Is honest with the child. Children can see through dishonesty. They need

straight, simple responses or an honest "I don't know."
- Is genuine. Caring cannot be contrived. Caring for a child requires knowledge of their developmental levels, of their emotional status, and of their social history. The genuine nurse displays spontaneous behaviors that seek to restore and protect the child.

As the nurse communicates with children, she must recognize that this is accomplished both verbally and nonverbally. Although many people think that spoken words convey our message, in actuality nonverbal communication conveys more than 80% of our message. Nonverbal communication includes our personal appearance. It is said that an opinion of us is formed by other individuals within the first 3 seconds of our first encounter. This opinion is developed before we ever say a word and is largely based on our dress, our posture, our facial expressions, and our gait.

Verbal communication is more than the words we say; it is also how we say them. The nurse can communicate a message effectively by speaking with enthusiasm, energy, and at a pace that indicates interest and not anxiety. Verbal communication should be easy to understand, clear, and as brief as possible.

The timing of verbal communication is also important. The message can go unheard if the child is not ready or willing to listen.

Children learn in different ways. Some must hear the information, whereas others must see it. Still others need to use their hands (e.g., write information or handle a stethoscope) before they can learn.

Developmental levels also influence how a child learns. For instance, a pre-

schooler enjoys learning by trial and error. An adolescent needs to learn independently.

The nurse must consider the child's vocabulary, education, psychomotor abilities, emotional status, societal values, and attention span when developing a teaching plan.

It is also important to choose an appropriate teaching strategy. The nurse can use demonstration to teach a skill and then ask the child to return demonstration. The nurse could also model specific behaviors. Teaching aids may assist the nurse in communicating the proper information. Written materials, posters, anatomic models, games, videos, computers, or dolls may be used in both formal teaching and informal teaching.

PLANNING AND IMPLEMENTATION

Development of a Nurse–Client Relationship

Prior to the child's appointment, the nurse reviews the child's chart, noting any medical or social history that would impact the behavior of the child. The nurse should note the child's age and recall information about the appro-

priate developmental age. The nurse should practice pronouncing the child's name and note any special likes or dislikes that are noted in the chart. For example, if the child likes a certain cartoon character, the nurse might be able to find a Band-Aid with that character on it or place the child in an exam room decorated with this character. Be sure to include this documentation in the child's chart and update as needed.

Social interaction at the beginning of the appointment is necessary to help ease the child's anxiety and to develop a trusting relationship. The nurse should be at eye level with the child when speaking directly to him or her (see Figure 13-1). Initially, the nurse should avoid touching the child until trust is established.

As the appointment progresses and the nurse seeks to understand the health care needs of the child, listening becomes vital. Active listening requires much energy and is vital in achieving trust. Listening behaviors include eye contact and body language that suggests a willingness to listen (e.g., relaxed body parts, a face-to-face position, a slight leaning toward the child). Listening also requires silence on the nurse's part. As the child speaks, the nurse must actively consider the child's words and not try to develop a wise or witty comeback while the child is speaking. Only after gathering all subjective and objective data can the nurse develop a plan of action. Plans developed before data collection is complete are likely to be ineffective.

Appropriate Communication Techniques

Pediatric nurses often choose brightly-colored uniforms that will appeal to children. Hair should be neat. Makeup should look natural, so as not to distract or frighten the child. Posture should be erect but not tense.

Children can read the thoughts of the nurse through the nurse's facial expressions. It is important for nurses to learn to control feelings of disgust, impatience, or boredom. The nurse's face needs to display interest, enthusiasm, and energy. If a child confides that he or she has been abused by an adult, the nurse must not express horror or anger. The nurse's face should convey interest and concern so the child will continue to share information.

When communicating verbally with children, the nurse should speak to the child in language and terms that they can understand. The nurse should use open-ended questions when trying to obtain information from a child. Questions such as "Tell me how your tummy feels" or "What happened to your leg?" will elicit more information than a question that can simply be answered "yes" or "no."

Appropriate Teaching Methods

The nurse needs to have a variety of teaching aids available in order to conduct formal or informal teaching for the child. A simple drawing of the

body can help the nurse describe a disease, procedure, or surgery. Dolls or puppets appeal to preschoolers.

In school settings, videos are often a way of providing information. If videos are used, the dialogue should be appropriate for the age group. Slides or photographs should also be age appropriate. For example, photographs of genitalia should not be shown in a classroom of mixed genders. The nurse should carefully assess readiness to learn and evaluate learning following the teaching session.

With diligence and continued effort, the nurse should be able to relate to the pediatric client and provide effective care.

SELF-REFLECTION

When a child reacts negatively to you, what feelings do you have? If a child has never acted negatively to you, imagine what the scenario might look like. Be honest about your feelings. When you encounter a strange environment, what factors make you feel more uncomfortable? What factors make you feel more comfortable? What do you need to change in your nursing practice to help develop trust with your clients? To communicate better with your pediatric clients? To be more effective in providing them with teaching as it relates to their health care?

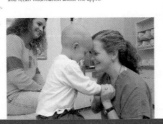

SUGGESTED RESOURCES

For the Nurse

www.ChildbirthGraphics.com The catalog available at this website can provide the nurse with posters, pamphlets, three-dimensional models, and videos to assist in health care teaching.

Blackwell, P., & Baker, B. (2002). Estimating communication competence of infants and toddlers. *Journal of Pediatric Health Care, 16*(1), 19–35.

Humphries, J. (2002). The school health nurse and health education in the classroom. *Nursing Standard, 16*(17), 42–45.

Sydnor-Greenberg, N., & Dokken, D. (2001). Communication in healthcare: Thought on the child's perspective. *Journal of Child and Family Nursing, 4*(3), 225–230.

Health Promotion Issues examine topical issues and show students how to move from problems to solutions as they care for clients.

Learn to prioritize nursing actions and deliver safe, effective nursing care as part of the health care team!

Nursing Care Nursing Care is presented in the five-step nursing process format, but emphasizing the scope of practice for the LPN/LVN. Rationales after each nursing intervention explain why the action is important and support evidence-based nursing process.

NURSING CARE
PRIORITIES IN NURSING CARE

When caring for individuals, remember to include family members as well. Focus your care on establishing a therapeutic relationship based on trust. Be careful to develop a nonthreatening, nonjudgmental attitude when family values and behaviors differ from yours. Use positive, supportive words of encouragement and provide a list of resources for family support.

Critical Thinking questions allow students to apply their new knowledge to a specific client.

Critical Thinking in the Nursing Process

1. What conditions may have led to the sickle cell crisis?
2. When performing physical interventions with this client, what concern will be most important?
3. What nonpharmacologic interventions can be used in this situation?

Note: Discussion of Critical Thinking questions appears in Appendix I.

Priorities in Nursing Care focus thinking on key assessments and interventions.

Nursing Care Plan Chart
Respiratory Syncytial Virus

GOAL	INTERVENTION	RATIONALE	EXPECTED OUTCOME
1. Ineffective Airway Clearance related to inflammation of the bronchioles			
The child's airway will be clear within 48 hours	Monitor vital signs every hour.	*The child's condition can change rapidly and therefore must be closely monitored*	The child will be able to breathe at a rate and depth considered within normal limits (see Table 12-1).
	Monitor oxygen saturation continuously. See Procedure 8-29 ⬀.	*Continuous monitoring of oxygen saturation will alert the nurse if the child's condition deteriorates.*	Oxygen saturation will be at 95%.
	Administer oxygen as ordered. See Procedure 8-28 ⬀.	*Oxygen is administered to maintain oxygen saturation above 95%.*	
	Anticipate worsening respiratory distress by monitoring breath sounds, respiratory effort, and level of consciousness.	*Anticipating a worsening of the child's condition allows the nurse time to prepare for airway maintenance.*	
	Reposition every ½ hour.	*Frequent position changes facilitate drainage of respiratory mucus*	
	Administer IV fluids via appropriate equipment.	*IV fluids are administered by infusion pump to prevent accidental fluid overload*	
	Administer medications with careful attention to dosage.	*Pediatric dosage is individualized based on body weight. If dosage is not calculated carefully, overdosage or underdosage could occur. To maintain medication blood level in a therapeutic range, medications must be administered on time*	
The family will be able to execute an effective plan of care for the child at home.	Teach the family to recognize changes in respiratory status.	*Prompt recognition of symptoms will facilitate treatment*	The family manages respirator
	Demonstrate and observe a return demonstration of postural drainage techniques.	*Learning is enhanced when procedures are demonstrated and correct learning can be documented by return demonstration*	

Nursing Process Care Plans and **Charts** illustrate nursing care in "real-life" scenarios and reinforce the progression from goals to interventions to outcomes.

NURSING PROCESS CARE PLAN
Client with Sickle Cell Anemia

An 8-year-old girl was admitted yesterday to the facility in sickle cell crisis. Her family was vacationing when the crisis began, and they drove several hours back by car in order to admit their daughter to her "home" hospital. A blood transfusion and fluids have been administered. She is receiving oxygen at 2 liters per minute. The parents state that their son has a cold, but that they "were sure Yolanda did not have it" when they started their trip. When you enter the room, Yolanda is moaning. She cries when you say it is time to reposition her in bed. She states she does not want to have a position change because "it hurts too much to move."

Assessment. When caring for Yolanda, the following data should be collected:

- Status of pain: location, intensity, duration, alleviating factors
- Vital signs
- Intake and output
- Skin (pallor, cyanosis, tenting)
- Review of lab work

Nursing Diagnosis. The following important nursing diagnosis (among others) is established for this client:

- Acute **P**ain related to sickle cell crisis resulting from vasoocclusion in lower extremities

Comprehensive reviews at the end of the chapter...

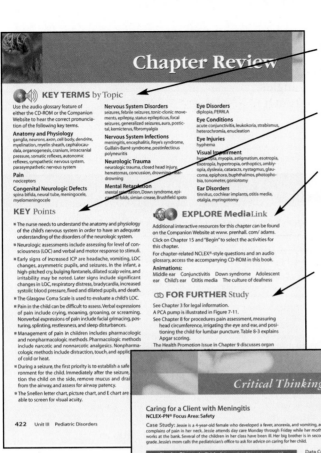

Key Terms by Topic link important new vocabulary to its content area in the chapter.

Key Points summarize need-to-know concepts from the chapter.

EXPLORE MediaLink encourages you to use the Prentice Hall MediaLink CD-ROM and Companion Website for a multi-modal review, regardless of your learning style.

For Further Study shows where related content areas are cross-referenced throughout the book.

Critical Thinking Care Maps prepare you for success on NCLEX-PN®, in clinical, and on-the-job with a focused review of a client problem, including:

- NCLEX-PN® Focus Area
- Case Study
- Nursing Diagnosis
- Data Collection
- Reporting
- Nursing Care
- Documentation

NCLEX-PN® Exam Preparation includes:

- A Test-taking Tip with a focused study hint
- NCLEX-PN® -style questions to review and practice taking tests with traditional and alternative question formats. Answers are found in Appendix I.

Prepare for your career as an LPN/LVN...

After each unit in this book, students can use the **Thinking Strategically About** pages as an opportunity to review topics in the context of important LPN/LVN curriculum themes. Short scenarios and project ideas spotlight the unit's content from a variety of angles. Review of concepts enables students to approach unit topics from a more integrated perspective.

Critical Thinking questions highlight specific challenges students will face as they become new nurses and assist them to provide the best possible care.

Collaborative Care challenges students to think about different health care settings and to envision the many health care workers who may participate in a client's care.

Delegating helps students determine which nursing interventions may be delegated to assistive personnel.

Management of Care highlights specific nursing interventions appropriate to the care of the client.

Communication and **Client Teaching** focus on communication methods and educational strategies necessary to teach the client and the family.

Time Management and **Priorities in Nursing Care** help students to organize care and to focus on the most important aspects of care first.

Documenting and Reporting helps students practice what and how to document and when to report their findings.

Cultural Care Strategies build confidence by providing information and scenarios to familiarize students with a variety of cultural patterns and differences.

UNIT III WRAP-UP

Thinking Strategically About...

You are employed by a pediatrician. Your responsibilities include obtaining client health histories, taking vital signs, weighing and measuring clients, vision and hearing screening, obtaining lab specimens, administering medications, assisting in procedures, and providing client teaching and discharge instructions. Today, there are 18 children scheduled.

CASE 1 SCENARIO
The first client of the day is Jeremy. He is 12 years old. He weighs 120 lb and is 5 ft tall. His vital signs are T 98.6, P 62, R 16, BP 106/76. Jeremy's mother relates that he is frequently fatigued. He is thirsty all the time, even during the night. He is also urinating many times a day and is always hungry. A review of the family history reveals that Jeremy's father has type I diabetes mellitus.

After conferring with the physician, you obtain a urine specimen and a blood specimen. A reagent strip is used to test the urine for glucose. The urine test is positive for glucose. Blood glucose reveals 210 mg/dL.

CRITICAL THINKING
Jeremy's mother tells you she just doesn't know what to do about her son and she is very worried. When considering the Essential Intellectual Traits (Box 2-3 (CD)), determine which trait applies to Jeremy's mother's current level of thinking.

The test results reveal that Jeremy does have diabetes mellitus. You are responsible for teaching Jeremy to self-administer his insulin, but he is afraid of "shots." What measures could you take to minimize the pain of injections?

COLLABORATIVE CARE
Jeremy and his parents will need to adjust his diet in order to manage his disease appropriately. Describe the report of Jeremy's condition you will give when you contact the nutritionist.

Jeremy's mother is concerned about how she will manage Jeremy's care and keep him healthy. What resources would you want to suggest to Jeremy's mother?

CASE 2 SCENARIO
Jackson, 4 years old, is admitted to the pediatric unit with a diagnosis of gastroenteritis. For the past 48 hours, Jackson has been vomiting and having diarrhea. He has been unable to keep any food or beverage down. Over the past few hours, he has been irritable and sleepy. You take his vital signs and review his admission orders. The physician orders an electrolyte profile, complete blood count, and urinalysis. He also orders an IV of D5 ½ NS to infuse at 1,000 mL in 8 hours,

daily weight, and full liquid diet. Phenergan 12.5 mg, rectal suppository every 4 hours is ordered for nausea.

DATA COLLECTED
Jackson's admission vital signs are T 99.9, P 110, R 18, BP 90/60. Skin turgor is poor. Hematocrit is increased. Urine-specific gravity is increased. Current weight: 45 lb.

DELEGATING
Which of the previous orders could be delegated to the certified nursing assistant?

MANAGEMENT OF CARE
Calculate the infusion rate for the previous order using a drop factor of 10 drops/mL.

COMMUNICATION AND CLIENT TEACHING
Jackson improves and is ready for discharge. His mother asks the nurse what foods are appropriate if Jackson should have a stomach virus again. Develop a teaching plan to provide this nutritional information.

CASE 3 SCENARIO
Janice is a 17-year-old who is admitted to the emergency room following a motor vehicle crash. Janice has facial abrasions and a fractured right clavicle. She is being evaluated for an abdominal injury due to the impact of the seatbelt.

DATA COLLECTED
Janice is oriented to person, time, and place. She complains of shoulder and abdominal pain, 6 on a scale of 10. She is able to move the fingers of her right hand. The abrasions are not actively bleeding. Vital signs include T 98.6, P 110 and thready, R 14, BP 100/70. Her skin is pale and moist. Her bowel sounds are decreased in all four quadrants.

TIME MANAGEMENT AND PRIORITIES IN NURSING CARE
List in order the nursing interventions that need to be implemented for Janice.

DOCUMENTING AND REPORTING
What findings about Janice are important to document? Which are important to report to the physician?

CULTURAL CARE STRATEGIES
Janice's admission information reveals she is a Jehovah's Witness. How will this affect care management? What strategies are appropriate if she needs blood replacement?

Pediatric Nursing Care will be a key resource as you progress through your nursing courses and become a nurse.

The nature of nursing—grow with it!

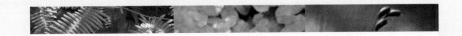

To the children in my life who taught me how to listen to, love, and protect the beautiful spirit within you all. To my two sons, David and Jonathan, God's best gift to my soul. To my nieces Mary Katherine, Sarah, Anna, Emma, Bailey, and Ansley, who taught my heart to dance; and my nephews Bill, Chris, Brian, Greg, Keith, and John, who give me energy every time I am with you.

■ *Ellise D. Adams*

To my God and my church family who provide me with spiritual energy to face life challenges.

■ *Mary Ann Towle*

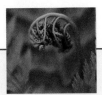

Preface

Pediatric Nursing Care is written to provide the LPN/LVN student with a foundation for providing safe, effective nursing care of the child within the community. Although the traditional role of the LPN/LVN has been in acute and long-term care, nursing practice is moving out of the hospital and into a variety of settings within the community. This shift has resulted in a more interdisciplinary approach to client care. The task of defining the role of the LPN/LVN in community-based nursing practice is in its early stages. The themes of this book have been developed to provide a basic understanding of community-based nursing practice and care of the child and the family in a variety of settings within the community. A strong emphasis is placed on understanding the role of the LPN/LVN and helping the student learn to make appropriate decisions within that role.

Organization

Pediatric Nursing Care is divided into three units. Unit One focuses on the foundations of pediatric nursing care. This unit will help the student make decisions, think critically, delegate activities, and provide care ethically and within the legal scope of practice for an LPN/LVN. Also included are chapters on the family, growth and development, and health promotion. Most pediatric texts present growth and development as a basis for nursing assessment, and many end with the adolescent. The authors feel that to make an accurate family assessment and to promote family health, the nurse must have an understanding of growth and development of all family members, including the adult and older adult. Therefore, growth and development across the life span is presented in its entirety.

Unit Two focuses on the ill child. These chapters provide the student with the tools to adapt nursing procedures for the pediatric client. The student will also learn how to recognize illness and to partner with the health care team caring for the ill child in both the hospital and community setting. Finally, this unit will assist the LPN/LVN in providing respectful, appropriate care to the dying child and the family.

Unit Three provides the student with up-to-date information about the care of the pediatric client facing a variety of disorders. The disorders are presented by body system. The student will review anatomy and physiology related to the body system, learn assessment skills related to the disorder, and learn about health promotion activities and nursing care of the child when illness occurs.

Features

Throughout each chapter the student will find consistent features to facilitate and reinforce learning.

- Each chapter begins with **Learning Outcomes** to help focus student learning.

- A **Nursing Care** section demonstrates the nursing process format and includes references to the role of the LPN/LVN in a variety of settings. Because time management and prioritizing tasks are such an important part of the student's day, this section begins with **Priorities in Nursing Care**, a summary of the areas on which the student must focus in order to provide quality nursing care. Nursing interventions are followed by rationales, to reinforce student understanding of why nursing actions are performed.

- **Case Studies** and **Critical Thinking** exercises are designed to bring the concepts to life and to engage students in problem-solving in situations they might encounter at work.

- **Health Promotion Issues** explore current issues in health care and provide a step-by-step solution for managing them.

- **Communicating Across the Life Span** offers practical examples of how development affects delivery of nursing care, as well as possible ways of addressing children at various ages.

- **Pharmacology** tables occur within clinical chapters to reinforce some of the most common medications students will administer.

- **Nursing Care Plan Charts** show how the process of nursing implementation works in relation to specific disorders.

- **Key Terms** and **Key Points** are reviewed at the end of each chapter.

- **NCLEX-PN® Review Questions** help students practice their test-taking skills.

- **Appendices** contain invaluable reference material including growth and development charts, normal laboratory values, and answers to Critical Thinking and NCLEX-PN® Review Questions.

Acknowledgments

A project such as this could not be accomplished without the contributions of many people. Without LPN/LVN students, there would not be a need for this book. Our students have been our inspiration and our motivation. Their enthusiasm for learning stimulates and challenges us to provide a quality textbook. It is our hope that this text will enhance students' knowledge and understanding of care of the child and will prepare them for success. We want to thank our students, past, present, and future, from whom we learn so much.

Many nursing professionals gave invaluable time and expertise to this project. Our contributors provided knowledge and writing skill in selected chapters and features of the book. Reviewers used their skill as educators to help maintain quality. They gave us ongoing assistance in deciding what students need to know and how to express our ideas for optimal learning. Contributors and reviewers for *Pediatric Nursing Care* are shown in a listing that follows this preface.

Health care is a team effort. This textbook is no different. Many intelligent individuals contributed their expertise to this work. Kelly Trakalo, Senior Acquisitions Editor, gave active support to reach our goals and deadlines. Our Development Editor, Rachel Bedard, was our visionary, our sounding board, our cheerleader, and most importantly, our nurse. When we were energy depleted, she gave us encouragement to just keep writing. This textbook is what it is because of Rachel. Her knowledge and endless attention to detail have kept us on track. Through our weekly conversations she helped us remain focused and not let the day-to-day issues of life prevent us from accomplishing our goal. Other important people in the production of this book were Yagnesh Jani (production editor); editorial assistant JulieAnn Oliveros; Patrick Walsh (managing production editor); Ilene Sanford (manufacturing manager); Carol Singer (GGS project manager) and the GGS staff; Mary Siener and Maria Guglielmo-Walsh, design; John Jordan and Stephen Hartner, in media; editorial assistant Teresa Himpsl; and Francisco Del Castillo and Michael Sirinides in marketing. Our thanks to all of you!

Finally, we want to thank our nursing colleagues, our friends, and our families for their support and encouragement. To all of you we are most grateful!

Nursing is an exciting, ever-changing profession. Advances in the medical management of clients have resulted in shorter length of stay in acute care hospitals and more clients being cared for in the home. Providing care in the home is a new challenge for many nurses and a new role for the LPN/LVN. To meet this challenge, the LPN/LVN must be more knowledgeable than ever before and be able to think critically in a variety of situations. With this text, we hope to prepare the LPN/LVN for these challenges.

About the Authors

Ellise D. Adams, CNM, MSN, CD (DONA), ICCE

Ellise D. Adams is an instructor of nursing at the University of Alabama in Huntsville where she serves as Clinical Assistant Professor. She enjoys lecturing, counseling students, and watching them learn and grow in the clinical setting. Ellise has been affiliated with Prentice Hall Publishers since 2000. The publication of this textbook fulfills a primary career goal.

Ellise is a member of the Association of Women's Health, Obstetric, and Neonatal Nurses (AWHONN) and serves as Alabama's co-chair for programs. She is an invited presenter to the national conventions, consultant to special projects, research grant recipient, and contributor to publications. In 2000, she was awarded the AWHONN Johnson and Johnson Pediatric Institute Marshal Klaus Award along with her colleague Ann L. Bianchi for their research entitled "Intrapartum Nurses as Doulas: Increasing Training in Supportive Behaviors to Aid in the Reduction of Cesarean Rates, Length of Labor, and Anesthesia and Analgesia Use."

Ellise obtained her Bachelor of Science in Nursing from the University of Alabama in Huntsville. Because her first son was born during her tenure in nursing school, she is especially sensitive to the concerns of students who attempt to balance school, children, and a marriage. She received her Master of Science in Nursing from Case Western Reserve University in Cleveland, Ohio, and her Certificate of Nurse-Midwifery from Frontier School of Midwifery and Family Nursing in Hyden, Kentucky. She feels especially privileged to have had the opportunity to learn nurse-midwifery in the hills of Kentucky where Mary Breckenridge left an amazing legacy.

Ellise views nursing as one of the noblest of professions. Someone once asked her why she did not just become a doctor. Her response was, "Because I want to be a nurse. I want to spend time with patients in their hour of need. I want to provide nursing care, not make medical decisions." Nursing also provides diversity. There are so many opportunities in nursing that the nurse can always find professional fulfillment.

Ellise has been married to her husband Tom for 27 years. They have two sons, David and Jonathan. She is proud that her daughter-in-law Karla is also a nurse. Ellise enjoys volunteering in a variety of capacities at her church, including serving as a short-term missionary to Mexico City, Mexico; Vienna, Austria; and Cuzco, Peru. She also enjoys leisure travel, especially tailgating on the campus of her favorite SEC team, the University of Alabama.

Mary Ann Towle, RN, MEd, MSN

Mary Ann Towle "always wanted to be a nurse," but teaching science in high school also seemed appealing. After graduating from Idaho State University with a baccalaureate degree in nursing, she moved to Boise, Idaho, where she accepted a position at St. Luke's Medical Center. Mary Ann felt confident with her entry-level knowledge but was unsure of herself when it came to performing nursing procedures. Several LPNs helped her gain the necessary skills and confidence. Within a few months, she was working in the Coronary Intensive Care Unit as the evening charge nurse.

Although Mary Ann enjoyed the direct client care of the CICU, she felt that something was missing in her career. She taught a few in-service programs and workshops to nurses as well as to Respiratory Therapy students from Boise State University. After three years, an opportunity became available to teach in the LPN program at Boise State University. Mary Ann jumped at the chance to combine her love for nursing with her desire to teach.

All faculty in the Vocational-Technical Education programs were required to take education classes in order to improve their teaching performance. With a husband and two young children to care for and while teaching full-time, Mary Ann attended classes two or three nights a week. In 1983, she completed a Master of Education degree with a specialty in Vocational Education. A proponent of lifelong learning, Mary Ann returned to school once her family was grown and completed a Master of Science degree in Nursing in 1998. Having taught the entire curriculum, Mary Ann sees herself as a generalist with experience in maternity, pediatrics, medical-surgical nursing, and geriatrics.

It has been 31 years since Mary Ann began her career as a nursing instructor at Boise State University. She has been recognized by the American Vocational association as vocational Teacher of the Year at the state and regional levels, and as first runner-up at the national level. Mary Ann's students have received state and national recognition by Vocational Industrial Clubs of America (VICA). Mary Ann is a strong advocate for the LPN/LVN. She works to advance their education and scope of practice within the health care community. Mary Ann feels that by reducing the stress involved in learning, providing positive feedback, and role modeling, she can help all students develop into quality nurses who can think critically and function in any situation.

Contributor Team

Chapter Contributors

Jeanne Hately, RN, MSN, PhD
President, Professional Nurse Consultants, LLC
Aurora, CO

Supplement Contributors

Student CD-Rom

Ann L. Bianchi, RN, MSN, ICCE, ICD
Clinical Assistant Professor
University of Alabama
Huntsville, AL

Companion Website (www.prenhall.com/adams)

Ann L. Bianchi, RN, MSN, ICCE, ICD
Clinical Assistant Professor
University of Alabama
Huntsville, AL

Terrilynn Quillen, RN MSN
Department of Environments for Health
Community Health Nursing
Indiana University School of Nursing
Faith Community Nurse
New Life in Christ Ministries
Indiana, IN

Also our thanks to the instructor resources writers from *Maternal-Child Nursing Care:*

Laura L. Brown, RN, MSN, CPN
Nursing Instructor
Asheville-Buncombe Technical Community College
Asheville, NC

Cheryl DeGraw, RN, MSN, CRNP
Faculty/Course Coordinator
Florence-Darlington Technical College
Florence, SC

Jane Headland, RNC, MSN
Nursing Instructor
Asheville-Buncombe Technical Community College
Asheville, NC

Reviewer Panel

Also out thanks to the reviewers of *Maternal-Child Nursing case*, from which material was used.

Priscilla Anderson, RN, MSN
Assistant Professor of Nursing
New Hampshire Technical Institute
Concord, NH

Janice Ankenmann-Hill, RN, MSN, CCRN, FNP
Faculty
Napa Valley College
Napa, CA

Margaret Batson, RN-cMSN
Nursing Instructor
San Joaquin Delta College
Stockton, CA

Laura L. Brown, RN, MSN, CPN
Nursing Instructor
Asheville Buncombe Technical Community College
Asheville, NC

Marti Burton, RN, BS
Instructor and Curriculum Designer/Developer
Canadian Valley Technology Center
El Reno, OK

Rebecca Cappo, RN, MSN
Coordinator
Lenape LPN Program
Ford City, PA

Traudel Cline, RN, MSN
Nursing Instructor
Milwaukee Area Technical College
Milwaukee, WI

Kathy Cochran, RN, MSN
Director of Practical Nursing
Coosa Valley Technical College
Rome, GA

Mary Davis, RN, MSN
Nursing Faculty
Valdosta Technical College
Valdosta, GA

Patricia M. Demers, RN, MS/MPH, CNA, BC
Associate Professor
Northern Essex Community College
Lawrence, MA

Gail Finney, MSN, RN
Nursing Education Specialist
Concorde Career College, Inc.
Mission, KS

Shari Gholson, MSN, RN
Associate Professor
West Kentucky Community and Technical College
Paducah, KY

Julie Hansen, RN, BSN, MA
LPN Program Instructor
Southeast Technical Institute
Sioux Falls, SD

Jeanne Hately, RN, MSN, PhD
President, Professional Nurse Consultants, LLC
Aurora, CO

Cynthia E. Hudson, DNSc, RN, APRN, BC
Assistant Professor of Nursing
University of Alabama
Huntsville, AL

Susie Huyer, MSN, RN
Nursing Education Consultants
Chantilly, VA

Julie Kay, RN, BSN, MSN
Nursing Instructor
San Joaquin Delta College
Stockton, CA

Pamela Kersey-McCandless, RN, MSN
Assistant Professor
San Diego City College
San Diego, CA

Tabatha R. Mauldin, RN, BSN, CPN
Faculty
Surry Community College
Dobson, NC

Kimberly McDonnell, RN
NICU Nurse
Lancaster General Hospital
Respiratory Home Care Nurse
Lancaster, PA

Jeffrey C. McManemy, PhD, APRN, BC
Associate Professor/Program Coordinator
St. Louis Community College at Florissant Valley
St. Louis, Missouri

Mary Pat Norrell, RNC, BSN, MS
Professor, Nursing Department
Ivy Tech Community College of Indiana
Seymour, IN

Noel Piano, RN, MS
Instructor/Coordinator
Lafayette School of Practical Nursing
Williamsburg, VA

Becki Quick, RN, BA, MAC
Director of Nursing VN Program
Maric College San Diego
San Diego, CA

Carolyn Reese, MSN, RN
Nursing Instructor
Blinn College, Bryan Campus
Bryan, TX

LuAnn Reicks, RNC, BS, MSN
Professor/PN Coordinator
Iowa Central Community College
Fort Dodge, IA

Betty Kehl Richardson, PhD, RN CS Psych-MH, BC
Professor Emeritus
Austin Community College
Private Practice Marriage and Family Therapy
Austin, TX

Russlyn St. John, RN, MSN
Coordinator, Practical Nursing

St. Charles Community College
St. Peters, MO

Marcia Scherer, RN, BSN, PHN, LSN
Nursing Faculty
Hennepin Technical College
Eden Prairie, MN

Patricia Schrull, RN, MSN, MBA, MEd
Assistant Professor and Program Director
Lorain County Community College
Elyria, OH

Molly Showalter, BS, RN
Vocational Nursing Program Coordinator
North Central Texas College
Gainesville, TX

Sue Smith, RN, MSN, MEd
Assistant Professor
Iowa Western Community College
Harlan, IA

Carlotta South, RN
Licensed Vocational Nursing Instructor
San Jacinto College North
Houston, TX

Cindy Steury Lattz, MSN, APRN, BC
Professor of Nursing
Kankakee Community College
Kankakee, IL

Claudia Stoffel, MSN, RN
Instructor
Paducah Community College
Paducah, KY

Angie Sutherland, RN, BSN, CPN
Faculty
Spencerian College
Louisville, KY

Elaine Tobias, RN, BSN, IBCLC
Maternity Nurse, Lactation Specialist

Heart of Lancaster Hospital
Lancaster, PA

Laura Travis, RN, BSN
Health Careers Coordinator
Tennessee Technology Center at Dickson
Dickson, TN

Cheryl S. Weidman, RN, BSN
PN Administrator
Brown Mackie College
Findlay, OH

Jan Weust, RN, MSN
Nursing Faculty
Ivy Tech Community College
Terre Haute, IN

Janice Wimbish, RN, CCRN
Instructor, Practical Nursing Program
Forsyth Technical Community College
Winston-Salem, NC

Contents

Contents **xxiii**

Introduction to Pediatric Nursing

UNIT I

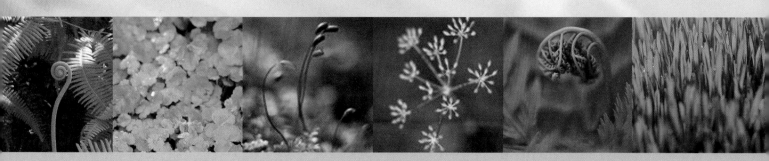

Chapter 1

Pediatric Nursing in the Community

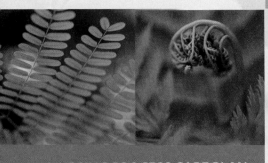

NURSING PROCESS CARE PLAN:
Caring for a Family That Desires Alternative Therapies

HEALTH PROMOTION ISSUE:
Male Circumcision without Anesthesia

BRIEF Outline

LEARNING Outcomes

After completing this chapter, you will be able to:
1. Define key terms.
2. Describe historical changes in pediatric care and in nursing care.
3. Describe the benefits of research-based pediatric care in nursing practice.
4. Describe community-based nursing practice.
5. Describe LPN/LVN roles in pediatric nursing.

In our mobile society, the LPN/LVN comes in contact with children in a variety of settings. The nurse might interact with children in the school, health clinic, church, or synagogue, as well as the emergency room or pediatric unit of an acute care hospital. The nurse might interact with children at playgrounds, parks, or entertainment centers. Some of these interactions might be as an employee of the health care agency. Other interactions might be on a personal level. In either case, the LPN/LVN must be prepared to provide assistance with health care as needed. The role of the LPN/LVN in these settings varies from assisting the RN and other health care providers in complex situations to providing first aid in a simple situation. The LPN/LVN must be prepared to provide direct care, teaching, and referral to the child and the family. This chapter introduces the role of LPNs/LVNs in providing pediatric care in the community setting.

History of Pediatrics

What is pediatrics? **Pediatrics** is the medical science related to the diagnosis and treatment of childhood illness. As a specialty, it is relatively young. Before the mid-1800s, health care focused on meeting the immediate needs of adults. The infant mortality rate was high, and epidemics could wipe out entire families. Infancy lasted until age 7, when the child entered adulthood and was expected to work and assist with the family income.

Scientific progress, such as the discovery of sanitation and immunizations, improved the life span of children. As infants survived longer, parents and society took more interest in the health of children. Child development specialists such as Erikson, Piaget, and others (see Chapter 5 ⬭) raised society's awareness of childhood as a separate stage of development. Their work altered the way we look at children.

In the 20th century, laws were passed to protect children's rights, including the right to health care. For example, Aid to Families of Dependent Children was established by the Social Security Act of 1935 to provide money for needy children without fathers. In 1965, Medicaid was established to reduce the financial barriers to health care for the poor. The Child Health Assessment Program is a major part of the Medicaid program. In 1974, the Women, Infants, and Children (WIC) program was started to provide nutritious foods and education to low-income pregnant, postpartum, and lactating women, and to infants and children up to age 5 years. Other interesting points about pediatric history are provided in Table 1-1 ■.

TABLE 1-1

Names and Events in Pediatric Care

DATE	NAME AND/OR EVENT	IMPORTANCE TO PEDIATRIC CARE
1796	Edward Jenner	His experiments mark the beginning of immunology. He infected people with cowpox in order to make them immune to smallpox. This procedure involves injecting harmless microbes to stimulate immunity to a more dangerous microbe. His contribution both enabled control of this dreaded disease and established the science of immunization.
1802	Pediatric hospitals	The first children's hospital was established in Paris, France. In 1855, the United States established its first children's hospital, known as The Children's Hospital of Philadelphia (still in existence today).
1842	Oliver Wendell Holmes	Published a paper on the contagious nature of puerperal fever that increased the survival rate of the mother and child during childbirth.
1853	New York City Children's Aid Society	This society was the first founded in the United States to care for homeless children.
1867	Joseph Lister	He adopted the use of carbolic acid as an antiseptic agent in the prevention of infections. This form of sterilization introduced the era of antiseptic surgery and dramatically reduced mortality rates following surgery.
1884	Karl Sigismund Franz Credé	Developed the method of placing drops of an antiseptic solution of silver nitrate in the eyes of the newborn to prevent blindness caused by gonorrhea.
1888	Arthur Jacobi	Recognized as the "Father of Pediatrics." He established pediatric units in several New York hospitals and was instrumental in the formation of the American Pediatric Society. He also initiated the boiling of milk to lower the incidence of diarrhea in children.

(continued)

TABLE 1-1

Names and Events in Pediatric Care (continued)

DATE	NAME AND/OR EVENT	IMPORTANCE TO PEDIATRIC CARE
1896	Incubators	These were first developed in1896 by a German physician. In 1903 the incubator was brought to the United States by Dr. Martin A. Couney, the "incubator doctor." He set up incubators at Coney Island as part of the carnival's exhibition. He also toured the country with his display, including the World's Fair in 1933. He reportedly saved 6,500 of the 8,000 babies who used his incubators. However, it was not until the 1940s that incubators were used in hospitals.
1912	Children's Bureau	Creation of this bureau marked the beginning of modern child-welfare programs and public recognition of children's special needs. Focused on infant and maternal mortality. Mandated birth registration in all states. It established the school hot lunch program in 1930.
1921	Sheppard Tower Act	Provides funds for state-managed programs for maternity care. It also provides federal grants-in-aid to states to promote better care for mothers and dependent children.
1930	White House Conference on Children and Youth, development of Children's Charter	Issued statements related to the needs of children in the areas of education health, welfare, and protection.
1930	American Academy of Pediatrics	Dr. Clifford Grulee, Dr. Isaac Abt, and Dr. William Lucas were key figures in the founding of the American Academy of Pediatrics, whose goals are to develop the scope and field of pediatrics and to have a positive influence on the life and health of its clients.
1932–1970	Neonate stimulation and maternal deprivation	Joseph Brennamen was the first to recognize the relationship between an infant's poor health and the lack of stimulation the infant received in the maternity wards. Over the years many physicians have studied mother and infant bonding and the effects of a long-term stay in the hospital on children. Today hospitals have modified their policies of visitation to reflect these findings.
1939	Mary Breckinridge	Opened the Frontier School of Midwifery and Family Nursing. After a family nursing curriculum was added to the school's program in 1970, the name was changed to the Frontier School of Midwifery and Family Nursing.
1956	La Leche League	Breastfeeding rates in the United States had dropped close to 20% when the first meeting of LLL was held. Their first publication was a loose-leaf edition of *The Womanly Art of Breastfeeding*.
1962	Child Protection Laws	Laws that require the reporting of incidents of child abuse. All states are required to have such laws.
1974	Women, Infants, and Children (WIC)	Program provides supplemental food and education to lower-income children under the age of 5 and women who are pregnant, postpartum, or breastfeeding.
1979	International Year of the Child	Focused attention to the critical needs of the world's children. Its stated mission was to consider how to provide food globally to children in need.
1992	Office of Alternative Medicine (OAM) within the National Department of Health	Agency developed to promote research and publicize information on complementary and alternative therapies. Emphasizes prevention, wellness, and a holistic approach to health care.
1996	Newborns' and Mothers' Health Protection Act	Provides for a postpartum stay of 48 hours following a vaginal birth and 96 hours for a cesarean birth.
2002	Best Pharmaceuticals for Children Act (BPCA)	Established a drug program that identifies drugs and clinical studies that are needed for children.
2003	Human Genome Map	Completion of 99% of human genome map has led to enhanced diagnosis of genetic disorders. The use of gene transfer therapy in curing some genetic conditions is a new and expanding field.

Developments in Nursing

Like pediatric care, the field of nursing has changed dramatically since its infancy. In Florence Nightingale's time, nursing involved providing for the sick person's activities of daily living. Nurses would cook, clean, stoke the coal stove, and trim the wicks on the kerosene lamps. The nurse was an assistant to the doctor, helping only as requested.

Until the mid-20th century, nursing care followed the medical model, focusing on the treatment of disease. The nurse worked "for" and was dependent on the doctor's medical orders. This was reflected in the way nurses talked about people who came for treatment. Because nurses' roles were limited to carrying out orders to treat an illness, it was quite common for nurses and hospital staff to refer to "the appendectomy in room 225" or "the C-section in room 20." Although medical advances (such as the development of antibiotics and laparoscopic surgery) had a tremendous impact on the medical care of individuals, they did little to change nursing practice.

Nursing has gradually evolved into a true profession with its own governing agencies. Today, *nursing* is described as a knowledge-based process discipline in which the licensed nurse's specialized education, professional judgment, and discretion are essential for quality nursing care (National Council of State Boards of Nursing [NCSBN], 1995). The American Nurses Association (ANA) defines nursing practice as "the nursing diagnosis and treatment of human responses to actual or potential health problems" (ANA, 1980, p 9). The ANA (1991) further identifies four essential features of nursing practice.

- Attention to the full range of human experiences and responses to health and illness without restriction to a problem-focused orientation.
- Integration of **objective data** (data that can be observed and measured by the senses or by mechanical instruments) with **subjective data** (knowledge gained from an understanding of the client's or group's subjective personal experience).
- Application of scientific knowledge to the process of diagnosis and treatment.
- Provision of a caring relationship that facilitates health and healing.

The nursing profession has grown to be interdependent with that of the physician. Nurses have clear areas of responsibility and knowledge. In contrast to many areas of medicine that have become narrower and more specialized, nursing has become **holistic** (inclusive of the physical, psychological, and spiritual aspects of the person). Through the work of nursing theorists such as Jean Watson, Martha Rogers, and others, nursing has come to recognize that health and illness are more than simple physical states. Instead, they reflect the whole person, including the person's level of development, mental status, physical health, coping ability, and more.

In pediatric nursing especially, the client is no longer just an individual. Instead the term *client* refers to the entire family. Nurses who obtain the vital signs of a child will also be actively involved in helping the parents promote the child's health. They will provide client teaching, because children are sent home from hospitals to recuperate as soon as an acute condition has stabilized. Nurses teach families to watch for complications and alterations in the healing process. This is done by observing parenting skills and by providing teaching to the parent to positively affect the child.

Nursing Process in Pediatric Care

The nursing process provides a systematic approach to planning and implementing nursing care. The LPN/LVN participates to some degree in every aspect of the nursing process. The depth of involvement depends on:

- The particular state's nurse practice acts
- The policies of the facility where the nurse works
- The nurse's skills and experiences

ASSESSING

The nursing process is a continuous, unbroken process (Figure 1-1 ■). During the assessment phase, the LPN/LVN collects data from the client and family. The LPN/LVN is not required to analyze and synthesize data to the same degree as the RN. Still, it is the LPN/LVN at the bedside who monitors changes in the client, compares the data with given normal ranges, and decides whether findings should be reported. Because the RN may be unable to be at the bedside constantly, the LPN/LVN plays a valuable role in the assessment and monitoring process.

DIAGNOSING AND PLANNING

When defining nursing as a distinct profession, it is important to identify actions the nurse performs independently of physicians or other members of the health care team. Names for client conditions that nurses are qualified and trained to treat independently (called **nursing diagnoses**) have been defined and developed by the North American Nursing Diagnosis Association (NANDA, 2008). The RN analyzes the assessment data and determines the appropriate nursing

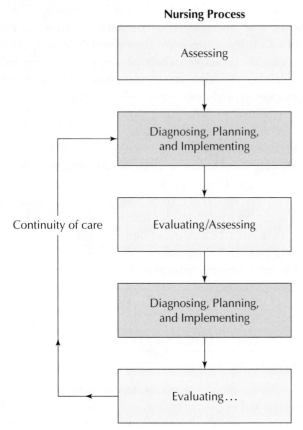

Nursing Process

Assessing

↓

Diagnosing, Planning, and Implementing

↓

Evaluating/Assessing

↓

Diagnosing, Planning, and Implementing

↓

Evaluating...

Continuity of care

Figure 1-1. ■ Nursing process model.

diagnosis and specific **desired outcomes** (or general goals) for the client. For example, when Pain is identified as the nursing diagnosis, the desired outcome for the client would be a client report of reduction in pain to tolerable levels, or perhaps an observation that the client was sleeping quietly.

Planning is the third step of the nursing process. The **care plan** (an organized and prioritized plan) addresses the nursing diagnoses and helps the client identify measurable outcomes. In some states, the LPN/LVN assists the RN in writing and updating the nursing diagnoses and nursing care plan.

Regardless of whether planning is a shared role with the RN, the LPN/LVN must understand and follow both the nursing diagnosis and care plan and the medical diagnoses and plan of care.

IMPLEMENTING

The experienced nurse can name several possible nursing actions to assist a client toward an improvement in health. In the case of a client with <u>P</u>ain, these nursing actions (called **interventions**) would include administration of prescribed analgesics, nonpharmacologic comfort measures such as a bath or backrub, or distractions such as a favorite

TV program. In performing these actions, the nurse is following both the medical and the nursing orders.

To implement the medical plan, the nurse would administer pain medication when needed, give antibiotics as ordered, and document administration promptly. To implement the nursing plan, the nurse would turn and position the client, provide adequate nutrition and fluids, and ensure adequate elimination. The nurse would also use diversion (such as soothing music) to help the client focus on something other than the pain.

In implementing medical and nursing care plans, the nurse must be aware of his or her limitations. States and facilities define which actions may be taken by LPNs/LVNs. Levels of experience, training, and skill also determine which actions are appropriate to take. For example, in some states the LPN/LVN can administer medication by the intravenous route into a central venous catheter. In other states, this route of medication administration is reserved for the RN. In a large, acute-care hospital the LPN/LVN may be expected to provide direct client care to four to six pediatric clients. In a long-term care facility for severely disabled pediatric clients, this same nurse might assume the responsibility of "charge nurse" for an entire unit. (Ideally, in the charge nurse role, the LPN/LVN would supervise the care, instead of providing the care.)

EVALUATING

Once nursing actions have been carried out, the nurse has the responsibility of evaluating those actions and determining whether they have moved the client toward identified goals. Data collected from ongoing assessments are compared with expected outcomes and with decisions about care. In the case mentioned earlier, the nurse would return to evaluate (and document) how well the medication has worked. If the client says the pain is reduced to 4 and he or she feels sleepy, then the goal has been met. If the client is moaning and still reports pain at 9, then the goal has not been met. The LPN/LVN would report this to the RN team leader or charge nurse. This report could lead to a medical solution (e.g., a change in medication) or to a nursing solution (e.g., increased use of nonpharmacologic methods to help reduce pain).

LPNs/LVNs work with a variety of care plans and care pathways, depending on the facility. This book provides Care Plan Charts in clinical chapters and Nursing Process Care Plans in each chapter. These two approaches to care plans provide realistic examples of situations in which LPNs/LVNs must make decisions. Questions following the Nursing Process Care Plans will help students practice critical thinking skills to prepare for everyday nursing practice. The following is a sample.

NURSING PROCESS CARE PLAN
Caring for a Family That Desires Alternative Therapies

A family brings their 10-week-old son to the pediatrician's office. The child is gaining weight appropriately. He is breastfed and has adequate output. The nurse discusses immunizations with the family. The mother and father express concern about the safety of immunizations. They have done some reading on the Internet that led them to believe that a child could be healthy without immunizations. There are no other children in the home. The mother reports allergies, and the father smokes regularly in the home.

Assessment

- Parents believe child could be healthy without immunizations.
- The stated resource is the Internet.
- Parents are unaware of the need for immunizations, especially in a high-risk environment (family history of allergies and smoking in the home).

Nursing Diagnosis.
The following important nursing diagnosis (among others) is established for this client:

- Deficient **K**nowledge related to misinterpretation of information

Expected Outcome

- Parents will demonstrate adequate knowledge about immunizations prior to giving informed consent.

Planning and Implementation

- Assess the parents' ability to learn. *If the parents have learning disabilities, it would be important for the nurse to know this prior to developing a teaching plan.*
- Clarify the knowledge the parents have about immunizations. *The nurse needs to understand what information should be confirmed and what should be corrected.*
- Collaborate with the supervising nurse and the physician prior to developing a teaching plan for these clients. *This situation will be best handled with a team approach.*
- Design an environment conducive to learning to present the teaching plan. *To maximize learning, the family should be comfortable and the area should be free of distractions.*
- Present information about the effects of disease for which immunizations are available. *It is important for the parents to understand the symptoms, treatments, and long-term effects of the diseases.*
- Present information about methods of immunizations and the side effects related to each. Include rates of occurrence. *Clear, concise, accurate information about the immunizations will give the parents an understanding of immunizations.*

- Encourage feedback and document understanding. *The nurse can assess learning better when the parents provide verbal feedback.*
- Provide the parents with printed literature. *This provides a way to reinforce the teaching the nurse has given and allows parents to review the material in their own home.*

Evaluation.
Verbal and written information provided to family. Father expressed surprise that items on the Internet might not be reliable. The Internet address to Centers for Disease Control and Prevention (CDC) site is offered, so the parents can pursue reliable sources and statistics. Mother wondered whether her allergies might affect her child. Both parents agreed to consider the possibility of immunizing the child at the 6-month visit.

Critical Thinking in the Nursing Process

1. Describe the alternative thinking of those who do not want to immunize their children.
2. Review the history of the polio vaccine.
3. How might you show support to a family who chooses not to immunize their child?

Note: Discussion of Critical Thinking questions appears in Appendix I.

Research-Based Pediatric Care

RECUPERATION SETTING

As medical science made dramatic improvements early in the 20th century, researchers began to note differences between care of adults and care of children. For example, as care improved and children survived illnesses that had once been fatal, children spent long periods of time recovering in hospitals. However, they did not thrive in that environment. Research studies determined that children recover faster in their own homes than in institutional settings (Krepper, Young, & Cummings, 1994). Today, children remain in the hospital until their condition stabilizes and are discharged at any time of the day or night.

Nurses in the hospital environment must be knowledgeable about the physiology of pediatric disorders and about family dynamics. They need to be ready to provide client teaching at every available opportunity and to work with a variety of family dynamics to promote the health of the child and the family (Figure 1-2 ■). They must be alert to potential complications and alterations in the healing process.

MORTALITY

The health of infants and children is of critical importance in assessing the current health status of a population and in predicting the health of the next generation. **Mortality** describes

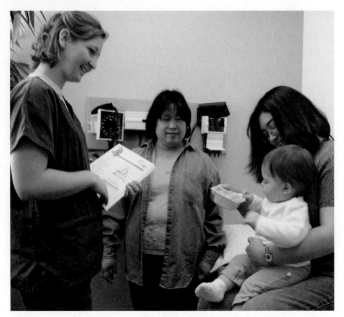

Figure 1-2. ■ In pediatric nursing, the LPN/LVN must be prepared to support the family and provide client teaching at every opportunity.

the number of deaths over a given period of time for a given population. The infant mortality rate is the number of deaths per 1,000 live births during the first year of life. The disparity in mortality rates among different races, areas of the country, or parts of the world is significant in reflecting the general health of the population. The infant mortality rate of 5.7 for White infants and 13.5 for Black infants demonstrates the disparity between health status of Black families and White families in the United States. This information can be used when seeking funding to provide prenatal care to Black women in poverty-stricken areas or when identifying target

groups for prenatal teaching. Infant mortality rates for the United States are illustrated in Table 1-2 ■.

Sudden Infant Death Syndrome

The leading causes of infant mortality are congenital anomalies, sudden infant death syndrome (SIDS), and low birth weight. Research into causes and prevention of these problems affects the nursing care provided to infants, parents, families, and communities. For example, until the mid-1990s, parents were taught to position infants on their abdomens to sleep. It was believed that if an infant vomited during sleep, this position would enable the infant to clear the airway and prevent aspiration. Through research led by the American Academy of Pediatrics, it was determined that infants positioned on their side or back during sleep had fewer incidents of SIDS (American Academy of Pediatrics, 2005). This information has changed not only the nursing care of infants, but also the teaching that nurses provide to parents (see Chapter 12 ⚭).

MORBIDITY

Morbidity is the prevalence of a specific disease or disorder in the population at a specific period of time. Data are collected from physician office visits, hospital admissions, and interviews. The data may not reflect the general population, but they do reflect those who are accessing health care in a given area. It is important, therefore, to look at trends rather than one-time numbers.

Childhood morbidity rates vary according to the age of the child. By studying the common causes of childhood illness or injury, plans for prevention can be made. For example, at one time polio was a leading cause of illness, disability, and death. However, through immunization

TABLE 1-2

Infant, Neonatal, and Postneonatal Deaths and Mortality Rates by Origin of Mother: United States, 2004

HISPANIC ORIGIN AND RACE OF MOTHER	LIVE BIRTHS	NUMBER OF DEATHS			MORTALITY RATE PER 1,000 LIVE BIRTHS		
		INFANT	NEONATAL	POSTNEONATAL	INFANT	NEONATAL	POSTNEONATAL
All origins[a]	4,090,007	27,936	18,593	9,343	6.79	4.52	2.27
Total Hispanic	912,331	5,151	3,573	1,579	5.65	3.92	1.73
Non-Hispanic White	2,321,921	13,228	8,797	4,431	5.70	3.79	1.91
Non-Hispanic Black	576,047	7,836	5,335	2,501	13.60	9.26	4.34
Not stated	28,609	448	368	80	N/A	N/A	N/A

Note: N/A, Category not applicable. Infant deaths are weighted so numbers may not exactly add to totals due to rounding. Neonatal is less than 28 days and post-neonatal is 28 days to less than 1 year.
[a]Origin of mother not stated included in "All origins" but not distributed among origins.
Source: National Vital Statistics Report, Vol. 54, No. 16, May 3, 2007.

against polio, this illness has nearly been eradicated worldwide. (It still exists in certain areas of Africa.)

Falls from playground equipment are a leading cause of injury in the preschool child. Knowing this, nurses can focus on parent teaching toward prevention. They can try to influence the design and selection of playground equipment and encourage community leaders to provide safe places for children to play.

Research-Based Nursing Practice

Nurses are educated to ask questions and to observe. Observations that begin to form a pattern are often the basis for nursing research. Research gives direction to nursing practice. When research indicates a need for change in current practice, the prudent nurse effects changes in the way care is provided. Over time these changes can have a tremendous impact on the quality of health.

The nurse must use every opportunity to improve health care. This is done through client and family teaching, conducting research to document quality of care (either by formal study or informal data collecting), and assisting in the revision of facility standards-of-practice policies. The Health Promotion Issue on pages 10 and 11 shows how observations and information gathered during the nursing process can lead to improvements in care of neonates. The issue of circumcision is presented here as an example of how data can be used to initiate change. Further information regarding circumcision is presented in Chapter 18 ⚭.

Community-Based Nursing Practice

In recent years, there has been a tremendous debate over health care reform. The United States government sponsored a proactive study of health, illness prevention, and positive steps for change called *Healthy People 2000* and its update *Healthy People 2010*. The "Issue and Trends" portion of *Healthy People 2010* indicates that effective community-based programs would have the following characteristics (U.S. Department of Health and Human Services, 2000):

■ Community participation with representation from at least three of the following areas:
  • Government
  • Education
  • Business
  • Faith organizations
  • Health care

  • Media
  • Voluntary organizations
  • Public

■ Community assessment of the community's health problems, resources, perceptions, and priorities for action. (The community decides together what problem areas should be addressed. It is not told what its problems are by an outside agency.)

■ Measurable objectives addressing at least one of the following:
  • Health outcomes
  • Risk factors
  • Public awareness
  • Services and protection

■ Monitoring and evaluation processes to determine whether goals have been reached.

■ Interventions that target several areas for change and that are culturally relevant. Interventions would address the community at several levels:
  • Individual (e.g., racial or ethnic, age, or socioeconomic group)
  • Organizational (e.g., schools, workplaces, faith communities)
  • Environmental (e.g., local policies and regulations)

AND

■ Interventions would include multiple approaches to change:
  • Education
  • Community organization
  • Regulatory and environmental reform

Community-based nursing is a response to the changes in health care. The philosophy of community-based nursing is that care should be provided to individuals, families, and groups wherever they are, including where they live, work, play, pray, or attend school (Zotti, Brown, & Stotts; 1996). Community-based care is vital to bringing health promotion initiatives to underserved populations. In an effort to implement *Healthy People 2010* guidelines, neighborhood health care clinics have become common. Education programs have been implemented to teach children the effect of lifestyle choices on health. Greater effort is being placed on providing care to those with limited financial resources. These advances have caused a necessary change in the way nursing care is provided. In response to political debates, the ANA and the National League for Nurses composed Nursing's Agenda for Health Care Reform (also known as Nursing's Agenda). Nursing's agenda for reform is "to provide primary health care services

(Text continues on p. 12.)

HEALTH PROMOTION ISSUE

MALE CIRCUMCISION WITHOUT ANESTHESIA

The staff in the newborn nursery has become increasingly concerned that their male clients are not given anesthesia during circumcision because they have observed painful reactions to the procedure. Parents are questioning more frequently why their children are not given anything for pain relief. Also, two of the nurses attended a national nursing convention where they learned that providing anesthesia during circumcision is common practice in many hospitals nationwide. At the monthly unit meeting, these nurses address their concerns to the unit manager.

DISCUSSION

The debate lingers: Is there pain associated with newborn circumcision? If so, how can we be sure? Pain can be assessed by looking at the behavioral parameters and physiologic parameters. Several assessment tools have been developed to assist health care practitioners in assessing pain in the newborn. These include the Neonatal Infant Pain Scale (NIPS); the CRying, Increased vital signs, Expression, and Sleeplessness scale (CRIES); and Pain Assessment In Neonates (PAIN). Each scale measures criteria associated with pain and awards a score indicating pain or lack of pain.

Behavorial parameters associated with pain in the newborn include furrowing of the brow, tightly closed eyes, a quivering chin, a high-pitched cry, increased motor movements, and withdrawal from painful stimulus. Physiologic symptoms indicating pain include tachycardia, tachypnea, hypertension, and sweating of the palms.

Pain Relief Options for Newborns

The American Academy of Pediatrics suggests that health care practitioners provide pain relief in the newborn during circumcision in the form of environmental, nonpharmacologic, or pharmacologic measures.

- Environmental measures would include decreasing the stimuli in the setting where the circumcision is performed. Music, increased room temperature, a soft surface, and dimmed lighting are environmental measures of pain relief.
- Nonpharmacologic measures include nonnutritive sucking on either a pacifier or the breast of the mother who has not begun to lactate. Nonnutritive sucking provides analgesia only during the period of sucking. Nutritive sucking in the form of breastfeeding has also been found to provide pain relief to the newborn. Nutritive sucking or ingestion of sucrose has been found to provide analgesia. Sucrose can be supplied to the infant via a specially designed pacifier,

nasogastric tube, or drops placed directly on the tongue.
- Pharmacologic measures for pain relief in the newborn include administration of acetaminophen preoperatively and postoperatively. Application of eutectic mixture of local anesthetic (EMLA) cream administered 60 minutes before the circumcision will give the newborn up to 3 hours of pain relief. Nerve blocks can also provide the newborn with pain relief during circumcision.

What is Evidence-Based Practice?

Evidence-based practice (EBP) can be defined as the use of current research to make decisions about client care. If a clinical procedure is not based on research, it is based on a commonly accepted tradition. Health care practitioners have the responsibility of providing the best care possible. This care must be based on scientific data. Evidence-based care provides benefits to the nurse, physicians, client, and administration.

Implementing Research into Practice

These eight steps have been suggested by Gennaro and associates (Gennaro, Hodnett, & Kearney, 2001):

1. Review the current literature related to the clinical issue.
2. Resolve to move forward only when you have gathered enough data to provide a rationale for the proposed change in practice.
3. Present your findings creatively. Use graphs, charts, posters, and so forth.

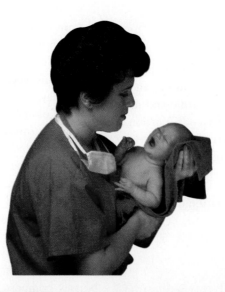

4. Include in your presentation a detailed clinical practice guideline. Develop a timeline for implementation.
5. Present a plan for evaluating client outcomes as they relate to the change in practice. Include how and when data will be reported.
6. Invite to the presentation each practitioner and administrator who might be affected by this change in practice. Discussing the idea with the opposition as well as with supporters is crucial for the plan to succeed.
7. Realize that small measures may need to be implemented prior to a full-blown change in policy.
8. Publish positive client outcomes and successful changes in practice in order to inspire others.

PLANNING AND IMPLEMENTATION

During the unit meeting, the nursing supervisor selected staff members and formed a committee to research the issue of pain relief during circumcision. The committee consisted of the two staff members who had recently attended the convention (one LPN and one RN), one pediatrician, one obstetrician, the nursing supervisor, and a parent who volunteers regularly in the nursery. Following is an outline of the committee's work.

1. They performed a literature search using the databases Cumulative Index to Nursing and Allied Health Literature (CINAHL) and MedLine. Key words used in the search were *pain, analgesia, anesthesia, newborn,* and *circumcision.*
2. Each committee member was responsible for outlining several research articles. Once in summary form, each article was reviewed by each member of the committee.
3. The information was developed into a PowerPoint presentation depicting the risks and benefits of using pain relief for newborn circumcision.
4. The committee also contacted several hospitals who had policies for using analgesia and anesthesia for newborn circumcision. After reviewing these policies, the committee developed a proposed policy for their own institution based on the literature review.
5. The committee also developed a cost analysis and client outcome evaluation method for implementing this change in practice.
6. All nursing staff, pediatricians and family physicians, obstetricians, nursing administration, and hospital administration were invited to hear the presentation of the literature review and proposed policy change.
7. After the presentation, it was decided that nonpharmacologic pain relief methods would be implemented

immediately. Pharmacologic pain relief methods would be reviewed carefully by each obstetrician. Obstetricians would meet with the committee in 6 months to discuss which pharmacologic method they would implement.
8. The committee planned to compare CRIES pain assessment scores in three situations:
   a. Prior to implementation of pain relief during circumcision
   b. Following implementation of nonpharmacologic pain relief methods
   c. Following implementation of pharmacologic pain relief methods

They planned to publish the results of this research.

SELF-REFLECTION

Have you ever heard the rationale for a procedure, "Because we've always done it that way?" What procedures or nursing interventions do you perform routinely without considering whether there is adequate research to support them? Could client safety be compromised because of your belief? Develop an action plan to review the literature as it related to this procedure. Develop a plan, if necessary, for changing your unit's policy and procedure for this procedure.

SUGGESTED RESOURCES

Brady-Fryer, B., Wiebe, N., & Landeer, J. (2004). Pain relief for neonatal circumcision. *The Cochrane Library*, issue 4.

Clifford, P. A., String, M., Christensen, H., & Mountain, D. (2004). Pain assessment and intervention for term newborns. *Journal of Midwifery and Women's Health, 49*(6), 514–519.

Gennaro, S., Hodnett, E., & Kearney, M. (2001). Making evidence-based practice a reality in your institutions: Evaluating the evidence and using the evidence to change clinical practice. *American Journal of Maternal/Child Nursing, 26* (5), 236–250.

Henry, P. R., Haubold, K., & Dobrzykowski, T. (2004). Pain in the healthy full-term neonate: Efficacy and safety of interventions. *Newborn Infant Nursing Review, 4*(2), 126–130.

Razums, I., Dalton, M., & Wilson, D. (2004). Practice applications of research. Pain management for newborn circumcision. *Pediatric Nursing, 30*(5), 414–417.

to households and individuals in convenient, familiar places" (ANA, 1991, p. 1). The "convenient, familiar places" are homes, schools, work sites, churches, and neighborhood clinics.

Policy makers have pressed for a cost-effective health care system. This cost-consciousness has resulted in decreases in the average length of stay for inpatient care, and community services are often required to fill the gap. Although clients may be discharged "sicker," a positive consequence has been an increased emphasis on the impact of lifestyle choices on individual health and illness prevention.

LEVELS OF CARE

Community-based nursing encompasses primary, secondary, and tertiary care.

- **Primary care** includes prevention activities such as immunizations, well-child checkups, routine physical examination, and use of infant car seats. Its purpose is to maintain health and prevent illness or injury from occurring.

- **Secondary care** refers to relatively serious or complicated care. Historically, this care was provided in acute-care hospitals, but with new techniques and procedures, much of this has been moved to community settings, including outpatient centers and home care. The purpose of secondary care is to help the client return to health after an acute disorder or disease. An example of this level of care would be care of a client after appendectomy.

- **Tertiary care** is the management of chronic, terminal, complicated, long-term health care problems such as cystic fibrosis or asthma. This level of care is frequently delivered in hospitals and community settings, including rehabilitation centers and home care. Its purpose is to help the client return to or maintain the highest possible level of functioning, and to adapt as necessary to the changes the condition requires.

CULTURALLY PROFICIENT CARE

During the end of the 20th and beginning of the 21st centuries, nurses have placed increased emphasis on understanding and responding to unique aspects of diverse groups of clients. At first, ethnicity was simply equated with culture and identified on the admission paperwork. Slowly, the concept evolved and the term *culture awareness* was used to describe knowledge of the similarities and differences among cultures. Unfortunately, many nurses focused on clients' differences instead of their similarities, so the quality of nursing care was not improved.

BOX 1-1	CULTURAL PULSE POINTS

Ways Institutions Can Respond to Cultural Diversity

- Hire interpreters when there is a sizable non-English-speaking population in an area.
- Post "Se habla español" signs at hospitals and clinics where Spanish is spoken.
- Provide teaching materials that are visual, not just written.
- Offer options on hospital menus for special diets (kosher, vegetarian, etc.).
- Open neighborhood clinics that cater directly to non-English-speaking populations.
- Purchase toys for children's hospitals that reflect a variety of racial and ethnic backgrounds.
- Offer regular in-service education to staff nurses on how to communicate with culturally diverse clients.

Since the 1990s, the nursing profession has been talking about **cultural competence,** or a set of skills, knowledge, and attitudes that include:

- Awareness and acceptance of differences
- Awareness of one's own cultural values
- Understanding of the dynamics of difference
- Development of cultural knowledge
- Ability to adapt practice skills to fit the cultural context of the client or patient

When these components become second nature to the nurse, **cultural proficiency** has been obtained (Leininger, McFarland, & McFarland, 2002).

The United States as a nation is becoming more aware of its variety of cultures. Colleges and universities are requiring that educational programs provide courses addressing cultural differences. Health care institutions are adapting to provide a better environment for people from many different backgrounds. Being bilingual or multilingual is becoming a requirement for employment in some areas. Box 1-1 ■ illustrates some ways that health care institutions are working to provide culturally proficient care. (Each chapter of this text contains further information about culture and culturally proficient nursing care.)

Roles of the LPN/LVN in Community Care

COLLABORATING WITH THE INTERDISCIPLINARY TEAM

As health care moves from the acute-care setting into the community, the members of the health care team must have a better understanding of how each role affects the quality

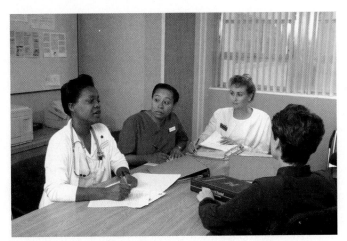

Figure 1-3. ■ Interdisciplinary team with LPN/LVN. (Pearson Education/PH College.)

of care provided. Collaboration with members of the health care team, in partnership with the family, is essential (Figure 1-3 ■). The health care team consists of physicians, social workers, psychologists, respiratory care professionals, physical therapy professionals, dietitians, and pharmacists, as well as nurses with a variety of educational backgrounds. Auxiliary workers and unlicensed assistive personnel and family members may be trained to perform selected tasks. As a result, nurses collaborate with a wide variety of individuals in delivering professional care.

To provide nursing care outside the acute-care setting, nurses once needed a bachelor's degree. Today, though, there are many opportunities for LPNs and LVNs in community-based nursing practice. With the move to community-based nursing practice, nursing roles are being redefined. The role of the LPN/LVN is no exception. The scope of practice for the LPN/LVN is more varied than that of the registered nurse from state to state and from facility to facility. Collaborative efforts with other health team workers are always based on the state's nurse practice acts, facility policy, and individual LPN/LVN capabilities.

PARTICIPATING IN THE NURSING PROCESS

In an acute-care setting, the LPN/LVN assists the RN and physician to provide direct client care. In most cases, this involves assisting in all aspects of the nursing process. The LPN/LVN collects data for assessment, contributes information toward naming nursing diagnoses and making a plan of care, implements nursing actions, and evaluates results of those interventions.

In community-based nursing practice, the LPN/LVN performs the same functions as in the acute-care facility. In this case, though, the client and the client's family are both the recipients of care. The LPN/LVN is responsible for keeping the registered nurse informed of changes in the client and family.

Communication and collaboration with other nurses and health care team members might be by telephone or electronic device instead of face to face. For example, an LPN/LVN providing care in the home to a child who was injured in an automobile accident may notice that a surgical incision site has become red and inflamed and is draining purulent fluid. The child's temperature is elevated. The LPN/LVN would instruct the mother and possibly other family members in the care of the wound and in the disposal of contaminated dressings. The LPN/LVN would then contact the nursing supervisor and provide input to revise the plan of care to include more frequent nursing assessments and dressing changes. The physician would be notified and appropriate medications would be obtained. The pharmacist might provide instructions about medication use and side effects.

PROBLEM SOLVING

Problem solving is a complex process that is at the heart of nursing. The LPN/LVN must collect data, evaluate the importance of the information to the care of the client, and take appropriate action. The nurse uses a variety of cognitive skills in the problem solving process. The nurse must be able to collect data, think rapidly, and make timely decisions. To do this the nurse uses inductive and deductive reasoning, critical thinking, and decision making skills. The problem-solving process includes critical thinking and decision making, which is discussed in Chapter 2 ⬭.

PRIORITIZING AND IMPLEMENTING CARE

Prioritizing care is something the LPN/LVN must do constantly. The most critical aspects of care must be initiated first. They include the ABCs of nursing (ensuring that the client has an open **A**irway, is **B**reathing, and has adequate **C**irculation). The next priority is to make the client safe and comfortable.

Nurses follow the established priorities in care plans. However, a change in the client's condition may cause the nurse to shift priorities suddenly in response. For example, the LPN/LVN assigned to care for a first-day postoperative client may be planning to bathe the client and then get her out of bed. While bathing the legs, the nurse notices a large, hard, red area behind the knee. The client states that the area hurts. The nurse does not get the client out of bed, because determining the cause of the hard, red area has a higher priority at this moment in time. If the cause is a

TABLE 1-3	
Priority-Setting Guidelines	
PRIORITY ACTIVITY	**RATIONALE**
1. Check sickest client or the one at most risk first. Assess ABC (airway/breathing/circulation), pain/safety. Check operation of all equipment.	The condition of this client may change rapidly, and he or she may not be able to call for help.
2. Check remainder of assigned clients in order of highest risk.	Ensures all clients are safe.
3. Return to complete assessments on each client.	Detailed assessments are needed to determine client problems and condition.
4. Update a written time line identifying what each client needs and at what time.	A written time line will provide a visual view of what will need to be completed at each time. The nurse can then decide what has priority at that time.
5. Administer medications within 30 minutes of scheduled time.	Medication administration is a high priority.
6. Review lab values and diagnostic study results as available.	Lab values/diagnostic study results may need to be called to the doctor. Some values may affect the administration of medication.
7. Provide all treatments, assessments, and basic care as ordered/scheduled.	Treatments generally have a higher priority than bathing, but the nurse may be able to do several things at one time.

blood clot, moving the client could cause the clot to move, resulting in life-threatening complications.

The LPN/LVN also establishes priorities when planning and implementing care for several clients at a time. The nurse must make priority decisions about each individual client and then about care of all the clients. The nurse decides which client to assess first, which ones to bathe first, and so on. Although each situation is different, Table 1-3 ■ identifies general guidelines that can help with priority setting.

DELEGATING

In today's health care environment, nurses have an increased responsibility to provide care to the individual client, to support the family, to develop health promotion activities, and to work to improve the health of entire communities. As a result there is an increasing use of Unlicensed Assistive Personnel (UAP) in direct client care activities. To maintain quality care, it is critical for the nurse to understand **delegation** (transferring to a competent individual the authority or right to perform selected nursing tasks in a selected situation). The nurse retains the accountability for the delegation. Delegation is discussed in more detail in Chapter 2 ⬭.

HEALTH PROMOTION TEACHING

A major role of LPNs and LVNs is client teaching. As mentioned earlier, the U.S. Department of Health and Human Services (1991) developed a systematic approach to health

with its sets of goals called *Healthy People 2000* and *Healthy People 2010* (U.S. Department of Health and Human Services, 2000). *Healthy People 2010* continues the effort to educate the public about ways in which they can positively affect their own health.

More and more people are recognizing the benefits of staying healthy. Health promotion activities emphasize nutrition, exercise, and stress reduction. Nurses often provide information about complementary or alternative therapies that can support a client's efforts to achieve or maintain health. Box 1-2 ■ lists some complementary therapies that are commonly seen today. Related topics such as immunizations, infection control, and identifying risk factors are directed toward illness prevention. Nurses are instrumental in health promotion and illness prevention by providing health teaching to individuals and groups. Because teaching is an important role of the LPN/LVN, health promotion activities are presented throughout the text.

Employment Opportunities for LPNs/LVNs in Community-Based Nursing

Pediatric clients are generally admitted to acute care hospitals only when they are extremely sick. Because of their acute status, care is complex, and employment opportunities for the LPN/LVN in these settings is becoming

BOX 1-2	COMPLEMENTARY THERAPIES

Selected Complementary and Alternative Therapies

- **Homeopathy**   A healing system that uses a small amount of a substance to produce the same symptom as the disorder. It stimulates the body's system to increase its immune response.
- **Naturopathy**   Natural medicines are used in the prevention and treatment of a disease. Naturopathy often employs a variety of approaches to solve a problem (e.g., changes in diet, increased ingestion of some vitamins, changes in activity).
- **Traditional Chinese Medicine**   Trigger points in acupressure and acupuncture, and breathing movements in T'ai Chi or Qi Gong, are used to achieve a balance of energy and promote well-being and harmony throughout the body.
- **Reiki (ray-key)**   Japanese energy healing employs a light laying on of hands from head to throat, heart, abdomen, knees, and feet. It is often used with people who have cancer or chronic health problems.
- **Mind-Based Therapies**   Guided imagery, hypnosis, visualization, biofeedback, music therapy, mediation, prayer, and chanting all help in the reduction of stress and can be helpful in the relief of chronic pain and some addictions. These therapies can also be combined with exercise forms of therapies such as yoga that use meditation, exercise, and diaphragmatic breathing to induce a relaxation response.

- **Massage Therapy and Therapeutic Touch**   Touch in the form of massage and reflexology is used to relax muscles, improve blood flow, and stimulate the immune system.
- **Chiropractic**   Manipulation to correct misalignment of the vertebrae can reduce the stress of pregnancy on the lower back. Client should be cautioned to use a fully qualified chiropractor.
- **Hydrotherapy**   Relaxation is achieved through the use of water. It is often used during labor and delivery in the form of a relaxing shower or to deliver the baby underwater. Cold compresses, hot compresses, and sweat baths are also types of hydrotherapy.
- **Herbal Therapies**   Plants have been used for medicinal purposes for thousands of years. Herbal therapies are often used to treat specific symptoms, such as to reduce menopausal symptoms.
- **Aroma Therapy**   Aroma therapy uses scented oil for relaxation and a psychological response. It is believed that different aromas can influence heart rate and blood pressure. They can also be used on the skin during massage therapy.

Note: Because there is little or no regulation of essential oils, pregnant women should be advised not to use essential oils during pregnancy.

limited. However, employment opportunities for the LPN/LVN have increased as more neighborhood clinics have opened. In some states, employment opportunities are also increasing in immunization clinics, home health, and school nursing. Because the LPN/LVN is unable to practice in an independent role, the employing agency should have clear policies identifying the RN or doctor who is responsible for directing and reviewing their work.

Note: The reference and resource listings for this and all chapters are compiled at the back of the book.

Chapter Review

KEY TERMS by Topic

Use the audio glossary feature of either the CD-ROM or the Companion Website to hear the correct pronunciation of the following key terms.

History of Pediatrics
pediatrics

Developments in Nursing
objective data, subjective data, holistic

Nursing Process in Pediatric Care
nursing diagnoses, desired outcomes, care plan, interventions

Research-Based Nursing Practice
mortality, morbidity

Community-Based Nursing Practice
community-based nursing, primary care, secondary care, tertiary care,

cultural competence, cultural proficiency

Roles of the LPN/LVN in Community Care
delegation

KEY Points

- The nursing care of children is evolving to include the entire family.
- The nursing process guides the care planning process.
- Community-based nursing practice is the provision of nursing care wherever the client lives, works, plays, or prays.
- Nursing includes health promotion and illness prevention activities as well as assistance in the medical management of illness.
- The terms *client*, *patient*, and *consumer* all refer to the recipient of health care services. The term *client* indicates that the person is actively involved in health care decisions.
- Being able to set priorities is essential in providing safe care.
- The state nurse practice act governs nursing practice. Facility policy regulates nursing practice within the specific clinical setting.

EXPLORE MediaLink

Additional interactive resources for this chapter can be found on the Companion Website at www. prenhall. com/ adams.

Click on Chapter 1 and "Begin" to select the activities for this chapter.

For chapter-related NCLEX®-style questions and an audio glossary, access the accompanying CD-ROM in this book.

FOR FURTHER Study

Cultural issues and competency are addressed in Cultural Care boxes throughout the text.

Delegation and critical thinking are discussed in detail in Chapter 2.

Standards of care and other legal and ethical issues are discussed in Chapter 3.

For a full discussion on child development, see Chapter 5.

See discussion of SIDS in Chapter 12.

Circumcision is discussed in Chapter 18.

NCLEX-PN® Exam Preparation

TEST-TAKING TIP Cover the answers and read the question. Try to answer the question without looking at the answers. Trust your first instinct, and do not try to rationalize why another given response might also be correct by reading into the question.

1 The nurse understands that primary nursing care is best identified as:
1. Helping a child with diabetes learn how to monitor blood sugar.
2. Teaching an 11-year-old with a sprained leg how to walk with crutches.
3. Screening for scoliosis in a school health room.
4. Administering eye drops into a child with acute conjunctivitis.

2 The nurse understands that tertiary nursing care is best identified as:
1. Obtaining a sterile urinary specimen for the purpose of determining the effectiveness of antibiotic therapy.
2. Immunizing a 3-year-old child for influenza.
3. Monitoring hematocrit each trimester during pregnancy.
4. Administering tracheostomy care to a 4-year-old with a permanent tracheostomy.

3 The LPN/LVN has many roles in the acute-care setting. Choose all of the following that apply to these roles:
1. Administering PO medications
2. Supervising unlicensed assistive personnel
3. Collecting data
4. Administering blood products intravenously
5. Developing a nursing diagnosis based on assessment data

4 Which of the following statements reflects current thinking about pediatric care?
1. "Your child will go home to complete recovery as soon as she is stable, so it is important for you to know about wound care."
2. "Your child will go home 2 weeks after surgery; this will give us time to watch the wound heal."
3. "We will keep your child here until we are sure there will be no complications."
4. "If the wound is puffy, red, and warm to the touch when you are changing the dressing at home, lance it with a sterilized sewing needle."

5 Which of the following comments by an LPN/LVN demonstrates that people under the care of an LPN/LVN are viewed as active participants in their own care?
1. "My patient in room 212 needs something for pain."
2. "My client would like to ask the doctor some questions now."
3. "Don't worry, the doctor will be able to make decisions for you."
4. "I will help the teenage mother feed her baby."

6 The nurse is concerned about a particular health issue for a client and has been given approval to research the issue to document if a change in practice is necessary. List the following steps for implementing research into practice in the correct order.
1. Develop a plan to evaluate client outcomes.
2. Create a presentation presenting the risks and benefits to support a change in practice.
3. Document approved changes to the clinical guidelines.
4. Invite practitioners and administrators to discuss the proposed new practice guidelines.
5. Review current literature.
6. Publish positive client outcomes relating to the new clinical practice guidelines.
7. Develop clinical practice guidelines and a time frame for possible implementation.
8. Gather data that provides rationales for a proposed change in practice.

7 The nurse has requested the LPN/LVN to assist her during a home visit. Which of the following agencies should the LPN/LVN refer to before collaborating with the nurse during a home visit?
1. Individual state's nurse practice act
2. Association of Women's Health, Obstetric and Neonatal Nurses
3. Nurse's Association of the American College of Obstetricians and Gynecologists
4. American Nurses Association

8 The LPN/LVN has been assigned to care for the following clients. Based on the morning report, which client should the LPN/LVN assess first?
1. A 1-hour-old newborn with acrocyanosis
2. A 2-year-old receiving oxygen for croup
3. A 7-year-old in Buck's traction
4. A 2-day-old with physiologic jaundice

9 During a home visit with a breastfeeding mother, the mother states that she is worried about bleeding from the base of the umbilical cord. Which of the following health care team members should the LPN/LVN contact first?
1. The unlicensed assistive personnel
2. The nursing supervisor
3. The child's father
4. The pediatrician

10 Which of the following tasks reflects the LPN/LVN role for pediatric nursing care?
1. Establishes a nursing diagnosis for a client recovering from surgery for umbilical hernia.
2. Independently plans care for clients in the home setting
3. Teaches the client about reasonable expectations for toilet training
4. Prescribes an antibiotic for a child with an ear infection

Answers for NCLEX-PN® Review and Critical Thinking questions appear in Appendix I.

Chapter 2

Critical Thinking in Pediatric Care

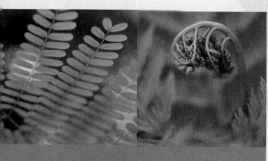

HEALTH PROMOTION ISSUE:
Applying Critical Reading to Evidence-Based Nursing Practice

CRITICAL THINKING CARE MAP:
Caring for a Client with Hyperbilirubinemia

BRIEF Outline

CRITICAL THINKING
Intellectual Standards
Elements of Thought
Critical Thinking Care Map
Essential Intellectual Traits or Values

DECISION MAKING AND DELEGATION
Decision Making
Delegation

LEARNING Outcomes

After completing this chapter, you will be able to:
1. Define key terms.
2. Discuss the critical thinking process and standards that define it.
3. Identify the elements of thought.
4. Discuss the intellectual traits that result from critical thinking.
5. Describe decision making and prioritizing as they relate to nursing scope of practice.
6. Describe the delegation process related to nursing scope of practice.

To provide quality pediatric care in today's complex world, nurses must be knowledgeable, flexible, and capable of making difficult decisions. The nursing process provides LPNs/LVNs with a systematic approach: collect data for assessment, report it so that the nursing diagnoses can be identified and a plan of care can be developed, implement the care plan by providing direct care to the client, and evaluate (critically review) the results of the care provided. Nurses use critical thinking skills to research each aspect of client care. To provide the best possible client care, critical thinking must occur before decisions are made. This chapter will help the student develop beginning critical thinking and decision-making skills.

CRITICAL THINKING

Although everyone thinks, much of human thought is biased, uninformed, incomplete, or prejudiced. Yet, the quality of nursing care depends on the quality of the nurse's thought. Shallow, incomplete thinking may be costly in both money and the health of the client. Poor or partial thinking might result in delays in treatment and complications in the client's condition. Biased thinking may mean that a client in pain is seen as a "complainer" and is not managed promptly.

Richard Paul and Linda Elder (2005, p. 1) state, "**Critical thinking** is, in short, self-directed, self-disciplined, self-monitored, and self-corrective thinking." To improve critical thinking skills, Paul and Elder teach critical thinkers to apply certain intellectual standards to the elements of reasoning in order to develop intellectual traits.

Intellectual Standards

Intellectual standards are concepts that guide the critical thinker to better and better reasoning (Box 2-1 ■). **Clarity** (clearness) is necessary to eliminate confusion. In order to address a client's question or problem adequately, the nurse must have a clear understanding of what the person asking the question considers the problem to be. Nurses ask questions ("Could you give me an example?" "Could you elaborate on that?"), restate what they hear the person saying, and ask the client to verify accuracy, in order to clarify the problem.

It is important to determine the **accuracy** (correctness) of the data being considered. A statement can be clear but inaccurate. For example, "Most women gain 100 pounds during pregnancy" is a clear statement, but not accurate. By thinking, "How can I find out if that is true?" the accuracy of data can be explored.

A statement could be both clear and accurate, but lack **precision** (scientific exactness). The statement, "The infant is overweight," is clear and may be accurate but lacks precision in identifying how much overweight the baby is. There is a big difference between being 1 pound and 5 pounds overweight. The nurse needs to ask, "Could you be more specific?" in order to have precise information.

At times, a great deal of information is collected about a client. The nurse must determine the **relevance** of the information (its connection to the matter in hand). For example, a mother may bring a child to the clinic with a sore throat. During the assessment, the mother may state that her husband had surgery. The nurse thinks, "How is this related to the sore throat?" While the husband's health may be important to the client's mental well-being, it is irrelevant to the child's sore throat. In this situation, the nurse would need to assess the sore throat, deciding that data about the husband's surgery is a separate problem.

Information can be clear, accurate, precise, and relevant, but be superficial. In order to think critically about an issue, the complexities or **depth** (complexity) of the issue must be explored. The nurse should think, "What are the related factors?" or, "What are the complexities of this question?" Sometimes the nurse must collaborate with others in order to explore complex issues thoroughly. For example, a couple

BOX 2-1

Intellectual Standards

Certain tools we can use improve our ability to think. The list below names intellectual standards (Paul & Elder, 2005) and ways the nurse can implement them:

- Clarity—Provide a clear explanation with examples.
- Accuracy—Provide back-up for checking facts or means of verifying data.
- Precision—Give specific, measurable details.
- Relevance—Show the relationship of data to the problem and the value of finding a solution.
- Depth—Identify the factors that make the problem complex or difficult.
- Breadth—View the problem from several perspectives; seek out new viewpoints.
- Logic—Determine whether the pieces of the solution make sense together.
- Significance—Decide whether the problem is important and the solution is well focused.
- Fairness—Assess whether the solution benefits one group over another or whether all viewpoints are considered.

HEALTH PROMOTION ISSUE

APPLYING CRITICAL READING TO EVIDENCE-BASED NURSING PRACTICE

A nurse working in a hospital is concerned that four young male clients who underwent surgical repair in the past year for leg fractures have developed infections in the wound. The hospital policy is to use a safety razor to shave the leg area prior to surgery. Nancy wonders if this extensive shaving is contributing to the number of infections. When she asks her peers how they know this intervention is best practice, they respond with, "No one is able to provide actual evidence. This is the way we have always prepared clients for surgery."

DISCUSSION

As stated in Chapter 1 ⬀, evidence-based practice (also called best practice) is the use of the best evidence currently available for clinical decision making in order to provide the most consistent and best possible care to clients. Most nurses, according to Estabrooks (1998), practice nursing according to what they were taught in nursing school. According to the National Sample Survey of Registered Nurses conducted by the U.S. Health Resources and Services Administration (HRSA) in March 2000, 70% of nurses graduated from nursing programs before 1990. The data raise the issue of whether nurses are using the most up-to-date information in providing care. The nurse must not only have accurate data, but also have the most up-to-date research in how to interpret the data and implement nursing care. In many instances, nursing practice has changed in response to data (evidence) that "the way we have always done it" is not always the best, most efficient, or safest practice. As data are collected, researchers publish their findings in professional journals with the hope that nursing practice will change accordingly.

Once a clinical practice problem is identified, searching for, finding, and evaluating appropriate evidence is critical. Professional literature is the most important source for change in nursing practice. However, professional literature may not be readily available in the workforce. Nurses who graduated before the wide use of computers and the Internet may not know how to access information technology. Few nurses are able to conduct a successful literature search using *CINAHL database* or *MEDLINE database* (the two most common databases of medical, nursing, and allied health literature). Some health care facilities do not allow access to the Internet in the workplace for fear the technology will be misused. Hospital libraries, if they exist, usually have limited hours and may not be readily available to the nursing staff.

Once professional literature is obtained, nurses may not be prepared to evaluate the validity of the content. More nurses are familiar with the Internet and the World Wide Web as sources of information than with the CINAHL and MEDLINE search engines. However, Internet searches may provide a great deal of information, not all of which is reliable.

---

who has a baby with severe physical disabilities may need assistance to provide for their child. The nurse working as a discharge planner might collaborate with the physical therapist, social worker, and social security advisor when assisting the family in making long-range plans for their child.

To examine the **breadth** (scope) of the issue, different points of view need to be considered. By asking, "Is there another way to look at the question?" all sides of the issue can be explored.

Active attempts to learn more about a situation promote **fairness** (impartiality). To reach this intellectual standard, the nurse asks, "Am I listening to the viewpoints of others the way I would want them to listen to mine?"

When we think critically, we use **reasoning** (process of forming conclusions, judgments, or inferences from facts or assumptions). When the thoughts are combined in an order that "makes sense" the thinking is **logical** (reasonable). An example of logical thinking is this: This person is pregnant; since only women become pregnant, then this person is a woman. If the combination is contradictory, it is not logical. **Inductive reasoning** is the process of making generalized statements from a limited set of facts. For example, if a client has dry skin, poor skin turgor, and dry mucous membranes, the nurse can induce that the client is dehydrated. **Deductive reasoning** is the process of making specific statements from a generalized concept. For example, the nurse reads in the

PLANNING AND IMPLEMENTATION

Nurses must make time in their busy schedules to read professional literature and take part in continuing education classes, in order to remain up-to-date. Ideally, time and resources will be available in the workplace. If that is not the case, the nurse must read during his or her personal time. The skill of performing literature searches using educational technology is an essential skill that nurses must acquire. Colleges and universities, technology assistants, and other resources are available to teach nurses these skills.

The nurse uses critical thinking skills to read critically. At times professional journal articles need to be read several times to ensure complete understanding. The first reading is used just to rephrase the author's words into your words. Writing down this paraphrasing helps in capturing the text's essential meaning. If the paraphrasing lacks

clarity, depth, breadth, logic, and fairness, the article should be read again. The nurse should be able to identify the question or problem being addressed, the assumptions and the implications being made, and the concepts (ideas) and conclusions of the article.

After the nurse has reviewed the literature, further data may need to be collected in the form of research. (This was true in the research case presented in Chapter 1 ⊂⊃ of this text.). Once data are collected, they should be shared with other nurses through professional journal articles. The nurse uses best practice evidence when writing the client's care plan, providing direct client care, supervising unlicensed personnel, and collaborating with other nurses in revising facility policy.

The LPN/LPN must critically read evidence-based practice in order to learn and remain up-to-date with research findings. If the LPN/LVN identifies best-practice evidence that contraindicates the

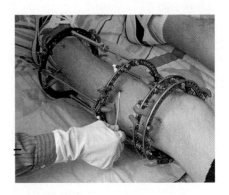

care provided in his or her facility, the nurse should share the research with the supervising RN and other nurses.

SELF-REFLECTION

When reading a journal article, do you accept the concepts at face value, or do you try to apply concepts of critical thinking in order to understand the issue better? What can you do to get a deeper understanding from your reading? How can you apply critical thinking concepts to other aspects of your life?

SUGGESTED RESOURCES

Estabrooks, C. (1998). Will evidence-based nursing practice make practice perfect? *Canadian Journal of Nursing Research, 30*(1), 15–36.

Pravikoff, D., Ranner, A., & Pierce, S. (2005) Readiness of U.S. nurses for evidence-based practice. *American Journal of Nursing, 105*(9), 40–51.

Spratley, E., Johnson, A., Sochalski, J., Fritz, M., Spencer, W. (2001). *The registered nurse population March 2000: Findings from the National Sample Survey of Registered Nurses.* Rockville, MD: U.S. Department of Health and Human Services.

---

chart that this same client has been vomiting much of her food and liquid for 2 weeks. The nurse knows that vomiting can cause dehydration. From this generalized information, the nurse can deduce that the client's mucous membranes will be dry, the urinary output will be low, and the urine will be dark amber. The nurse will expect these findings in the client. The use of evidence-based thinking and research to improve nursing practice is illustrated further in the Health Promotion Issue on pages 20 and 21.

The nurse must look at the information and determine the **significance** (importance) to the client's health at this point in time. By asking, "Is this the most important problem to consider?" the nurse sets priorities in providing care.

In the case previously mentioned, dehydration is very significant because it will affect the health of the client.

Elements of Thought

To do critical thinking, it helps to identify the different elements of thought (Paul Elder, 2005). Box 2-2 ■ reviews these elements. All critical thinking has a **purpose** (an end, aim, or result), which should be stated clearly and specifically. In nursing, each step of the nursing process contains at least one purpose. For example, the purpose of assessment is to collect and analyze data in order to determine the client's health status. The nurse must determine the

BOX 2-2

Elements of Thought

Our thoughts include all of the following components:

- Purpose of our thinking
- Question at issue
- Available information
- Point of view
- Interpretation and inference
- Concepts
- Assumptions
- Implications and consequences

Source: Data from Paul, R., & Elder, L. (2005). *The miniature guide to critical thinking concepts & tools.* The Foundation for Critical Thinking. Dillon Beach, CA: Foundation for Critical Thinking.

accuracy and precision of the data, and then determine their relevance to the client's condition.

All critical thinking is an attempt to figure out something or settle some problem or question. The problem should be stated clearly and precisely. In many instances in nursing, the problem may be the client's presenting health issue. The problem may be broken down into several underlying subproblems. For example, when a client is short of breath, has an increased respiratory rate, has wheezy lung sounds, and has a nonproductive cough, the nurse would determine that the client has an alteration in respiratory function (the problem). However, underlying problems are bronchial constriction (which causes the wheezing) and inability to clear the airway (which results in nonproductive cough). The nurse states the problem in terms of nursing diagnoses (in this case, Ineffective **B**reathing Pattern" and "Ineffective **A**irway Clearance" (NANDA, 2008).

The critical thinker bases decisions on accurate, complete, and relevant **information** (knowledge gained through research or observation). The nurse would ask, "What information am I using to reach this conclusion?" "What more information do I need?" and, "What experience do I have that supports my conclusion?" At times it is important for the critical thinker to consider different **points of view** (perspectives). By asking, "Is there another point of view I should consider?" the critical thinker maintains an open mind to other alternatives or actions.

Before taking action, the critical thinker would explore **interpretations** (ways of clarifying the meaning), **inferences** (deductions), and **assumptions** (ideas taken for granted). The results would be used to reach informed **conclusions** (decisions based on prior thought). By asking questions such as, "Is there another way to interpret this information?" "What am I taking for granted?" and, "Are these inferences consistent with the data?" the nurse can reach accurate conclusions.

The critical thinker uses **concepts** (theories, laws, and principles) from many disciplines to further understand the

problem and address possible solutions. For example, the nurse uses gas laws identified by the chemist to understand the transport of oxygen from room air to the blood. Principles of microbiology are used in infection control practices. Education theory is applied when the nurse provides infant care instruction to new mothers.

The critical thinker explores the **implications** (consequences) of actions or decisions. By asking, "If someone accepted my position, what would be the implications?" or, "What would be the consequences of this action?" the critical thinker develops sound judgment.

These elements of thought are an important part of the nursing process, because the nurse must reach accurate conclusions about the client's health problem, about which interventions to try first, and about the effectiveness of treatments. Learning to apply these elements of thought and standards of critical thinking to the care of clients takes practice. The nursing student may be asked to demonstrate critical thinking through written care plans, examinations, and clinical performance. Each chapter of this book will provide the student with exercises to improve critical thinking skills applicable to the care of children.

Critical Thinking Care Map

This text provides an interactive tool for practicing critical thinking. At the end of each chapter of this book, critical thinking exercises are presented in the form of a Critical Thinking Care Map. The care map presents a clinical situation related to the content of the chapter. It identifies the NCLEX-PN® focus area related to the case study, to help the student think in terms of the categories needed for licensure. An **NCLEX-PN® focus area** is one of 11 areas of client needs around which the NCLEX-PN® test is constructed. The care map then identifies one appropriate NANDA nursing diagnosis for the client. A list of data is shown. Some of it is relevant to the identified nursing diagnosis. Some of it is not. The student selects and organizes the relevant information under the subjective and objective data headings. Irrelevant data are omitted.

The student then decides if any of the information needs to be reported. Are any values outside of normal ranges? Is there an acceptable explanation for the data outside the normal range? For example, if a client is receiving an IV infusion to correct hypercalcemia, it would not be necessary to report the calcium imbalance unless the condition was not improving with therapy, or unless it appeared that the client's calcium level was decreasing.

The student needs to decide who should get the report. For example, the nurse might report to the team leader or charge nurse if a postsurgical client complains that pain medications are not effective. However, if a client complains of pain 4 days after an operation for scoliosis, and the client also has bright red bleeding from the wound site, the nurse would immediately inform the surgeon of the possibility of a wound *dehiscence* (separation of the wound.)

The next step in the care map is for the student to select relevant interventions. Again, the student would select *only* those interventions that relate to the nursing diagnosis identified for this exercise. Other interventions, even though they might be suitable for the client, would not be chosen from the list provided.

Finally, the student practices documenting pertinent information. The date, the time, the pertinent data, the intervention performed, the results of the nursing actions, and the nurse's signature are all essential elements of narrative notes in the client chart. Sample documentations for the Critical Thinking Care Maps and the answers to the questions posed in the exercise are provided in Appendix I. A sample Critical Thinking Care Map is provided below.

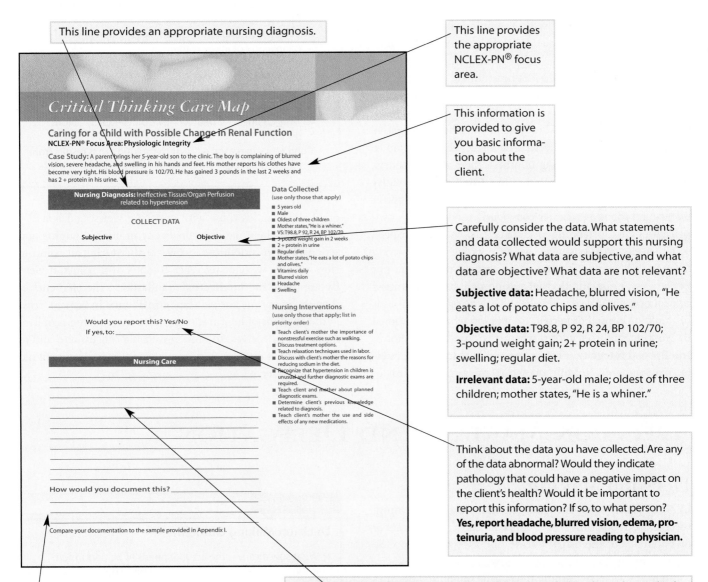

This line provides an appropriate nursing diagnosis.

This line provides the appropriate NCLEX-PN® focus area.

This information is provided to give you basic information about the client.

Critical Thinking Care Map

Caring for a Child with Possible Change in Renal Function
NCLEX-PN® Focus Area: Physiologic Integrity

Case Study: A parent brings her 5-year-old son to the clinic. The boy is complaining of blurred vision, severe headache, and swelling in his hands and feet. His mother reports his clothes have become very tight. His blood pressure is 102/70. He has gained 3 pounds in the last 2 weeks and has 2 + protein in his urine.

Nursing Diagnosis: Ineffective Tissue/Organ Perfusion related to hypertension

COLLECT DATA

Subjective   Objective

Would you report this? Yes/No
If yes, to: _____

Nursing Care

How would you document this? _____

Compare your documentation to the sample provided in Appendix I.

Data Collected
(use only those that apply)

- 5 years old
- Male
- Oldest of three children
- Mother states, "He is a whiner."
- VS: T98.8, P 92, R 24, BP 102/70
- 3-pound weight gain in 2 weeks
- 2 + protein in urine
- Regular diet
- Mother states, "He eats a lot of potato chips and olives."
- Vitamins daily
- Blurred vision
- Headache
- Swelling

Nursing Interventions
(use only those that apply; list in priority order)

- Teach client's mother the importance of nonstressful exercise such as walking.
- Discuss treatment options.
- Teach relaxation techniques used in labor.
- Discuss with client's mother the reasons for reducing sodium in the diet.
- Recognize that hypertension in children is unusual and further diagnostic exams are required.
- Teach client and mother about planned diagnostic exams.
- Determine client's previous knowledge related to diagnosis.
- Teach client's mother the use and side effects of any new medications.

Carefully consider the data. What statements and data collected would support this nursing diagnosis? What data are subjective, and what data are objective? What data are not relevant?

Subjective data: Headache, blurred vision, "He eats a lot of potato chips and olives."

Objective data: T98.8, P 92, R 24, BP 102/70; 3-pound weight gain; 2+ protein in urine; swelling; regular diet.

Irrelevant data: 5-year-old male; oldest of three children; mother states, "He is a whiner."

Think about the data you have collected. Are any of the data abnormal? Would they indicate pathology that could have a negative impact on the client's health? Would it be important to report this information? If so, to what person? **Yes, report headache, blurred vision, edema, proteinuria, and blood pressure reading to physician.**

This question allows you to practice your documentation. It is not necessary to document all the data or interventions for this exercise. For example, the assessment documentation might be.

(date/time) Client seen in clinic with c/o severe headache, blurred vision, and swelling in hands and feet. Mother states, "He has been eating a lot of potato chips and olives." BP 102/70. 2+ protein in urine. Weight up 3 lb in two weeks. M. Towler, LPN

Consider the client's and the mother's deficient knowledge about the medical condition and its consequences. Make a decision about which interventions are relevant and which are not. Place relevant interventions in priority order.

Relevant interventions: Recognize that hypertension in children is unusual and that further diagnostic exams are required. Determine client's mother's previous knowledge related to diagnosis. Teach client and mother about planned diagnostic exams. Discuss with client's mother the reasons for reducing sodium in the diet. Teach client's mother the use and side effects of any new medications.

Irrelevant interventions: Teach client's mother the importance of nonstressful exercise such as walking. Discuss treatment options. Teach relaxation techniques.

Essential Intellectual Traits or Values

As with any skill, critical thinking develops with practice. However, critical thinking is especially valuable because it can improve virtually every area of one's life. As one thinks about thinking and gains strength in these skills, it is helpful to keep in mind what the best critical thinking would be (Paul & Elder, 2005). Standards of excellence in critical thinking (also called essential intellectual traits for critical thinking) are provided, with examples, in Box 2-3 ■. **Intellectual humility** is having a consciousness that one's knowledge base, prejudices, biases, and point of view have limitations. It implies the lack of boastfulness, arrogance, and conceit. **Intellectual courage** is facing and fairly addressing ideas, beliefs, or viewpoints that might, on a superficial level, seem absurd or false, or toward which we might have negative emotions. Through intellectual courage, we may come to have a deeper understanding of others, their ideas or beliefs, and the environment in which they live. **Intellectual empathy** is imagining oneself in the place of others in order to better understand them. It requires consciously ignoring one's own perceptions, long-standing ideas, or beliefs. At times, we need to remember occasions when we were wrong despite strong feelings that we were right, and understand that this might be the present case. **Intellectual autonomy** is having a rational control over one's ideas and beliefs. The critical thinker learns to think for himself or herself, to question when it is rational to question, and to conform when it is rational to conform. **Intellectual integrity** is being true and consistent with intellectual standards, holding oneself to the same standards of

proof as one holds those with opposing views, and honestly admitting when one is inconsistent in one's thoughts and actions. **Fair-mindedness** is consciously treating all points of view equally, without reference to one's own points of view. By applying the intellectual standards to the elements of thought, over time one develops **confidence in reason** (trust in the outcome of logical thought). By encouraging people to think for themselves, to draw reasonable conclusions, and to persuade each other with reason, the interests of humankind will best be served.

BOX 2-3

Essential Intellectual Traits

When critical thinking is occurring, certain positive intellectual traits surface (Paul & Elder, 2005). The sentences next to each intellectual trait provide a way of rephrasing the traits in everyday terms:

Intellectual humility—I know that I do not know everything.
Intellectual courage—I dare to consider other points of view.
Intellectual empathy—I try to learn about and understand others.
Intellectual autonomy—I can think something even if people do not agree with me.
Intellectual integrity—I hold myself to the same standard as I hold others.
Intellectual perseverance—I will continue to think until I understand.
Fair-mindedness—I treat all viewpoints equally before deciding.
Confidence in reason—I trust the solution that results from logical thinking.

DECISION MAKING AND DELEGATION

Decision Making

LPNs/LVNs are faced with daily decisions about performing specific acts. Sometimes they will be asked to perform acts or tasks outside of the usual routine, and they need to decide whether or not to perform them. New graduates or inexperienced nurses who are learning the routine might find decision making challenging. (Legal and ethical aspects of decisions are discussed in the following chapter.) LPNs/LVNs working in community agencies may face more decisions than nurses working in a structured environment, such as an acute or long-term care agency. In all cases, however, the nurse will be held to the standards of reasonable and prudent care.

LPNs/LVNs have guidelines to follow when making decisions about performance of specific acts. Box 2-4 ■ provides these guidelines. By specifically identifying the act and

---

BOX 2-4

Decision Making Guidelines

- What specifically is the act that needs to be performed?
- Is the act expressly permitted/prohibited by the state's nurse practice act, board of nursing rules, or board of nursing position statements?
- Is the act expressly permitted or prohibited by agency policy?
- Is the act something that was taught in your basic nursing education program, and do you possess current clinical skills?
- Is the act consistent with positive and conclusive data in nursing literature and supported by research?
- Can you document successful completion of additional education that includes instruction and supervised clinical practice?

collecting data through client assessment, the nurse has a clear picture of what needs to be done. Once the nurse understands the act and the client's condition, a series of questions should be answered.

1. Is the act expressly permitted or prohibited by the state's nurse practice act, board of nursing rules, or position statements? The registered nurse and LPN/LVN need to be familiar with the state nurse practice act and the Board of Nursing rules and regulations. Copies of these documents can be obtained by contacting the state board of nursing or, in most states, by accessing its website. If the act is prohibited by law, the LPN/LVN must inform a nursing supervisor or physician.

2. Is the act expressly permitted or prohibited by agency policy? A review of the agency policy book reveals whether the act is sanctioned by the agency. Agency policy can be more restrictive than the board of nursing rule, but it cannot be more lenient. If the nurse performs an act against agency policy and the client outcome is not positive, the nurse might not be supported by the agency.

3. Once it is determined that the act may be performed per the foregoing standards, the nurse needs to examine her or his own competence to perform the act. Is the act something that was taught in the nursing education program, and does he or she possess current clinical skills? Even if the act was taught in the basic nursing education program, if the nurse has not performed the act for a long time, it may not be wise to proceed unassisted or unsupervised. It is expected that even an experienced nurse would need assistance when confronted with an unfamiliar act.

As advances are made in health care, new techniques will be found and new equipment will be produced. Before performing a new procedure the nurse should ask, "Is the act consistent with positive and conclusive data in nursing literature and supported by research? Have I been trained in performing this procedure, and if so is documentation of that training on file?" Most agencies provide in-service programs where new equipment and techniques are demonstrated and supervised practice is offered. Documentation of completion of these programs becomes part of the continuing education file.

When these questions are answered, the correct decision about performing the act will become clear (Figure 2-1 ■).

Delegation

The shift to community-based nursing has resulted in increased responsibility for nurses to provide care to the individual client, support the family, develop health promotion activities, and work to improve the health of entire communities. Consequently, there has been an increase in use of Unlicensed Assistive Personnel in direct client care

activities. In order to maintain quality care, it is critical the nurse understands the delegation process. **Delegation** is transferring to a competent individual the authority or right to perform selected nursing tasks in selected situations. To help the nurse make wise decisions regarding delegating tasks, the National Council of State Boards of Nursing published a list of Premises or explanatory statements. These premises are listed in Box 2-5 ■.

BOX 2-5

National Council of State Boards of Nursing Premises for Delegating Tasks

The following premises constitute the basis for the delegation decision-making process.

1. All decisions related to delegation of nursing tasks must be based on the fundamental principle of protection of the health, safety and welfare of the public.
2. Boards of Nursing are responsible for the regulation of nursing. Provision of any care which constitutes nursing or any activity represented as nursing is a regulatory responsibility of Boards of Nursing.
3. Boards of Nursing should articulate clear principles for delegation, augmented by clearly defined guidelines for delegation decisions.
4. A licensed nurse must have ultimate responsibility and accountability for the management and provision of nursing.
5. A licensed nurse must be actively involved in and be accountable for all managerial decisions, policy making and practices related to the delegation of nursing care.
6. There is a need and a place for competent, appropriately supervised, unlicensed assistive personnel in the delivery of affordable, quality health care. However, it must be remembered that unlicensed assistive personnel are equipped to assist—not replace—the nurse.
7. Nursing is a knowledge-based process discipline and cannot be reduced solely to a list of tasks. The licensed nurse's specialized education, professional judgment and discretion are essential for quality nursing care.
8. While nursing tasks may be delegated, the licensed nurse's generalist knowledge of client care indicates that the practice-pervasive functions of assessment, evaluation and nursing judgment must not be delegated.
9. A task delegated to an unlicensed assistive personnel cannot be redelegated by the unlicensed assistive person.
10. Consumers have a right to health care that meets legal standards of care. Thus, when a nursing task is delegated, the task must be performed in accord with established standards of practice, policies and procedures.
11. The licensed nurse determines and is accountable for the appropriateness of delegated nursing tasks. Inappropriate delegation by the nurse and/or unauthorized performance of nursing tasks by unlicensed assistive personnel may lead to legal action against the licensed nurse and/or unlicensed assistive personnel.

Source: National Council of State Boards of Nursing, Incorporated. (1995). *Delegation: concepts and decision-making process.* Chicago: Author.

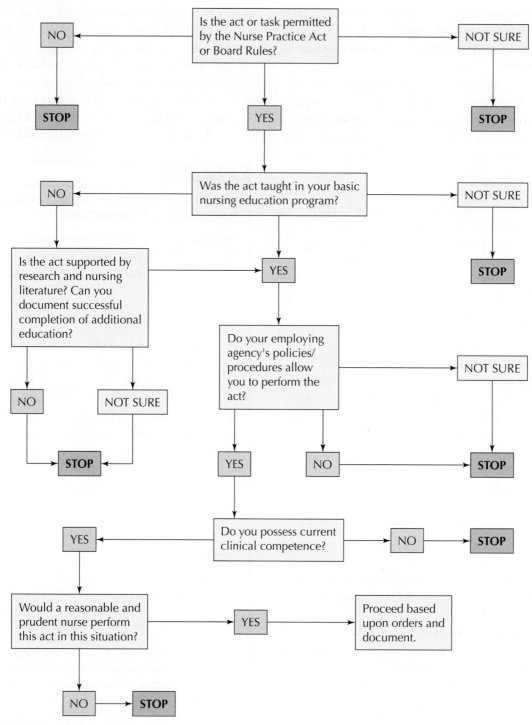

Figure 2-1. ■ Decision-making model.

All decisions related to delegation of nursing tasks must be based on the fundamental principle of protection of health, safety, and welfare of the public. State boards of nursing have established through each state's nurse practice act the standards of delegation. Because the scope of practice varies from state to state, it is important for the LPN/LVN to read and follow the state nurse practice act. Five Rules of Delegation are presented in Box 2-6 ■ as a basis for understanding the role of the LPN/LVN in community-based nursing practice. Figure 2-2 ■ illustrates steps to take in preparing to delegate tasks.

When delegating, the nurse is accountable for the delegation. Key words in the definition must be further described. **A competent individual** is a person who has received training, including instruction and clinical practice, to perform certain tasks and can demonstrate safe performance. Before

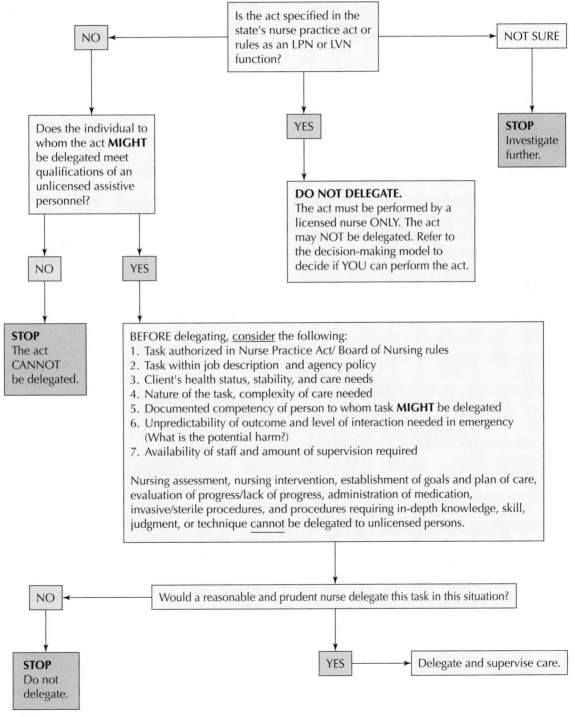

Figure 2-2. ■ Delegation model.

BOX 2-6

Five Rules of Delegation

- RIGHT TASK: One that is delegated for a specific client
- RIGHT CIRCUMSTANCES: Appropriate client setting, available resources and other relevant factors considered
- RIGHT PERSON: <u>Right person</u> is delegating the right task to the <u>right person</u> to be performed on the <u>right person.</u>
- RIGHT DIRECTION/COMMUNICATION: Clear, concise description of the task, including its objective, limits, and expectations
- RIGHT SUPERVISION: Appropriate monitoring, evaluation, intervention as needed, and feedback

---

care is delegated to an unlicensed assistive person, the nurse must verify that the unlicensed person is competent to perform the task. Many health care agencies hire only unlicensed assistive personnel who have completed a Certified Nursing Assistant course and are listed on the state registry. In this case, the nurse needs to observe the Certified Nursing Assistant performing the desired tasks in order to evaluate his or her competence. If the unlicensed assistive person has not completed formal instruction, the nurse must provide instruction and clinical supervision prior to allowing the unlicensed person to provide care independently. In either case, periodic evaluation of the unlicensed person's competence is necessary to assure the health and safety of clients.

The nursing task being delegated must be selected based on client assessment, the individual situation, and the skill of the individual unlicensed person. For example, assisting a client in ambulating might be delegated if the client's condition is stable, but if the client has been in bed for some time, has been unstable, or has just had surgery, then it might not be wise to delegate this task to an unlicensed person. In addition, the nurse must keep in mind that "while nursing tasks may be delegated, the licensed nurse's generalist knowledge of client care indicates that the practice-pervasive functions of assessment, evaluation, and nursing judgment must not be delegated" (National Council of State Boards of Nursing, 1995, p. 3). Therefore, if the purpose is to assess the client's stability or progress, the task should not be delegated. For example, if the client's strength needs to be evaluated to determine whether the client is ready for discharge or able to care for himself, the ambulation should not be delegated.

Once the nurse decides to delegate specific tasks to a competent unlicensed person, the nurse must give specific directions. Directions should include the following:

- What is to be done
- The expected outcome of the task

- Possible complications
- The actions to take if a complication should occur

In some circumstances such as acute care where the licensed nurse is readily available, the directions may be given verbally with close supervision by the LPN/LVN. In other circumstances such as home care where the LPN/LVN is not readily available but may be reached by telephone, both verbal and written directions should be given. For example, if the unlicensed person will be assisting the home-bound elderly client with administering ear drops, the licensed nurse should provide the unlicensed person with written directions on how to administer ear drops, the name of the medication, the reason for the medication, the dose, the side effects, and the actions to take in case of emergency. The licensed nurse should visit the client with the unlicensed person and observe the unlicensed person administering the medication.

Once the unlicensed person has accepted the delegation, he or she may not redelegate the task to someone else. For example, if the LPN/LVN delegates the obtaining of a blood sugar measurement by finger stick, and for some reason the unlicensed assistive person cannot complete the task, the unlicensed assistive person should inform the LPN/LVN instead of asking another unlicensed assistive person to do the task. Because it is the responsibility of the LPN/LVN to determine the competence of the individual performing delegated tasks, the unlicensed assistive person is not qualified to delegate nursing care.

LPN/LVNs are accountable for the outcome of the tasks they delegate. Therefore, it is essential that the LPN/LVN provide supervision to the unlicensed assistive personnel to whom the tasks have been delegated. **Supervision** means to give directions and inspect the tasks performed.

The LPN/LVN must provide appropriate monitoring of the unlicensed assistive person's work, to evaluate the performance and provide feedback as needed. If the unlicensed assistive person is not performing to an acceptable standard of care, the LPN/LVN needs to make provisions for review of instructions, further education, clinical practice, and reevaluation. This process might involve others such as agency nurse educators, or it might be the responsibility of the individual LPN/LVN. In either case, documentation of the evaluation, education, clinical practice, and reevaluation must become part of the unlicensed assistive person's employment file.

Note: The reference and resource listings for this and all chapters have been compiled at the back of the book.

Chapter Review

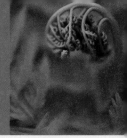

 KEY TERMS by Topic

Use the audio glossary feature of either the CD-ROM or the Companion Website to hear the correct pronunciation of the following key terms.

Critical Thinking
critical thinking

Intellectual Standards
intellectual standards, clarity, accuracy, precision, relevance, depth, breadth, fairness, reasoning, logical, inductive reasoning, deductive reasoning, significance

Elements of Thought
purpose, information, points of view, interpretations, inferences, assumptions, conclusions, concepts, implications

Critical Thinking Care Map
NCLEX-PN® Focus Area

Essential Intellectual Traits or Value
intellectual humility, intellectual courage, intellectual empathy, intellectual autonomy, intellectual integrity, fair-mindedness, confidence in reason

Delegation
delegation, competent individual, supervision

KEY Points

- Critical thinking is done to improve our ability to understand situations more fully. It provides ways to overcome the limits each person has, resulting from our unique experience, upbringing, and education.

- Critical thinking does not mean that we give up what we believe. It means that we respect and value the experiences and thinking of others without having to think the same way.

- Critical thinking explores options to find the best possible outcome.

- LPNs and LVNs must use critical thinking for their increasing responsibilities in the workplace.

- Making decisions, setting priorities, and delegating tasks are just some of the ways that LPNs/LVNs use critical thinking.

- The person who does the delegating is always responsible for the results.

- Delegated jobs should not be redelegated.

- A delegated job is not complete until evaluation and follow-up have occurred.

 EXPLORE MediaLink

Additional interactive resources for this chapter can be found on the Companion Website at www.prenhall.com/adams. Click on Chapter 2 and "Begin" to select the activities for this chapter.

For chapter-related NCLEX®-style questions and an audio glossary, access the accompanying CD-ROM in this book.

FOR FURTHER Study

Evidence-based practice was discussed in Chapter 1.

Legal and ethical aspects of decisions are discussed in Chapter 3.

Jaundice is discussed in detail in Chapter 17.

Critical Thinking Care Map

Caring for a Client with Hyperbilirubinemia*
NCLEX-PN® Focus Area: Physiologic Integrity

Case Study: A 4-day-old infant was discharged from the hospital following a diagnosis of hyperbilirubinemia (physiologic jaundice). His pediatrician ordered that he spend time each day wrapped in a *BiliBlanket* (a fiber-optic phototherapy blanket designed to provide light therapy and to keep the baby warm). An LPN was assigned to make a home visit to reassess the infant. On the first home visit, the LPN found that the parents were accurately using the BiliBlanket. The baby's urine output was only four wet diapers a day. She also noted that his mucous membranes were dry and that he was lethargic. The mother stated that the baby was rarely hungry and drank about 5 ounces of formula every 5 to 6 hours.

Nursing Diagnosis: Deficient Fluid Volume related to inadequate fluid intake and exposure to BiliBlanket

COLLECT DATA

Subjective	Objective
_____	_____
_____	_____
_____	_____
_____	_____
_____	_____
_____	_____
_____	_____

Would you report this? Yes/No

If yes, to: _____

Nursing Care

_____

_____

_____

_____

_____

_____

_____

_____

_____

_____

How would you document this? _____

_____

Data Collected
(use only those that apply)

- Decreased urine output (4 diapers daily when typically should be 6 to 8)
- Dry mucous membranes
- Father states the baby smiled yesterday
- Umbilical cord drying
- Lethargy
- Decreased oral intake
- Mother states infant rarely hungry
- Intake of 5 ounces every 5 to 6 hours

Nursing Interventions
(use only those that apply; list in priority order)

- Contact the registered nurse to report findings.
- Encourage parents to also place infant in the sunlight several times a day.
- Teach parents the importance of adequate fluid intake during the use of the BiliBlanket.
- Teach parents symptoms of dehydration.
- Obtain vital signs every 1 to 2 hours.
- Closely monitor vital signs.
- Obtain a daily electroencephalogram (EEG).
- Provide fluid replacement per order.
- Teach parents to obtain and record vital signs.

Compare your documentation to the sample provided in Appendix I.

*This care map gives students the chance to apply critical thinking concepts and prior knowledge in a real situation. Hyperbilirubinemia is discussed in detail in Chapter 17.

1 An LPN/LVN has recently graduated from nursing school and has a first job in labor and delivery. The LPN/LVN is alone in a client's room when the physician says, "I want you to apply a fetal scalp electrode." Which decision below is appropriate for the LPN/LVN to make?

1. Apply the fetal scalp electrode as the LPN/LVN had seen the RN do yesterday.
2. Read the policy and procedure for applying the fetal scalp electrode and then go ahead with the procedure.
3. Contact the RN and ask the RN to complete the physician's order.
4. Tell the physician, "I do not know how to perform that procedure. Ask someone else."

2 The LPN/LVN appropriately applies the Five Rules of Delegation. When she or he evaluates the care given by the unlicensed assistive personnel, which of the following rules is being applied?

1. Right task
2. Right circumstances
3. Right direction
4. Right supervision

3 The LPN/LVN needs to delegate a finger-stick blood sugar (FSBS) on a client who is hospitalized for management of diabetes mellitus. Which of the following is an appropriate individual to perform this skill?

1. Unlicensed assistive personnel in his or her first week on the job
2. The unit secretary who is also a diabetic
3. The client's husband
4. A certified nursing assistant with 5 years' experience

4 The LPN/LVN delegated the skill of blood glucose testing. The client's blood sugar is found to be elevated. Which of the following scenarios is appropriate nursing care?

1. Ask the client's husband to administer the insulin.
2. The UAP gives the insulin and then notifies the LPN/LVN.
3. The LPN/LVN notifies the RN and works collaboratively to administer the insulin.
4. The UAP notifies the physician about the client's blood sugar.

5 The LPN/LVN determines that the CNA instructed the client to obtain a 24-hour urine specimen by adding the first voided urine to the container. Which nursing action, in a supervisory role, is appropriate?

1. Praise the CNA.
2. Review the procedure with the CNA.

3. Recommend that the CNA be reassigned to another unit.
4. Recommend that the CNA receive a raise.

6 A child's mother calls and states that the child is complaining of a backache. The LPN/LVN gathers the following assessment: exact location of the pain, any recent injuries, other accompanying symptoms, length of time the client has experienced the pain, use of relief measures. Which of the following intellectual standards is the LPN/LVN using in this situation?

1. Relevance
2. Clarity
3. Accuracy
4. Precision

7 The nurse uses _____ reasoning to determine that a child who says he or she has a stomachache may experience nausea, other viral symptoms, or constipation. (Fill in the blank.)

8 The LPN/LVN reviews the EKG of a child with a cardiac condition and considers the consequences of each possible nursing action prior to implementing care. Which of the following elements of thought is the LPN/LVN using in this situation?

1. Points of view
2. Assumptions
3. Implications of actions
4. Concepts

9 Which of the following statements by the LPN/LVN demonstrate the intellectual standard that refers to clarity? Select all that apply.

1. "Could you be more specific about the type of pain you have?"
2. "How would you describe the sensation you feel?"
3. "Give me an example of how it feels."
4. "Are there any related factors that might contribute to your pain?"
5. "Tell me more about your pain."

10 The LPN/LVN has received an order to hang IV fluids using the new IV pump. After evaluating the situation, the LPN/LVN may decide not to proceed because:

1. An unlicensed assistive personnel can hang the fluids.
2. Proper training has not been completed by the LPN/LVN.
3. Only RNs can hang IV fluids.
4. Certified nursing assistants can hang IV fluids.

Answers for NCLEX-PN® Review and Critical Thinking questions appear in Appendix I.

Chapter 3

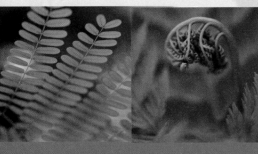

Legal and Ethical Issues in Pediatric Nursing

HEALTH PROMOTION ISSUE:
Sexually Transmitted Infection Education

NURSING PROCESS CARE PLAN:
Client with Hodgkin's Lymphoma

CRITICAL THINKING CARE MAP:
Caring for a Teen Desiring Pregnancy Termination

BRIEF Outline

Federal Programs Affecting Children

Legal and Ethical Issues Affecting Children

Legal and Ethical Issues Affecting Teens

The Role of the LPN/LVN

Complementary Therapies

Nursing Care

LEARNING Outcomes

After completing this chapter, you will be able to:

1. Define key terms.
2. Describe federal initiatives to protect children.
3. Describe parents' rights as they relate to the care of children.
4. Describe client's rights as they relate to children.
5. Name situations in which the nurse must legally report to public agencies.
6. Describe common legal and ethical issues that can affect a mother, child, and family.
7. Describe the role of LPNs or LVNs in legal and ethical issues.

Pediatric care, like other areas of nursing, may sometimes present nurses with challenges to their worldviews and values. Nurses may disagree with laws or policies but still be required to uphold them. They may also disagree with a person's **ethics** (system of values and ideas that shape a sense of right and wrong). In fact, it is certain that every nurse will some day face a situation in which his or her personal standards of right and wrong are challenged. The challenge may come from a client, a supervisor, a facility regulation, or a state or federal law. The nurse may also encounter situations in which there is no "right" decision because all solutions will involve some negative outcomes. At these times, the nurse will need to act professionally and without bias to support the client and family and help them come to a decision. Because the nurse may need to relate not just to children but also to pregnant females who are still in their teens, the content presented in this chapter will address both maternal and pediatric legal and ethical issues.

Federal Programs Affecting Children

Since the early 1900s, the White House Conference on Children and Youth has met at the federal level to discuss the health care of children. Following these meetings, recommendations and some federal laws have been passed to improve children's care. The U.S. government established programs such as Medicaid's Early and Periodic Screening, Diagnosis, and Treatment (EPSDT); the Women, Infants and Children's (WIC) program; and the National School Lunch Program (NSLP) to assist low-income families (Table 3-1 ■).

TABLE 3-1	
Federal Programs Affecting Children	
ACRONYM OF FEDERAL PROGRAM	**FULL NAME OF FEDERAL PROGRAM**
EPSDT	Early and Periodic Screening, Diagnosis, and Treatment
NCLB	No Child Left Behind
NSLP	National School Lunch Program
SCHIP	State Children's Health Insurance Program
SFBSP	Summer Food Service Breakfast Program
SF/SC	Strong Families/Safe Children
VFC	Vaccination Funding for Children
WIC	Women, Infants and Children

HEALTHY PEOPLE 2000 AND *HEALTHY PEOPLE 2010*

In 1990, the U.S. Department of Health and Human Services (USDHHS) released *Healthy People 2000: National Health Promotion and Disease Prevention Objectives*. This document presented an opportunity for Americans to take responsibility for their health. It recommended access to health care for all, particularly the most vulnerable. (USDHHS, 1992). Figure 3-1 ■ illustrates factors from the more recent *Healthy People 2010* that determine an individual's health (USDHHS, 2000).

Some of the objectives in the *Healthy People 2000* document that related to maternal health include the following:

- Reducing disparities in key maternal, infant, and child health indicators so that all could have access to quality care
- Understanding issues related to preconception, prenatal, and obstetric care
- Preventing birth defects and developmental disabilities

Some of the objectives in the *Healthy People 2000* document that related specifically to children included the following:

- Increased participation in school physical education programs
- Reduced use of drugs, alcohol, and tobacco by children
- Reduced teen pregnancy
- Reduced prevalence of dental cavities

In 2000, the U.S. Department of Health and Human Services updated goals and objectives for health care for the next 10 years. *Healthy People 2010* contains 467 objectives divided into 28 focus areas. One of these is Maternal, Infant, and Child Health. Important topics in this area include:

- Reducing infant, child, and maternal mortality
- Increasing the proportion of women who receive early and adequate prenatal care

---

Healthy People 2010 **Leading Health Indicators**

- Physical Activity
- Overweight and Obesity
- Tobacco Use
- Substance Abuse
- Responsible Sexual Behavior
- Mental Health
- Injury and Violence
- Environmental Quality
- Immunization
- Access to Health Care

Figure 3-1. ■ *Healthy People 2010* identifies objectives for each health indicator. (USDHHS, 2000)

- Increasing the percentage of healthy full-term infants who are put down to sleep on their backs
- Reducing the occurrence of developmental disabilities
- Increasing abstinence from alcohol, cigarettes, and illicit drugs among pregnant women (USDHHS, 2000)

Achieving maternal-child objectives involves both research and teaching. The government publishes weekly reports on various topic areas of *Healthy People 2010*.

Legal and Ethical Issues Affecting Children

Even when laws and programs ensure health care for children, legal and ethical issues will still exist. For example, a 16-year-old girl is pregnant and wants an abortion. Because she is a minor, does she need parental consent? If she delivers, can she make decisions about the health care of the infant? At what age can a minor make decisions to accept or refuse treatment? Answers to these questions differ from state to state, so the nurse should understand the general guiding principles and obtain legal advice for complex family issues.

PARENTS' RIGHTS

In most situations, parents or legal guardians have the authority to make decisions for their minor children. There are a few exceptions:

- If the parent(s) is (are) incapacitated and cannot make a decision
- If there is actual or suspected child abuse or neglect
- If the parent's choice does not permit lifesaving procedures for the child

Even though the nurse may not agree with the parent's decision about treatment, nursing care must be provided in an unbiased manner. The LPN/LVN should report all concerns to the supervising RN. Legal counsel might be necessary to settle disputes.

Usually it is the parent or legal guardian who gives **informed consent** (written approval for a treatment or procedure, following explanation of pros and cons by the physician or other professional who is performing the procedure). Procedure 3-1 ■ reviews important steps and rationales for witnessing informed consent.

CHILD'S RIGHTS

There are some exceptions to parents giving informed consent. Some states have a **mature minor act** (an act that permits adolescents age 14 or 15 to make decisions about their treatment). In some cases, self-supporting adolescents are emancipated by court decision. Such minors, who include minors who marry, are called **emancipated minors.** They

are responsible for their own health care decisions and expenses.

The "Patient's Bill of Rights," a fundamental document of health care, is illustrated in Box 3-1 ■. These rights, with some modifications, apply both to the pediatric client and to adults. For example, young children may not be able to understand the diagnosis and treatment of a disorder in order to provide an informed consent, yet they should still be included in the process. Explanations in age-appropriate language should be given, and every attempt should be made to acquire their cooperation. It is important to give children as much control as possible over what happens to them by including them in decisions about their welfare. (However, do not attempt to give them a choice when there is really no option.)

It is reasonable to expect parents and older children to participate in health care in the following ways:

- By providing accurate and complete information about health issues
- By increasing their knowledge about diagnosis and treatment
- By being responsible for their own actions
- By reporting changes in client condition
- By keeping appointments
- By meeting financial obligations for health care

It is the responsibility of the nurse to help the client and family understand how to participate in their care.

PRIVACY AND CONFIDENTIALITY

The child has as much right to privacy and confidentiality as an adult. On the physical level, privacy means screening from view: closing curtains and draping the client to prevent a third party from seeing the body or body parts. At the legal level, privacy also means keeping the client's chart screened from a third party. **Confidentiality** means keeping secret any privileged information.

For a young child, these rights may not pose a problem. The young child usually does not have requests or needs that may conflict with his or her parents' choices.

In an older child or adolescent, maintaining confidentiality may cause some conflict for the nurse. For example, an adolescent may request treatment for a sexually transmitted disease, birth control, pregnancy, or drug and alcohol treatment without notifying the parents. If the nurse breaches confidentiality and informs the parents, the client may lose trust in the nurse and possibly in the entire health care system. However, if the parents learn about the health problem from another source, they may accuse the nurse of withholding information from them. As parents, they may have the right to access the dependent child's medical record.

PROCEDURE 3-1 | Witnessing Informed Consent

Purpose

- To document informed consent (agreement by a client, client's parent, or guardian to accept a course of treatment or procedure after complete information has been provided by the health care provider).

Equipment

- Copy of the agency informed consent form
- Black pen

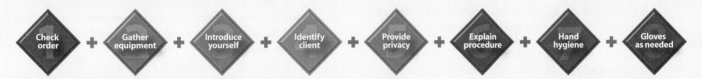

Check order + Gather equipment + Introduce yourself + Identify client + Provide privacy + Explain procedure + Hand hygiene + Gloves as needed

Interventions and Rationales

1. Perform preparatory steps (see icon bar above).

2. Stamp the agency informed consent form with the client's addressograph plate. *The addressograph information identifies the form as a part of the legal record.*

3. Complete all information requested on the form. *Note:* The informed consent form may be computer generated in some facilities. Complete the information requested before printing out the form. *This ensures that complete, accurate information is obtained.*

4. Write the procedure for which consent is being given in the space provided. Use proper medical terminology with no abbreviations. Include "right" or "left" as appropriate (e.g., "Right inguinal herniorrhaphy" not "fix R inguinal hernia"). *For accuracy in communication, the legal record must contain appropriate medical terminology and identification of appropriate body part when more than one exists.*

5. Listen to the information the primary care provider gives to the client, client's parent, or guardian. *When you witness an informed consent, you are witnessing the exchange between the primary care provider and the client, client's parent, or guardian. You are establishing that they really did understand (were informed).*

6. Have the client or his or her parent or guardian sign the form. The nurse should sign as a witness. *Note:* Some schools of nursing do not allow student nurses to serve as witness for informed consent. *Signatures document that information was provided and the client, client's parent, or guardian understood and agreed to the procedure.*

7. If the primary care provider is not present and you did not hear the information provided, ask the client, client's parent, or guardian to tell you what they were told. Ask if they have any questions. If they have accurate information and no questions, have them sign the consent form. Sign on the witness line with the statement "witnessing signature only" written under your signature. *Because you did not hear the information provided by the physician, you cannot witness that interaction. If they have accurate information and no questions, you can be reasonably assured they have been informed. When you write "witnessing signature only," you are not held accountable for the information.*

8. If the information they tell you is incorrect or they have questions, do not have the consent signed. Instead, notify the primary care provider. *It is the responsibility of the primary care provider to obtain informed consent. If more teaching is needed, the primary care provider should provide it.*

9. Place the signed informed consent form in the client's chart. *The informed consent form is part of the legal record and should be kept with the client's chart.*

SAMPLE DOCUMENTATION

(date/time)   Dr. R. Jones talked with parents regarding need to repair R inguinal hernia, including benefits, risks, and possible complications. Informed consent form for right inguinal herniorrhaphy signed and witnessed. _____
L. Lopez, LPN

BOX 3-1

Patient's Bill of Rights

A Patient's* Bill of Rights was first adopted by the American Hospital Association (AHA) in 1973. The Bill of Rights below incorporates the AHA update as well as Bill of Rights information from the American Academy of Pain Management and the National Institutes of Health.

Bill of Rights

These rights can be exercised on the client's behalf by a designated surrogate or proxy decision maker if the client* lacks decision-making capacity, is legally incompetent, or is a minor.

1. The client has the right to considerate and respectful care.
2. The client has the right to and is encouraged to obtain from physicians and other direct care givers relevant, current, and understandable information about diagnosis, treatment, and prognosis. Except in emergencies when the client lacks decision-making capacity and the need for treatment is urgent, the client is entitled to the opportunity to discuss and request information related to specific procedures and treatments, the risks involved, the possible length of recuperation, and the medically reasonable alternatives and their accompanying risks and benefits.

   Clients have the right to know the identity of physicians, nurses, and others involved in their care, as well as when those involved are students, residents, or other trainees. The client also has the right to know the immediate and long-term financial implications of treatment choices insofar as they are known.
3. The client has the right to make decisions about the plan of care prior to and during the course of treatment and to refuse recommended treatment or plan of care to the extent permitted by law and hospital policy and to be informed of the medical consequences of this action. In case of such refusal, the client is entitled to other appropriate care and services that the hospital provides or to be transferred to another hospital. The hospital should notify the client of any policy that might affect client choice within the institution.
4. The client has the right to have an advance directive (such as a living will, health care proxy, or durable power of attorney for health care) concerning treatment or designating a surrogate decision maker with the expectation that the hospital will honor the intent of that directive to the extent permitted by law and hospital policy.

   Health care institutions must advise clients of their rights under state law and hospital policy to make informal medical choices, ask if the client has an advance directive, and include that information in client records. The client has the right to timely information about hospital policy that may limit the hospital's ability to implement fully a legally valid advance directive.
5. The client has the right to have every consideration of privacy. Case discussion, consultation, examination, and treatment should be conducted to protect each client's privacy.
6. The client has the right to expect that all communications and records pertaining to his/her care will be treated as confidential by the hospital, except in cases of suspected abuse or public health hazard when reporting is permitted or required by law. The client has the right to expect that the hospital will emphasize the confidentiality of this information when it is released to any other parties entitled to review information in these records.
7. The client has the right to review the records pertaining to his/her medical care and have information explained or interpreted as necessary, except when restricted by law.
8. The client has the right to expect that, within its capacity and policies, a hospital will make reasonable response to request of a client for appropriate and medically indicated cares and services. The hospital must provide evaluation, services, and/or referral, as indicated by urgency of the case. When medically appropriate and legally permissible, or when a client has so requested, a client may be transferred to another facility. The institution to which the client is to be transferred must first have accepted the client for transfer. The client must also have the benefit of complete information and explanation concerning the need for, risks, benefits, and alternatives to such a transfer.
9. The client has the right to ask and be informed of the existence of business relationships among the hospital facility, educational institutions, other health care providers, or payers that may influence the client's treatment and care.
10. The client has the right to consent to or decline to participate in proposed research studies or human experimentation affecting care and treatment or requiring direct client involvement, and to have those studies fully explained prior to consent. A client who declines to participate in research or experimentation is entitled to the most effective care that the hospital can otherwise provide.
11. The client has the right to expect reasonable continuity of care when appropriate and to be informed by physicians and other caregivers of available and realistic client care options when hospital care is no longer appropriate.
12. The client has the right to be informed of hospital policies and practices that relate to client care, treatment, and responsibilities. The client has the right to be informed of available resources for resolving disputes, grievances, and conflicts such as ethics committees, client representatives, or other mechanisms available in the institution. The client has the right to be informed of the hospital's charges for services and available payment methods.
13. The client has the privilege to examine and receive an explanation of the bill.
14. The client has the right to expect that medical information about him or her discovered at the clinical center, as well as an account of his or her medical program there, will be communicated to the referring physician.
15. The client has the right, at any time during the medical program, to designate additional physicians or organizations to receive medical updates. The client should inform the outpatient department staff of these additions.

*Note: This book uses the word *client* instead of *patient* to indicate that the person is an active participant in the process of achieving or maintaining health.
Data from: American Hospital Association, Chicago, IL; American Academy of Pain Management, Sonoma, CA; National Institutes of Health, Washington, DC.

REPORTABLE SITUATIONS

In certain instances, the decision about reporting the health concern of a child is made by law:

- If the child has a **reportable disease** (a disease that poses a public health hazard), the health care provider must file a report with the appropriate agency (usually the public health department). See more about this topic in Chapter 10 ⊘ .
- Suspected cases of child abuse or neglect must be reported to state law enforcement officers (local police, child protection services, and the department of health and human services).
- Threats to injure one's self must be reported to the supervisor in charge. This must be done even if a child asks the nurse to "promise" not to tell anyone. In this case, the nurse would tell the child that the nurse's job requires him or her to report anything that might cause harm to a client.

It is important for the nurse to be clear with clients about the limits of confidentiality and the mandatory reporting requirements.

Reportable Diseases

Reportable diseases may include, but are not limited to, sexually transmitted infections, some food-borne infections, and some viral or airborne infections such as measles, whooping cough, and tuberculosis. (Information about these illnesses—including pathology, signs and symptoms, and treatment—is included in later chapters of this book. See Chapter 10 ⊘ and appropriate chapters by body system.) The LPN/LVN might contact the health care provider or report the condition directly to the local health department. Infections must be reported immediately so that investigation, diagnosis, and treatment of others can be made in a timely manner. The nurse would be provided with reporting forms either from the employing agency or from the health department. Documentation should also be included in the client chart.

Suspicion of Abuse

Every state has child abuse laws that define different types of abuse and the agency to which abuse issues should be directed. Any professional who reasonably suspects that abuse has occurred is required to report the suspicion to the local authorities. The LPN/LVN should follow facility policy and always be careful to ensure privacy during the interview (Figure 3-2 ■). Questions should be referred to the registered nurse.

Reports of suspected abuse that are made in good faith are not liable for countersuits. However, professionals who fail to report suspicions may be held responsible by the courts. Signs of abuse and related nursing care issues are

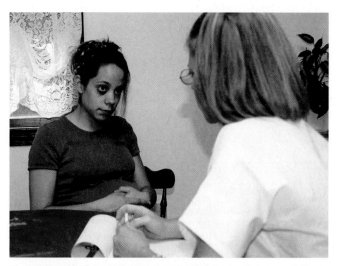

Figure 3-2. ■ Privacy is always a client right, but it is especially important when asking a client questions about abuse.

discussed in Chapters 16 ⊘ and 20 ⊘ of this text. The nurse must record detailed information in the client's chart and complete any report forms provided by the investigating agency.

clinical ALERT

Reports of child abuse must be made immediately in order to protect the child from further harm. The child <u>should not be left alone</u>. In some cases, a child is admitted to the hospital for "observation" while authorities are notified and an investigation is conducted.

PATIENT SELF-DETERMINATION ACT

The federal Patient Self-Determination Act requires health care institutions to inform clients of their rights to treatment, including advanced directives or "living wills" (Figure 3-3 ■). Nurses frequently discuss these issues with adult clients and families. The pediatric nurse may need to discuss them with minor children and their parents.

When it becomes apparent a child will not recover, an open discussion about treatment and terminal care should take place. This discussion should involve key decision makers in the family, as well as the child.

"Do not resuscitate" orders for a child can raise a more emotional response than the same order for an older adult. Also, conflict can arise when the child wants to stop treatment but the parent(s) is (are) not ready to allow the child to die. It is important for the nurse to use effective therapeutic communication in all situations, including group meetings, to help resolve the conflict. (Care of the dying child is discussed in Chapter 9 ⊘ of this text.)

POWER OF ATTORNEY FOR HEALTH CARE

(1) **DESIGNATION OF AGENT:** I designate the following individual as my agent to make health care decisions for me: _____

_____
(Name of individual you choose as agent)

_____
(address) (city) (state) (zip code)

_____
(home phone) (work phone)

OPTIONAL: If I revoke my agent's authority or if my agent is not willing, able, or reasonably available to make a health-care decision for me, I designate as my first alternate agent:

_____
(Name of individual you choose as first alternate agent)

_____
(address) (city) (state) (zip code)

_____
(home phone) (work phone)

OPTIONAL: If I revoke the authority of my agent and first alternate agent or if neither is willing, able, or reasonably available to make a health care decision for me, I designate as my second alternate agent:

_____
(Name of individual you choose as second alternate agent)

_____
(address) (city) (state) (zip code)

_____
(home phone) (work phone)

(2) **AGENT'S AUTHORITY:** My agent is authorized to make all health care decisions for me, including decisions to provide, withhold, or withdraw artificial nutrition and hydration, and all other forms of health care to keep me alive, **except** as I state here:

(3) **WHEN AGENT'S AUTHORITY BECOMES EFFECTIVE:** My agent's authority becomes effective when my primary physician determines that I am unable to make my own health care decisions unless I mark the following box. If I mark this box [ ], my agent's authority to make health care decisions for me takes effect immediately.

(4) **AGENT'S OBLIGATION:** My agent shall make health care decisions for me in accordance with this power of attorney for health care, any instructions I give below, and my other wishes to the extent known to my agent. To the extent my wishes are unknown, my agent shall make health care decisions for me in accordance with what my agent determines to be in my best interest. In determining my best interest, my agent shall consider my personal values to the extent known to my agent.

(5) **AGENT'S POSTDEATH AUTHORITY:** My agent is authorized to make anatomical gifts, authorize an autopsy, and direct disposition of my remains, except as I state here or elsewhere in this form:

INSTRUCTIONS FOR HEALTH CARE
Strike any wording you do not want.

(6) **END-OF-LIFE DECISIONS:** I direct that my health care providers and others involved in my care provide, withhold, or withdraw treatment in accordance with the choice I have marked below: **(Initial only one box)**
[ ] (a) **Choice NOT To Prolong Life**
I do not want my life to be prolonged if (1) I have an incurable and irreversible condition that will result in my death within a relatively short time, (2) I become unconscious and, to a reasonable degree of medical certainty, I will not regain consciousness, or (3) the likely risks and burdens of treatment would outweigh the expected benefits, **OR**
[ ] (b) **Choice To Prolong Life**
I want my life to be prolonged as long as possible within the limits of generally accepted health care standards.

(7) **RELIEF FROM PAIN:** Except as I state in the following space, I direct that treatment for alleviation of pain or discomfort should be provided at all times even if it hastens my death:

DONATION OF ORGANS AT DEATH
(8) Upon my death: (mark applicable box)
[ ] (a) I give any needed organs, tissues, or parts,
OR
[ ] (b) I give the following organs, tissues, or parts only: _____
[ ] (c) My gift is for the following purposes:
(strike any of the following you do not want)
(1) Transplant
(2) Therapy
(3) Research
(4) Education

(9) **EFFECT OF COPY:** A copy of this form has the same effect as the original.

(10) **SIGNATURE:** Sign and date the form here:

_____ | _____
             (date) | (sign your name)

_____ | _____
        (address) | (print your name)

_____ | _____
           (city) | (state)

(11) **WITNESSES:** This advance health care directive will not be valid for making health care decisions unless it is either: (1) signed by two (2) qualified adult witnesses who are personally known to you and who are present when you sign or acknowledge your signature; or (2) acknowledged before a notary public.

Figure 3-3. ■ This sample power of attorney for health care includes end-of-life decisions and an organ donor form.

Legal and Ethical Issues Affecting Teens

A few ethical and legal issues that affect the child have been introduced. There are some ethical and legal issues that affect teens in particular. There are no easy answers to these issues, and they are addressed here for discussion purposes only. Each person's situation will be different, and at times, the courts will make the final decisions. The nurse must be able to look at each situation with an open mind, and provide the necessary care for the teen and family. Box 3-2 ■ reviews steps in making ethical decisions.

Nurses who frequently work with these families must become familiar with the state and federal laws governing these situations.

PREGNANCY AFTER RAPE

Many teenage women are sexually assaulted every year. The rapist could be a stranger, a friend, or a relative. At times, pregnancy results from these crimes. If the teen seeks health care immediately, measures may be taken to prevent pregnancy. However, even with medical care, pregnancy could result. The teen could choose to abort the pregnancy, put the child up for adoption by another person, or keep the

---

BOX 3-2	NURSING CARE CHECKLIST

Steps in Making Ethical Decisions

☑ **Step 1: Review the situation to determine:**
1. Health problems—physical, spiritual, mental, psychosocial
2. Decision/actions needed immediately and in near future
3. Key individuals potentially affected by the decision/action and outcomes
4. Any potential human rights violations in the situation?

☑ **Step 2: Gather additional information to clarify and understand:**
1. Legal constraints, if any
2. Limited time to thoroughly explore
3. Decision capacity of individual(s)
4. Institutional policies that affect choices in situation
5. Values inherent in choice of information

☑ **Step 3: Identify the ethical issues or concerns in the situation:**
1. Ethical components/concerns of situation and decision/action
2. Explore historical roots of each
3. Identify current philosophical/religious positions on each issue
4. Discuss societal/cultural views on each issue

☑ **Step 4: Define personal and professional moral positions on ethical concerns:**
1. Review personal biases/constraints on issues raised
2. Understand personal values affected by situation/ethical issues raised
3. Review professional codes of ethics (moral behavior) for guidance
4. Identify any conflicting loyalties and/or obligations of professionals and family in the situation
5. Think about your level of moral development operant in the situation
6. Identify the virtues needed for professional action

☑ **Step 5: Identify moral positions of key individuals in the situation:**
1. Think about levels of moral development operant in each participant
2. Identify any communication gaps or misunderstandings

3. Provide guidance in clarifying varying levels of moral development

☑ **Step 6: Identify value conflicts, if any**
1. Provide guidance in identifying potential conflicts, interests, competing values
2. Work toward possible resolution of conflict based on respect for differences
3. Seek consultation if needed to resolve key conflicts

☑ **Step 7: Determine who should make needed decision:**
1. Clarify your role in the situation
2. Who "owns" the problem/decision?
3. Who stands to lose or gain the most from the decision/action?
4. Is the decision to be made by single individual or group?

☑ **Step 8: Identify the range of actions with anticipated outcomes of each:**
1. Determine the moral justification for each potential action
2. Identify the ethical theory that supports each action
3. Apply concepts of beneficence and fairness to each potential action
4. Attach outcomes to each potential action and determine best outcome
5. Are more actions/decisions required as a result of each action?

☑ **Step 9: Decide on a course of action and carry it out:**
1. Understand why a given action was chosen
2. Help all involved understand these reasons
3. Establish a time frame for review of the decision/action and expected outcomes
4. Determine who can best perform the chosen action/decision.

☑ **Step 10: Evaluate/review outcomes of decisions/actions:**
1. Determine whether expected outcomes occurred
2. Is a new decision or action needed?
3. Was the decision process fair and complete?
4. What was the response to the action by each key individual?
5. What did you learn from this situation?

Note: Adapted from Thompson, J. B., & Thompson, H. O. (1981). *Ethics in nursing.* New York: Macmillan Publishing. Updated July 2006.

infant. Regardless of whether she chooses to keep the child, some ethical and legal questions exist. If a dependent teen was raped but decides she wants to keep the infant, can the parents overrule her? If she keeps the child and the rapist is identified by DNA testing, can he be forced to pay child support? Would he have rights as the biologic father?

ABORTION

At times a pregnancy will end before the due date. Although medically, any termination of pregnancy is termed **abortion,** a spontaneous occurrence is more commonly called a **miscarriage.** The term *abortion* most often refers to the planned (elective) termination of pregnancy. The legalization of abortions has resulted in great debate. Each state has laws pertaining to the stage of pregnancy at which an abortion can be performed. Other legal and ethical questions are also under discussion. For example, if a teen desires an abortion, do her parents need to give consent? What are the rights of the grandparents? Do parents of minors, including the parents of the minor father, have any rights and responsibilities? Abortion is usually discussed in more detail in a maternal-newborn textbook.

BARRIER-BREAKING TECHNOLOGIES

Increased capability with DNA testing and therapy has raised a host of ethical issues. Stem cell therapy can be viewed as a huge medical breakthrough, similar in importance to the discovery of penicillin in the last century. Stem cell therapy (discussed also in Chapter 14 ⬯) may have potential to correct heart defects, cure inherited diseases such as sickle cell anemia, and prevent degenerative diseases such as Parkinson's. However, it can also be viewed as the intrusion of humans into the very process of life. When more genes and gene markers are identified, it may be possible to know with near certainty that a child will be born with a crippling condition. What effect will result if insurance companies refuse to cover the needs of this child? What controls will there be to ensure quality of life for those who cannot afford advanced and expensive gene therapy?

Parents may now be presented with the option of "banking" their child's umbilical cord blood after birth. The frozen stem cells from the cord could be used in later years if the child needed therapy, such as for leukemia. However, it is not clear who owns the blood. Would the parent have the right to sell this cord blood for cash? Would the hospital have the right to keep the blood and use it to help others who have an immediate need for it? Could a child sue a parent or a facility because his or her cord blood was disposed of without his or her consent?

Fetal research is another broad area of ethical conflict. Some believe that unused embryos from *in-vitro* fertilization

should be used to aid research. Others believe equally strongly that these embryos are alive and that no human has the right to terminate that life. Advances in neonatal care and equipment only further the controversy, as neonates survive from increasingly premature stages of development.

Medical advances can also raise ethical issues from the maternal side. Consider the case of the dying pregnant woman who asked to be maintained on life support to bring her child to term. Is it right to maintain life support on someone who is brain dead? Does the family have the right to demand life support? Is it right to stop life support, knowing that the fetus will not survive? What might the effects be on an infant if most of its development has occurred inside a cadaver? These and other questions will become more common as technology continues to advance.

Role of the LPN/LVN

LPNs and LVNs are not ultimately responsible for resolving legal or ethical issues. However, they need to have a basic understanding of the issues in order to be supportive of the client, the family, and other health care professionals. The health care team discussing legal and ethical issues will need to use the critical thinking skills discussed in Chapter 2 ⬯. The Code of Ethics for LPNs and LVNs is shown in Box 3-3 ■.

BOX 3-3

Code of Ethics for the LPN/LVN

The Licensed Practical and Licensed Vocational Nurse shall:

- Consider as a basic obligation the conservation of life and the prevention of disease.
- Promote and protect the physical, mental, emotional, and spiritual health of the client and his/her family.
- Fulfill all duties faithfully and efficiently.
- Function within established legal guidelines.
- Accept personal responsibility for his/her acts, and seek to merit the respect and confidence of all members of the health team.
- Hold in confidence all matters coming to his/her knowledge, in the practice of his/her profession, and in no way at no time violate this confidence.
- Give conscientious service and charge just remuneration.
- Learn and respect the religious and cultural beliefs of his/her client and of all people.
- Meet the obligation to the client by keeping abreast of current trends in health care through reading and continuing education.
- As a citizen of the United States of America, uphold the laws of the land and seek to promote legislation that will meet the health needs of its people.

Source: Reprinted by permission of the National Association of Practical Nurse Education and Service.

FOLLOWING THE SCOPE AND STANDARDS OF PRACTICE

In pediatric nursing, as in any other area, the nurse must know and abide by the scope and standards of practice. Familiarity with a procedure does not give the nurse the right to perform it. State practice acts and facility policies provide the framework for nursing practice. The facility's policies can be more restrictive than state nurse practice acts; however, they cannot be more lenient.

PROVIDING TESTIMONY

When the courts decide legal issues, the LPN/LVN may be required to provide documentation or testimony. Therefore, it is critical for the nurse to provide accurate and complete documentation of the care provided, the client response, and family interactions. Box 3-4 ■ illustrates the principles

| BOX 3-4 | NURSING CARE CHECKLIST |

Accurate Documentation

When documenting, remember the following guidelines:

☑ Make documentations correct and accurate.
☑ Show the timing and the sequence of actions.
☑ Identify the dose, route, and time of medications.
☑ Indicate equipment or materials used.
☑ Use accepted terminology and abbreviations.
☑ Label late entries and continued notes on charts.
☑ Provide facts, not opinions.

Note the two examples below. The underlined portions of Example 2 make the second documentation much more accurate and measurable than the first.

Example 1:

(date)On admission ulcerated area noted on lower, inner aspect of right leg. No apparent dressing. Moderate amount of drainage observed. Foul odor noted. Pedal pulses present but weak, foot slightly cyanotic with edema. Wound edges red, surrounding skin hot. Charge nurse notified. Wound cleansed, dressing applied. Acetaminophen 320 mg given PO per physician's order. Teaching done. M. Penn, LVN

Example 2:

(date) 0830 On admission ulcerated area noted on lower, inner aspect of right leg. No apparent dressing. Moderate amount of thick yellow-green drainage observed. Foul odor noted. Area 15 cm long, 6 cm wide, 1.5 cm deep. Pedal pulses present but weak, foot slightly cyanotic with +2 edema. Wound edges red, surrounding skin hot. States wound has "stinging pain." Charge nurse notified. Wound cleansed with sterile normal saline, wet-to-dry dressing applied. Foot placed in dependent position, with blanket for warmth. Acetaminophen 320 mg given PO per physician's order. Teaching about wound contamination done. M. Penn, LVN

and importance of accurate documentation. If the nurse is called to provide testimony in court, professional grooming and behavior will be required. The nurse should answer questions honestly and without bias. The nurse should not try to protect other health care personnel, but should relate facts exactly as they occurred.

DO NO HARM

LPNs/LVNs often witness parents struggling with treatment options. Because children often are not capable of making decisions that affect them, ethical issues in pediatrics are more complex. Ethical decisions are based on respect for the child and his or her ability to make decisions independently. The underlying principle is to "do no harm." Sometimes consultation with other health care professionals is necessary to determine whether responsibility is limited to care of the child or includes the wishes of the parents.

ETHICS COMMITTEES

Health care institutions generally have ethics committees that make treatment recommendations or decisions. LPNs and LVNs may be asked to serve on these committees (see Health Promotion Issue on pages 42 and 43). Work on ethics committees would require the nurse to increase his or her knowledge in several areas such as:

- The specific health care problem
- The makeup of the family
- The religious and cultural beliefs of the family
- State and local statutes that relate to the legal and ethical choice of the client

Through group decision by nonfamily members, an unbiased, objective decision can be made.

REFERRAL TO SUPPORT GROUPS

Many community agencies and groups exist to support the family. Some of these agencies are federally funded, whereas others are privately funded. The LPN/LVN should be aware of community support groups that can help families cope with pediatric issues. For example, local churches or hospice may be the site of support groups for parents of terminally ill children. Schools may offer evening seminars on health topics that affect school-age children.

SUPPORT GROUPS FOR STAFF

Many facilities have staff support groups to assist nurses and other health care workers to adjust to difficult situations in pediatric care. For example, when a chronically ill child has received care at the same hospital for several years, the staff may become attached to both client and family. If the child dies, the staff may need time and a safe place away from work to share their feelings of loss. They may also experience feelings of failure because the child died despite their care.

HEALTH PROMOTION ISSUE

SEXUALLY TRANSMITTED INFECTION EDUCATION

The nurse works for a family planning clinic and has provided sex education in the public school system for 11th graders for the past 5 years. Recently, the state regulations for sex education have changed and her curriculum needs to be revised. She now needs to promote abstinence and provide information about contraception. She will also need to include detailed information about sexually transmitted infections (STIs). She needs to understand her state laws, as well as neighboring state laws, related to consent to care in pregnancy, contraception, abortion, and STI treatment. She seeks the assistance of her nurse manager on this project.

DISCUSSION

There is a great need to approach the issue of teenage pregnancy and teenage STI prevalence. In the United States, more than 800,000 women under the age of 20 become pregnant every year. Nine million teenagers will acquire an STI each year. Although these rates seem staggering, they are down for the first time in many years. Data seem to support the use of abstinence in sex education and the increased use of condoms as effective in this decline.

Although the decline is encouraging within our own nation, when compared to other nations American teens still become pregnant more often, have more abortions, and contract more STIs. Data from the Alan Guttmacher Institute suggests that American teens do not have more sex than teens in other nations, but they are less likely to use effective contraception and have more sexual partners. The countries with lower pregnancy, abortion, and STI rates are more accepting of teenage sex but strongly condemn teenage parenthood. These countries also provide greater access to contraception and have more developed sex education programs, including STI prevention.

Sex education curricula should include comprehensive information about physical and emotional changes of adolescence, pregnancy and conception, the emotional effects of sexual intercourse, decision making related to sexual intercourse, the risks of sexual intercourse including pregnancy and STIs, and contraception methods including abstinence.

Each state has particular regulations that must be followed related to the content taught in sex education programs. States regulate whether sex education and HIV/STI prevention is mandated in the school setting. The content is also regulated. For sex education and HIV/STI prevention alike, abstinence and contraception may be stressed, covered, or not allowed. Each state also regulates the parental role in sex education as it relates to consent. The regulations may require consent, not require consent, or allow the parent who is religiously or morally opposed to sex education for their children to ask that their children be placed in another class.

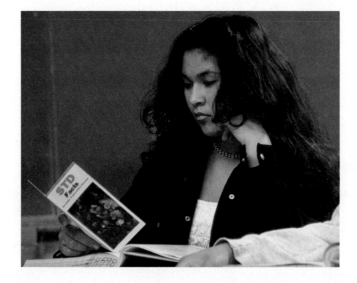

Complementary Therapies

There is a movement toward integrating complementary therapies into health care. Research into the use and safety of complementary and alternative treatments has grown dramatically in recent years. The use of complementary therapies raises some legal and ethical issues. What standards are used to ensure public safety in placebo-controlled clinical trials? What are the legal and ethical responsibilities when health care professionals administer controversial complementary therapy instead of conventional treatment? The LPN/LVN

PLANNING AND IMPLEMENTATION

The LPN and her nurse manager decide that a committee needs to be developed to redesign this curriculum. The committee members are a teacher in the public school system, a physician, a certified nurse-midwife, the LPN and her nurse manager, and several parents from the community.

The community carefully reviews the existing curriculum for age and development appropriateness. They also review the teaching methods for applicability to all learning styles. They take care to include the state regulations for abstinence.

It is decided that all content should be presented in a nonjudgmental, risk-benefit manner. The nature of this content requires students to make life decisions that may be at times life altering. Therefore, a course will be presented prior to this one on how to make sound decisions. The LPN can then incorporate those methods into the content on sex education and HIV/STI prevention.

Audiovisual (AV) aids are discussed in the committee. All posters, videos and slides are reviewed for age appropriateness and content. AV aids chosen include images of teenagers of this era that are simple and easy to understand. There was much discussion about the use of graphic, realistic images of STIs. Some committee members were concerned that teens would ignore the images, thinking they were too graphic to look at. Other committee members rationalized that these images presented a reality that discussion alone could not afford. The committee decided that the benefits of these slides were important and that the LPN should use her judgment regarding the appropriateness from class to class.

There also was some discussion among the committee members about whether the class should include males and females or should separate them into different sections. There was discussion about whether the female LPN would be as effective with the male students. It was decided that separate classes would be best and that they would hire a male nurse to teach the male students. These decisions were made to encourage students to discuss the issues presented.

The committee was pleased with the final product. They have expanded the curriculum and added a section with a new male instructor. Long-term evaluations will be conducted to determine the effectiveness of this program.

SELF-REFLECTION

What are your personal beliefs about teenage sexuality and pregnancy? Where did you learn information regarding sex during your teenage years? What information do you wish you had during that time frame? Was there any education or support system that would have influenced your sexual behavior during adolescence?

Why do you think the rates of teenage sexuality and pregnancy in America are so high? Do you think the promotion of abstinence in sex education is a good idea? Why or why not? Should school clinics distribute contraceptive devices to students? What is the parents' responsibility? Devise a plan you believe would be effective in decreasing the teenage pregnancy rate. Approach a school system and offer to present this program in the school system.

SUGGESTED RESOURCES

Centers for Disease Control. (2005). National surveillance data for Chlamydia, gonorrhea, and syphilis. *Trends in reportable sexually transmitted diseases in the United States, 2005.* The Centers for Disease Control website offers several downloads related to STI prevention, including slides containing realistic images of STIs.

Guttmacher Institute. An overview of minors' consent laws. Guttmacher Institute State Policies in Brief. (April 2007). Accessed online. The Guttmacher website provides information concerning state policies and requirements for minors related to pregnancy, contraception, abortion, and STIs.

may be involved in this clinical research by assisting with the administration of the complementary therapy and collecting data. It is important for the LPN/LVN to understand the purpose of the research, as well as the legal and ethical responsibilities for reporting adverse client reactions.

NURSING CARE

PRIORITIES IN NURSING CARE

When providing nursing care to a client who has legal or ethical issues, the priorities are therapeutic listening, critical thinking, and awareness of the law. Using skills such as reflecting, asking open-ended questions, and listening, the nurse can support the client and family in exploring their reactions to the situation, whether it is a teen pregnancy or the death of a child. The nurse can practice critical thinking by teaching the family about treatment options and by helping them to shape questions to ask the care provider. In situations such as suspected child abuse, the LPN/LVN will know that the law requires a report to social services.

ASSESSING

The data the nurse gathers in legal and ethical situations will likely relate to psychosocial factors. Does the 2-year-old flinch when the mother turns suddenly toward her? Does the family argue in the visitors' lounge about treatment decisions for their boy with leukemia? Has the teenager been yelling at the staff since he heard the diagnosis of cancer? The nurse would document these findings in objective, nonjudgmental terms. In situations that have legal or ethical difficulties, the LPN/LVN would collaborate with other members of the health care team to see that client needs were met.

DIAGNOSING, PLANNING, AND IMPLEMENTING

Some common nursing diagnoses in legal and ethical client situations are:

- Deficient **K**nowledge related to [details, such as beginning pregnancy]
- Altered **F**amily Processes, related to [details, such as learning a child was born with cerebral palsy]
- **G**rieving, related to [details of terminally ill child]
- Risk for **I**njury, related to physical abuse
- Risk for **V**iolence (parent), related to inability to manage anger

The expected outcomes for these clients and their families might include:

- Client/family will express a clearer understanding of the condition and treatment options.
- Client/family will confer with social services to establish a plan of care and to obtain referrals.

Nursing interventions for clients with legal and ethical issues are based on the particular situation. The following interventions may apply:

- Always practice within the limits of the nurse practice acts of your state and the guidelines of your facility. *It is your responsibility to learn the laws of the state in which you practice and the guidelines (which may be more strict) of your workplace.*
- Become familiar with the laws of your state as they relate to health care. *It will be useful for you as a professional to know more about legal or ethical situations you may encounter in your job.*

- Think about your own values, and imagine positive ways of responding to those whose values are different from your own. Never advise clients to choose one option over another. *Your job is to provide quality care, no matter what the client decides. Your own decisions and choices must be left aside.*
- Uphold client confidentiality. *Violation of HIPAA regulations can lead to severe penalties. Your standing as a professional and the trust of your clients and colleagues depend on your integrity.*
- Use other members of the health care team as a resource when you are unsure of an answer or the correct action. Do not try to answer what you do not know. *Your facility will have a person or persons trained to answer difficult legal questions, or will have referrals to qualified people in the community.*
- Remember to practice culturally sensitive nursing care. *Most communication occurs through nonverbal "language." By paying attention to cues and showing genuine concern for clients, nurses can provide culturally proficient, individualized care.*
- Always provide quality nursing care using the "six rights and three checks." Box 3-5 ■ provides these as a reminder. *The most common reason for lawsuits is improper administration of medications. Be careful and consistent in order to ensure client safety.*
- Be prompt and accurate in reporting any incidents. Remember that the nurse who delegates a task is responsible for the successful completion of that task. Figure 3-4 ■ shows an incident report form. *Prompt reporting can prevent further problems from occurring and supports quality care for the client.*

BOX 3-5

Six Rights and Three Checks of Medication Administration

The most common reason for legal action against a nurse can be avoided by remembering and practicing these safety measures:

Six Rights	Three Checks
Right Client	Compare the drug to the Medication Administration Record (MAR) when removing the drug from the drawer.
Right Drug	
Right Dose	
Right Route	Compare the drug to the MAR when pouring it into the cup.
Right Time	
Right Documentation	Compare the drug to the MAR when returning the container to the drawer.

Source: Adapted from Ramont, R., Niedringhaus, D. (2008). *Fundamental nursing care.* (2nd ed.). Upper Saddle River, NJ: Prentice Hall, p. 639.

CONFIDENTIAL REPORT OF UNUSUAL OCCURRENCE
NOT a part of the Medical Record - Please forward to RISK MANAGEMENT

I. (COMPLETE IF ADDRESSOGRAPH UNAVAILABLE)

CLIENT/VISITOR _____ PHYSICIAN _____

MEDICAL RECORD #_____ DATE OF BIRTH _____

ADDRESSOGRAPH

II. DATE OF OCCURRENCE _____ TIME OF OCCURRENCE _____ LOCATION (ROOM OR FLOOR) _____

NAME OF M.D. NOTIFIED_____ CLIENT AWARE OF OCCURRENCE: YES___NO___ FAMILY AWARE OF OCCURRENCE: YES___NO___

REPORT COMPLETED BY_____ OTHERS FAMILIAR WITH OCCURRENCE _____

III. ADMITTING DIAGNOSIS _____

CLIENT CONDITION PRIOR TO OCCURRENCE: ALERT _____ ASLEEP _____ ANESTHETIZED _____ DISORIENTED _____ OTHER _____

IF SEDATIVE/NARCOTICS/DIURETICS GIVEN IN LAST 12 HOURS (WHERE APPLICABLE) PLEASE COMPLETE: (MED, DOSE, TIME)

IV. EVENT

FALLS

100 Unobserved Fall
101 Assisted to Floor
102 Fell from Bed
103 Fell from Table/Equipment
104 Fell in Bathroom
105 Walking/Standing/Slip & Fall
106 Sitting Commode/Wheelchair
107 Restrained Prior to Fall
108 Restrained After Fall
109 Bed Rails Up (1 2 3 4)
110 Bed Rails Down (1 2 3 4)
112 Visitor Fall
113 Outpatient Fall
119 Other_____

BURNS

120 Electrical/Chemical Burn
121 Spill
122 Fire
129 Other_____

ALTERCATION/COMPLAINTS

130 Pt/Family/Employee/Visitor
131 Complaint-Waiting Time
132 Complaint-Billing Services
133 Complaint-Food Services
134 Complaint-Housekeeping/Ancillary
135 Complaint-Nursing
136 Complaint-Medical Staff
137 Complaint-Security
139 Other_____

MISCELLANEOUS

140 Suicide/Attempt
141 Left AMA/Elopement
142 Equipment-Struck/Failure
143 Property Loss/Damage
144 Unexpected Death
145 Non-Compliant Smoking
148 Development of Pressure Ulcer
149 Other_____

MEDICATIONS Drug_____

150 Order (Computer Entry)
151 Wrong Time
152 Wrong Dosage
153 Wrong Route
154 Wrong Drug
155 Wrong Patient
156 Omission
157 Adverse Drug Reaction
158 Prescribing Error
159 Other_____

INTRAVENOUS Sol._____

160 Infiltration
161 Wrong Rate
162 Wrong Solution
163 Wrong Time
164 Order (Computer Entry)
165 Infected Site/Phlebitis
169 Other_____

BLOOD TRANSFUSION

170 Allergic/Adverse Reaction
171 Delay in Administration
172 Incorrect Flow Rate
173 Infiltration
174 Omitted/Client Refusal
175 Wrong Amount
176 Wrong/Omitted Filter
177 Wrong Component
178 Biological Product Deviation
179 Other_____

PATHOLOGY

180 Reference Laboratory Error
181 Lost/Mishandled Specimen
182 Specimen Collection Error
183 Cytology/Biopsy Discrepancy
184 Biopsy/Resection Discrepancy
185 Autopsy Suggests Serious Clinical Discrepancy
186 Frozen Section/Pathological Discrepancy
187 Error Performing Test/Error Reporting Results
188 Delayed Draw
189 Hematoma Following Draw
190 Other_____

OR/PACU/OPS/WOR

200 Removal Foreign Body
210 Incorrect Count-Sponge/Needle/Instr
202 X-rays Taken/Deferred
203 Arrest
204 Wrong Pt/Side/Site/Procedure
205 OPS Pt Admitted Post-Op
206 Unplanned Organ Repair/Removal
207 Lac/Tear/Puncture-Organ/Body Part
208 Canceled Surg-Prep/Equipment Problem
209 Unplanned Return to OR
210 Surgery Delayed
211 Consent Incorrect/Incomplete/Not Done
212 Reddened Area
213 Unsterile Situation
214 Specimen Problem
215 Eye Irritation/Injury
216 Post Arterial Hematoma
217 Improper Discharge
219 Other_____

ANESTHESIA

220 Unexpected Arrest
221 Canceled Surgery After Induction
222 Injury/Death Post Induction
223 Tooth/Face/Lip/Mandible Damage
224 CNS Injury/Brain Damage
225 Unplanned Transfer to Special Care Unit
226 Aspiration
229 Other_____

EMERGENCY DEPARTMENT

230 Arrives DOA After Discharge/Seen in ED within Past 7 Days
231 Seen for Complication Post Treatment/ Procedure from Prev. Hospitalization
232 Left AMA
239 Other_____

OB/GYN/INFANT CARE

240 Delivery Occurred Outside L&D Area
241 Mother Transferred to ICU
241 Unplanned Return to Surgery
243 Stirrup Related Injury
244 Delivery Unattended by any Physician
245 Blood Loss > 1500 cc
246 Cord Blood Gas pH <7.0
247 Cardiac/Respiratory Arrest
248 Infant Seizures in Delivery Room
249 Apgar Score 5 or Less at 5 Minutes
250 Unusual Condition - Child
251 Infant Injury-skull fx/paralysis/palsy
252 Transfer From NB Nursery to ISC/NICU
253 Instrumented Delivery-Injury
259 Other_____

ADULT/PEDIATRIC CARE

260 Unexpected Tx – Higher Care Level
261 Significant Neurosensory/Functional Deficit/ Intractable Pain not Present upon Admit
262 Acute MI/CVA within 48 hours of Surgery/Procedure
263 Death within 48 hours of Surgery/Procedure
264 Nosocomial Infection Prolonging Stay or Complicating Pt's Condition > 5 days
265 Client Found Unresponsive
266 Self Extubation
267 Arrest – Code Team Activation
268 Soft Tissue Injury
269 Other_____

TESTS/TREATMENTS

270 Wrong Client
271 Wrong Test/Treatment
272 Treatment Delayed
273 MD Ordered-Not Done
274 Complication Resulting in Injury
275 Computer Entry
276 Infection Control issue
279 Other_____

RADIOLOGY/RAD ONC/IMAGING

280 Complication Requiring Surgical Correction
281 New Onset Nerve Deficit
282 Reaction to Contrast Agent
283 Overexposure to Radiation
284 Cardiac/Respiratory Arrest
285 Treatment Delayed Worsening Condition
286 Unplanned Repeat Diagnostic Procedure
287 Monitored Inadequately
288 X-ray Inaccurately Read
289 Equipment Failure
290 Lack of Prep-Cancel Procedure
291 Wrong Pt/Side/Site/Prodedure
299 Other_____

V. OUTCOME

SEVERITY OF OUTCOME
350 No Injury/Unaffected
*351 Minor Injury
*352 Major Injury/Consequential

*_SPECIFY INJURY BELOW –

GENERAL

300 Delay in Therapy
301 Embolism
302 Reaction/Toxic Effect
303 Death
304 Prolonged Hospital Stay
305 Neurological Sensory
306 Decubitus
307 Arrest/CPR
309 Other_____

OBSTETRICAL

310 Unusually Low Apgar
311 Fetal Injury
312 Fetal Death
313 Maternal Injury
314 Maternal Death
319 Other_____

SKELETAL

320 Fracture
321 Dislocation
322 Teeth
323 Sprain
329 Other_____

TISSUE

330 Hematoma/Contusion
331 Necrosis
332 Laceration
333 Fistula
334 Dehiscence
335 Abrasion/Blister
336 Swelling
337 Reddened Area/Ecchymosis
338 Skin Tear
339 Other_____

VI. BRIEF COMMENTS IF NECESSARY _____

1004952 (9/01)

Figure 3-4. ■ An incident report form.

EVALUATING

In evaluating legal and ethical issues, the nurse would collect data about whether the specific interventions were effective. For example, the client's questions have been answered sufficiently for the time. The parents state that they have met with social workers. The nurse would ensure that reports and referrals have been made, and that written materials have been provided if possible. The nurse would also note any conclusions about treatment the family has reached.

NURSING PROCESS CARE PLAN
Client with Hodgkin's Lymphoma

Jean, a 16-year-old girl, is admitted to a pediatric unit with a diagnosis of recurrent Hodgkin's lymphoma. Jean has been fighting this disease for 4 years. She has been in remission three times, each one shorter than the time before. This time, she had been in remission only 3 months. During the admission process, Jean tells the nurse she does not want any more treatments. She says, "They make me so sick. They are not working anyway, I just want to die and get it over with." Jean is requesting all treatment be stopped.

Jean's parents are sure the treatments will "work this time and she will get well."

Assessment. The following data should be collected as soon as possible after admission:

- Strength of marital relationships
- Character of parent-child relationships
- Knowledge of illness and treatments
- Jean's feeling about illness and treatments
- Parent's feelings about illness and treatments.

Nursing Diagnosis. The following important nursing diagnosis (among others) is established for this client:

- Dysfunctional **F**amily Processes related to terminal illness of a child

Expected Outcomes. The family will:

- Develop methods of communication and problem solving related to terminal illness of the child.
- Come to an agreement concerning Jean's treatment that is satisfying for both parties.

Planning and Implementation

- Provide opportunities for the family and the client to express fears and expectations both privately and collectively. *Therapeutic communication will enhance family dynamics and facilitate decision making.*

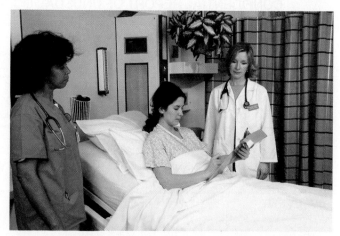

Figure 3-5. ■ Obtaining informed consent is the responsibility of the person performing the procedure. The nurse may be asked to witness the consent signature.

- Promote understanding and empathy among family members. *Understanding of feelings, concerns, and viewpoints will promote respect and trust.*
- Encourage family members to set appropriate goals as they work through the decision-making process. *Goal establishment helps the family with organization and provides a framework for decision making.*
- Ask questions to be sure client and family understand procedures for which they must give written consent. Obtain answers to questions if necessary, or report the need for more information. Witness informed consent (Figure 3-5 ■). *If they cannot answer questions, they might not really be informed. By asking questions, the nurse can document that they are informed about the procedure.*
- Provide referrals as necessary. *These provide the family with information and assistance as they work through the issues.*

Evaluation. The nurse would review client outcomes to determine whether they have been met. The nurse might also assess the following: Have the client and family members verbalized their fears? Do client and family members verbalize appropriate goals for health care? Have client and family members been in contact with support groups/agencies?

Critical Thinking in the Nursing Process

1. Explore Jean's legal rights in your state to refuse treatment.
2. If Jean's parents are unaware of her desires to stop treatment, what should the nurse do?
3. What type of resources would be helpful to Jean and her family?

Note: Discussion of Critical Thinking questions appears in Appendix I.

Note: The reference and resource listings for this and all chapters have been compiled at the back of the book.

Chapter Review

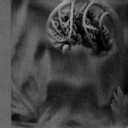

 KEY TERMS by Topic

Use the audio glossary feature of either the CD-ROM or the Companion Website to hear the correct pronunciation of the following key terms.

Introduction
ethics

Legal and Ethical Issues Affecting Children
informed consent, mature minor act, emancipated minors, confidentiality, reportable disease

Legal and Ethical Issues Affecting the Mother
abortion, miscarriage

KEY Points

- Nurses should be familiar with the agencies and groups in their community.
- The pediatric client is guaranteed the same rights as any other client, but it is often the parent who will make decisions about treatment(s).
- Depending on the state, teens may have the legal right to make decisions about their own treatment.
- Emancipated minors have the legal right to make their own decisions about health care.
- Conflicts may arise when the wishes of the child are different from the wishes of the parent(s). LPNs and LVNs may seek assistance from the shift supervisor or from legal counsel.
- Legal and ethical issues related to sexually active or pregnant teens must be handled with sensitivity and care.
- If any client has a health problem that puts the community at risk, or if child abuse or neglect is suspected, the nurse must notify the appropriate public health or law enforcement agency.

 EXPLORE Media Link

Additional interactive resources for this chapter can be found on the Companion Website at www.prenhall.com/adams.

Click on Chapter 3 and "Begin" to select the activities for this chapter.

For chapter-related NCLEX®-style questions and an audio glossary, access the accompanying CD-ROM in this book.

⬭ FOR FURTHER Study

Critical thinking skills are discussed in Chapter 2.

Reportable infectious diseases are discussed in Chapter 10.

Care of the dying child is discussed in Chapter 9.

Stem cell therapy is discussed in Chapter 14.

Reportable sexually transmitted diseases, signs of abuse, and related nursing are discussed in Chapter 16.

Box 20-7 provides assessment data to determine the possibility of child abuse.

Critical Thinking Care Map

Caring for a Teen Desiring Pregnancy Termination

NCLEX-PN® Focus Area: Safe and Effective Care Environment: Coordinated Care

Case Study: Susan, a 15-year-old-female, comes to the school nurse stating she is 12 weeks pregnant. Her parents are unaware of her pregnancy. Susan states she just does not know what to do. There is no way she can raise a baby, but she does not think abortion is right for her either. She is crying inconsolably.

Nursing Diagnosis: Hopelessness related to unwanted pregnancy

COLLECT DATA

Subjective	Objective
_____	_____
_____	_____
_____	_____
_____	_____
_____	_____
_____	_____

Would you report this? Yes/No

If yes, to: _____

Nursing Care

_____
_____
_____
_____
_____
_____
_____
_____

How would you document this? _____
_____
_____
_____
_____

Compare your documentation to the sample provided in Appendix I.

Data Collected
(use those that apply)

- Concerned that her father will be physically abusive if he finds out she is pregnant
- States unable to care for a baby
- Crying
- LMP (date/month/year)
- Urine dipstick negative for protein and glucose
- Reports breast tenderness and nausea
- No eye contact with nurse
- Current weight: 135 pounds
- States family incapable of financial support
- Reproductive history: no previous pregnancies
- "My boyfriend says I have to abort the baby or he won't have anything to do with me."
- 24-hour diet recall: six soft drinks
- States lack of sleep times 3 days

Nursing Interventions
(use only those that apply; list in priority order)

- Explore options available to this client and the pros and cons of each.
- Encourage client to express feelings and concerns openly.
- Discuss importance of prenatal care.
- Teach client about signs and symptoms of early pregnancy.
- Encourage client to explore personal strengths.
- Encourage client to engage parents in decision-making process.
- Encourage client to register for childbirth classes and a tour of the birth facility.
- Address client in a nonjudgmental fashion.
- Explore client's past successes in difficult circumstances.

TEST-TAKING TIP Identify the key words in the stem of the test question before trying to answer the item. Key words often place the scenario in a time frame. These words may be *early, late, immediately,* or *initial.* They will assist you in eliminating information that is nonessential. Key words will often clarify exactly what the question is asking.

1 A 4-year-old girl is seen in the clinic with complaints of burning on urination. The nurse notices two large bruises on her inner thigh. The child's stepfather states she fell on the bar of her brother's bicycle. The LPN/LVN should:

1. believe the stepfather.
2. call the police.
3. keep the stepfather's comment confidential.
4. report the information to the RN.

2 A 10-year-old boy is diagnosed with acute leukemia and requires a blood transfusion. His mother agrees, but his father refuses because of religious beliefs. The nurse should:

1. side with the mother to save his life.
2. side with the father because the man is the head of the household.
3. provide care for the boy without taking sides.
4. refuse to provide care for the child until the parents resolve the conflict.

3 Which of the following is NOT a breach of confidentiality?

1. The nurse talks with her neighbor about the boy with acute leukemia, his condition, and his parents' conflict.
2. The nurse leaves the client chart open on the counter in the hall.
3. The nurse talks with the hospital chaplain about the parents' conflict.
4. An off-duty nurse from the adult unit, a friend of the child's mother, reads the child's chart.

4 A 14-year-old girl confides in the nurse that she is sexually active with several partners who are 15 to 17 years old and states she does not want her parents to know. She states she cannot get pregnant because she only has sex during her menstrual period. The most appropriate nursing response would be to:

1. call her parents.
2. provide instruction on use of condoms and contraceptives.
3. tell her she is breaking the law and you will not help her.
4. ask her the names of her partners so you can call the authorities.

5 A 12-year-old boy is in the final stage of muscular dystrophy. His family asks the nurse what to do in planning for his death. The best nursing response would be:

1. "It would be best to keep him from knowing he is in the final stages."
2. "I will notify the charge nurse and set up a meeting with him, the entire family, and the doctor."
3. "He is not old enough to have a 'Do not resuscitate' order so we must put him on life support."
4. "We will let you know when it is time to make funeral arrangements."

6 A 3-year-old is scheduled to have a myringotomy. Her mother signed the consent for surgery. When providing preoperative care, the nurse should ask the child:

1. "Do you want an IV in your right arm?"
2. "Is it OK if I start your IV?"
3. "Do you want your ears to feel better?"
4. "Do you want to take your doll with you?"

7 A parent states, "I understand this hospital does lots of research. I don't want you experimenting on my daughter or giving her experimental drugs." The best nursing response should be:

1. "I don't know which drugs are experimental and which are sugar."
2. "You must sign a consent to participate in research studies, so you can be assured no experimental treatment would be done without your knowledge and permission."
3. "Only the doctor knows when experiments are being done. You need to talk with him."
4. "You are wrong; only prisoners are used for experiments."

8 Which of the following are appropriate expectations for clients and families regarding their participation in health care decisions? Choose all that apply.

1. Complete and accurate health information will be provided to health care personnel.
2. Families and clients have a responsibility to seek information regarding their medical condition and required treatments.
3. Health care personnel have the sole responsibility to ensure that families and clients understand their medical condition and required treatments.
4. Health care personnel are responsible to ensure that families and clients keep all appointments.
5. Families and clients are financially responsible for health care.

9 The newborn nursery nurse is concerned about privacy issues in the nursery. Which of the following would be of most concern to her?

1. Crib cards visible to the public through the nursery windows.
2. Client charts stay in the nursery instead of on the crib when infant is taken to mother's room.
3. Procedures such as circumcisions are performed in a closed procedure room.
4. Consent forms are signed by parents prior to releasing information to hospital website.

10 A mother brings her 36-month-old to the physician's office with bronchitis. The child is 50th percentile for height but only 20th for weight. The mother states that she often does not have money for food. The nurse must tell her about the federal program that provides milk and other food products for children. The mother needs information about _____. (Hint: Use initials.)

Answers for NCLEX-PN® Review and Critical Thinking questions appear in Appendix I.

Introduction to Care of the Family

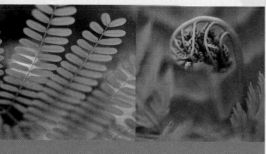

BRIEF Outline

LEARNING Outcomes

After completing this chapter, you will be able to:

1. Define key terms.
2. Describe the characteristics of family systems.
3. Describe the normal changes a family undergoes over time.
4. Describe the effect of cultural and religious beliefs on family functioning.
5. Describe family assessment techniques such as genogram and ecomap.
6. Identify the role of the LPN/LVN in family assessment and care.
7. Describe the characteristics of a family under stress.
8. Apply the nursing process to care of the family.

When planning care for the individual client, it is also important to consider the needs of the family. This is most obvious in the areas of maternal/infant care, pediatrics, geriatrics, and mental health. Individuals rarely live alone or in isolation. The quality of the interactions and relationships between the individual and others is important to the health of the individual. **Family-centered care** is treatment to a designated client with recognition that the family system or unit may also need intervention. The practical/vocational nurse must have a basic understanding of how a family functions and how to assess that functioning. The practical/vocational nurse must be able to identify characteristics of families under stress and understand when to seek assistance and guidance from the supervising registered nurse.

The Family Unit

What is a **family?** The classic definition of family is two or more people related by blood or marriage who reside together. In recent years, the definition has been broadened to two or more individuals who come together for the purpose of nurturing. The structure of families traditionally is linked to the relationship between parent and child, between spouses, or both.

NUCLEAR FAMILY

The traditional family type is the **nuclear family**, consisting of parents and biologic offspring. At one time, the majority of nuclear families in America were made up of a married father and mother with two to four children. The father was the breadwinner, working 9 a.m. to 5 p.m. to provide for his family. The mother remained at home, caring for the children and completing the household chores. Today this traditional nuclear family makes up only 23% of the American family units (Simmons & O'Neil, 2001).

EXTENDED FAMILY

The **extended family** was traditionally described as a network of relatives including grandparents, aunt, uncles, and cousins who lived within a 50-mile radius and took an active role in the emotional support of the family. Today, the makeup of the family is changing. For reasons of employment, income, or living conditions, nuclear families have moved away from extended families. Some individuals now include close friends as part of their extended family unit. Individuals may even consider pets as vital family members. It is important to remember that the family, not the nurse or society, identifies its members (Figure 4-1 ■).

The dividing of the family structure is believed by many social scientists to be the cause of the breakdown of American society. This book does not address global issues

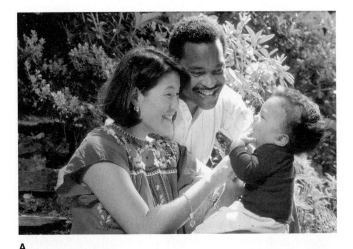

A

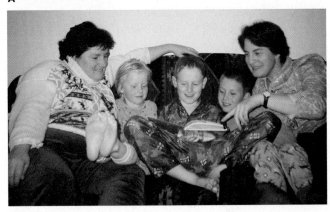

B

Figure 4-1. ■ **(A)** Families come in many different sizes, racial or gender mixtures, and types. **(B)** Evidence indicates that children raised in a homosexual family are at no greater developmental or dysfunctional risk than a child raised in a heterosexual family (Ariel & McPherson, 2000). (A. Lawrence Migdale/Lawrence Migdale/Pix.)

of family functioning. Instead, the functioning of the family in neighborhoods or communities is the focus.

SINGLE-PARENT FAMILY

Today we see many types of families. With the high divorce rate and an increasing number of unwed mothers, single-parent families are becoming more commonplace. In a **single-parent family**, either a mother or a father raises the children alone. There may be support from extended family, but the second parent does not play an active role. At times conflict can arise over custody, visitation rights, or restraining orders. The nurse has the responsibility of ensuring the child's safety. Social workers and law enforcement officers may be needed if conflicts could endanger the child.

OTHER FRAMEWORKS FOR FAMILY

The rise in the divorce rate since the mid-1950s has meant that a majority of children do not spend their developing years in nuclear families. In a **binuclear family**, both

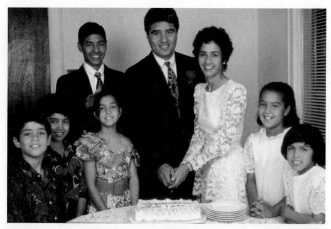

Figure 4-2. ■ Blended families are a regular part of U.S. culture in the 21st century. (PhotoEdit, Inc.)

parents share custody of the children, and the children move between two households. Conflicts can arise between the parents about different rules and methods of discipline at each house. When parents remarry, they find themselves in a **stepfamily** situation, meaning there is a new marriage that creates family relationships between people who were previously in a different family.

The term **blended family** describes a situation in which one or both adults have had a previous relationship and have children from that relationship (Figure 4-2 ■). Blending of families can cause major changes for children in the midst of other developmental challenges. Often, the blending of families brings greater financial and emotional stability to a family, as well as "ready-made" siblings. The struggle to become a larger functioning family can encourage tolerance and understanding. Occasionally, however, the blending of families results in child abuse (when new parents and children clash) or in sexual abuse (by the stepparent, or by a stepbrother or stepsister). The nurse needs to be aware of the potential for these situations.

There is an increase in the number of families in which grandparents are raising their grandchildren. Guardians, foster care, and adoptions provide a family for almost 2 million children in this country.

Interracial families are an ever-growing part of family groupings. In 2000, nearly 7 million Americans of all ages were identified as more than one race.

Unmarried partners with or without children form a **cohabiting family.** In the 2000 census in the United States, the number of these families had increased 72% in the previous decade (including same-sex and heterosexual couples).

Another family type is the **communal family.** This family includes several adults and children, who may or may not be related, who live in the same household. In this type of family, family decisions and responsibilities are shared. A communal

family should not be confused with a **cult family**, a group in which a leader makes all decisions and controls the actions of those who live there.

Theoretical Framework for Working with Families

As stated in Chapter 1 ⟳ of this book, theory guides nursing practice. As part of community-based nursing practice, family theories and culture theories are used to determine the health of the family unit. This section briefly examines several theories that are beneficial in understanding and assessing the family functioning.

FAMILY SYSTEMS THEORY

The *general systems theory* was developed by Ludwig von Bertalanffy in 1936. He felt that several disciplines had parallel characteristics that would allow researchers to identify laws and principles which would apply to many systems. With a common framework, researchers could better communicate their findings and build on each other's work. The understanding of systems has evolved to the point that many concepts are part of everyday language. For example, we understand what is meant by *health care system*, *body system*, *information system*, and *banking system*. A **system** is defined as an organized group of entities which can perform a particular function in the face of change from within or without. The **family system**, therefore, is a group of individuals (as defined by its members) who establish a relationship for the benefit of nurturing, supporting, educating, and providing for the needs of each individual.

In **family systems theory** (a set of concepts to describe the functioning of families in the larger society), the family system maintains a flexible boundary with the world. A **boundary** is an imaginary border beyond which the members of the system come in contact with others outside the system. Boundary maintenance is healthy when the family can adjust the boundary to the needs of its members. For example, at times the family allows friends to visit, have dinner, and interact with the family members. At other times, friends are not allowed to participate in family business. The family chooses when to allow friends into the interaction and when to keep them out.

How well the family changes when problems arise is called **adaptability.** A family that has an open boundary is able to adapt to problems by accepting new ideas. It can reach out for help from available resources. The family that has a closed boundary resists input and has more difficulty adapting to change. When illness occurs, a closed family's stress increases because it is forced to allow health care providers to participate in family decisions. Even when the family as a whole is not closed, the nurse needs to understand that some family members may need time to adjust to help from an "outsider."

FAMILY DEVELOPMENT THEORY

Family development theory describes the changes the family undergoes over time. Family restructuring will occur several times over the parents' life span. People have children and form a family knowing that, in time, the children will leave the home. The family unit changes with the addition of each child, the death of grandparents or parents, and the departure of grown children. The flexibility of boundaries with each of these events is expected, although stressful. The maturing of the family unit brings strength through adaptation. The mature family may be better prepared to make decisions than the young family. Therefore, it may need less assistance from the nurse.

For the individual to have a healthy development, the family must progress through predictable stages of a family life cycle. Table 4-1 ■ provides a snapshot of stages in the family life cycle. By being familiar with each stage of

TABLE 4-1			
Stages of Family Development			
STAGE	**FAMILY TASKS**	**FAMILY ROLES**	**PARENTAL TASKS AND CLIENT TEACHING**
I. Beginning family (no children)	■ Learning to live together ■ Relating harmoniously to three families (families of origin and newly established family) ■ Family planning (whether to have children) ■ Satisfactory sexual and marital role adjustment	Husband Wife Parent of adults In-laws	**Tasks:** Partners establish patterns of communication and problem solving. Roles at work and home are set. **Teaching:** Nurses should use every opportunity to encourage open, healthy communication techniques. For example, this formula can be used for discussing conflicts: "When _____ [something happens], I feel _____ because _____." It is much easier to problem-solve with a statement like, "When the kitchen counter gets left messy, I feel frustrated because I have to clear a place to make my sandwich," than with a blaming statement like this, "You always leave messes around so that I'll have to clean them up!"
II. Early childbearing (birth of first child until infant reaches 30 months of age)	■ Develop a stable family unit with new parent roles ■ Reconciling conflicting developmental tasks of family members ■ Facilitating development needs of family members to strengthen the family unit ■ Accepting new child (children's) personality	Husband Wife Parent Child In-law Parent of adults Grandparent	**Tasks:** Bonding with the child. Learning to understand the child's cues. Supervising safety and development. Adjusting roles to fit new responsibilities. **Teaching:** Teach all caregivers (parents, siblings, grandparents) methods of holding, feeding, cleaning, and dressing. Identify actions, reflexes, appearance, and behavior that can be expected at each stage. Encourage a calm but watchful response to exploration.
III. Families with preschool children (first born 2½ to 5 years)	■ Child explores environment ■ Establish privacy, housing, and adequate space ■ Husband-father more involved in household responsibilities ■ Preschooler assumes responsibilities of self-care ■ Socialization of children ■ Integration of new family members ■ Separation from children as they enter school	Husband Wife Parent Child In-law Parent of adult Grandparent Sibling	**Tasks:** Accepting child's beginning independence. Supporting learning. Establishing behavioral norms. **Teaching:** Provide information about limit setting, "time-out" sessions, usual attention span of children (e.g., some suggest 1 minute of time-out per year of life as a guide). Stress the value of consistent expectations. Encourage "play groups" that can provide support for both the child and the parent. Support the parents as primary decision makers for their children.

(continued)

TABLE 4-1

Stages of Family Development (continued)

STAGE	FAMILY TASKS	FAMILY ROLES	PARENTAL TASKS AND CLIENT TEACHING
IV. Family with school-age children (first born 6 to 13 years)	■ Promote school achievement of children ■ Maintain satisfying marital relationship ■ Promote open communication in family ■ Accept approaching adolescence	Husband Wife Parent Child In-law Parent of adult Grandparent Sibling	**Tasks:** Letting children participate consistently in group settings for education and socialization. **Teaching:** Teach that children need to learn from positive and negative experiences. The parents' role is not to ensure that the child always "feels good," but to help the child learn how to deal with life's ups and downs. The parent should guide but should not make all decisions for the child. Grandparents can often provide useful support and perspective.
V. Families with teenagers	■ Maintain satisfying marital relationships while handling parental responsibilities ■ Maintain family ethical and moral standards while teens are searching for their own beliefs and values ■ Allow children to experiment with independence ■ Begin to become involved in care of aging parents	Husband Wife Parent Child In-law Parent of adult Grandparent Sibling Adolescent	**Tasks:** Recognizing the importance of peers. Allowing the child to make independent decisions and to accept the consequences of his or her actions. **Teaching:** Humor and empathy may be valuable when discussing changes in teens. Emphasize that teens are beginning to view the world through their own eyes, not as they have been taught to see it. Teach that some rejection of parental habits or life choices is normal and not always permanent.
VI. Launching center families (first child through last child leaving home)	■ Expand the family circle to include new members by marriage ■ Accept new couple's own lifestyle and values ■ Devote time to activities and relationships other than with children ■ Reestablish the wife-husband roles as children achieve independence ■ Assist aging and ill parents of husband and/or wife	Husband Wife Parent Child In-law Parent of adult Grandparent Sibling Young adult	**Tasks:** Assisting children to leave the parental home. Adapting to and incorporating people children choose as mates. Readjusting life in the home to fewer people. Parents beginning to take on some care of older generation. **Teaching:** Support parents in considering life problems from a broader perspective and in beginning to plan for their future without children in the home and with needier parents.
VII. Families of middle years ("empty nest" period through retirement)	■ Maintain a sense of well-being psychologically and physiologically by living in a healthy environment ■ Attain and enjoy a career or other creative accomplishments by cultivating leisure-time activities and interests ■ Sustain satisfying and meaningful relationships with aging parents and children ■ Adopt new role of grandparent ■ Sometimes provide housing and/or support for a grown child who returns home	Husband Wife Parent Child In-law Parent of adult Grandparent Grandchild Sibling Young adult Great-grandparent	**Tasks:** Finding mutually acceptable ways to keep connected with grown children. Being caring listeners while respecting that children will solve their own problems. Assisting grandparents to adapt to changes of old age or to death of spouse. **Teaching:** Support parents to separate from grown children and to explore their own interests. Encourage parents to seek information about activities they can enjoy independently of their children.

TABLE 4-1			
Stages of Family Development (continued)			
STAGE	FAMILY TASKS	FAMILY ROLES	PARENTAL TASKS AND CLIENT TEACHING
VIII. Families in retirement and old age (begins with retirement of one or both spouses, continues through loss of one spouse to death, and terminates with death of other spouse)	■ Maintain satisfying living and extended family relationships ■ Maintain marital relationship ■ Adjust to reduced income ■ Adjust to loss of spouse, family member, or friend	Husband Wife Parent Child In-law Parent of adult Grandparent of adult Grandchild Sibling Great-grandparent	**Tasks:** Welcoming grandchildren. Accepting children's life style and choices. Accepting the loss of loved ones. **Teaching:** Encourage participation to create a bond with grandchildren. Encourage acceptance of differences and a focus on positive aspects of child or situation. Provide information on activities and support groups to keep the survivor from becoming isolated in his or her loss.

development, the LPN/LVN can assess the family more accurately and report areas of concern.

CULTURE THEORY

Cultural and religious beliefs have an impact on the interaction of family members. It is vital for the nurse to have an understanding of these beliefs and the importance the family places on them. **Culture** is a style of behavior patterns, beliefs, and *products of human work* (e.g. art, music, literature, architecture) within a given community or population. Patterns of behavior include dress, language, and patterns of person-to-person interaction. Beliefs include **religion,** the belief in a superhuman power recognized as creator or governor of the universe, and other ideas accepted as true or factual.

An understanding of cultural background can give clues to assessment and implementation of care. The nurse must be careful not to engage in **stereotyping** (expectation that all members of a group will think and behave the same). This kind of generalized thinking is not appropriate.

Ethnicity is identity based on common ancestry, race, religion, and culture. Ethnicity is deeply rooted in the family and is transmitted by family values. For example, food preparation and family recipes are handed down from generation to generation. Religious beliefs influence food preparation and avoidance. The specific combination of seasoning, cooking, and presenting the food is part of the family's ethnicity.

Race should not be confused with ethnicity. **Race** is defined by biologic deviations shown in physical features, such as skin color, hair texture, and facial features. People of one race can have different cultures and ethnicity. For example, the Black race living in the African rain forest differs in culture and ethnicity from the Black race living in the southern United States.

Cultural family groups are an important consideration in planning and implementing family-centered care. In the United States, there are four main cultural groups: Rasa

Latina, Asian Pacific, American Black, and White. Box 4-1 ■ provides some insight into these cultural groups. Detailed description of all cultural and religious beliefs is not possible within this chapter. However, it is important for the nurse to become familiar with the cultural and religious beliefs of families in the immediate community. Family roles, views, and expectations may vary widely among these groups.

Culture theory describes factors of culture that should be considered when working with families. These factors include:

■ Communication
■ Space
■ Time
■ Role.

Communication

Communication can be problematic when the nurse is working with families of a different cultural background. We know that communication includes verbal language and dialect. Yet, more of what we "mean" is expressed nonverbally through touch, gestures, eye contact, and volume of speech than through words themselves. (Consider the rolled-up eyes and sarcastic tone a teenager might use with the words "Thanks a lot!" when a parent will not let him use the family car.) The words "Thanks a lot" have a very positive meaning. However, when the nonverbal rolling of eyes and tone of voice are added to the communication, the result is a negative meaning.

Expression and interpretation of communication vary from culture to culture. For example, a person who is raised in a family with Japanese ancestry might not be comfortable speaking loudly or requesting more analgesics, even when in pain. In contrast, a person from a Mediterranean culture might be quite vocal, both about the pain and about the need for more medication. The nurse who cares for these

MediaLink   What Is Cultural Competence?

| BOX 4-1 | CULTURAL PULSE POINTS |

Major Cultural Groups and Traits

Rasa Latina Group

Rasa-Latina families are those whose native language is Spanish and whose religion, most commonly, is Catholic. The family is led by a male head of the household, who is strong but distant, especially with father-son relationships. Mothers and daughters have a very close relationship. In the traditional family, the mother's role is to care for the home and children and to teach daughters to do the same. The Rasa-Latina family functions in the here and now. Customs, ethnic foods, and music are important and they are passed on, especially during celebrations. The family may follow native health care practices rather than seeking medical care. This is frequently related to lack of access to medical care. Health care professionals frequently become frustrated with Rasa-Latina mothers who are reluctant to make health care decisions, especially for their children. Before she can make a decision, the Rasa-Latina woman must often discuss it with the head of the household. (Note: Modern Rasa-Latina women are changing. Many are seeking education and job training. Attempts to increase their independence may cause resentment and family disruptions.)

Asian Pacific (or Pacific Rim) Group

The Asian Pacific or Pacific Rim group includes Japanese, Chinese, Vietnamese, Filipinos, Pacific Islanders, and others. These cultures do not have a common language or religion. The one common thread with this culture is the fact that they are not time limited. When Asian Pacific individuals speak of family, they are including many generations of ancestors. The family is a continuation of those who have gone before. An individual who brings shame upon him- or herself brings shame on the entire family. Many times a young Asian female who becomes pregnant prior to marriage may be reluctant to confide in her family because of the disgrace she perceives she has brought on her family. When young people marry, they do not form a new family. Instead, the young wife is absorbed into the family of the new husband. Although the Westernization of young Asian individuals has precipitated change, many families continue to arrange marriages. Health practices may involve Eastern medical treatment with the acceptance of some alternative medical practices in this country. Asians are more comfortable using Western medicine along with the native health care practices. In the Asian Pacific family, the father is the head of the household. His main responsibility is providing for the family. Traditionally, he leaves all household and childbearing responsibilities to the wife. An Asian Pacific mother would seek medical care for the children and herself, and make decisions in this area independently.

American Black Group

The American Black (or African American) family is traditionally a matriarchal family. This is a result of husbands and fathers being separated from the family during the slavery period in the United States. Today there continues to be an alarming number of fatherless Black American families. This is especially true in lower socioeconomic areas. Middle-class Black American families are frequently two-parent families. Many of them also are two-income families. Black American children often have the advantage of care by extended family members. Children contribute to the household early on by learning to do chores. They often seek employment as soon as they are of age. Family, as well as the church, is the center of the Black American family social support system. Health-seeking behaviors in the lower socioeconomic area continue to be a problem. Access is difficult, and many Black American children are without a primary health care provider. In many urban areas, hospital emergency rooms have become the primary provider for Black children. This fact is frightening when it is noted that the highest infant mortality rates in this country are in three of our largest urban areas (Philadelphia, Detroit, and Washington, D.C.).

White Group

The White family in the United States has changed dramatically since the mid-1970s. Once, the middle-class family was provided for by the husband, and the wife was the homemaker and primary caregiver for the children. Now, a second income is often required, and child care is provided outside the home. White women are better educated than other groups and often seek a career. Women are no longer completely dependent on the status of their husbands. For Whites, the "American dream" not only includes a house and one or more cars, but also health care. Good health care is viewed as a right by middle-class White families. They also believe that health care should be paid for by their employer and that they should have a choice in who delivers the care. White workers may turn down a career opportunity because of benefits that do not equal those of the present job. The White American family differs from other family groups in that individual needs frequently take precedence over the needs of the family.

Source: Ramont, R. P., Niedringhaus, D. M., & Towle, M. A. (2006). *Comprehensive nursing care.* Upper Saddle River, NJ: Prentice Hall, p 457.

clients must be able to perceive the differences in the ways they communicate. Otherwise, the nurse might miss the needs of the first client and feel "yelled at" by the second.

clinical ALERT

Nursing measures that comfort one person may seem intrusive or wrong to another. The best way for you to know what the client wants is to ask.

Space

Personal space and feelings of territory are developed in a cultural setting. Although the environment can have an impact on personal space, the need to have some personal space is consistent. For example, the person living in a two-room apartment with 10 other people still has a need for a small area in which to keep belongings. Personal space also includes the area around the individual. Invading personal space or moving someone's personal belongings decreases a sense of security and causes stress.

Time

The element of time varies greatly among cultures. Members of a cultural group may be past, present, or future oriented. Those who focus on the past generally work to maintain traditions. They may have difficulty setting goals. Those who focus on the present may also have difficulty setting goals and may not save for the future. Those who focus on the future will put off rewards and work today to accomplish future goals.

The importance each member of the family places on time can have a great effect on health care decisions. For example, the family who is focused on the past may not bring a child to the clinic for immunizations to prevent future illness. The family who is focused on the present may be late to an office visit because a good friend dropped by. The family who is working for future goals may have difficulty dealing with a family crisis that causes them to move away from their set plans.

Role

The **family role** (expectations or behaviors associated with a person's position in the family, e.g., mother, father, grandparent, child) is affected by the family's culture. Distinct roles based on gender may be stressed by the culture and are taught to the children. For example, in some cultures the husband makes all decisions for the family. When pregnancy occurs, the husband would decide between breastfeeding and bottle feeding. These roles may conflict with the health care provider's expectation that female clients will make decisions for themselves.

The LPN/LVN must be observant of the family, take clues offered by family interactions, and ask direct questions to identify specific aspects of the family's culture and religious beliefs.

Roles and Functions of the Family

The functions of the family are to:

- Provide economic support for other family members
- Satisfy emotional needs for love and security
- Provide a sense of place and position in society

Roles play an important part in healthy family functioning. Clear roles within a family are directly connected to the family's ability to deal with day-to-day life.

Individual members occupy specific roles. As family members mature, they take on new roles. Children grow, mature, leave home, marry, and become parents. Parents become grandparents. A person's role is always expanding or changing, depending on age and family stage. Family expectations are closely connected to roles. Parents are expected to teach, discipline, and provide for their children. Children are expected to cooperate with and respect their

TABLE 4-2			
Parenting Styles			
STYLE	CONTROL	WARMTH	DESCRIPTION
Authoritative	High	High	Give-and-take communication; clear expectations for behavior. Children are mature, resilient, and achievement oriented. "We can talk about it."
Authoritarian	High	Low	Highly directive, value obedience. Children show lower internalization of prosocial values and ego development. "Because I said so."
Permissive	Low	High	Parents make few demands, allow children to regulate self, and avoid confrontation of behavior. "Do whatever you want."

parents. See Health Promotion Issue: Grandparents Raising their Grandchildren on pages 58 and 59.

Parenting styles play an important part in family expectations. Two important factors to consider when analyzing parenting styles are:

- **Demandingness,** which relates to the demands that parents make on the children, their expectations for mature behavior, the discipline and supervision they provide, and their willingness to confront behavioral problems.
- **Responsiveness,** which relates to how much parents foster individuality, self-assertion, and self-regulation, and how responsive they are to special needs and demands.

Table 4-2 ■ lists types and descriptions of parenting styles.

Family Assessment Techniques and Tools

ASSESSMENT OF RELATIONSHIPS

Each family member is continually growing and developing. The stage of growth and development of these members needs to be identified and recorded so appropriate care can

HEALTH PROMOTION ISSUE

GRANDPARENTS RAISING THEIR GRANDCHILDREN

Jim, 52, and Kathy, 50, have two daughters, Kim, 22, and Janet, 25. They have been looking forward to their children becoming adults and moving away from home. They plan to retire within 5 years and travel. Janet is unmarried with two young children. Their father is in prison for child abuse and has relinquished all responsibility for them. Janet has decided she is unable to care for the children and has left them for Jim and Kathy to raise.

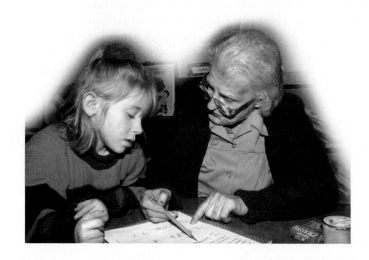

DISCUSSION

Throughout history grandparents have cared for their grandchildren while parents worked outside the home. Although grandparents were ideal babysitters, the parents remained responsible for supplying the basic needs for survival, teaching, and disciplining their children. In recent years, more grandparents are assuming total responsibility for their grandchildren. According to the U.S. Census Bureau (2000), in 2.5 million households grandparents are responsible for raising their grandchildren. In 57% of these households, the grandparents are working outside the home, and 17% are below the poverty level.

What is the reason for the shift in parenting? The answer to this question is not an easy one. It appears that a shift away from the nuclear family to "live-in" relationships coupled with an increase in adolescent pregnancy, crime, and drug abuse have contributed to the problem. Many adolescents and young adults become pregnant without the commitment to a long-lasting relationship. The couple may not have planned for a child and may not have adjusted their previously self-centered lifestyles into a child-comes-first attitude. Without a commitment to each other and the child, couples are not taking responsibility for their actions by raising their children.

In such situations, grandparents can feel trapped. Because they love their grandchildren, it is difficult to see their children shirking their parental responsibilities. In an attempt to provide for the safety of the grandchildren, grandparents are assuming more and more responsibility. The parents allow (and in many circumstances encourage) grandparents to raise their grandchildren. Many times, the only other option is for the children to be placed in foster care or adopted by another family. Grandparents, fearing they will not being able to have any contact with the grandchildren, begin to provide the child care.

When grandparents begin to raise their grandchildren, questions of legal responsibility arise. The parents are legally responsible for their children unless the parents have transferred legal responsibility through guardianship or legal adoption. Therefore, grandparents are unable to obtain social services to help provide health insurance and financial assistance. If the child becomes ill, it is the parent who must give informed consent for treatment. If the parent cannot be contacted, health care may be delayed.

Who financially supports the child? Grandparents may be on a fixed or limited income. Grandparents may have their own health problems that require medical attention and create a financial drain. Unless the parents provide finances, grandparents may struggle to pay all the bills. Many social programs will not provide income unless the parent qualifies. Some parents take the money for their own income, instead of giving it to the care of the child.

How much support can grandparents provide? Although grandparents may want to care for their grandchildren, they may not be the best persons to be totally responsible for their care. As grandparents age, they naturally slow down. They may not have the stamina to keep up with a growing child. Grandparents may not have the knowledge or resources to keep up with an adolescent.

Are there any positive reasons for parents raising their grandchildren? Yes. The relationship between grandparents and grandchildren is a very special one. Grandparents may have more time and patience with children than parents do. Grandparents have experience in raising children and may be able to provide stability in the home environment.

PLANNING AND IMPLEMENTATION

Before grandparents assume responsibility for raising their grandchildren, a lot of discussion and planning needs to occur. A clear understanding should be reached about who will be the legal guardian for the child. Arrangements for insurance and financial support must be made. In some circumstances, visitation must be discussed and arrangements made for the protection of the child.

For grandparents, raising their grandchildren is not easy. They may need to discuss their frustrations about reaching this point of their lives and still being "tied down" to the care of a child. Grandparents may worry that they will die before the grandchild is raised, and what will happen in that event.

Many communities have support groups for grandparents raising their grandchildren. Support group information and other available resources can be obtained on the Internet, from health and social services and the American Association of Retired Persons (AARP). The nurse can be instrumental in helping the family to explore all issues and identify resources prior to the grandparents assuming the responsibility for their grandchildren. In some circumstances, it might be better for a non–family member to take over child-rearing activities and for grandparents to visit the child on a regular basis. In working with this family, it is important to document all plans. It may be necessary for the court to make a ruling regarding custody and guardianship of the child. In all cases, it is the welfare of the child (children) that must be the priority.

SELF-REFLECTION

How would you feel if you suddenly had to have your parents raise your children? How would you feel if you suddenly had to raise grandchildren? How would you feel if you were raised by your grandparents instead of your parents?

SUGGESTED RESOURCES

American Association of Retired Persons. (2007). *Help for grandparents raising grandchildren*. Retrieved April 11, 2007.

Simmons, T., & Dye, J. L. (2003). Grandparents living with grandchildren: 2000. *Census Brief 2000*. Washington, DC: U.S. Department of Commerce, Economics, and Statistics Administration. U.S. Census Bureau.

be given. For example, the infant must meet milestones such as sitting and crawling to be prepared for walking. The adolescent, striving for independence, may not understand or follow parents' requests to "be home early." Grandparents, becoming self-actualized, take pride in watching their children become parents. For review of normal growth and development, see tables in Chapter 5 ⬭.

Family assessment is an ongoing process of examining the relationships and functioning of family members. These relationships need to be identified in order to understand the individual family.

The first step in family assessment is to ask the client to identify the members of the family and their relationships to each other. To do this, a genogram is often used. A **genogram** is a diagram of relationships among family members. Figure 4-3 ■ illustrates an uncomplicated genogram. Symbols are used to represent family members. For example, a square is used for males, and a circle is used for females. The client is identified by a double circle or square. Small marks inside the circle or square represent deceased members. Straight lines are used to identify the relationships. Slash marks represent broken relationships, such as separation and divorce. A dotted line is drawn around all members living in the same household. As more information is learned about the family members, it is added to the genogram.

The second step in family assessment is to develop an **ecomap.** An ecomap provides a diagram of family member

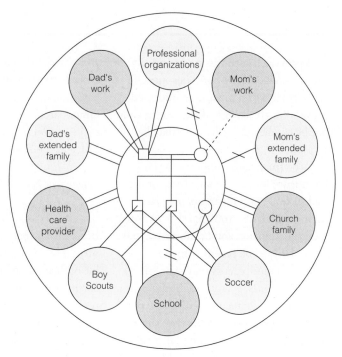

Figure 4-4. ■ Ecomap.

interactions with the immediate environment. Figure 4-4 ■ shows an uncomplicated ecomap. The family is located in the center with significant people, organizations, and agencies placed in circles around the family. Different lines are used to show relationships between family members and those outside influences. Straight lines represent strong relationships, dotted lines represent tenuous relationships, and slashed lines represent stressful or conflicted relationships.

ASSESSMENT OF ENVIRONMENT

Assessment of the family would not be complete without an assessment of the family's environment. A complete environmental assessment is necessary in a community-based approach to nursing care. The practical or vocational nurse assists the RN with the environmental assessment. Only general topics are discussed here.

Assessing the home is essential in planning care for children. Figure 4-5 ■ suggests some questions to use in assessing the home. Key areas to assess are:

- The condition of housing, both inside and outside
- The availability of sanitary conditions, running water, toilet facilities, and garbage disposal
- The kitchen area, including cooking and refrigeration facilities
- Sleeping arrangements for each member of the family
- Presence or absence of safety hazards

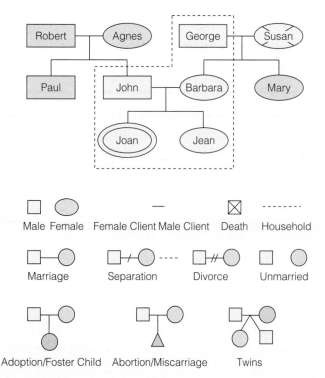

Figure 4-3. ■ Genogram.

When assessing the home, the following should be considered:

Dwelling Type	Own:	Rent:
House	Apartment	# Bedrooms
Year constructed _____ (Note: older homes may contain lead-based paint)		

Condition of Exterior			
Paint/Siding	Intact	Detached	Flaking/peeling
Yard	Clean/trimmed	Unkempt	Fenced
Hazards	Sand box	Play equipment	Swimming pool

Condition of Interior			
Paint	Intact	Flaking	Notes:
Furnishings	Safe	Notes:	
Floors/stairs/railing	Safe	Notes:	
Heating/cooling	Adequate	Notes:	
Lighting	Adequate	Notes:	
Telephone access	Adequate	Notes:	
Water supply	Hot/cold	Notes:	
Cleanliness/sanitation	Good	Vermin Infestation	Notes:
Pets	Clean	Sanitation	Notes:
Kitchen	Clean	Water	Sanitation
	Refrigeration	Cooking facilities	Notes:
Bathroom	Clean	Shower/tub	Toilet function
	Towels	Soap	Safety rails
Bedrooms	Adequate #	Clean	Private

SAFETY ISSUES	Medication storage	Toxic substance storage	Toys
Notes:	Electric cords	Smoke/fire detector	Hobby supplies

Figure 4-5. ■ Home assessment.

Certain aspects of the neighborhood or community must also be assessed. Figure 4-6 ■ offers sample questions used to assess the neighborhood. The major topics to examine here are:

- Availability of shopping for clothes and groceries
- Location of schools and churches
- Availability of health care, including doctors' offices, clinics, and hospitals
- Opportunities for employment.

The gathering of data in family assessment is quite time consuming. Relationships between family members and the environment change. Although the nurse might think the family is stable with working, healthy relationships, outside stressors can threaten the stability of the relationships.

The nurse will use active listening and therapeutic communication to obtain assessment data. At times, the nurse talks with individual members. At other times, group meetings are best in order to see family interaction. The nurse must always keep an open mind and a nonjudgmental attitude. The nurse's

In assessing the neighborhood or community, the following should be considered:

Type of neighborhood	Rural	Suburban	Urban	Inner city
Types of buildings	Residential	Agrarian	Industrial	Combined
Condition of buildings	Excellent	Good	Poor	Unsafe
Condition of streets	Paved Unpaved	Curbs	Sidewalks	Kept up Deteriorating
Traffic	Congested	Stop signs/ lights	Public transportation	
Environmental hazards	Soil	Air	Water	Noise
Population	Young families	Older families	Sparsely populated	Densely populated
Facilities available	Market Shopping	Church	School	Parks & playgrounds
Health care facilities	Doctor office Clinics	Hospital Long-term care	Home health	Other
Distance from home to health care facility				

Figure 4-6. ■ Neighborhood or community assessment.

role is not to take sides or show preference to individuals, but rather to facilitate a move toward healthy relationships.

ASSESSMENT OF POTENTIAL ABUSE

The nurse, working with families, must be alert for signs of possible family violence. Family violence includes spousal abuse, child abuse and neglect, and elder abuse. While in the home, children learn behaviors they will practice as adults. In homes where spousal or child abuse occurs, children grow up believing that this behavior is acceptable, and the cycle continues. Abusive parents may have a knowledge deficit about the needs of their children and how to meet these needs best. Abusive parents are often without a support system. They may be alone, angry, in crisis, or have unrealistic expectations.

Indicators of abuse may include:

- Changes in appointments with health care provider (increased appointments with vague somatic complaints or missed appointments)
- Depression, attempted suicide, self-directed abuse
- Severe anxiety, insomnia, violent nightmares
- Alcohol and/or drug abuse
- Unexplained bruising or other injuries.

Questions that need to be addressed during family assessment are included in Box 4-2 ■. As you recall (see Chapter 3 ◯◯),

if the nurse suspects abuse or neglect, a report must be filed with law enforcement agencies. The LPN/LVN must also notify the supervising RN or health care provider. Complete documentation of the nurse's observations must be made in the client record.

LPN/LVN Role in Family Care

The role of the LPN/LVN is to assist with data collection, report findings, and implement the written plan of care. For example, the practical or vocational nurse can assist in collecting information about family members and can diagram relationships on a genogram and ecomap. When interacting with family members, the nurse identifies healthy functioning patterns as well as characteristics of stress, documents this information, and reports observations to the registered nurse.

Family Under Stress

Many factors can put stress on the family unit. Financial problems, drug and alcohol use, and extramarital relationships are but a few. Chronic illness of family members places a huge, long-term burden on a family and requires many adjustments. The child who is chronically ill may never leave home, and there may be no end to the parents' financial care of the child. Dealing with such stress can strengthen family ties and promote a healthy family unit, or it can cause additional stress and lead to a breakdown in family unity.

When family unity is severely disrupted, divorce is the most likely outcome. Divorce has become a common stressor for families; it involves all family and extended family members. Although divorce is no longer considered a stigma, it is a difficult transition that causes stress and that can adversely affect the health of family members. The LPN/LVN helps identify signs of the unhealthy family unit and communicates this information to the caregiver in charge.

In most instances, parents use the same or similar strategies to reduce stress that their parents used. Healthy families tend to work together to reduce stress, whereas unhealthy families tend to become defensive and blame others for their problems. In healthy families, individuals

---

BOX 4-2	ASSESSMENT

Abuse in Women or Children

Actions Suggestive of Abuse in Adults
- Inappropriate laughing
- Crying
- No eye contact (may be usual in some cultures)
- Searching eye contact (look of "fear")
- Comments about emotional abuse (of self or of "friend")

Questions for Pregnant Women
- Are you in a relationship with a person who hurts you?
- Does the person threaten to abuse you?
- Has the person hit, slapped, kicked, or hurt you since you have been pregnant?
- If yes, has the abuse increased since you became pregnant?
- Do you know where you can go for help?

Actions Suggestive of Abuse in Children
- Failure to thrive
- Poor hygiene, unclean, inappropriate dress
- Frequent injuries, unexplained injuries and bruising
- Dull, inactive, passive behavior
- Begging or stealing food
- Frequent absences from school, poor or declining grades
- Drug and/or alcohol abuse
- Vandalism, shoplifting

Questions for Children
- Has someone hurt you?
- Did they hit, slap, kick, or hurt you in some other way?
- Are you left alone?
- Has someone touched you in your "private parts"?
- How did your get this bruise (and other injuries)?

BOX 4-3	ASSESSMENT

Signs of an Unhealthy Family
The following signs of an unhealthy family should be reported to the registered nurse
- Denial of problem(s)
- Active overt exploitation/scapegoating
- Use of threat
- Abandonment
- Drug or alcohol abuse
- Violence including
  - Spouse or partner abuse (all relationships)
  - Child abuse
  - Sibling abuse
  - Elder abuse
  - Parent abuse
  - Child abuse related to alternative lifestyles

---

learn to use effective communication and problem-solving techniques to reduce stress and promote emotional stability. In unhealthy families, individuals use ineffective communication and place blame on others, causing those individuals to feel unwanted, unloved, and worthless. These negative feelings tend to block communication and lead to additional stress. Box 4-3 ■ lists some signs of an unhealthy family that should be reported to the charge nurse.

NURSING CARE

PRIORITIES IN NURSING CARE

When caring for individuals, remember to include family members as well. Focus your care on establishing a therapeutic relationship based on trust. Be careful to develop a nonthreatening, nonjudgmental attitude when family values and behaviors differ from yours. Use positive, supportive words of encouragement and provide a list of resources for family support.

ASSESSING

The LPN/LVN follows state nurse practice acts and facility policies to help the RN or care provider collect the individual's data and identifying signs of healthy and unhealthy family units. The LPN/LVN documents and reports findings to the registered nurse and implements the plan of care to help the family achieve a healthier level of functioning.

DIAGNOSING, PLANNING, AND IMPLEMENTING

Families cope with health events together throughout their lives. They may be excitedly awaiting the birth of their first child. They may be trying to decide whether a family member should have surgery, chemotherapy, and/or radiation for cancer. They may be exhausted from years of caring for a chronically ill child or spouse.

Certain NANDA diagnoses that relate particularly to families are the following:

- **C**aregiver Role Strain
- Compromised, Disabled, or Readiness for Enhanced Family **C**oping:
- Interrupted or Readiness for Enhanced **F**amily Process
- Impaired or Readiness for Enhanced **P**arenting
- Parental **R**ole Conflict
- Ineffective **T**herapeutic Regimen Management: Family

Client outcomes for these diagnoses would address the particulars of the family situation. For example, a family with a chronically ill child with a worsening condition of cystic fibrosis may have a nursing diagnosis of Caregiver Role Strain. The nurse would be sure to inform the family of all groups and services that might be able to provide some support for the primary caregivers. In a new family in which the mother has just had a cesarean delivery, the nursing plan might indicate that the father is eager to learn to help (Readiness for Enhanced Parenting). The nurse could demonstrate diaper care and burping techniques to the father so the mother could get more rest.

Situations with Compromised Family Coping are more challenging for the nurse because they often involve working with family members who are in conflict. The movement from unhealthy to healthy functioning takes time and patience. Once the plan of care is established, all health care providers must be consistent in their approach to individual family members. For example, the nurse may observe a mother who continually tells a child he is "a brat" and "nothing but trouble." The nurse could suggest that the child might listen better if the parent focused on his good attributes and if the parent was specific and matter-of-fact when correcting undesirable behaviors. The LPN/LVN, working with families in the care of the maternal or pediatric client, has the opportunity and responsibility to promote a healthier family unit.

Nursing interventions could include:

- Provide instructions (on topics specific to the situation). *An important role of the LPN/LVN is teaching. In stressful situations such as health crises, it is useful to repeat or explain information that has been given. This may allow the family to ask questions about the disorder or about treatment options. If nurses do not know the answer, they can either obtain it and tell the family or refer the family to the appropriate professional.*
- Provide a list of support groups and agencies. *Continuity of care includes having information about follow-up after leaving the facility.*

- Support the family in decision-making processes. *The nurse provides information, answers questions, encourages the family to explore options, and shows respect for family processes and decisions.*
- Observe family relationships, watching for signs of abuse. *Thankfully, abuse is not common. However, the nurse must be vigilant in noting injuries or actions that suggest abuse may have occurred.*

clinical ALERT

Signs of abuse or neglect must be reported to law enforcement agencies.

EVALUATING

Working from the care plan laid out for the family, the LPN/LVN would ask questions to determine whether desired outcomes had been met. Progress and unmet outcomes are documented and reported as necessary. The nurse would report any suspicions of abuse to the appropriate agency (see Chapter 3 ☛).

DISCHARGE CONSIDERATIONS

The nurse should ensure that the client and family are prepared for discharge. The new mother must be given instruction in both self-care and infant care. The parents (or care providers) will need home care instructions specific to the care of the individual child. Printed information should include:

- Use, action, and side effects of medication
- Use and care of any equipment
- Signs of complications that need to be reported to the health care provider
- The date and time of follow-up appointments
- Name, address, and phone number of any referral agency (WIC, abuse shelters, counseling services, etc.)

Documentation of client and family understanding of instructions should be included in the client chart.

NURSING PROCESS CARE PLAN
Stressful Family Situation

Jean, a 5-year-old girl, was injured in an automobile accident on June 10. She sustained a ruptured spleen, a compound fracture of her left arm, and a traumatic amputation of the left leg. Her parents and baby sister were also in the accident but received only minor injuries. The nurse is preparing the client for discharge.

Assessment.   The following data should be collected:

- Family knowledge of extent of traumatic event
- Family knowledge of care necessary for family member
- Coping mechanisms used by the family
- Support systems available to the family
- Resources available to the family.

Nursing Diagnosis.   The following important nursing diagnosis (among others) is established for this client:

- Compromised Family <u>C</u>oping, related to traumatic event.

Expected Outcome.   Family members will identify the effect of the traumatic event on the family unit and identify resources to assist with coping.

Planning and Implementation

- Assess past family coping to include strengths and weaknesses. *Past coping is a predictor of future coping.*
- Identify symptoms of family stress to include fatigue, insomnia, and depression. *Stress symptoms would further compromise family coping.*
- Identify support system and outside resources available to the family. *Support and resources assist with coping. Family coping is compromised by lack of support and resources.*
- Assist the family in developing a plan for coping with the traumatic event. *The nurse provides suggestions and resources and then supports the family's decisions in coping with the traumatic event.*
- Offer assistance in contacting resources if accepted by the family. *Following periods of illness or trauma, families usually require outside assistance in managing these events.*

Evaluation.   Parents were instructed in care of the wound and given written information about signs of infection or other reasons to contact the physician. Follow-up visits were scheduled. Parents were provided with referrals for physical therapy, occupational therapy, and an amputees' support group. Parents reported that their church would provide dinners for the family for the first 2 weeks.

Critical Thinking in the Nursing Process

1. What information would be important to include in an ecomap for this family?
2. In assessing the family home, what areas would be most important?
3. What community or neighborhood resources should be assessed and included in Jean's care?

Note: Discussion of Critical Thinking questions appears in Appendix I.

Note: The reference and resource listings for this and all chapters have been compiled at the back of the book.

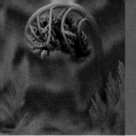

Chapter Review

 KEY TERMS by Topic

Use the audio glossary feature of either the CD-ROM or the Companion Website to hear the correct pronunciation of the following key terms.

Introduction
family-centered care

The Family Unit
family, nuclear family, extended family, single-parent family, binuclear family, stepfamily, blended family, cohabitating family, communal family, cult family

Theoretical Framework for Working with Families
system, family system, family systems theory, boundary, adaptability, family development theory, culture, religion, stereotyping, ethnicity, race, culture theory, family role

Roles and Functions of the Family
demandingness, responsiveness

Family Assessment Techniques and Tools
family assessment, genogram, ecomap

KEY Points

- The LPN/LVN who works with families in an acute-care setting or home/community setting must be alert for signs of healthy and unhealthy family functioning.

- Tools such as a genogram and ecomap are useful in assessing the family.

- Cultural and religious beliefs affect the functioning of the family members.

- By understanding the characteristics of family systems, the nurse can more accurately assess family functioning.

- The family develops and changes over time.

- Identifying the characteristics of the family under stress enables the nurse to make appropriate referrals.

FOR FURTHER Study

For a complete discussion on community-based nursing practice, see Chapter 1.

For information about reporting abuse, see Chapter 3.

For review of normal growth and development, see tables in Chapter 5.

EXPLORE MediaLink

Additional interactive resources for this chapter can be found on the Companion Website at www. prenhall. com/adams.

Click on Chapter 4 and "Begin" to select the activities for this chapter.

For chapter-related NCLEX®-style questions and an audio glossary, access the accompanying CD-ROM in this book.

Animations:
Defining Family
What Is Cultural Competence?

Caring for a Child Following the Divorce of His Parents
NCLEX-PN® Focus Area: Health Promotion and Maintenance

Case Study: Ms. Jacobs brings her 7-year-old son, Sam, to the pediatrician's office. She reports that he is not eating, sleeps frequently, complains of a stomachache daily, and refuses to go to school. Ms. Jacobs reports that she and her husband have recently finalized their divorce. She and her ex-husband are finding it difficult to be civil to one another. Sam is living with her but sees his father weekly, sometimes spending several nights at his father's house. His father has a girlfriend who also spends the night.

Nursing Diagnosis: Interrupted Family Processes related to parents' recent divorce

COLLECT DATA

Subjective	Objective
_____	_____
_____	_____
_____	_____
_____	_____
_____	_____
_____	_____
_____	_____

Would you report this? Yes/No

If yes, to: _____

Nursing Care

_____
_____
_____
_____
_____
_____
_____
_____
_____

How would you document this? _____
_____
_____
_____
_____

Data Collected
(use only those that apply)

- Weight 35 pounds
- Bowel sounds active in all four quadrants
- Sam's responses barely audible
- No masses or tenderness noted following light abdominal palpation
- Complaint of daily stomachache
- Sleeping 10 hours plus a 2.5-hour nap daily
- Refuses to go to school
- Parents recently divorced
- Parental relationship strained
- Some days spent with mother, some spent with father
- Pulse 55 bpm
- Dark circles under eyes
- Father has new female relationship

Nursing Interventions
(use only those that apply; list in priority order)

- Assist the family in setting realistic goals.
- Encourage the use of stimulation to keep Sam awake during the day.
- Refer to community resources as needed.
- Encourage Sam and his mother to express concerns and fears.
- Explore negative feelings of anger, worry, sorrow, and so on.
- Evaluate family strengths and weaknesses.
- Administer antidepressant as ordered.
- Encourage each family member to try to understand the other's feelings.

Compare your documentation to the sample provided in Appendix I.

NCLEX-PN® Exam Preparation

1 A couple's 6-month-old son has been diagnosed with cystic fibrosis. In assessing the dynamic of this family, the nurse completes a genogram. This assessment tool is useful in:

1. understanding the family member's relationships in the community.
2. understanding the relationships of family members.
3. identifying the genetic link for cystic fibrosis.
4. identifying the physical characteristics of family members.

2 A family of five is new to the area. They have come to the health clinic for an introductory visit. To understand each family member's relationship to the community, the nurse would complete the assessment tool called a(n)_____.

3 A Chinese family is in the United States as tourists when their 10-year-old daughter develops appendicitis and requires emergency surgery. The emergency room nurse notes that the child's mother never makes eye contact with the doctor. The nurse should:

1. request that the woman look at the doctor when spoken to.
2. understand the behavior is consistent with her culture.
3. ignore the mother and ask the doctor to speak with the father.
4. determine that this behavior could indicate guilt over child abuse, and contact social services.

4 A pediatric client is discharged following an acute episode of muscular dystrophy. You have been asked by the RN to make a home visit and collect data for an environmental assessment. Choose the following assessments that would be appropriate.

1. lawn maintenance
2. condition of the floors
3. exterior color
4. number of televisions and their locations
5. availability of hot and cold water

5 A client has leukemia. Her mother says to you, "I just need to pray with my minister in order to make my daughter well." The most appropriate response would be:

1. "The medicine ordered by the doctor will make her well."
2. "Why do you think only prayer will make her well?"
3. "May I call her minister for you?"
4. "When she goes home, you can take her to church."

6 It is important to be aware of a family's religion and culture because:

1. differences in care should not be based on culture or religion.
2. aspects of care might be adapted to meet cultural and religious beliefs.
3. reimbursement is based on cultural and religious beliefs.
4. some cultures and religious groups are more numerous than others.

7 Which of the following statements would indicate the family is coping well and does not need additional help?

1. "People tell us we need help since the death of our children, but we are fine."
2. "It is nice having my aunt and uncle living so close. We talk with them daily, and they have been so supportive."
3. "If my wife had been home like a good wife should be, the house would not have burned down! It is her fault!"
4. "Look, missy, you might be 16, but I'm your dad and if you try sneaking out again, you won't live to be 17. Do you hear me?"

8 If the LPN/LVN suspects the family is under undue stress, he or she should:

1. set up a meeting with a family counselor.
2. meet with the family as a group to solve the problem.
3. tell the supervising RN.
4. ignore the problem; it is not your concern.

9 A mother and father ask the nurse why she is so interested in how their family functions. The nurse responds:

1. "I'm very interested in the differences between families. I like to compare notes."
2. "I have a responsibility to identify factors that might affect the health of a child."
3. "I have a legal responsibility to search out illegal behavior and alert the police."
4. "I am the only person trained to search out wrongdoing."

10 An LPN/LVN, caring for a child with a progressive terminal illness, is looking for local resources to help a family that needs financial support. Choose all the interventions that would be appropriate.

1. Perform a web search.
2. Look in the local yellow pages.
3. Contact social services.
4. Take a quick survey of other clients.
5. Consult with the registered nurse.

Answers for NCLEX-PN® Review and Critical Thinking questions appear in Appendix I.

Chapter 5

Life Span Growth and Development

BRIEF Outline

Principles of Growth and Development

Theories of Development

Standards of Physical Growth and Development

Stages of Physical and Cognitive Growth and Development

LEARNING Outcomes

After completing this chapter, you will be able to:

1. Define key terms
2. List factors that influence growth and development.
3. Describe Piaget's stages of cognitive development.
4. Describe Erikson's levels of psychosocial development.
5. Describe Freud's stages of psychosexual development.
6. Describe Kohlberg's levels of moral development.
7. Describe normal growth and development for each age group, as well as deviations from the norm.

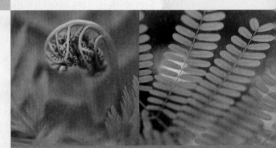

HEALTH PROMOTION ISSUE:
Internet Safety for Children

NURSING PROCESS CARE PLAN:
Infant with Delayed Growth and Development

CRITICAL THINKING CARE MAP:
Caring for Client with Risk for Injury

Growth and development are continual processes of change. These processes begin at the moment of conception and continue until the moment of death. **Growth** is the process of increasing in physical size. **Development** is the process of maturation, including the refinement of body systems, thought processes, and judgment.

Principles of Growth and Development

Growth and development progress uniquely in each individual but follow a general pattern from simple to complex. These processes, although orderly, are usually uneven, with growth spurts followed by periods of little or no growth. Changes are often gradual and blur or blend together instead of having definite starting and ending points. Box 5-1 ■ identifies the principles of growth and development. (Note: This chapter includes all stages of the life span, just as all phases of the family are included in Chapter 4 ●●.)

PATTERN OF DEVELOPMENT

The directional patterns of development are fundamental to all humans and occur bilaterally. Development is **cephalocaudal,** proceeding from head to toe (Figure 5-1 ■). For example, the infant must be able to raise his or her head before sitting up, and control his or her trunk before walking (Figure 5-2 ■). Development is also **proximodistal,** meaning from the center of the body to the periphery and proceeding from general to specific. For example, the infant can close its hand and grasp before it can finger pinch. The child has gross motor control before fine motor control.

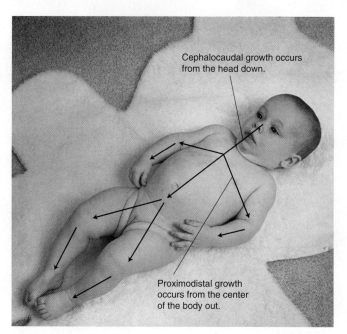

Figure 5-1. ■ Illustration showing growth and development direction in a small child.

Cephalocaudal growth occurs from the head down.

Proximodistal growth occurs from the center of the body out.

BOX 5-1

Principles of Growth and Development

- Growth and development are continuous, bilateral processes.
- Not all parts of the body mature at the same time.
- Growth and development are individualized.
- Growth and development are orderly and proceed from simple to complex.
- Growth and development are uneven at times, with growth spurts followed by plateaus.
- Growth and development changes are insidious, blurring and blending together.
- Growth and development proceed from head to toe (cephalocaudal).
- Growth and development proceed from center to periphery (proximodistal).
- Growth and development proceed from general to specific.

FACTORS THAT INFLUENCE GROWTH AND DEVELOPMENT

Heredity

There are many factors that influence normal growth and development (Box 5-2 ■). Heredity plays an important role. Characteristics of ancestors are passed on to future generations at conception through countless combinations of genes. Characteristics may be dominant or recessive. Dominant characteristics are more frequently manifested. Eye and hair color and physical stature are examples of hereditary characteristics. If both parents are tall with blond hair and blue eyes, the children will probably be the same. If one parent is tall and blond with blue eyes and the other parent is short with brown hair and brown eyes, the children will probably show a mixture of these characteristics.

Nationality, Race, and Culture

One's nationality, race, and cultural customs can influence the rates of growth and development. To some extent this might appear to be genetic, but researchers are finding that growth and development are more complex. In the past, both parents came from the same town, were of the same race and nationality, and had the same cultural customs. Children from these towns grew and developed at similar rates. As our world has become more mobile, and race and cultural customs have blended, growth and development patterns have changed. As these changes are studied, it has been discovered that cultural customs affecting diet, activity, and family dynamics influence childhood development.

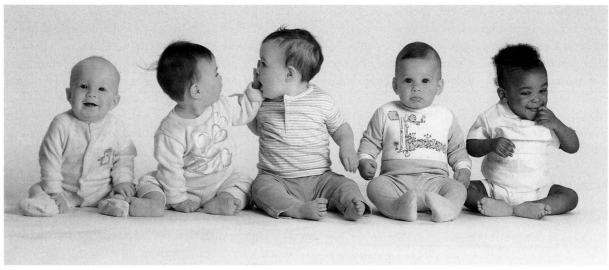

Figure 5-2. ■ Infants learn to sit up by about 6 months. They communicate with body language long before they speak. (Barbara Campbell/Getty Images, Inc.)

For example, it was once believed that people of Asian descent were short in stature. Today, a person of Asian descent who is born in the United States grows to a height comparable to other U.S. children. Box 5-3 ■ discusses the importance of viewing a client's culture as only one aspect of the whole person.

Order of Birth

The order of birth **(ordinal position)** in the family can influence development. The oldest child's greatest influence is parents who are just learning to parent. The middle child is influenced by parents who have some experience and also by the older child. The youngest child may develop more quickly in some ways because he or she learns from the older children. In other ways, the youngest child may develop more slowly because of the family's tendency to do things for "the baby." An only child might mature faster intellectually because of the amount of time spent with adults instead of other children. However, parents of

| BOX 5-3 | CULTURAL PULSE POINTS |

Thinking Clearly About Clients of Other Cultures

When culture is an issue in the delivery of client care, the nurse must make use of his or her critical thinking ability. Cultural awareness does not take the process far enough. Cultural awareness can be used to categorize, rather than to individualize, care. It may cause too great a focus on race, culture, and ethnicity.

Nurses must not label people by culture and race. We must not assume that the characteristics of a certain group are true for every client who belongs to that racial, ethnic, or cultural group. Assumptions close our minds to the real information we can obtain through our senses and through insightful questions addressed to the client.

The information we learn about cultural groups is no more than an overview. Nurses must always be aware of what people may be thinking that may differ from our own thoughts. We must also recognize that other sources outside the traditional medical community exist to help clients.

Source: Adapted from Ramont, R. P., Niedringhaus, D. M. (2006). *Comprehensive nursing care.* Upper Saddle River, NJ: Prentice Hall, Box 4-2, p. 53.

| BOX 5-2 | |

Factors Influencing Normal Growth and Development

- Heredity
- Nationality, race, and culture
- Ordinal position in family
- Gender
- Family function or dysfunction
- Physical environment

an only child may also "spoil" the child or slow the development in an attempt to "hold on to their baby."

Gender

The gender of the person influences growth and development. Males are usually longer and weigh more at birth. This growth difference continues into adulthood. Development and **maturation** (the process of becoming fully developed) also occur at different rates. In addition to biologic reasons for these differences, they are also influenced by different expectations of the genders.

Culture has a significant influence on gender role. For example, a cultural expectation that girls should be protected and should care for the house and that boys should go out and confront the world could easily lead to the assumption that girls are weaker and that boys are stronger. Children who live out those expectations may find them to be self-fulfilling.

Family Structure

The family structure influences the development of the child. The traditional roles of the mother and father have changed. In many families, both parents are employed outside the home, so the children spend a lot of time interacting with other children and adults in child care facilities. Some families consist of one parent, homosexual parents, or grandparents assuming the role of parents. Families with support from only one parent may spend more time alone while the single parent manages parenting roles. Single gender parents also do not provide the gender role influence from the opposite sex. Children may live in poverty, lack proper nutrition, and have limited access to health care. The function or dysfunction of the family affects the development of the child. Family systems are discussed later in this chapter.

Physical and Emotional Environment

The physical environment in which the child lives will influence the development of the child. A clean, secure, and stable environment with adequate nutrition and health care allows a child to focus energy toward healthy growth and development. A tense environment, in which the child feels unloved, or an insecure environment, where there is limited nutrition and health care, interferes with the developmental process.

Theories of Development

Theories provide a framework for studying the world around us. Many individuals have devoted their life's work to understanding the process of human growth and development. They have developed theories to organize their "systems approach," believing that everyone in the system or family is influenced by everyone else in the family. Others have studied various aspects of the individual such as physical growth, cognitive ability, or moral development. The LPN/LVN must have a basic understanding of these theories in order to assist in the assessment of the growth and development of the child and individual members of the family. These theories will be applied to each stage of development.

COGNITIVE DEVELOPMENT

The intellectual ability of an individual is called cognition or **cognitive development.** Children are born with an innate cognitive ability that must be developed. Jean Piaget, a Swiss psychologist, was a pioneer and a well-respected authority on cognitive development. Piaget believed that intelligence is defined by levels of interaction and the ability to cope within one's environment. He proposed four interrelated stages of cognitive development. These are shown in Table 5-1 ■.

Sensorimotor Period

The first stage, the **sensorimotor,** is from birth to 2 years of age. During this stage, the baby and young child begin interaction with the environment by reflex response and progress to experiencing the environment through sensimotor skills. The sensorimotor stage consists of five substages.

1. Use of Reflexes: The infant from birth to 1 month experiences his or her environment through reflexes. For example, with the sucking reflex, the infant responds to the touch of the mother's nipple and tastes breast milk. Likewise, when the Moro reflex causes the infant's hand to move, he or she touches objects accidentally and experiences sensations of hardness, softness, cold, or warmth.

2. Primary Circular Reactions: From 1 to 4 months of age, the infant purposely attempts to repeat pleasurable behaviors that were first experienced through reflex activity. For example, the palmar grasp allows the infant to cause a rattle to move. The infant will attempt to repeat this action to hear the rattle make noise again.

TABLE 5-1		
Piaget's Stages of Cognitive Development		
STAGE	**AGE (YEARS)**	**DEMONSTRATION OF INTELLIGENCE**
Sensorimotor Period	Birth–2	Interacts with the environment by reflex response
Preoperational Period	2–7	Begins to use language and progresses to use of numbers and letters
Concrete Operations Period	7–11	Sees everything in "black and white," "right or wrong" terms
Formal Operations Period	11–16	Interactions include abstract thought, able to predict future outcomes of today's behavior

3. Secondary Circular Reactions: From age 4 to 12 months, the infant begins to understand that actions have a cause and effect. Peek-a-boo becomes a favorite game as he or she understands that mother's face is only temporarily hidden behind her hands. Prior to this sub-stage, the infant forgets about objects that are not visible. During this substage, **object permanence** develops. Object permanence is an understanding that unseen objects still exist. A favorite toy can be hidden under a blanket and the infant will enjoy trying to uncover it. However, an understanding of object permanence does not keep the infant from being anxious when the parent is absent.

4. Tertiary Circular Reactions: The 12- to 18-month old fully explores his or her environment using all of the senses. Most objects end up in the toddler's mouth as he or she attempts to taste them. Objects are thrown to explore the sound they make as they hit the ground.

5. Mental Combinations: From age 18 to 24 months the child develops language, and object permanence is fully developed. Knowledge and previous experiences have been stored as mental images; the child can retrieve these images to solve simple problems. For example, a child who has toys in both hands and who wants another soon learns to set the first toy down to get the new one. The 18- to 24-month-old child also begins to develop the ability to pretend. Playing with toys now becomes more purposeful.

Preoperational Period

As children learn to interact with members of the environment, they move into the **preoperational** stage, ages 2 to 7 years. The child at age 2 begins to use symbolism (mainly in the form of language) and progresses to the use of other symbols, such as numbers and letters, by age 7. For example, the child learns to display the number of fingers related to his age. During the preoperational stage the child is said to be egocentric. **Egocentrism** is the tendency to view things only from one's own point of view. If a caregiver pours milk into two cups, the preoperational child will usually pick the one that appears to have more. This child also has **magical thinking.** The child believes that ideas and mental images become reality. The child may believe that he or she caused a sibling's illness by wishing that the sibling would go away.

Concrete Operations Period

In the next stage, the **concrete operations period,** the child from ages 7 to 11 is oriented in the here and now. Everything in the environment is "black and white," "right or wrong." The child has difficulty with "gray" areas or abstractions. The child understands that even when an object changes shape, it is the same object. For instance, when molding clay is formed into a different shape, it is the original piece of clay. In the concrete operational period, the child is also able to categorize objects and place them into series. These skills are necessary for the child to learn mathematical principles.

Formal Operations Period

From ages 11 to adulthood, abstract comprehension develops. This includes being able to predict future outcomes of today's behavior. In this final stage, called the **formal operations period,** the adolescent gradually completes the intellectual development that is necessary to function as an adult. In this period, the child is able to understand that cigarette smoking causes health problems, that companies may promote activities such as smoking despite their bad effects, and that peer pressure may lead some of their friends to smoke cigarettes anyway.

PSYCHOSOCIAL DEVELOPMENT

Psychosocial development is a much more complex process, and more theorists have contributed to our understanding. Although there are differences in the theories, there are also many similarities.

Erikson's Stages of Development

Erik Erikson's theory is widely used and is described here. (Psychosocial issues are also discussed in Chapter 16. ⚭) Erikson described eight stages of development in which the individual must accomplish specific tasks. These stages are listed in Table 5-2 ■.

TABLE 5-2

Erikson's Eight Stages of Development

STAGE	AGE (YEARS)	TASK
Infancy	0–1	Trust versus mistrust
Early childhood	1–3	Autonomy versus shame and doubt
Late childhood	3–6	Initiative versus guilt
School age	6–12	Industry versus inferiority
Adolescence	12–18	Identity versus role confusion
Young adult	20–40	Intimacy versus isolation
Middle adult	40–65	Generativity versus self-absorption/stagnation
Elder adult	Older than 65	Ego integrity versus despair

TRUST VERSUS MISTRUST. The first stage is infancy. In this stage, infants (from newborn to 1 year) are developing trust. For example, when infants are hungry, they cry in an attempt to make their needs known. There is a brief period of mistrust as they wait for satisfaction. As caregivers respond by holding and feeding them, infants learn to trust that their needs will be met. Over time, they will become less stressed in time of need. The task at this stage is to establish trust instead of mistrust. Children who do not have their basic needs met often have difficulty trusting anyone later in life.

AUTONOMY VERSUS SHAME AND DOUBT. The second stage is early childhood, from ages 1 to 3 years. In this stage, toddlers must learn autonomy instead of shame and doubt. As children become more mobile, they explore their environment independently. When they are unsuccessful, or when they are scolded for exploring, they feel shame and doubt about their ability to be independent.

Children gradually develop confidence through repeated tries and eventual successes. For example, toddlers develop autonomy by learning to use the toilet. If parents focus on "accidents" and scold them for soiling themselves, toddlers will learn shame and doubt, and they may not try as hard. Feelings of "being a failure" may affect them throughout their lives. However, if parents praise their efforts and calmly accept the times when they are not successful, their feelings of trust (from stage 1) will be compounded by a sense of autonomy. Their bowel and bladder control will develop over time, and eventually they will become successful.

INITIATIVE VERSUS GUILT. The third stage is one of initiative versus guilt. In this stage, ages 3 to 6 years, children learn to take initiative to meet their own needs. If they do not receive praise for their efforts, they will feel guilt about being a failure or about not giving pleasure to those they love. They may become quite creative in an effort to accomplish what they set out to do. For example, if their hair is hanging in their face, they might get scissors and cut it instead of combing it. If the parent reacts by yelling or punishing, they will feel guilty. If the parent quietly explains the reasons for not cutting their own hair, they will not experience guilt. Through positive reinforcement of initiative, they will continue to develop a positive attitude.

INDUSTRY VERSUS INFERIORITY. The fourth stage, school age, from 6 to 12 years, is a time for developing industry versus inferiority. As children progress through school and apply what they learn to a variety of life experiences, they become more industrious. They seek praise beyond their own parents, from teachers, other adults, and peers. If they are unsuccessful or do not receive praise, they feel inferior and may become withdrawn. They may become quiet, have few friends, and not participate in any outside activities, or the effect may be quite the opposite. They might act out in groups, become bullies, or become physically or verbally abusive in an attempt to feel better about themselves. Children who do receive praise for things they do well are able to generalize the positive effects of their industriousness and work for improvement in difficult areas. They eventually learn that everyone has areas of strength and areas that need improvement. They learn to emphasize their areas of strength and manage their areas of weakness.

IDENTITY VERSUS ROLE CONFUSION. The fifth stage is adolescence. This stage, ages 12 to 20 years, is the time of identity versus role confusion. Teenagers are developing their sexual identity, becoming more independent, and beginning the process of separation from their parents. Teenagers have a strong desire to make their own decisions and "live their own life," but at the same time they have a real need to know the boundaries or rules. Teenagers are examining the world and trying to decide where they fit, what their life's work will be, and how they can accomplish their goals. They are beginning to use peers for support instead of relying on parents for help in making decisions. With positive reinforcement of their progress, they can develop a strong identity. However, with continual negative feedback, coupled with feelings of inferiority and guilt, they can become confused, ambivalent, and withdrawn. If the parents do not allow them to separate from their influence, develop peer relationships, and make their own decisions, they will remain dependent because they have not developed a clear identity.

INTIMACY VERSUS ISOLATION. The sixth stage, young adult, ages 20 to 40 years, is a time of intimacy versus isolation. Young adults have made some decisions regarding their life's work and are now interested in finding a companion, someone with whom to share a life. This is a time when many people marry and begin a family. The relationships developed in this stage are usually meaningful, long-lasting bonds. If young adults have difficulty finding a companion, they fear a life of loneliness and isolation. This fear can either be a motivating force or be immobilizing. If motivated, the young adult settles into a life of companionship, special friends, and/or raising children. Marriage is not the only method of obtaining intimacy. Many single adults find intimacy with friends and family without ever marrying. If immobilized by the fear of loneliness, however, young adults settle for a life of few or no close friends, where leisure time is spent alone. These young adults live lives of isolation.

***GENERATIVITY VERSUS SELF-ABSORPTION AND STAGNA-
TION.***   The middle years, ages 40 to 65, constitute the
seventh stage. This is a time of generativity versus self-
absorption and stagnation. *Generativity* comes from the
same root word as *generation*, *generator*, and *generous*. This is
the time in life when adults become great generators of
ideas and beliefs. They think of what they have contributed
or want to contribute to society and future generations.
They are generous in sharing their resources and what they
have learned from their life experiences. This is a time
when most adults become grandparents and are proud to
see their life's work carried on by their offspring. The
middle adult's contributions may be in the form of writing,
inventions, science, art, or social causes. Sometimes,
though, adults become absorbed in their own lives. People
who do not complete this stage successfully become stagnant and lack creativity. They have difficulty seeing any
value and meaning in their lives. Bitterness and emptiness
may begin to develop.

EGO INTEGRITY VERSUS DESPAIR.   The eighth state is the
older adult, older than 65 years. This time is devoted to ego
integrity versus despair. Most adults have learned to trust
as infants, have developed a sense of identity during adolescence, and have enjoyed an adult life with rich relationships. If older adults have had these positive life experiences, they will probably enter old age with a strong
identity. They can look at their lives and know the world
was a better place because of their contributions. They can
truly say, "I've had a good life." However, if they have had a
life of mistrust, guilt, and feelings of inferiority, or if they
have been isolated and stagnant, they will enter old age in
despair. They will find no joy in life and may describe their
lives as useless. They may become preoccupied with the
past. They become angry and bitter in their old age and
drive others away, leading to more isolation. Ultimately,
they must face the inevitability of death. Older adults
either fear death or accept the fact that it is a basic part of
living and face it with grace.

PSYCHOSEXUAL DEVELOPMENT

Sigmund Freud (1856–1939), an Austrian physician,
worked with adults who were experiencing nervous disorders. By studying the results of psychoanalysis, he developed
the belief that early childhood experiences unconsciously
motivate actions in later life. He believed that sexual
instincts were important to the development of the personality. He termed the need for sensual pleasure **psychosexual.**

Freud viewed the personality as having three parts: id,
ego, and superego. The **id** is the basic energy that drives the
individual to seek pleasure and satisfy needs. The **ego** is the
realistic part of the personality that searches for acceptable

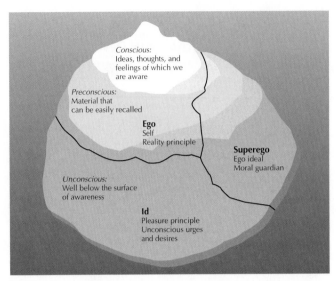

Figure 5-3. ■ Freud saw the vast importance of the unconscious
in people's lives. He said that most actions are motivated by subconscious thought. He viewed the personality in three parts: the *id*
(the basic energy that drives the individual to seek pleasure), the
ego (the realistic part of the personality that searches for acceptable ways of obtaining pleasure), and the *superego* (the moral
system that contains learned values and conscience). People are
aware of their conscious thoughts, but it is often the subconscious
that drives them. (Reprinted from Morris, C. G., & Maisto, A. A. [2001]
Understanding psychology [5th ed.]. Upper Saddle River, NJ: Prentice Hall.)

methods of meeting pleasure needs. The **superego** is the
moral system that contains learned values and conscience.

Freud emphasized that much of what people experience is
governed by the subconscious parts of the mind. In other
words, we are often not aware of the feelings and buried
thoughts that motivate us and cause us to respond the way
we do. As illustrated in Figure 5-3 ■, he believed that our
conscious thoughts are like the tip of an iceberg, and that
most of our actions are motivated by the unconscious mind.

Freud described five stages of psychosexual development. Table 5-3 ■ identifies these stages. He introduced
the idea that a client could uncover problems by talking,
remembering dreams, and *free association* (linking thoughts
as they come to mind). Although many of Freud's theories
have been refuted by later theorists, two aspects of his
thinking still prevail:

1. Behavior is motivated, often by the unconscious, and is
   not accidental.

2. People have ways of "protecting the ego from threatening impulses or painful realities of life experiences"
   (Eby, 2005). These ways of protecting oneself are called
   defense mechanisms. Common defense mechanisms
   are described in Chapter 16 ○○. Four defense mechanisms that are commonly used by children are shown in
   Table 5-4 ■.

TABLE 5-3

Freud's Stages of Psychosexual Development

STAGE	AGE (YEARS)	DESCRIPTION
Oral	Birth–1	Baby obtains comfort and pleasure through the mouth.
Anal	1–3	Child achieves pleasure through control of waste elimination from the body.
Phallic	3–6	Child works out relationships with parents and relatives of the same and opposite genders.
Latency	6–12	Sexual energy is at rest.
Genital	12–Adulthood	Mature sexuality develops and the person establishes relationships with others.

TABLE 5-5

Kohlberg's Levels of Moral Development

STAGE	APPROXIMATE AGE (YEARS)	DESCRIPTION
Preconventional	4–7	Decisions are based on desire to please others and avoid punishment.
Conventional	7–11	Rules are important and must be followed. Conscience begins to develop.
Postconventional	12 and older	Individual has internalized ethical standards and recognizes social responsibility.

MORAL DEVELOPMENT

Lawrence Kohlberg (1927–1987) focused his theoretical study on the moral development of people. Kohlberg was born in New York and served as a professor of education and social psychology at Harvard University. To develop his theory, he presented stories involving a moral dilemma and asked children and adults to solve the problem. He then analyzed their expressed motives for the decisions they made. In this way, Kohlberg established three levels of moral development. He noted that the age guidelines he presented are approximate and that many people never reach the highest level. Table 5-5 ■ describes these levels of moral development.

Standards of Physical Growth and Development

Physical growth is usually measured by height, weight, and head circumference. Before children can stand, length is measured horizontally rather than vertically. The standard measurements for height and head circumference are inches or centimeters. Weight is measured in pounds and ounces or in kilograms or grams. See Chapter 8 ⬀ for more information about the procedures for obtaining these measurements. Height and weight measurements are recorded on a growth chart (see Appendix II ⬀). The growth chart has lines to correspond to 5th, 10th, 25th, 50th, 75th, 90th, and 95th percentile. **Percentile** is a statistical measure in which a value on a scale of one hundred indicates the portion of the overall population that is the same. For example, a child who is at the 75th percentile for height is taller than 75% of the population and shorter than 25% of the population. The use of growth charts is valuable for the following reasons:

- The child's growth can be compared to the average for his age. A difference of 2 or more percentiles between height and weight may indicate the child is overweight or underweight and should be further evaluated.

TABLE 5-4

Defense Mechanisms Commonly Used by Children

DEFENSE MECHANISM	DEFINITION	EXAMPLE
Regression	Returning to an earlier stage of behavior	A 7-year-old who does not suck his thumb suddenly begins to suck his thumb when hospitalized.
Repression	Involuntary forgetting of hurtful situations	A child who witnessed the brutal death of her parent cannot consciously recall the incident.
Rationalization	Attempting to make unacceptable feelings acceptable	A child explains pulling another child's hair by saying, "She won't give me my doll."
Fantasy	Creating a story in the mind to help deal with unacceptable fears	A child with a history of abuse pretends to be Cinderella.

■ The current measurements can be compared to the child's previous measurements. If the child's growth falls outside the normal pattern, or if there is a sudden unusual change in the pattern, further evaluation may be suggested.

Stages of Physical and Cognitive Growth and Development

It is important for the nurse to know and understand the stages of physical and cognitive development. Although development occurs in a predictable pattern, the nurse must carefully assess each child to determine progress through the stages. See Chapter 6 ⚭ for more information about psychosocial development as it relates to illness prevention, health promotion, and nutrition issues.

INFANT (BIRTH TO 1 YEAR)

At no time is rapid change as notable as during the first year of life. The infant enters the world totally dependent but by year's end can walk and communicate.

Years of study of growth and development have allowed researchers to develop tables showing standard milestones for each age group. It is important to compare the progress of the growing child with these standards. By referring to these tables, problems can be identified early and intervention begun. Table 5-6 ■ illustrates the milestones the infant should reach during the first year of development.

Physical Growth

With good nutrition, the infant gains weight rapidly, doubling its birth weight by 5 months and tripling the birth weight by 12 months. The child grows about 12 inches

---

TABLE 5-6

Growth and Development Milestones During Infancy

AGE (MONTHS)	PHYSICAL GROWTH	FINE MOTOR SKILLS	GROSS MOTOR SKILLS	SENSORY ABILITY
Birth–1	Gains 5–7 oz (140–200 g)/ week Grows ½ inch (1.5 cm) in first month Head circumference increases ½ inch (1.5 cm)/month	Holds hand in fist (1) Draws arms and legs to body when crying Tight grasp	Inborn reflexes such as startle and rooting are predominant activity May lift head briefly if prone (2) Alerts to high-pitched voices Comforts with touch (3) Has jerky arm/leg movement	Prefers to look at faces and black-and-white geometric designs Follows objects in line of vision (4)

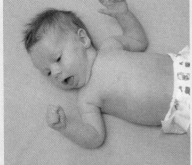

(1) Holds hand in fist

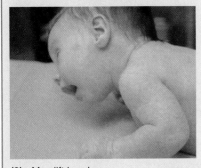

(2) May lift head

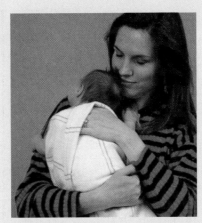

(3) Comforts with touch

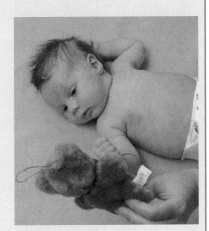

(4) Follows objects

(continued)

TABLE 5-6

Growth and Development Milestones During Infancy (continued)

AGE (MONTHS)	PHYSICAL GROWTH	FINE MOTOR SKILLS	GROSS MOTOR SKILLS	SENSORY ABILITY
2–4	Gains 5–7 oz (140–200 g)/week Grows ½ inch (1.5 cm)/month Head circumference increases ½ inch (1.5 cm)/month Posterior fontanel closes Eats 120 mL/kg/24 hr (2 oz/lb/24 hr)	Holds rattle when placed in hand (5) Looks at and plays with own fingers Readily brings objects from hand to mouth	Moro reflex fading in strength Can turn from side to back and then return (6) Decrease in head lag when pulled to sitting; sits with head held in midline with some bobbing. When prone, holds head and supports weight on forearms (7)	Follows objects 180° Turns head to look for voices, sounds

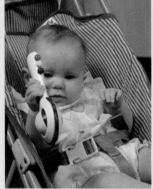
(5) Holds rattle

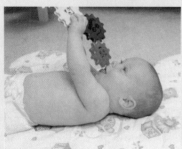
(6) Can turn from side to back

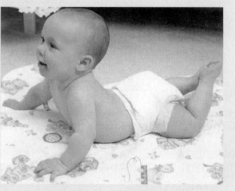
(7) Holds head up and supports weights with arms

AGE (MONTHS)	PHYSICAL GROWTH	FINE MOTOR SKILLS	GROSS MOTOR SKILLS	SENSORY ABILITY
4–6	Gains 5–7 oz (140–200 g)/week Doubles birth weight by 5–6 months Grows ½ inch (1.5 cm)/month Head circumference increases ½ inch (1.5 cm)/month Teeth begin to erupt by 6 months Eats 100 mL/kg/24 hr (2 oz/lb/24 hr)	Grasps rattle and other objects at will; drops them to pick up another offered object (8) Mouths objects Mouths feet and pulls to mouth Holds bottle Grasps with whole hand (palmar grasp) Manipulates objects (9)	Holds head held steady when sitting Turns from abdomen to back by 4 months and then back to abdomen by 6 months When held standing supports much of own weight (10)	Examines complex visual images Watches the course of a falling object Responds readily to sounds

(8) Grasps objects at will

(9) Manipulates objects

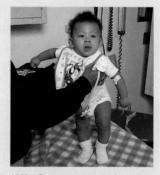
(10) Supports most of weight

AGE (MONTHS)	PHYSICAL GROWTH	FINE MOTOR SKILLS	GROSS MOTOR SKILLS	SENSORY ABILITY
6–8	Gains 3–5 oz (85–140 g)/week Grows ⅜ inch (1 cm)/month Growth rate slower than first 6 months	Bangs objects held in hand Transfers objects from one hand to other Beginning pincer grasp at times	Has lost most newborn reflexes Sits alone without support by 8 months (11) Likes to bounce on legs when held in standing position	Recognizes own name and responds by looking and smiling Enjoys small and complex objects at play

AGE (MONTHS)	PHYSICAL GROWTH	FINE MOTOR SKILLS	GROSS MOTOR SKILLS	SENSORY ABILITY

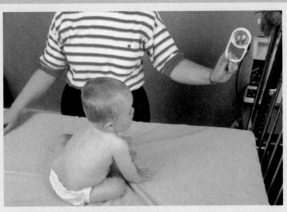

(11) Sits alone without support

AGE (MONTHS)	PHYSICAL GROWTH	FINE MOTOR SKILLS	GROSS MOTOR SKILLS	SENSORY ABILITY
8–10	Gains 3–5 oz (85–140 g)/week Grows ³/₈ inch (1 cm)/ month	Picks up small objects (12) Uses pincer grasp well (14)	Crawls or pulls body along floor by arms (13) Creeps by using hands and knees to keep trunk off the floor Pulls self to standing and sitting by 10 months Recovers balance when sitting	Understands words such as "no" and "cracker" May say one word in addition to "mama" and "dada" Recognizes sound without difficulty

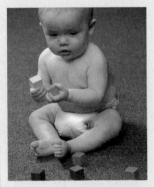

(12) Picks up small objects

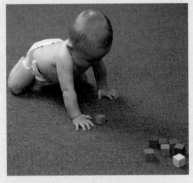

(13) Crawls or pulls body by arms

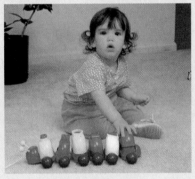

(14) Uses pincer grasp well

AGE (MONTHS)	PHYSICAL GROWTH	FINE MOTOR SKILLS	GROSS MOTOR SKILLS	SENSORY ABILITY
10–12 months	Gains 3–5 oz (85–140 g)/week Grown ³/₈ inch (1 cm)/ month Head circumference equals chest circumference Triples birth weight by 1 year	May hold crayon or pencil and make mark on paper Places objects into container through holes (15)	Stands alone (16) Walks holding on to furniture Sits from standing (17) May walk alone for short distance	Plays peek-a-boo and pattycake

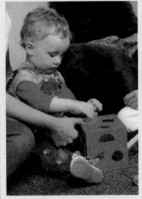

(15) Places objects in container

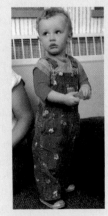

(16) Stands alone

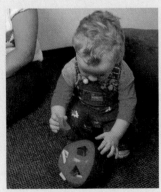

(17) Sits down from standing

during the first year of life. With this growth comes a change in body proportion (see Figure 6-13 ⬭). The head, growing rapidly during fetal development, now slows its growth, while the torso and limbs become longer and stronger.

Organs and body systems are completely formed early in the fetal development process, though they are not fully mature for several years. The liver and kidneys begin to mature and are able to detoxify and excrete drugs and other chemicals. Liver maturation is usually complete by the end of the first year and kidney maturation is accomplished after 6 months of life. The nervous system is able to coordinate muscle movements. The senses are able to discriminate visual images, sounds, and tastes. Teeth eruption begins at about 6 months. With the intake of more solid food, the stomach and intestines are also able to digest more complex foods.

Cognitive Development

The infant's behavior provides clues to cognitive development. Initially, reflexes govern a newborn's actions. By 12 months, however, the infant is interacting with the environment and interpreting sights and sounds. The 2-month-old learns to make noise in response to voices, and by the end of the year can understand many words and usually say a few. During the course of a child's first year, the brain registers and stores information for future reference.

Three behavioral states have been identified to describe the normal newborn: sleep state, quiet alert state, and crying state. The newborn sleeps for 20 to 22 hours a day. Over the next few months, the infant will gradually stay awake for longer periods of time. By 4 months, the infant will normally sleep through the night and be awake for 2 to 3 hours at a time during the day.

During hours of wakefulness, it is important for infants to begin to explore the environment. With little mobility, their "world" is the area within their reach (Figure 5-4 ■).

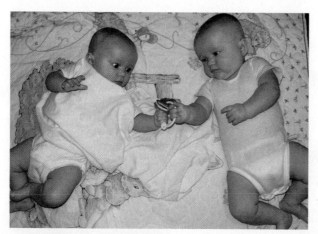

Figure 5-4. ■ In the first year, reflex actions gradually evolve into deliberate actions. Until the infant becomes mobile, the "world" of the infant consists of things within his or her reach.

As they move and stretch to explore, infants learn to turn over and roll. They explore by touch and taste. They learn to manipulate things in their grasp and produce pleasure, thus developing the foundation for play. As their strength grows, infants learn to sit up by themselves, to crawl, and finally to stand. With mobility comes a wider and wider environment to explore.

TODDLER (1 TO 3 YEARS)

The word *toddle* means to walk with short unsteady steps. Children in this age group fit this definition well. As they learn to walk, toddlers are unsteady, falling frequently. Their steps are short, with feet far apart to broaden their base of support. Once toddlers gain security and practice in walking, they begin to walk faster and finally to run. At the same time, toddlers are learning to climb and want to stand on everything. By age 3, toddlers can stand briefly on one foot and can ride a tricycle.

Physical Growth

During the second year of life, the toddler's growth slows, but body proportions continue to change. Their legs become longer and their head smaller in relation to body size. At first, they appear potbellied because their abdominal muscles lack strength. Over time, their activity strengthens these muscles, and the abdomen becomes flatter (see Figure 20-3 ⬭).

Toddlers continue to cut teeth, with complete eruption of 20 deciduous teeth by 34 months (Figure 5-5 ■). This helps them eat a broader variety of foods. Toddlers want to be independent and try to feed themselves; they should be encouraged to do so.

During the second year, toddlers begin to gain control of their elimination. Box 5-4 ■ provides some guidelines

---

BOX 5-4   CLIENT TEACHING

Determining Readiness for Toilet Training

Bladder and bowel control is physiologically possible between 18 and 24 months. However, other factors must be in place for toilet training to be successful. The nurse can use the following questions with parents who are considering toilet training:

- Does the child stand and walk?
- Can the child pull his or her pants up and down?
- Does he or she show interest in mimicking the toileting behavior of parents and siblings?
- Does the child recognize the need to "go"?
- Can the child wait to reach the bathroom?
- Are there noticeable indications that the child is defecating or urinating?
- Does the child have genital awareness?
- Does the child report that defecation or urination has occurred?

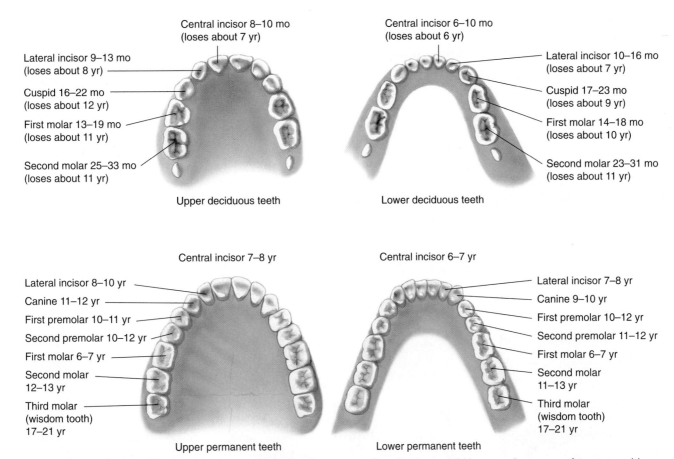

Central incisor 8–10 mo (loses about 7 yr)

Lateral incisor 9–13 mo (loses about 8 yr)

Cuspid 16–22 mo (loses about 12 yr)

First molar 13–19 mo (loses about 11 yr)

Second molar 25–33 mo (loses about 11 yr)

Upper deciduous teeth

Central incisor 6–10 mo (loses about 6 yr)

Lateral incisor 10–16 mo (loses about 7 yr)

Cuspid 17–23 mo (loses about 9 yr)

First molar 14–18 mo (loses about 10 yr)

Second molar 23–31 mo (loses about 11 yr)

Lower deciduous teeth

Central incisor 7–8 yr

Lateral incisor 8–10 yr
Canine 11–12 yr
First premolar 10–11 yr
Second premolar 10–12 yr
First molar 6–7 yr
Second molar 12–13 yr
Third molar (wisdom tooth) 17–21 yr

Upper permanent teeth

Central incisor 6–7 yr

Lateral incisor 7–8 yr
Canine 9–10 yr
First premolar 10–12 yr
Second premolar 11–12 yr
First molar 6–7 yr
Second molar 11–13 yr
Third molar (wisdom tooth) 17–21 yr

Lower permanent teeth

Figure 5-5. ■ (*Top*) Typical eruption of deciduous ("baby") teeth. (*Bottom*) The school-age child loses teeth at a rate of 4 a year and, by age 12, has 26 of the 30 permanent teeth. The remaining molars appear during adolescence.

for assessing readiness for toilet training. Many children prefer their own "potty" chair to using the adult toilet (Figure 5-6 ■). Fear of falling into the water may prevent successful toileting. Toddlers should be placed on the toilet for a few minutes at regular intervals during the day and should be rewarded for success. If they seem uninterested or confused about what is expected of them, parents should wait a few weeks and try again.

Cognitive Development

Toddlers are moving from the sensorimotor to the preoperational level of cognitive development (see Table 5-1). Table 5-7 ■ illustrates the major milestones during toddlerhood. Toddlers learn to associate words with things in the world around them. Their vocabulary expands rapidly, gaining 1,000 words by age 3. They can use words in short sentences. Their attention span is lengthening and they enjoy play. Toddlers enjoy socialization with other children but usually engage in **parallel play,** playing beside others rather than with them. Play with a variety of toys encourages both gross motor and fine motor development.

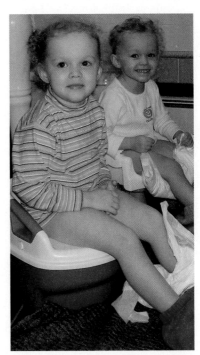

Figure 5-6. ■ Toilet training requires consistency and commitment on the part of the caregiver to schedule regular trips to bathroom.

TABLE 5-7

Growth and Development Milestones During Toddlerhood

AGE (YEARS)	PHYSICAL GROWTH	FINE MOTOR SKILLS	GROSS MOTOR SKILLS	SENSORY ABILITY
1–2	Gains ½ lb (227 g) per month Grows 3.5–5 inches (9–12 cm) during this year Anterior fontanel closes All deciduous teeth present by 33 months	By end of 2nd year, builds tower of four blocks (1) Scribbles on paper (2) Can undress self (3) Throws a ball	Runs Walks up and down stairs (5) Likes to push toys	Visual acuity 20/50 Increasing vocabulary of 200 words by 2 years
2–3	Gains 3–5 lb (1.4–2.3 kg)/year Grows 2–2.5 inches (5–6.5 cm)/year	Draws a circle and other rudimentary forms Learns to pour Learning to dress self (4)	Jumps Kicks ball (6) Throws ball overhand Rides tricycle	Communication improves Uses short three- to five-word sentences Vocabulary 1,000 words Displays frustration by temper tantrums

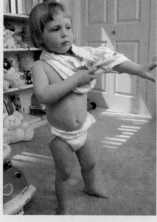

(1) Tower of four blocks

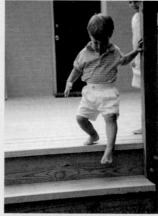

(2) Scribbles on paper

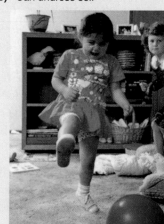

(3) Can undress self

(4) Learning to dress self

(5) Walks up and down stairs

(6) Jumps and kicks ball

Closeness to parents is important in helping toddlers feel safe and secure. Infants and toddlers experience a state of extreme discomfort when separated from loved ones. This **separation anxiety** results in many negative feelings including anger, fear, grief, and revenge. There are three phases of separation anxiety:

- The first phase, *protest*, is the expressed need for parents, characterized by screaming, clinging to parents, and prolonged crying. The child fears being deserted.
- The second phase, *despair*, is seen by less activity. The child is not crying but is in deep mourning. He or she

may appear sad or depressed, does not respond to others, and withdraws into his or her own world.

- The third phase is *denial*. This is a defense mechanism against the anxiety he or she is feeling. The infant or toddler represses the mental image of and feelings for the parents and does not protest when separation occurs. This quietness may be interpreted as recovery, because the child seems to take an interest in the environment, eats, plays, and accepts other adults. Anger and disappointment at parents are so deep that, on their return, the child acts as if he or she does not need them, showing revenge by rejecting them. However, it is important for the parents to understand that the child needs them more than ever at this point. If this phase is not identified, developmental delays may occur.

Toddlers use gestures and acting out to help communicate their needs. They may cry, stamp their feet, or lie down and kick their feet. These temper tantrums can be frustrating to parents. It is best to acknowledge the toddler's feelings and then to set limits. For example, "I know you are upset because you cannot have a cookie now. When you stop crying, you can come out of your room." When the child stops crying and comes out of his or her room, the parent should not bring up the bad behavior but should focus on some positive activity. For example, the parent could say, "I am glad you are ready to help me set the table for dinner."

PRESCHOOL CHILD (3 TO 6 YEARS)

Preschool children are becoming more independent. They are learning to obey rules and are becoming self-disciplined. They are very curious and are developing an imagination. Table 5-8 ■ illustrates growth and development milestones during the preschool stage of development.

Physical Growth

Preschool children continue to grow steadily, averaging an increase of 2 to 2½ inches (5–6 cm) and 4 to 5 pounds (about 2 kg) a year. The growth is mainly in the long bones of the arms and legs. Muscles are gaining strength and coordination.

Cognitive Development

Preschool children continue to progress in the preoperational level of cognitive development. They know their name and age. They are developing an understanding of relationships and gender identification. By age 5, they have a better concept of time, day, week, month, and year. They know their primary colors and can count to 10. Their attention span is getting longer, and they can spend 30 minutes at one activity.

Preschoolers' vocabulary continues to increase, with more than 2,000 words by age 5. Their sentence structure is also increasing to 7 to 8 words. They can describe drawings in detail. They can follow three simple commands given at the same time. They talk a lot, often asking "why?" and "what?"

SCHOOL-AGE CHILD (6 TO 12 YEARS)

The school-age years are a time of exciting growth and development. By this point, children have reached many milestones that allow them to explore their ever-expanding world. Table 5-9 ■ illustrates the milestones during the school-age years.

Physical Growth

The school-age child continues to grow about 2 inches and 2 pounds a year. Although the rate of growth is generally even, there may be a prepubescent growth spurt. The "childlike" appearance is replaced by a more adult appearance as the body proportions continue to change. Curvature of the spine (scoliosis) may be detected at this time (see Chapter 20 ⚭).

The school-age child loses teeth at a rate of 4 a year and, by age 12 has 26 of the 30 permanent teeth. The remaining molars appear during adolescence (see Figure 5-5).

Cognitive Development

School-age children are moving into the concrete operations stage of cognitive development. They can be expected to complete tasks, working both independently and in groups. They are learning to compromise and cooperate with others. Their confidence is developing, but they can be disappointed with their skills at times. If they feel left out or behind their peers, they may develop "attention-getting" behaviors.

As children move through the school-age years, they learn to be more logical and coherent. By studying a variety of school subjects, they learn reasoning skills, cause and effect, and reversibility. (For example $2 + 2 = 4$ and $4 - 2 = 2$ teaches not only a mathematical computation but also a concept of reasoning.) The vocabulary of school-age children increases to more than 2,500 words, and they use increasingly complex grammar in sentences. They are able to understand multiple meanings of words and they have the ability to learn complex physical-mental skills.

During these years, school-age children begin to question family rules and traditions. They move away from fantasy, giving up Santa Claus, the Easter Bunny and the Tooth Fairy. As they look to adults other than their parents as role models, they may begin to question family values, religious beliefs, and culture.

TABLE 5-8

Growth and Development Milestones During Preschool Years

AGE (YEARS)	PHYSICAL GROWTH	FINE MOTOR SKILLS	GROSS MOTOR SKILLS	SENSORY ABILITY
3–6	Gains 3–5 lbs (1.5–5 kg)/year Grows 1½–2½ inches (4–6 cm)/year	Uses scissors (1) Draws circle, square, cross (2) Draws at least a six-part person Enjoys art projects such as pasting, stringing beads, using clay Learns to tie shoes at the end of preschool years (3) Buttons clothes (4) Brushes teeth (5) Eats three meals with snacks Uses spoon, fork, and knife	Throws a ball overhand Climbs well (6) Rides tricycle May learn to ride bicycle with/without training wheels (7)	Visual acuity continues to improve Can focus on and learn letters and numbers (8) Begins to write letters, numbers Begins to write letters, numbers

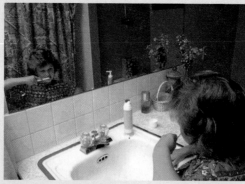

(1) Uses scissors

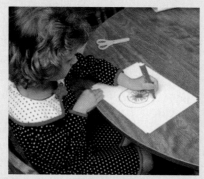

(2) Draws circle, square, cross

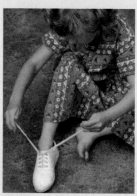

(3) Ties shoes

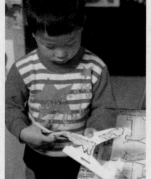

(4) Buttons clothes

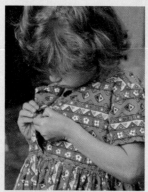

(5) Brushes teeth

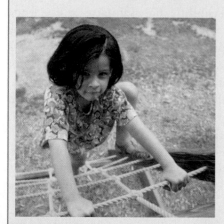

(6) Climbs well

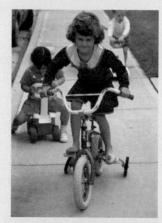

(7) Rides bicycle or bicycle with training wheels

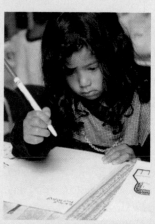

(8) Learns letters and numbers

TABLE 5.9

Growth and Development Milestones During School Age Years

AGE (YEARS)	PHYSICAL GROWTH	FINE MOTOR SKILLS	GROSS MOTOR SKILLS	SENSORY ABILITY
6–12	Gains 3–5 lb (1.5–5 kg)/year Grows 1½–2½ inches (4–6 cm)/year Loses teeth	Enjoys craft projects Plays cards, board games, and computer games	Rides two-wheeler (1) Plays musical instruments (2) Roller skates/blades or ice skates Balance and muscle strength increase Group sports (i.e. football, soccer, basketball, gymnastics, dance)	Can read Able to concentrate for longer periods on activities by filtering out surrounding sounds (3) Knowledge increases through school subjects

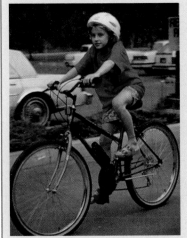
(1) Rides two-wheeler

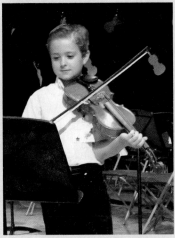
(2) Plays musical instruments

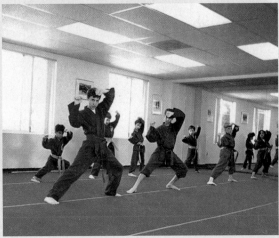
(3) Concentrates on activities for longer periods

Group play becomes important, and the school-age children often join clubs and teams. Through group play and team effort they learn "fairness." At about age 10, gender differences become more apparent in play activities.

ADOLESCENT (12 TO 20 YEARS)

The term *adolescence* comes from the Latin for "to grow up." Indeed, this is a time of maturation, where the individual moves from childhood to adulthood. Table 5-10 ■ illustrates the growth and development milestones for adolescence.

Physical Growth

Adolescence is the second-fastest growth period. It is the first stage in which patterns differ by gender. Both height and weight increase earlier in females than in males, but gains in both measurement are ultimately greater in males than in females. Table 5-11 ■ sketches height and weight information for normal adolescent physical growth.

As mentioned, females usually start to mature earlier than males. At puberty, increases in four primary sex hormones cause physical changes in girls. These hormones are follicle-stimulating hormone (FSH), luteinizing hormone (LH), estrogen, and progesterone. There is an increase in the rate of skeletal growth, a widening of the pelvis, and a change in fat distribution. Breast tissue begins to develop, and coarse hair forms under the arms and over the mons pubis. At about 13 years, females experience **menarche**, the beginning of the menstrual cycle. Menarche can begin as early as age 8 and as late as age 16. A few months later, ovulation begins. These changes take several years to complete. The female usually reaches full physical maturation by age 16, but it might be as late as 18 years of age. Sexual maturity can be documented in stages (called *Tanner's stages*), as shown in Table 5-12 ■.

Male development usually begins 2 years later than female development. Changes in hormones guide physical

TABLE 5-10

Growth and Development Milestones During Adolescence

AGE (YEARS)	PHYSICAL GROWTH	FINE MOTOR SKILLS	GROSS MOTOR SKILLS	SENSORY ABILITY
12–18	Variation in age of growth spurt, girls gain: 15–55 lb (7–25 kg) and grow 2–8 inches (2.5–20 cm); boys gain approximately 15–65 lb (7–29.5 kg) and grow 4½–12 inches (11–30 cm) Puberty results in body changes	Skills are well developed (1)	New sports activities attempted and muscle development continues (2) Some lack of coordination common during growth spurts	Fully developed

(1) Motor skills are well developed

(2) New sports activities attempted

changes in males, as in females. FSH and LH trigger the increase of testosterone. There is rapid growth with an increase in height, lengthening of the jaw, and a doubling of muscle mass. The penis and testicles mature, and coarse hair forms on the face, axillae, and pubis. The voice deepens. Ejaculation signals the beginning of spermatogenesis. Although these changes are usually apparent by age 16, the male may not reach his adult height until 19 to 21 years of age.

Cognitive Development

Although emotional and physical maturity is usually reached sooner in females, cognitive development progresses equally. The adolescent moves from the concrete operations level to the abstract comprehension (formal operations) level of cognitive development. Cognitive milestones include the following:

- Ability to examine hypothetical situations and apply the concepts to current issues

TABLE 5-11

Normal Adolescent Physical Growth Patterns

AGE	HEIGHT—FEMALES (INCHES)	HEIGHT—MALES (INCHES)	WEIGHT—FEMALES (LB)	WEIGHT—MALES (LB)
12	55–64	54–63.5	68–136	66–130
14	59–67.5	59–69.5	84–160	84–160
16	60–68	63–73	94–172	104–186
18	60–68.5	65–74	100–178	116–202

TABLE 5-12	
Tanner's Stages of Sexual Maturity	
STAGES OF SEXUAL MATURITY	DESCRIPTION
1	The adolescent has no pubic hair except for a fine "peach fuzz" body hair.
2	There is a sparse growth of long, slightly darkened, downy hair mostly along the labia in females or at the base of the penis and sometimes on the scrotum in males. This hair is usually straight or only slightly curled.
3	The pubic hair becomes darker, coarse, curlier. It now grows sparsely over the mons veneris area in females; it remains in the Stage 2 area in males.
4	The hair grows in more densely. It becomes as course and curly as in the adult, but there is not as much of it.
5	Pubic hair is the classic coarse and curly hair that extends onto the inner thighs.
6	The final amount, color, and distribution of pubic hair is quite variable.

Source: Data from Tanner, J. M. (1966). *Growth at adolescence.* New York: Appleton; Tanner, J. M. (1962). *Growth of adolescents.* Oxford: Blackwell; Marshall, W. A., & Tanner, J. M. (1970). Variations in the pattern of pubertal changes in boys. *Archives of Disease in Childhood, 45*(239), 13–23; Marshall, W. A., and Tanner, J. M. (1969). Variations in the pattern of pubertal changes in girls. *Archives of Disease in Childhood, 445*(235), 291–303.

- Ability to examine philosophical ideas and compare real-world situations to the ideal
- Ability to plan for the "what-if"
- Development of adult proficiency with language (although adolescents frequently use slang to "fit in" with their peer group).

In the early years (13 to 14), adolescents may be self-centered, but they gradually mature and develop a strong identity. This is a difficult transition, however. A changing body and an increase in hormones bring about confusion and doubt. Adolescents want to feel attractive, but they may feel ugly because of skin changes, the awkwardness of a rapidly changing body, and mood changes. Hormonal changes and a physiologic drive to reproduce put many pressures on development of sexuality. Peers are most important at this time and can have a positive or negative influence on behavior. Strong peer pressure and feelings of immortality ("it won't happen to

me") can lead to unwise choices and risk-taking behaviors (Figure 5-7 ■).

Parents often look for guidance at this period in their children's lives. The simple rules of the family are giving way to larger societal influences. Educational, religious, and health care professionals can offer valuable information to help parents provide guidelines for their teens. (See Health Promotion Issue box on pages 88 and 89.)

ADULT (18 TO 65 YEARS)

The adult years are subdivided into young adult, middle adult, and older adult. Young adults are adjusting to the "loss" of their place in the family. They move out of the home to attend school, begin a career, and/or start a family. This move causes a change in the organization of the family (see Table 4-1 ◯◯). They seek intimacy and a long-term relationship. Without intimacy, they face isolation.

As members of the family become young adults, the parents become middle-aged. This is a time for them not only to "let go" but also to take pride in their children as they become independent adults.

Physical Growth

Young adults (20–40 years) are resilient, and their bodies function at peak efficiency. Their posture is erect, with optimal muscle tone and coordination. Their skin is taut and smooth. They have a high reproductive capability, and sexuality is a powerful response. Sexual performance peaks for males at age 18 and for females at age 30.

As the years pass and people become middle-aged (40–65 years), the body gradually decreases in its abilities. With a slowing of metabolism, there can be an increase in weight and a change in fat distribution, and people generally need to pay more attention to diet and exercise to maintain

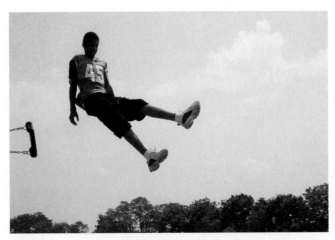

Figure 5-7. ■ Teens typically engage in high-risk behaviors and exhibit an attitude of "it can't happen to me."

HEALTH PROMOTION ISSUE

INTERNET SAFETY FOR CHILDREN

The school nurse conducts a parents' meeting with the eighth-grade parents each year as school is beginning for these junior high students. She discusses the issues that she will present during health class throughout the year. These issues include personal health, disease prevention, sexual behavior, and peer pressure. She describes for the parents some of the things they may expect from a child this age. She ends the parents' meeting with time for questions and answers. This fall, a father of a 13-year-old daughter asks her what she thought about the dangers of the Internet. The father also asked for the nurse's help in setting guidelines for his daughter related to the Internet. The nurse decided that this topic required more than a quick response and planned another parents' meeting to adequately address the issue.

DISCUSSION

A survey of 19,000 students, conducted by i-SAFE America (a government-funded Internet safety program), reviewed their online behavior. The survey found that 80% of students spend at least 1 hour per week on the Internet. Thirty percent say e-mail, chat rooms, or instant messaging is the main way they stay in contact with their friends. Fifty-five percent of the students admit giving out personal information such as name, gender, and age over the Internet. Almost half of the students say they have visited inappropriate sites on the Internet. It's frightening, but 10% of students have met someone face-to-face following an encounter on the Internet.

One in five children in the United States has been solicited sexually online, according to the Justice Department. This includes teenagers such as a 16-year-old girl lured into a face-to-face meeting by a 24-year-old parolee previously convicted of sexual assault. This young woman's parents claim they were vigilant in monitoring her online behavior. However, they are now searching for their daughter after she met with this parolee she encountered online.

How are teens accessing the Internet? They can e-mail, get into discussions in chat rooms, enter newsgroups, or engage in instant messaging. Web sites can be accessed not only by computer, but also by cell phones, pagers, personal digital assistants (PDAs), and video game systems. Cell phones allow teens to exchange digital photographs or videos, instant messages, or text messages, or to contact websites. They can engage in file sharing of music, videos, pictures, and other data over the Internet. These services may contain spyware that tracks Internet activity and that can share this information with others. Interactive gaming sites allow participants to play a game with an unknown individual on a computer at another location.

Many aspects of an adolescent's growth and development make him or her susceptible to engaging in risky behaviors online. Adolescents are attempting to separate from their family and are seeking independence. This makes them seek privacy and rebel when their privacy is invaded. The Internet provides teens with a way to figuratively venture away from their family. Fear of rejection and developing confidence can cause them to conform to the risky actions of their peers. A teen who wants to become independent, but who also wants to be loved and accepted, may not be able to discern the difference between the luring of a sexual predator and the true adoration of someone who loves him or her.

The unsupervised, unchecked use of the Internet can lead to many dangers. Unhealthy relationships can develop. These relationships can lead to physical, emotional, and sexual abuse. There are many instances when these relationships have led to the death of a teenager.

Many predators online seek important information so they can steal another person's identity. Predators may tap directly into financial information that

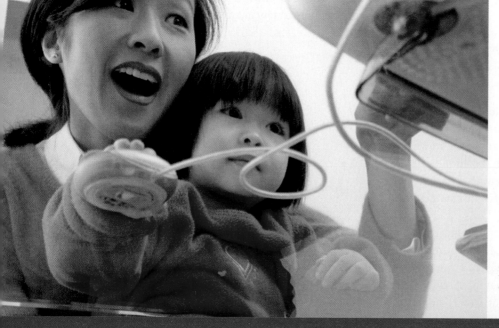

can be used to delete bank accounts and ruin credit. Teens need to learn the dangers of identity theft before they open a bank account.

The nurse can be effective in assisting families to safeguard against the dangers of the Internet. Parents need to be able to assess the online behaviors of their teens, set guidelines, and take swift action if risks are identified. The nurse can provide teaching and suggest resources to assist the family.

PLANNING AND IMPLEMENTATION

The nurse discusses with parents how to manage Internet use in their home. These are the teaching points the nurse uses:

- Learn to use your computer as efficiently as your child. Regularly review your web browser's history to see exactly where your child has gone while surfing the web. Be sure your child knows that you are going to do this.
- Learn the lingo (shortcuts and acronyms) for instant messaging and text messaging. Comprehensive lists of chat abbreviations are available on some Internet sites including the i-SAFE website.
- Screen names should be gender neutral and never contain sexual innuendos or personal descriptive information.
- Chat sites, instant messaging, and e-mail profiles should never contain personal information that a predator could use to make a connection. Personal information would include gender, age, address, phone number, likes, dislikes, hobbies, and interests. (Some parents have discovered that their child's "away

message for instant messaging contained their cell phone number.)
- Free e-mail accounts are simple to obtain. Children could have numerous ones without the parents' knowledge. The computer's web browser history would give a clue if the child has been to these sites.
- Create some clear house rules with clearly defined parameters for time spent on the computer, what is allowed, and what is not allowed. Remember also that it is not just the home computer that a teen uses. They can also access the Internet at Grandma's, or a friend's house. Discuss how the rules apply to these sites as well.
- Use a filtering program to block the computer from a predetermined set of websites, block e-mail except from a preset list, or block individual web pages with offensive words.
- Install a "firewall" and antivirus software that is updated regularly to protect your computer from unwanted intrusions.
- Software can be added to the computer to ensure that teens cannot share pictures online, set certain profiles, or use a webcam (camera).
- The teen's privacy can be respected when trust is earned. However, computer access should be in a common area of the home.
- Use a search engine to search weekly for your child's name, screen names, address, and telephone numbers. This assists in discovering postings that predators or even personal enemies may have posted.
- The computer should be password protected. If the teen has a password, it should be known to the parents. Change passwords frequently.

- Search recently downloaded file folders for more information about where the teen is surfing. Regularly review their other files and folders, not secretively but with their knowledge and perhaps in their presence.
- Sharing music, digital, and video files increases the risk of viruses that can infect the computer. It could also be illegal. Parents should learn about and discuss recent cases in which teens have been charged with theft when sharing digital files.
- Regularly review your child's cell phone bill to monitor calls received and sent. Many services allow records to be reviewed online for more frequent monitoring.

The nurse also decides to include a class on Internet safety in her health class. She invites law enforcement officials to discuss the hazards of the Internet, a student who was solicited online to discuss personal dangers, and an Internet/computer expert to discuss technical issues.

SELF-REFLECTION

How often do you access the Internet? What methods do you use for access? Carefully review your Internet practices. Do you participate in any risky behaviors that might compromise your safety or personal information? Do you know about the Internet practices of other family members in your home? Do you have any cause for concern? List three ways you could improve your Internet practices or those of family members within your home.

SUGGESTED RESOURCES

Criddle, L., & Muir, N. (2006). *Look both ways: Help protect your family on the Internet*. Redmond, WA: Microsoft Publishers.

Gralla, P. (2006). *The complete idiot's guide to Internet privacy and security*. Indianapolis, IN: Alpha.

Leavitt, J., & Linford, S. (2006). *Faux Paw's adventures in the Internet: Keeping children safe online*. New York: Wiley.

NAC Corner statistics and tips for our young messengers. (2007, March). *i-Parent Times*. Retrieved April 17, 2007.

National Center for Missing and Exploited Children. (2007). *Child safety on the information highway*. Office of Juvenile Justice and Delinquency Prevention. Washington, DC: U.S. Department of Justice. Retrieved April 17, 2007.

Roddel, V. (2007). *Internet safety family guide*. Rochester, NY: Lulu.

strength and mobility (Figure 5-8 ■). **Presbyopia** (farsightedness) and **presbycusis** (loss of hearing) are common with age. At about age 50, women enter menopause, the ovaries stop releasing ova and estrogen, and progesterone levels fall. Men also experience a change in hormone levels that causes a decrease in sperm production. As middle-age adults struggle to cope with these changes in body function, they may become depressed. This depression may be expressed in a variety of ways, such as a change in jobs, infidelity in the marriage relationship, or a total physical makeover. The emotional struggles of this period are rightly called a *midlife crisis*. Middle-age adults may also experience empty-nest syndrome. When their children no longer live with them, parents may experience feelings of sadness and loss.

Cognitive Development
Young and middle-age adults have all the cognitive skills necessary for a productive life. Their main challenges are adjusting to life's crises (career, marriage, purchasing a home, raising a family, coping with an empty nest, and participating in the lives of grandchildren or great grandchildren). Middle-age adults plan for retirement by reviewing their financial situations, their need to be productive, and their personal desires and goals.

SANDWICH GENERATION.   Middle-age adults have often been called the *sandwich generation*. This term describes their simultaneous responsibilities to children who are not quite established outside the home and to aging parents who begin to rely on them for physical, emotional, and/or cognitive support.

OLDER ADULT (OLDER THAN 65 YEARS)
The average life expectancy in the United States is 75 years. With the technologic advances in health care, improved nutrition, and health promotion activities at all ages, the

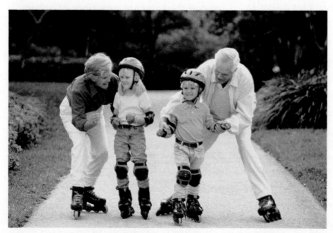

Figure 5-8. ■ Today's more health-conscious middle and older adults may be more than just observers of their grandchildren's activities. (Paul Barton/CORBIS.)

quality of health in the elderly has been much improved. Chronic disorders are often seen in this age group.

Physical Growth
When the body ages, there is a slowing or decreased function of all organ systems. As the skin ages, it becomes dry, thin, and pigmented. A loss of elasticity causes wrinkles. The hair becomes thin, dry, brittle, and gray. Male pattern baldness, a hereditary condition evident in younger men, usually has stopped progressing. The skeletal system undergoes changes in degree of calcification. Some bones become porous and more subject to fracture. Other bones degenerate, forming uneven edges and/or spurs. This process results in decreased mobility of joints. The spine (especially the low cervical and thoracic vertebrae) may develop compression fractures that result in curvature of the spine and shorter stature. The costal cartilage attaching the ribs to the sternum becomes hard and fixed. The result is a decreased expansion of the chest cavity and decreased respiratory ability. Years of smoking and inhaling air pollutants damage the bronchi, alveoli, and capillary bed and result in progressive lung disease.

One of the most significant changes associated with aging is a decrease in function of the heart and blood vessels. If fat deposits build up inside the blood vessels, the lumen narrows, blood pressure increases, and blood supply to distal tissues decreases. These changes can lead to heart attack, stroke, hypertension, and other vascular disease.

The number of functioning nephrons decreases by about 50% by age 75, so the kidney is less able to produce urine. As tissues lose their elasticity, there might be a decrease in capacity of the bladder, a prolapse of the bladder, and incontinence. Changes in the prostate can result in difficulty urinating.

The sense organs show a slow decline with age. Vision is affected by a clouding of the lens called *cataracts*. A hardening of the lens affects accommodation, resulting in farsightedness. In the ear, a decrease in the number of hair cells in the organ of Corti causes a significant decline in hearing. There is also a decrease in taste and smell that may affect appetite and food preferences.

Although both men and women may remain sexually active, a decrease in hormones affects the ability to reproduce. In men, erections may be more difficult to obtain and sustain, and sperm count decreases. In women, symptoms commonly seen with menopause include cessation of menstruation, a thinning and drying of the vaginal wall, and a decreased libido.

Cognitive Development
Cognition shows some decline with age. This is due in part to decreased circulation, decreased oxygenation, and disease processes. Most seniors can process mentally as

they did in younger years. However, there is a slow loss of memory, with recent memory affected more than distant memory. Seniors can also experience extreme cognitive deficits. Although parents need to exercise judgment in leaving small children with seniors who have cognitive deficits, most families value interaction among generations.

The main task in this stage of development is to "age gracefully." Seniors want to feel that they have made a contribution to the world and that their lives have had meaning. Without meaning, they can easily sink into despair and depression.

NURSING CARE

PRIORITIES IN NURSING CARE

Nursing priorities for clients throughout the life span include establishing a therapeutic relationship with the client and communicating appropriately for the client's age level. The nurse determines stage of development and cognitive level and validates teaching through appropriate means to ensure client understanding. This section will focus on care of the pediatric client and family.

ASSESSING

The role of the LPN/LVN is to assist in the assessment of the pediatric client and the family. Several preprinted tools are available to guide the data collection and assessment. While there are differences among the tools, the kinds of information collected are the same. Measurements of height, weight, and head circumference (for a small child or neonate) are taken and recorded on a growth chart. Other observations, such as activity, gross and fine motor control, and language development, are compared to the normal milestones for the age group. Parents and grandparents may supply information about development and maturation of children. The LPN/LVN documents these observations and reports any deviations from normal to the registered nurse or care provider.

DIAGNOSING, PLANNING, AND IMPLEMENTING

Nursing diagnoses for clients with growth and development delays, and their families, might include, among others:

- Impaired **P**arenting, related to developmental delay
- Delayed **G**rowth and Development, related to inadequate bonding
- Situational Low **S**elf-Esteem, related to rapid physical growth associated with adolescence

Outcomes for these clients might include the following:

- Parent provides for child's physical, emotional, cognitive, and social needs.
- The child will accomplish milestones of physical, cognitive, and psychosocial tasks expected for age group.
- The adolescent will verbalize acceptance of new physical characteristics.

When planning and implementing care, the nurse may use the following interventions:

- Encourage parents to consider the client's age and stage of development. *An understanding of what is normal is crucial when parenting.*
- Be sensitive to developmental issues and teach the parents what normal findings to expect. *Parents of children with growth or developmental delays may be very anxious about what these delays might mean for the child. Establish a therapeutic relationship by asking open-ended questions and allowing opportunities for the client to express feelings.*
- Encourage age-appropriate communication. The guidelines in Table 5-13 ■ will help the nurse understand how to communicate with children at different stages of development. *The way the nurse communicates with children and parents will have a great effect on their understanding, learning, and cooperation. The nurse can also teach parents these guidelines. Like other factors, the child's communication level develops over time. The nurse can improve communication and learning by gearing body language and verbal communication to the appropriate age.*
- Refer family to parenting support groups and parenting classes. *Organized programs can assist the parent to develop appropriate parenting skills and provide positive role models.*
- Assist the family in developing realistic expectations for the child. *Realistic expectations prevent discouragement.*
- Offer age-appropriate toys to the child. *Age-appropriate toys can encourage children to act in an age-appropriate manner.*
- Explore the child's feelings regarding physical changes. *Discussing the child's feelings allows for opportunities to provide further teaching and is often therapeutic for the child.*
- Set limits about negative self-comments. *Allowing negative self-comments may serve to reinforce the child's low self-esteem.*

EVALUATING

In order to evaluate the outcomes for the child with developmental delays the nurse must carefully assess the child's current growth and developmental stage. Parenting skills need to be evaluated as the child ages. Careful attention must be given to the adolescent's self-esteem.

TABLE 5-13

Communicating Across the Life Span: Providing Age-Appropriate Communication

	INFANT (BIRTH TO 1 YEAR)	TODDLER (1 TO 3 YEARS)	PRESCHOOLER (3 TO 6 YEARS)	SCHOOL AGE CHILD (6 TO 12 YEARS)	ADOLESCENT (12 TO 20 YEARS)
Nurse or parent	Speak softly. Communicate through touch. Avoid overstimulation. Comfort by holding or rocking. Encourage parents to participate. Be aware that older infants may be fearful of strangers.	Avoid frightening discussions. Say specifically what you want the child to do. Do not offer a choice if there really is none. Speak at the child's eye level. Have as few teachers as possible (one nurse). Use parallel play or toys to teach. Encourage parents to participate. Expect that the child will not understand time or "why."	Keep instruction brief for short attention span. Use simple, direct language. Speak with a simple vocabulary. Make learning fun. Allow the child to act out or express thoughts or feelings. Reinforce learning immediately. Use body outlines or drawings to explain illness. Separate fantasy from reality.	Determine the child understands about illness, treatment, and prognosis. Dispel myths and fears. Allow and encourage children to communicate their needs. Provide information in clear terms; they are able to learn more about body parts. Be aware that children may respond to third-person prompts: "I know a boy who is afraid of the x-ray machine."	Show respect by listening and explaining clearly. Give adolescent privacy and opportunity for confidentiality. Help adolescents trust adults by being honest about their treatment. Use peer support when possible. Never use a "baby" voice; speak as to another adult, but be sure language is clear. Provide space for questions.
Parent	Take time for bonding.	Allow the child to complete a thought without interruption.		Give child the opportunity to speak for himself or herself.	Allow for more independence.

NURSING PROCESS CARE PLAN:
Infant with Delayed Growth and Development

Jim, a 9-month-old infant, is brought to the clinic by his single, 19-year-old mother for his first well-baby checkup. His mother states that he weighed 7 pounds at birth. She states that he takes 6 to 8 ounces of formula three times a day, but he does not take solid food. She states that Jim spends most of the day in his crib, so she can work from her home.

Assessment

- Weight 15 pounds
- Height 26½ inches
- Skin pale
- Makes limited verbal response
- Smiles only occasionally.

Nursing Diagnosis. The following important nursing diagnoses (among others) are established for this client:

- Delayed **G**rowth and Development, related to nutritional deficits
- Impaired **P**arenting, related to lack of knowledge regarding child health maintenance

Expected Outcomes. The expected outcomes are:

- Height and weight will be at 5th percentile by 1 year of age.
- Demonstration of effective parenting skills such as:
  - Providing meals appropriate for age daily.
  - Providing toys appropriate for age daily.
  - Verbalizing appropriate parenting skills.

Planning and Implementation

- Teach mother about nutrition and the need for social interaction. *Mother cannot be expected to provide needed care without instruction.*

■ Monitor infant's height, weight, and social skills monthly. *Generally, single assessments do not reveal problems as well as repeated assessment. This infant is obviously delayed, and progress must be monitored frequently.*

■ Encourage mother to attend parenting classes. *This mother will need parenting skills and in-depth instruction in child care in order for infant to progress and maintain normal pattern of growth and development.*

Evaluation. It is critical to evaluate this child's progress. If further slowing of growth and development occurs, the child's life could be in danger. Evaluation by social services may be necessary to ensure the child is not being neglected. Because the child is 9 months old and has not had well-baby checkups prior to this visit, other health care issues may be present. For example, immunizations may be off schedule. It may important for the nurse to maintain contact with the mother to help ensure compliance and return visits to the health care practitioner.

Critical Thinking in the Nursing Process

1. What questions should the nurse ask Jim's mother to determine if other health issues are present?
2. What other information would have been helpful in this situation?
3. What data would indicate a need to call social services to protect Jim?

Note: Discussion of Critical Thinking questions appears in Appendix I.

Note: The reference and resource listings for this and all chapters have been compiled at the back of the book.

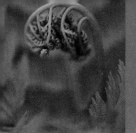

Chapter Review

KEY TERMS by Topics

Use the audio glossary feature of either the CD-ROM or the Companion Website to hear the correct pronunciation of the following key terms.

Introduction
growth, development

Principles of Growth and Development
cephalocaudal, proximodistal, ordinal position, maturation

Theories of Development
cognitive development, sensorimotor, object permanence, preoperational, egocentrism, magical thinking, concrete operations period, formal operations period, psychosexual, id, ego, superego, defense mechanisms

Standards of Physical Growth and Development
percentile

Stages of Physical Growth and Development
parallel play, separation anxiety, menarche, presbyopia, presbycusis

KEY Points

- Growth and development are influenced by genetics and environment. Development begins at conception and continues until death.
- Growth and development have five major components: physiologic, psychosocial, cognitive, moral, and spiritual.
- Health assessment and promotion activities assist the client in meeting developmental milestones.

EXPLORE MediaLink

Additional interactive resources for this chapter can be found on the Companion Website at www.prenhall.com/adams. Click on Chapter 5 and "Begin" to select the activities for this chapter.

For chapter-related NCLEX®-style questions and an audio glossary, access the accompanying CD-ROM in this book.

Animations:

Infancy: A major life transition

Communicating with toddlers

Handling temper tantrums

Health maintenance for school-age children

Teens: Mental & spiritual health

Health promotion & health maintenance

The importance of physical activity

Ovulation

FOR FURTHER Study

See Table 4-1 and Chapter 4 for discussion of family development.

Figure 20-3 shows some body proportion changes.

Nursing adaptations for children of different ages are discussed in depth in Chapter 8.

Information about typical infant reflexes appears in Chapter 15.

Defense mechanisms and other psychosocial information is provided in Chapter 16.

Appendix II shows growth charts for ages birth to 20 years.

Caring for Client with Risk for Injury
NCLEX-PN® Focus Area: Safety

Case Study: Jane, a 4-month-old, has been brought by her 17-year-old mother to the well-child clinic. When you enter the room, Jane is lying on the exam table with her mother at her side. Jane's vital signs are T 98, P 120, R 30, Wt 15 lb. Ht 22½ in. Head circumference is 16 inches. Her history indicates she weighed 7 lb 3 oz at birth and was 20 inches long with a 13½-inch. head circumference. Jane's mother tells you Jane rolls from front to back and enjoys putting her toys in her mouth. Jane drops her rattle on the floor. Her mother walks away from the exam table to pick it up.

Nursing Diagnosis: Risk for Injury, related to inappropriate parenting skills

COLLECT DATA

Subjective	Objective
_____	_____
_____	_____
_____	_____
_____	_____
_____	_____
_____	_____
_____	_____

Would you report this? Yes/No

If yes, to: _____

Nursing Care

_____
_____
_____
_____
_____
_____
_____
_____
_____

How would you document this? _____
_____
_____
_____

Data Collected
(use only those that apply)

- 11-month-old child
- VS: T 98.0°F, -P 120-R 30
- Weight 15 lb
- Height 22½ inches
- Head circumference 16 inches
- Activity: turns front to back, puts toys in mouth
- Observed mother not providing safe environment for the child

Nursing Interventions
(use only those that apply; list in priority order)

- Instruct mother to keep activated charcoal in first aid kit.
- Teach parent to avoid foods that could cause choking (raisins, peanuts, whole grapes).
- Instruct mother to begin adding soft pureed food to child's diet.
- Teach mother need for close supervision because the child is becoming mobile.
- Instruct mother on toys appropriate for age.

Compare your documentation to the sample provided in Appendix I.

NCLEX-PN® Exam Preparation

1 A woman has brought her 2-year-old to the well-child clinic. Which of the following would be recommended to encourage autonomy in a toddler?

1. Help the toddler complete tasks.
2. Provide the toddler opportunities to play with other children.
3. Help the toddler learn the difference between right and wrong.
4. Encourage the toddler to do things for herself when she is capable.

2 A 5-year-old child is in the hospital and is becoming bored. The best activity for this child would be:

1. Books.
2. TV.
3. Puppets.
4. Oil painting by number.

3 In terms of cognitive development, which of the following would a 5-year-old be expected to do?

1. Use magical thinking.
2. Think abstractly.
3. Understand conversation about matter.
4. Comprehend another person's perspective.

4 Which of the following would the nurse reasonably expect a 2-year-old to be able to do?

1. Jump rope.
2. Ride a bicycle.
3. Skip on alternate feet.
4. Balance on one foot for a few seconds.

5 The parents of an 8-year-old tell you that their daughter wants to join a soccer team. Which suggestions about participation in sports at this age should be made?

1. Organized sports such as soccer are not appropriate at this age.
2. Competition is harmful in establishing a positive self-image.
3. Sports participation is a good idea if the sport is appropriate to the child's abilities.
4. Girls should compete only against girls because at this age boys are larger and have more muscle mass.

6 The mother of a 13-year-old tells you that her daughter is a good girl but does not seem to do what she is told anymore. Your response would be guided by the knowledge that the adolescent is most influenced at this stage by her _____ (HINT: one word).

7 A disruptive 10-year-old is having difficulty with other children at school. Which nursing action would be best for the school nurse to use first?

1. Have a meeting with the teachers and discuss strategies to solve the problem.
2. Talk with the child about the behavior that is causing the problem and identify possible solutions.
3. Tell the other children to stop teasing the client and observe the changes in behavior.
4. Tell the child's parents that they need to take care of the problem.

8 A 52-year-old woman talks about her changing family. She is upset that her "baby girl" recently married and moved to New Jersey, and her son lives far away with his wife and three children. This woman is experiencing _____ (HINT: 3 words).

9 Exploratory abdominal surgery is planned for tomorrow on a 3-year-old girl. How would the nurse best prepare this child for the procedure?

1. The evening before the procedure, demonstrate by pointing on the child's body where the incision will be made.
2. Ask the child's parents to leave the room while the preoperative medication is given.
3. Ask the parents to hold the child down while sedation is given.
4. Explain the procedure to the child in simple terms just before giving preoperative medication.

10 An 18-year-old is upset about his 83-year-old grandfather, who is dying of lung cancer. The boy says, "I don't understand how he can be so calm and accepting about death." Which of the following is the best response, based on an understanding of development?

1. Your grandfather is just trying to be brave for your sake.
2. When we are young it is hard to understand that we can be content with our life's accomplishments and be ready to die.
3. It is the pain medication that is keeping your grandfather calm.
4. We will keep him comfortable, and this will be over soon.

Answers for NCLEX-PN® Review and Critical Thinking questions appear in Appendix I.

Chapter 6

Illness Prevention, Health Promotion, and Nutrition in Children

BRIEF Outline

Role of the Nurse in Illness Prevention and Health Promotion

Client and Family Teaching

Illness Prevention

Health Promotion

Nursing Care

Infant

Toddler

Preschooler

School-Age Child

Adolescent

Nursing Care

LEARNING Outcomes

After completing this chapter, you will be able to:

1. Define key terms.
2. Describe techniques for client and family teaching.
3. Describe illness prevention activities.
4. Describe health promotion activities for children in each age group.
5. Discuss important aspects of nutrition for each age group.

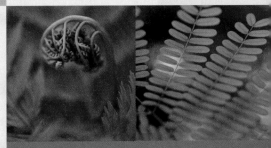

HEALTH PROMOTION ISSUE:
Types of Learning

NURSING PROCESS CARE PLAN:
Client with Unintentional Poisoning

CRITICAL THINKING CARE MAP:
Caring for a Client with Inadequate Nutrition

In community-based nursing practice, nursing care is not just the treatment of illness. It also includes teaching of good health practices in order to prevent illness and injury. Publications such as *Healthy People* (U.S. Department of Health and Human Services [USDHHS], 1979), *Promoting Health/Preventing Illness: Objectives for the Nation* (USDHHS, 1980), *Healthy People 2000* (USDHHS, 1991) and *Healthy People 2010* (USDHHS, 2000) have documented the need for activities to help Americans become healthier. This program was discussed in Chapter 1 ⚭.

Role of the Nurse in Illness Prevention and Health Promotion

As described in previous chapters, the role of the LPN/LVN is diverse. The nurse collects data from the client and family, reports to the charge nurse, assists in establishing the plan of care, and helps implement quality care. The nurse follows good health practices and acts as a role model for the client and family. Once a formal teaching plan has been established, the nurse implements the teaching plan and reports back to the charge nurse. Informal teaching occurs with each family interaction (Figure 6-1 ■). Client teaching techniques can be reviewed in a nursing fundamentals textbook. This chapter reviews client teaching principles as they apply to illness prevention and health promotion in the care of children.

Client and Family Teaching

Every interaction between the nurse and client and/or family needs to be one of assessment and teaching. Through the assessment process, the nurse determines specific areas of

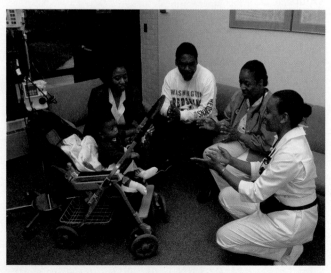

Figure 6-1. ■ The nurse begins assessment of the infant's family when they are seen in the waiting room and called in for care.

BOX 6-1   NURSING CARE CHECKLIST

Guidelines for Teaching

The following guidelines should be used for client and family teaching:

- ☑ Be a role model.
- ☑ Maintain a distraction-free environment.
- ☑ Use age-specific communication techniques.
- ☑ Have accurate and complete information.
- ☑ Be familiar with printed material.

---

needed instruction and the effectiveness of prior teaching. Some teaching needs to be a planned, formal event that might take several hours or days to complete. Other teaching is a spontaneous informal event, with one-to-one dialogue. Box 6-1 ■ outlines teaching guidelines the nurse should use in order to be efficient and effective with client and family teaching.

The nurse is a role model for good health practices. It is difficult to convince a client or family to be compliant with good health practices and instruction if the nurse does not practice them. For example, if the nurse is providing instruction on insulin administration and does not keep the needle sterile, the client or family will not see the need to use sterile technique either. If the nurse teaches about the effects of smoking on health and then is seen having a cigarette, the family will not view the nurse as credible.

For the client and family to get the most out of the instruction, the environment must be free from distraction. For example, if cast care instruction needs to be given to a mother who has her four other children with her at the pediatrician's office, one of the office staff members can take the other children to the playroom, providing the mother with a distraction-free environment. If the instruction is to be given in the home primarily to older children and adults, the nurse should turn off the television, request no telephone calls, and ask family members to leave the room so that privacy can be provided.

The nurse must use age-specific communication techniques, audiovisual aids, and vocabulary (see Table 5-13 ⚭). If instruction is too simplistic, an older child might feel "put down" and not pay attention to or follow it. If the instruction is too advanced, the client might be confused and will either do nothing or be poorly equipped to perform the needed care. If the client and/or family speak a language different from the nurse, an interpreter may be needed to ensure accurate communication.

The instruction provided must be accurate and complete. The nurse must keep up to date with the latest research, techniques, and technology. The nurse might use an outline or other notes so important points are not forgotten, resulting in incomplete instruction.

If questions arise that the nurse cannot accurately answer, she should say she does not know but will find out the answer. Then the nurse should be diligent in getting the information to the client. No instruction is better than inaccurate instruction.

The nurse needs to be familiar with the printed material provided to the client and family. By reviewing the printed material in its entirety prior to the client interaction, the nurse can discuss the content, using eye contact and a relaxed approach. Printed material should be individualized so the client and family will have complete written instructions at home. The nurse never assumes that the parents or the clients know, understand, and will practice good health promotion activities. The nurse must validate whether the pediatric client and his or her caregiver understand the teaching before ending the interaction.

Illness prevention and health promotion activities are designed to help the client regain and maintain the highest level of health possible for as long as possible. The health of the mother and father has an impact on the health of the developing infant. Therefore, both parents should practice a healthy lifestyle prior to pregnancy.

Parents are responsible for helping to maintain their children's health. Parents do this by providing a healthy environment and nutritious food, and by teaching their children healthful behaviors. The nurse encourages the parents by providing information and by being a positive role model. (See the Health Promotion Issue on pages 100 and 101 for different types of learning among pediatric clients.)

Illness Prevention

Illness prevention is encouragement of specific behaviors that can prevent illness and injury. Illness prevention can be divided into three categories: primary, secondary, and tertiary prevention.

LEVELS OF PREVENTION

Primary Prevention

Primary prevention includes activities to keep the individual from developing health problems. This includes activities such as immunizations to prevent communicable disease, wearing a seat belt to protect from injury during a motor vehicle accident, and learning about proper preparation of infant formula to avoid disease.

Secondary Prevention

Secondary prevention involves activities directed at early detection and treatment of health problems. Secondary prevention might be seen in such activities as voluntary drug screening in the school system or checking each child in a classroom for lice if one child is found to have lice. Screening for developmental delays using the Denver Developmental Screening Test (DDST) is also a type of secondary prevention, because it seeks to identify and address developmental problems at an early stage.

Tertiary Prevention

Tertiary prevention includes treating existing diseases to prevent the disease from developing complications. Tertiary prevention activities include antibiotics to prevent the spread of an infection, range of motion to prevent the effects of immobility, and rehabilitation after a car accident.

Many health disorders can be prevented by a healthy lifestyle. Children learn from their parents, and when the parents practice healthy behaviors, the children are more likely to practice good health as well. Health-promoting behaviors include exercising regularly, eating a balanced diet, obtaining adequate rest, limiting caffeine and alcohol consumption, and omitting the use of illicit drugs.

Not only is cigarette smoking harmful to the smoker's lungs and blood vessels, but the exhaled smoke can also stimulate respiratory disorders in children who live with the smoker. Children are more likely to begin smoking when one or both parents smoke. When a pregnant woman smokes, there is a greater risk that the baby will have a low birth weight. For these reasons, every family member should be encouraged to stop smoking. For those smokers who need assistance to quit, help is available through prescription medication, and support groups. Nurses should become familiar with the groups in their community.

Alcohol use during pregnancy can damage the infant's growing brain, resulting in mental and physical deficiencies (see Figure 16-5). When parents drink alcohol, they are teaching their children that drinking is accepted. Although an occasional drink may not be harmful, frequent consumption can lead to liver, heart, and behavior issues. The amount of alcohol needed to intoxicate varies from individual to individual. Intoxication leads to poor judgment, unpredictable behavior, and, sometimes, criminal actions. Adults need to consider the effects of alcohol on their children and families before choosing to drink.

WELL-CHILD VISITS

The child should be assessed at regular intervals by a pediatrician, family practice physician, or family nurse practitioner. An accepted schedule is 2 weeks, 2 months,

HEALTH PROMOTION ISSUE

TYPES OF LEARNING

The LPN works for a family practice office. Her job responsibilities include health promotion teaching for all ages of clients. She teaches the importance of immunizations, health screening, contraception control, sexually transmitted infection prevention, cardiac health, and so forth. The content for the teaching plan has been carefully researched and written in collaboration with the entire health care staff, including the physician and the supervising registered nurse.

Although she is knowledgeable about the content, the LPN has noticed that some clients respond enthusiastically while others seem to only tolerate the teaching. She has become increasingly concerned that the teaching may be ineffective for some clients. She discusses her concerns with the supervising nurse.

DISCUSSION

People learn in many different ways. Dr. David Kolb developed the following categories of learning styles:

- The Accommodator. This learner is flexible and needs an overview of the content prior to having the details. In fact, this learner will get lost if the teacher begins with the details. The accommodator also learns by trial and error. He or she needs activities such as games, written exercises, or role play.
- The Assimilator. This learner is a logical, structured, and task-oriented individual. The content should be presented in a practical manner with clear application of the principles. The teacher should provide concrete methods so the learner can put the principles into practice. This learner learns best through lectures, questioning, watching, and doing reasoning-type exercises such as thought questions.

This learner desires an organization to the teaching, including expected time frame and an outline of goals or objectives. The teacher must be diligent or this learner will become frustrated.

- The Diverger. This learner looks for multiple solutions to the topic being taught. He or she needs to own the content, to feel it, and to attach emotion to the subject. The teacher can assist this learner by relating personal stories. Using audiovisual aids will assist this learner. The teacher should also allow the diverger to participate in the learning experience by expressing his or her opinion.
- The Converger. This learner is task-oriented and loves to handle the content him- or herself. He or she enjoys researching the content, and will take notes and learn better when the teacher has prepared a handout. Much of this learner's learning occurs on his or her own time as he or she continues to dig into the content. Homework assignments work well for this learner. The teacher must be available outside the teaching session for this learner to discuss the content further.

Other theorists have defined learning styles as visual, auditory, and kinesthetic:

- The visual learner needs to see the content. The teacher will assist this learner best by providing visual material.
- The auditory learner needs to hear the content, and he or she also needs to verbalize the content. The teacher can lecture to this learner, but also needs to allow this learner to discuss the content.

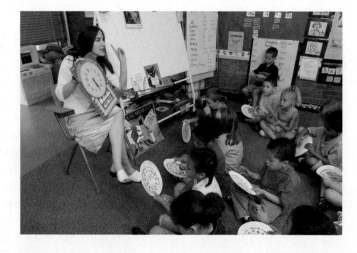

4 months, 6 months, 9 months, 12 months, 15 months, 24 months and yearly thereafter. Well-child visits (see Table 6-1 ■) gather data about physical health, including growth and development, nutritional health, emotional health, and neurologic status. These visits would also include immunizations, health promotion teaching, and assessment of parent-child relationships. During a visit with the toddler, information about toileting should

- The kinesthetic learner needs to touch the content. The teacher should provide a physical activity for this learner, such as handing him or her a syringe or an anatomical model.

The teacher must also keep in mind that a typical learner needs a variety of teaching methods to grasp the content. Learners will retain 10% of what they read, 20% of what they hear, 30% of what they see, 50% of what they hear and see, 70% of what they say, and 90% of what they say and do.

PLANNING AND IMPLEMENTATION

The supervising nurse and the LPN spent time reviewing different learning styles. They then reviewed their teaching plans and discovered that they were basically designed for an auditory learner. They decided that it was necessary to rework the health promotion teaching plans. They first wanted to assess the learning styles of their clients. They obtained a learning style inventory tool and asked clients to complete it while waiting for their appointments. The results of this inventory were then attached to each client's chart so the nurse providing health promotion teaching could adapt his or her content appropriately.

Second, they redesigned the health promotion teaching plans to accommodate each type of learner. They developed teaching and learning activities that would best meet the needs of each learning style. For example, when teaching cardiac health the nurse will:

- For the accommodator, present an overview of cardiac risks and prevention methods, followed by written activities about diet, exercise, and risk factors.
- For the assimilator, present a written agenda of the teaching, followed by a short lecture on cardiac risk and prevention methods. Then, together with the client, the nurse will help outline a very specific plan that fits his or her lifestyle.
- For the diverger, present the content in a visual format using pictures of people and objects rather than graphic drawings. The nurse will also incorporate personal stories of success and failure with cardiac health prevention.
- For the converger, present the content in a logical, straightforward manner with a handout to give the client. She will also suggest several websites and other resources where the client may learn more about the content.

Last, the supervising nurse and the LPN realized the need to add an evaluation tool to their teaching plan. It became apparent that they needed to know whether learning had occurred. They incorporated a variety of methods such as verbal reviews of the content, written reviews of the content, quizzes, and crossword puzzles and matching games for younger clients.

SELF-REFLECTION

What is your particular learning style? When you encounter teaching that is not presented in your learning style, how do you adapt so you can learn? When you teach, do you accept responsibility for the learning that occurs? What expectations do you have for those you teach? Are they realistic? Why or why not? What teaching methods do you use most often when presenting health content to clients? Are these methods always effective? Do you vary your teaching methods according to your client's needs? List five things you could do to improve your teaching style.

SUGGESTED RESOURCES

de Young, Sandra. (2002). *Teaching strategies for nurse educators.* Upper Saddle River, NJ: Prentice Hall.

Fuller, Cheri. (2001). *Opening your child's nine learning windows.* Grand Rapids, MI: Zondervan.

Wilkinson, B. (1983). *The 7 laws of the learner: How to teach almost anything to practically anyone.* Sisters, OR: Multnomah Press.

be gathered. Health screenings such as vision, hearing, urinalysis, hematocrit, and tuberculosis are usually initiated in the preschool years. Screening for scoliosis is done during the school years. The adolescent should be screened for involvement in sexual activity, and appropriate health care should begin when the teen is sexually active. Table 6-1 provides a summary of these well-child visit activities.

TABLE 6-1

Well-Child Visits

AGE	IMMUNIZATIONS	HEALTH PROMOTION TEACHING	HEALTH SCREENING
2 weeks		Breastfeeding or formula feeding; recognizing the sick newborn; SIDS prevention Safety in holding, feeding, bathing, transporting	Height, weight Head circumference PKU; jaundice if indicated
2 months	DTaP, Hib, IPV, PCV		Height, weight, head circumference Review developmental milestones
4 months	*HepB*, DTaP, Hib, IPV, PCV	Safety (related to turning over)	Height, weight Head circumference Review developmental milestones
6 months	DTaP, *Hib*, PCV	Introducing solid foods Safety (related to sitting up and grasping)	Height, weight Head circumference Review developmental milestones
9 months		Safety (related to standing, "cruising" with hands holding furniture, climbing)	Height, weight Head circumference Review developmental milestones
12 months	Hib, MMR, Varicella, PCV, start HepA Series	Dental health Safety (related to standing, walking, climbing)	Height, weight Head circumference Review developmental milestones
15 months	DTaP	Safety (prevention of poisoning)	Height, weight Head circumference Review developmental milestones
24 months		Toilet training Safety (related to increased mobility and exploration of environment)	Height, weight Head circumference Review developmental milestones
3, 4 and 5 years		Hand washing and hygiene Safety (related to drowning, burns, choking, wheeled vehicles) Teaching about strangers	Height, weight Review developmental milestones Vision, hearing, hematocrit, and tuberculosis
6 years	DTaP, IPV, MMR	Hand washing and hygiene Fire and emergency plans	Height, weight Review developmental milestones Urinalysis
7–14 years		Puberty Safety at school and after school	Height, weight Review developmental milestones Scoliosis Onset of puberty
15 years	Tetanus	Pregnancy and STI prevention Substance abuse prevention Motor vehicle safety	Height, weight Review developmental milestones Sexual activity

Source: Data from American Academy of Pediatrics. (2000). Recommendations for preventive pediatric health care. *Pediatrics, 105(3)*, 645–646; Centers for Disease Control and Prevention. (2006). *Recommended childhood and adolescent immunization schedule United States; Guidelines for health supervision of infants, children, and adolescents.* (2nd ed., rev.). (2001). Bright futures at Georgetown University. Washington, DC: National Center for Education in Maternal and Child Health. Georgetown University Public Policy Institute.

HYGIENE

Children are at high risk for contracting communicable diseases. This risk can be lowered through careful attention to matters of hygiene. Hand washing (Figure 6-2 ■) is an important measure for the nurse to teach parents. Children need to understand the importance of washing their hands vigorously before and after meals and after toileting. Germs are also spread among children by sharing toys and snacks. Children in church nurseries, day care centers, and schools should be monitored for hand-to-mouth activities and encouraged to wash their hands frequently.

The child who is ill can spread germs to other children by coughing, sneezing, and indiscriminately disposing of used tissues. The nurse can teach parents and children the importance of covering their mouth and nose when coughing or sneezing (see Figure 6-2B ■). School officials are now encouraging children to sneeze and cough into their elbows rather than their hands. This will prevent germs from getting onto the child's hands, where they can be more easily passed to others. Children should be taught to dispose of used tissues in trash receptacles and avoid leaving them where others may come in contact with them.

IMMUNIZATIONS

To prevent dangerous illnesses, vaccines have been developed. By injecting dead or weakened organisms, inactivated toxins, or toxoids, active immunity is produced. To be effective, repeat injections (immunizations) must be given on a schedule. The American Committee on Immunization Practices, the American Academy of Pediatrics (AAP), and the American Academy of Family Practitioners annually update the immunization schedule. A copy of the current schedule can be obtained from the client's local health department. Figure 6-3 ■ illustrates an immunization schedule. Table 6-2 ■ lists routine pediatric immunizations. See Chapter 10 ⬭ for more information on childhood diseases and prevention methods.

The nurse is responsible for reviewing the medical record and determining the need for immunization. Federal legislation requires written informed consent from the parent or guardian prior to administering a vaccine. The nurse must provide literature about the vaccine and its possible adverse effects. Parents should be given a copy of the child's immunization record because schools may require proof that immunizations are up to date before admitting a child.

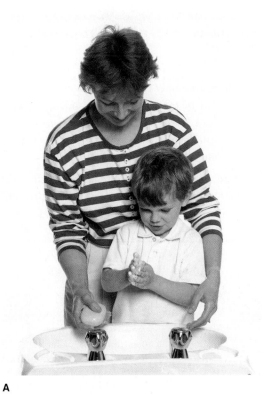

A

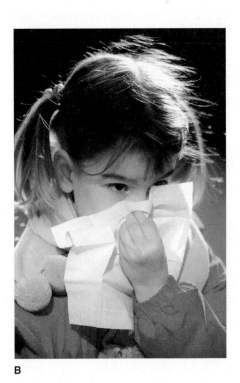

B

Figure 6-2. ■ (**A**) Adults teach children the proper technique for washing and drying hands. They can also teach children that this action is the single most effective way to prevent transmission of infection. (**B**) Many respiratory infections are transmitted by droplets from person to person. Children need to learn to completely cover the nose and mouth when coughing or sneezing. Some now recommend coughing into the sleeve at the elbow, so that hands are not contaminated.

DEPARTMENT OF HEALTH AND HUMAN SERVICES • CENTERS FOR DISEASE CONTROL AND PREVENTION

Recommended Childhood and Adolescent Immunization Schedule UNITED STATES • 2006

Vaccine ▼ Age ▶	Birth	1 month	2 months	4 months	6 months	12 months	15 months	18 months	24 months	4–6 years	11–12 years	13–14 years	15 years	16–18 years
Hepatitis B[1]	HepB	HepB		HepB[1]		HepB					HepB Series			
Diphtheria, Tetanus, Pertussis[2]			DTaP	DTaP	DTaP		DTaP			DTaP	Tdap	Tdap		
Haemophilus influenzae type b[3]			Hib	Hib	Hib[3]	Hib								
Inactivated Poliovirus			IPV	IPV		IPV				IPV				
Measles, Mumps, Rubella[4]						MMR				MMR	MMR			
Varicella[5]						Varicella				Varicella				
Meningococcal[6]											MCV4	MCV4		
								Vaccines within broken line are for selected populations		MPSV4		MCV4		
Pneumococcal[7]			PCV	PCV	PCV	PCV				PCV	PPV			
Influenza[8]						Influenza (Yearly)				Influenza (Yearly)				
Hepatitis A[9]										HepA Series				

This schedule indicates the recommended ages for routine administration of currently licensed childhood vaccines, as of December 1, 2005, for children through age 18 years. Any dose not administered at the recommended age should be administered at any subsequent visit when indicated and feasible. ▨ Indicates age groups that warrant special effort to administer those vaccines not previously administered. Additional vaccines may be licensed and recommended during the year. Licensed combination vaccines may be used whenever any components of the combination are indicated and other components of the vaccine are not contraindicated and if approved by the Food and Drug Administration for that dose of the series. Providers should consult the respective ACIP statement for detailed recommendations. Clinically significant adverse events that follow immunization should be reported to the Vaccine Adverse Event Reporting System (VAERS). Guidance about how to obtain and complete a VAERS form is available at www.vaers.hhs.gov or by telephone, 800-822-7967.

▨ Range of recommended ages   ▨ Catch-up immunization   ▨ 11–12 year old assessment

Figure 6-3. ■ Recommended childhood and adolescent immunization schedule.

clinical ALERT

The National Childhood Vaccine Injury Act of 1986 provides compensation if a link between immunization and serious adverse effect is found (Hay, Hayward, Levin, & Sondheimer, 2002). It is important, therefore, that the nurse record the date, the vaccine given, the lot number, and the expiration date of the immunization; the site and route of administration; and the name and address of the person administering the vaccine.

There are many reasons why a child's immunization schedule may be interrupted. Well-meaning parents can forget to schedule appointments. Parents may not see the need for immunization. The following guidelines can be used to prevent missing immunization opportunities:

■ Several immunizations can be given at the same visit.
■ Immunizations can be given when the child has a minor illness with or without low-grade fever.

TABLE 6-2

Pharmacology: Routine Pediatric Immunizations

DRUG (GENERIC AND COMMON BRAND NAME)	USUAL ROUTE/DOSE	SELECTED SIDE EFFECTS	DO NOT GIVE IF
Diphtheria, tetanus toxoid and acellular pertussis vaccine (Acel-Immune, Tripedia)	IM 0.5 mL[a]	Erythema and induration at site; fever; malaise	Children have symptoms of infection; seizure activity
Measles, mumps, rubella vaccine (M-M-R II)	SQ 0.5 mL[a]	Arthralgia; pain at injection site	Children have allergy to eggs
Hepatitis B vaccine (Engerix-B, Recombivax HB)	IM 10 mcg Engerix-B; IM 2.5 mcg Recombivax HB[a]	Soreness at site	Children have hypersensitivity to yeast

[a]See immunization schedule

- Immunizations can be given when the child is receiving antibiotics.
- Immunizations can be given even if the child has been exposed to an infectious disease.
- Premature infants have the same requirement for immunization as full-term infants.
- Immunization can be given when there has been a local reaction to previous immunizations.

For parents who refuse immunization of their children, it is important to teach about the development of immunity. Box 6-2 ■ provides information about alternative ways to strengthen the immune system.

Contraindications to immunization are anaphylactic reactions to the vaccine, moderate to severe acute illness, or pregnancy. Nonimmunized women of childbearing age are at risk not only for becoming infected, but also for exposing an unborn child to infection. Because immunization is contraindicated during pregnancy, it is important for women of childbearing age to remain current with the recommended immunization schedule.

When preparing and giving immunizations, the nurse should check the expiration date on the vaccine. Outdated vaccines may be weak and ineffective. Vaccines must be stored properly in the refrigerator. Some vaccines must be mixed with the solution provided. These vaccines usually have a short shelf life, so it is important to put the date the solution was mixed on the bottle. Once the vaccines have been prepared, they should be given quickly and efficiently. Allow the child to select the site where the injection will be given. The site needs to be gently restrained to prevent injury from the needle. This is best done by obtaining help from a colleague and allowing parents to give emotional support only. It is important for the parent-child relationship that the parent not be associated with the pain of injections. Give the child honest answers, and do not say that the needle will not hurt. Children become anxious, so do not hesitate in giving the injection even if the child begins to cry or scream. After the injection, allow the parent to comfort the child. Compliment the child for being brave, for holding as still as possible, or for other positive behavior. A token reward such as a sticker is appropriate for children preschool age and older.

Health Promotion

Health promotion is the encouragement of lifestyle changes that result in a healthier state for the individual. **Health,** a sense of physical, psychological, emotional, and spiritual well-being, is not just the absence of disease. Activities that promote health include eating a proper diet, getting adequate rest, and exercising. Activities such as chiropractic care, massage, taking herbs or nutritional supplements, meditation, and religious services can also promote a healthier individual. (*Note*: Encourage parents to discuss any complementary health care practices with their care provider, especially herbal and nutritional supplements.) Health promotion encourages the individual to take charge of personal health by making lifestyle changes.

Because of their broad knowledge base and experience in assisting in medical treatment of illness, nurses are the obvious choice for directing health promotion activities. (See also Chapter 5 ⬤ for health promotion in children.) This chapter introduces illness prevention and health promotion concepts through the stages of growth and development. Additional topics related to health promotion are addressed by body system in the remaining chapters of Unit III ⬤ .

BOX 6-2   COMPLEMENTARY THERAPIES

Boosting the Immune System

Some parents may choose not to immunize their children. They may be fearful of the negative effects of childhood immunizations. When parents make an informed decision, the nurse can assist parents in keeping their children healthy. The following are suggestions for boosting a child's immunity:

- Teach children to be diligent about washing their hands before and after meals, after handling pets, after blowing their nose, and after using the bathroom.
- Quarantine children from other children who have known illnesses.
- Give the child a diet containing plenty of foods with vitamin C and carotenoids such as carrots, green beans, oranges, and strawberries.
- Ensure that the child gets adequate sleep each night. The newborn should sleep 18 hours a day. The toddler should sleep 12 to 13 hours a day, and the preschooler should sleep at least 10 hours a night.
- Encourage regular exercise to boost immunity.
- Decrease exposure to secondhand smoke, which lowers immunity.
- Consider acupuncture during the cold and flu season. (Improved immunity may be linked to use of acupuncture.)
- After consultation with the physician, give vitamin and mineral supplementation to boost immunity.
  - Vitamin C can be given to children under 6 years at a dose of 250 mg per day and for children older than 6 at 500 mg a day.
  - Zinc supplements can be given to children under 6 at 10 to 20 mg a day and for children older than 6 at 20 to 40 mg a day.
- Provide the herbal product echinacea to improve immunity. During the cold and flu season, consult physician for proper dosage.

ENVIRONMENTAL SAFETY

Injuries resulting from accidents are a leading cause of death in children ages 1 to 19 (Anderson & Smith, 2005). Although accidents occur and not all injuries can be prevented, striving to keep the family as safe as possible is an important nursing intervention. As the child grows and becomes more mobile, keeping the environment safe becomes a greater challenge. Key safety issues are discussed for each age group.

PSYCHOSOCIAL HEALTH

Promoting Self-Esteem

The child growing up in today's American culture will have challenges never faced by previous generations. To face those challenges in a healthy manner, the child will need to have a strong sense of self. Promotion of self-esteem begins early in child development. By praising accomplishments, the parent gives positive feedback for hard work. This teaches the child that hard work will result in positive outcomes. For example, as the infant tries and tries to turn over, and finally accomplishes the task, parents can smile, clap, and praise the infant. Infants will learn that certain behaviors cause parents to smile. They will continue to try to elicit this response. The toddler learns to use the toilet through praise for his or her efforts and success. When parents emphasize the positive work the preschooler does in trying to make the bed and compliment that behavior, they build the child's self-esteem and pride in the task. If they add ways to improve, the child will be more willing to try to make it nicer. But if the parents repeatedly criticize the child because the bed is not made perfectly, the child will become discouraged and may stop trying to do the task at all.

Soon-to-be parents and new parents also need encouragement. If adults enter parenthood with a high level of self-esteem, they will generally have skills to help them be supportive parents. However, if parents have low self-esteem, they will need teaching and support to strengthen their self-esteem in order to be better parents. The nurse provides information about illness prevention and health promotion activities, and then praises the parents for their effort in making changes. By being a role model, the nurse helps the parents understand the effect of praise for good behavior and success.

Providing Discipline

To function in society, the child needs to learn rules and the consequences for breaking rules. The key to effective discipline is consistency. Both parents need to agree ahead of time on the family rules and the consequences of breaking the rules. The American Academy of Pediatrics (2004)

defines **spanking** as one or two flat-handed swats on a child's wrist or buttocks and states that corporal punishment is of limited effectiveness and has potentially dangerous side effects. The AAP recommends that parents develop methods other than spanking for managing undesired behavior. Striking the child, other than spanking as defined here, is considered to be child abuse. For ideas about the best way to discipline a child, see Box 6-3 ■.

More acceptable forms of discipline for the young child include "time-out" in the child's room or a corner (Figure 6-4 ■). For the older child, restricting the use of the computer, telephone, or outside activities may be effective. Discipline becomes ineffective when the parent does not allow the child to experience the consequences of his or her actions. The nurse needs to help parents explore different methods of discipline and work toward setting effective consequences for undesired behavior. The nurse must continually be alert for signs of child abuse. Child abuse is discussed in Chapter 16 of this text.

Promoting Play

Children play together wherever they gather. Play occurs in the home with siblings or friends, in the neighborhood at parks or backyards, at day care or other formal programs such as mother's morning out, and in the nursery at church. Play can be spontaneous, encouraged, or organized.

BOX 6-3

Child Development Experts' Views on Discipline

T. Berry Brazelton, M.D., a well-known expert in pediatric care, clinical professor of pediatrics at Harvard Medical School, and professor of psychiatry and human development at Brown University, views spanking as an unnecessary and potentially harmful method of discipline.

William Sears, M.D., associate clinical professor of pediatrics at the University of California, Irvine, School of Medicine, pediatrician in practice, and author of more than 30 books on parenting, does not advocate spanking. He sees this form of punishment as a method of teaching children that it is okay to hit and strike out at one another when a wrong has been done.

John Rosemond, a family psychologist who writes for 225 newspapers nationwide on parenting issues, believes children should be spanked only in an immediate response to an unacceptable behavior. He teaches that the spanking should be followed by a short explanation and an additional consequence if the unacceptable behavior is repeated.

James Dobson, a clinical psychologist with a Ph.D. in child development, former clinical professor of pediatrics at the University of Southern California School of Medicine, and current chairman of Focus on the Family, believes that if spanking is delivered in anger and with intimidation, negative outcomes may occur. However, he teaches that spanking can be used effectively, for willful disobedience.

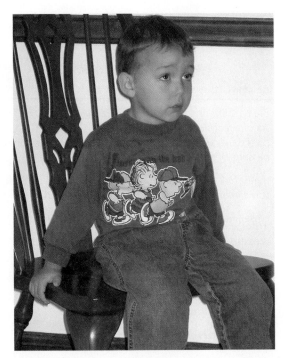

Figure 6-4. ■ One effective discipline method is to remove the child to an isolated area where no interaction with children and adults can occur and no toys are present. This is used to demonstrate that there is a consequence to misbehavior. For older children, consider the loss of phone, computer, or other privileges for a set period of time.

"To play" has many meanings, but in general it means to take part in an activity for entertainment and recreation. For the young child, play also has a valuable purpose. Through play, the young child learns and practices many skills that will be necessary in adulthood. For example, when preschoolers play with chalk and a chalkboard, they develop eye-hand coordination. For 6-year-olds, playing a board game is practice in "taking turns" and "cooperating." Adolescents also need time to play. Engaging in sports activities such as golf, tennis, fishing, and swimming can help both adolescents and adults stay fit, gain confidence, and receive positive feelings through competition. Adolescent play is also an opportunity to interact socially.

NUTRITION

A full-term infant needs 50 to 55 kcal/lb (110 to 120 kcal/kg), which equals 20 oz (600 mL) of breast milk or formula per day. At birth, the newborn's stomach will hold 20 mL or slightly less than an ounce. Because the newborn is initially unable to consume enough nutrition to meet its needs, the infant will lose weight during the first few days. By the end of the first week of life, the newborn can retain 2–3 ounces (60–90 mL) with each feeding. The infant will need to be fed every 2 to 4 hours in order to meet nutritional needs.

It is important for parents to receive information about the benefits of both breast- and bottle-feeding. Table 6-3 ■ illustrates benefits for each method of feeding. Some women may choose to breastfeed in the privacy of their homes and bottle feed when they are in public or with visitors. Once the parents have decided how to feed the baby, the nurse should support the decision. It is not appropriate to make the parents feel guilty about their decision.

Breastfeeding

Breastfeeding provides optimal, complete nutrition for infants and is recommended by the American Academy of Pediatrics for "all infants in whom breastfeeding is not specifically contraindicated" (2005). Some mothers, however, have difficulty breastfeeding because of low milk production or latch-on issues. Many hospitals have lactation consultants to assist new mothers in learning to breastfeed their infants and manage difficulties as they arise.

Breast milk is produced to meet the newborn's needs and changes as the infant grows. Breast milk contains easily digested nutrients as well as antibodies. *Colostrum*, the first fluid produced by the breast, is a thin yellow fluid, rich in protein, calories, and immune globulins. Colostrum protects the newborn from intestinal infections. Colostrum also contains a laxative that assists in the passage of *meconium*, the first feces of the newborn (Figure 6-5 ■).

Breast stimulation and emptying of the mammary glands stimulates the secretion of prolactin by the mother's anterior pituitary gland. Prolactin increases milk production. As the newborn nurses more frequently and for longer periods of time, more milk is produced.

The breastfeeding mother needs a balanced diet in order to provide nutritious breast milk and maintain her own nutritional needs. The breastfeeding mother needs to consume an extra 500 calories and 1000 mL of fluid per day to support breastfeeding.

The mother and newborn do not automatically know how to breastfeed. Teaching and support will be needed during the learning process. Several positions (Figure 6-6 ■) can be used for breastfeeding. The *cradle hold*, with the infant's head in the bend of the mother's elbow and the infant's body resting against the mother's abdomen, is the most common. Another position is a *football hold*, with the infant's body tucked beneath the mother's axilla and the infant's head positioned against the breast. A *side-lying position* is frequently used in bed. The mother lies on her side with pillows supporting her head and back. The newborn is positioned next to her with the infant's head against the breast and the body parallel to the mother's body. It is important to use a pillow under the mother's forearm to support the weight of the infant.

TABLE 6-3		
Reasons for Breastfeeding and Bottle Feeding		
METHOD OF FEEDING	**BENEFIT TO MOTHER**	**BENEFIT TO INFANT**
Breastfeeding	Decreases incidence of ovarian, uterine, and breast cancer	Breast milk enhances maturation of the GI tract; it is *species-specific* (human milk for human babies) so it supplies the exact nutrients needed by the infant; it assists in passage of meconium and stools
	Promotes involution	Breast milk contains antibodies that can protect against some infections
	Return to pre-pregnant weight sooner	Lower incidence of allergies among breastfed infants
	Unique bonding experience	Breastfed infants have lower incidence of SIDS
	Convenient, no formula and bottles to carry	
	Saves money	
Bottle Feeding	Personal preference	Bonding still can occur
	Provides a good option if mother has breast scarring or HIV infection or if maternal medication precludes breastfeeding	Others besides mother can feed infant
	Is good choice if mother's place of employment (such as hair salon) contains chemicals that could contaminate expressed milk	Provides adequate nutrition
	Provides solution if mother's workplace is intolerant of breastfeeding	Commercial formula comes in three forms for convenience
	Allows several people to share bonding experience while feeding infant	Commercial formula comes in cow's milk and soy milk
	May allow mother to get more rest if others take night feedings	WIC program provides iron-fortified formula

Once the newborn is positioned against the breast, the infant must open wide enough to take the nipple and areola into the mouth. To help the newborn to latch onto the breast (Figure 6-7 ■), the mother holds the breast in her hand with the thumb and forefinger in the shape of a "C" around the breast and well behind the areola. She tickles the infant's lips with the nipple. The infant will open its mouth (part of the sucking reflex). When the mouth is wide open,

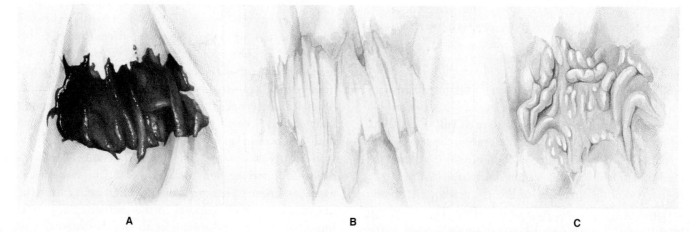

Figure 6-5. ■ Newborn stool samples. (**A**) Meconium stool. (**B**) Breast milk stool. (**C**) Cow's milk stool.

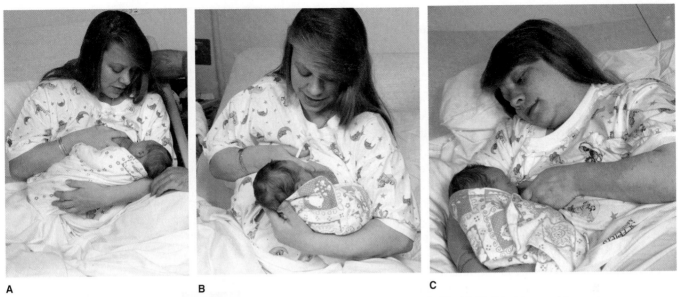

A   **B**   **C**

Figure 6-6. ■ Three positions are often used for breastfeeding. (**A**) Cradle hold. (**B**) Football hold. (**C**) Side-lying position.

and the tongue is down, the infant is brought rapidly to the breast. When "latched on" properly, the nipple and areola will be in the mouth, with the tongue under the nipple and the lips flared outward. The suction will be strong, but there

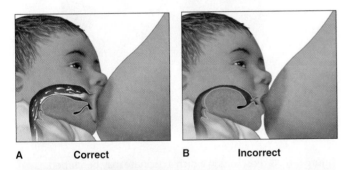

A   Correct   **B   Incorrect**

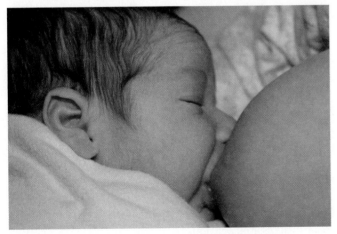

C

Figure 6-7. ■ Latching on. (**A**) Correct position with tongue over gum ridge. Nipple is down far into mouth and milk flows. (**B**) Incorrect position with tongue behind the lower gum ridge. Only the tip of the nipple is in the mouth. The nipple is pinched, and milk cannot flow. (**C**) Newborn properly latched onto mother's breast.

will be no discomfort. When the infant latches on properly, milk is sucked easily from the nipple. If the mother experiences discomfort, the infant should be removed from the breast, repositioned, and allowed to latch on again. There are a variety of positions for breastfeeding (see Figure 6-6). In the traditional cradle position, the baby and mother are belly-to-belly, chest-to-chest, and the infant's nose and chin should touch the breast. This close position helps the infant to latch on; it also helps prevent nipple soreness.

When removing the newborn from the breast, the mother should gently insert a finger into the corner of the infant's mouth to break the suction. If the nipple becomes sore, cracks, or bleeds, or if blisters form, the nipple needs treatment. Leaving a small amount of milk on the nipple after feeding helps to heal sore nipples. Also, the tannic acid obtained by gently rubbing the nipple with a cool wet tea bag can help with healing. A light film of an approved emollient (such as Eucerin) may be applied after feedings.

Breastfeeding may range from 10 to 30 minutes a side, depending on the size and health of the infant. Frequency is at least 8 to 12 times a day. However, it is more important to know when the infant is full than to follow the clock. Infants will nurse vigorously at first, and then slow as they become full. The breast will become soft when empty. Infants should be allowed to empty one breast and then be moved to the other breast until they are full. At the next feeding, the infant is started on the breast used last at the previous feeding. This technique allows each breast to be emptied completely every other feeding. As infants grow, both breasts may be emptied with each feeding. Breastfed infants generally do not swallow as much air as bottle-fed infants, but they still should be burped halfway through and again at the end of the feeding.

Bottle Feeding

To bottle-feed the infant, parents should be taught to position the infant with the head higher than the stomach. The infant should be burped when about half of the feeding is consumed and again at the end of the feeding.

Bottle feeding will take some forethought and preparation. Bottles and nipples should be cleaned regularly with a brush and soapy water and thoroughly rinsed. If there is question about the safety of the water supply, both bottles and nipples should be boiled.

A variety of nipples are available. Generally babies will feed well from any bottle and nipple, but they may eventually prefer one style. Formulas are available in ready-to-feed, concentrated liquid, or powder forms. There is a great range of prices for formula, and finances should be a factor in choosing what type of formula to use. Accurate mixing is essential to provide the necessary nutrients, the proper number of calories, and an easily digested concentration. If the water is contaminated, it must be boiled to remove harmful bacteria. Leftover formula needs to be refrigerated or discarded because it is a rich medium for bacteria growth. Formula is given throughout the first year. Because of the possibility of milk allergy, the use of cow's milk is generally not recommended until after 1 year of age.

The physician orders the brand of formula. It is important to note that, if the woman is participating in the Women, Infants and Children (WIC) program, some brands of formula may not be funded. Adjustments can usually be made between the physician and the WIC program. Most newborns will take 20 mL (1/2 ounce) per feeding for the first few days but gradually increase the amount of each feeding over time. To avoid wasting formula, only a few ounces should be made until the infant is taking higher volumes.

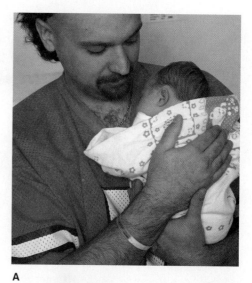

A

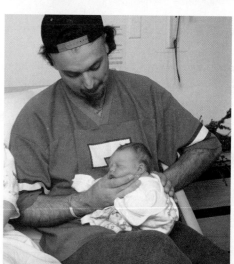

B

Figure 6-8. ■ Positions in which a neonate may be burped. **(A)** Upright. **(B)** Sitting, leaning forward. The infant may also be laid across the lap.

clinical ALERT

The microwave oven is not appropriate for heating infant formula. Burns could occur because of uneven heating. Also, the rubber used in bottle nipples can deteriorate with frequent microwave use (Pediatric Nutrition Practice Group of the American Dietetic Association, 2003).

Burping

To facilitate burping, the infant can be held upright against the feeder's shoulder (Figure 6-8 ■), leaned forward in a sitting position with the head and chest supported, or laid prone across the feeder's lap. Gently rubbing or patting the infant's back can also facilitate burping.

Preventing Poor Nutrition

Malnutrition is often associated with emaciated-looking children with protuberant abdomens from underdeveloped countries. However, malnutrition in the United States presents more often as obesity. According to Carmona (2003), 15.3% of American children are considered to be clinically obese. For the most part, improper nutrition is not due to a lack of finances but to a lack of knowledge coupled with readily accessible convenience food.

The goal of *Healthy People 2010* is to reduce the prevalence of obesity in children and adolescents to 5% (USDHHS, 2000). Proper nutrition is the first line of defense against obesity. The standard American diet is high in fat, carbohydrates, and sodium, and deficient in fruits, vegetables, fiber, and water. Oversized portions are a cause of obesity, providing excessive calories. A typical fast-food meal is a double patty hamburger with cheese, super-sized French fries, and an extra large soft drink. This meal contains approximately 1,480 calories. For the 9- to 13-year-old whose recommended daily caloric intake is 1600–2200 kcal/day, this diet would lead to the consumption of excessive calories. The nurse can assist clients in making more appropriate choices. For example, the following is a healthier lunch: 2 cups green salad with low-fat dressing, 3 ounces grilled chicken breast with the skin removed, and unsweetened iced tea or diet soda. This meal contains approximately 250 calories.

The foundation fat cells are established in childhood. When parents choose high-fat diets for their children, the lifelong struggle to maintain normal weight begins. The nurse can teach parents the importance of serving healthy foods. The U.S. Department of Agriculture's Center for Nutrition Policy and Promotion has improved the food pyramid (Figure 6-9A ■). My Pyramid is a helpful tool that can be used to individualize (by age, gender, and activity level) the number of servings needed daily in each food group. A portion plate (see Figure 6-9B ■) helps give children an easy way to remember how much of each food type to consume.

NURSING CARE

PRIORITIES IN NURSING CARE

When caring for pediatric clients with nutrition problems, it is important for the nurse to focus care on the client's weight and height, nutritional status, nutritional intake, and environmental factors that might impact the client's diet.

ASSESSING

To determine adequate nutritional status, the nurse must obtain height and weight measurements. These measurements are then compared with previous values to determine growth patterns. The nurse uses a graph to plot these measurements (see Appendix II 🔗). A 24-hour nutrition diary can provide information about the child's intake and identify deficits in the diet. With infants, it is optimal for the nurse to observe a feeding in order to observe difficulties in breastfeeding, swallowing, or feeding techniques. If the mother is bottle-feeding, the nurse can provide information and teaching. Box 6-4 ■ discusses bottle-propping in formula-fed infants.

DIAGNOSING, PLANNING, AND IMPLEMENTING

Nursing diagnoses for pediatric clients with nutritional problems might include:

- Ineffective **B**reastfeeding related to poor latch-on
- Imbalanced **N**utrition: Less than Body Requirements related to poor nutritional choices
- **S**elf-Care Deficit: Feeding related to developmental age

Some outcomes for pediatric clients with nutritional problems are provided. The client and/or parent will

- Establish proper latch-on during breastfeeding and obtain adequate nutrition from breastfeeding.
- Demonstrate balanced nutrition as evidenced by healthy food choices and maintenance of appropriate weight.
- Obtain adequate nutrition from caregiver until able to feed self independently.

The nurse's role in providing support to these clients would include the following:

- Assess for adequate intake of breast milk by evaluating urine output and infant weight. *This assessment provides data used to prevent dehydration and imbalanced nutrition.*
- Determine child's adequate body weight. *The data will assist the caregiver in planning for appropriate interventions.*
- Obtain a nutrition history from parent and/or child. *Provides information about nutritional elements that are deficient.*
- Teach parent and child the benefits of adequate nutrition and risks of inadequate nutrition. *Compliance to prescribed nutritional regime may be improved with knowledge of risks and benefits.*
- Instruct the parent and/or child about the number of calories needed and healthy food options (see Figure 6-9), etc.

EVALUATING

The care plan is revised until expected outcomes are achieved. To evaluate the effectiveness of interventions, the nurse would gather data concerning:

- Adequate urination following breastfeeding
- Maintenance of body weight appropriate for age and height
- Adequate nutrients consumed daily

Infant

HEALTH PROMOTION

Environmental Safety

Because the infant has limited mobility, it is easy to think that falls are not a risk. However, when left unattended on a high surface, such as a changing table or a

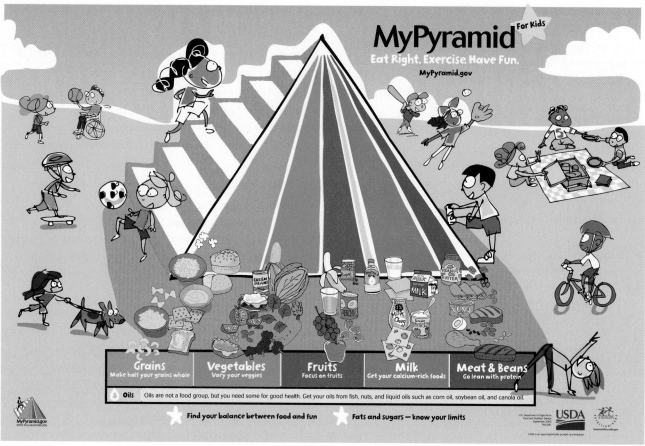

A

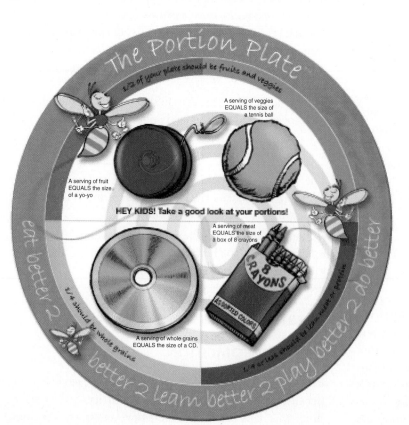

B

Figure 6-9. ■ (A) Food pyramid. (B) A pediatrics portion plate, showing the right amounts of food to consume as one serving. *Note:* (A) From the U.S. Department of Agriculture and U.S. Department of Health and Human Services. (B) The child's Portion Plate product design and name is registered to beBetter Networks. To learn more about how the plate teaches portion control, or to order the plate, please visit www.theportionplate. com.

BOX 6-4   CLIENT TEACHING

Dangers of Bottle-Propping

- Decreases bonding due to lack of physical contact with caregiver
- Increases risk for dental caries or bottle mouth syndrome because the formula or juice in the bottle contains high amounts of sugar, which coats the deciduous teeth and may erode enamel
- May lead to overfeeding from ingestion of large amounts of formula
- Increases risk for otitis media, because the formula can pool in the eustachian tube and become a medium for bacterial growth
- Increases risk for aspiration, because the infant may fall asleep with a mouthful of formula and be unable to swallow properly

---

BOX 6-5   CLIENT TEACHING

Guidelines About Physical Injury and Safety

- Support the infant's head carefully when carrying the infant or picking him or her up.
- Never leave the infant unattended on any surface other than the floor. He or she may fall.
- Never leave the child unattended in the bathtub or near any other source of water such as swimming pools or spas. Swimming pools and spas should have locked gates surrounding them. Children may also drown in water left in buckets.
- Raise the siderails on the crib and lock them into place.
- Position safety gates at the top and bottom of staircases, no matter how few steps. Gates are also appropriate in entrances to areas such as the kitchen or laundry room where dangerous products are stored.

Burns
- Carefully test the temperature of heated formula or breast milk before giving it to the infant.
- Carefully test the temperature of bathwater before immersing the child.
- Never place the child close to fireplaces, space heaters, or stoves.
- Do not smoke or carry hot beverages when holding an infant.
- Cover electrical outlets.
- Adjust the temperature of hot water heater to 120° F (48.8° C)

Car Safety
- Never leave a child unattended in a motor vehicle. Temperatures inside of cars can quickly become dangerous.
- Only use age-appropriate, approved car safety seats.
- Place an infant in the back seat to avoid injury from airbags.

Choking
- Never place the infant's crib near drapes or blinds because the child could choke on the cords.
- Secure electrical cords out of reach.
- Remove pillows and plastic from an infant's reach. Do not place an infant on a bean bag, feather bed, or sheepskin rug.
- Be diligent about keeping small objects out of the infant's reach.
- Do not give infants small foods such as hard candy, grapes, hot dogs, or popcorn.
- Do not prop bottles.

Poisoning
- Keep toxic products in locked areas.
- Keep houseplants out of reach.
- Keep prescribed and over-the-counter medicines in locked cabinets.
- Ensure that the child is not exposed to paint containing lead.
- Keep the local Poison Control Center phone number by the phone.

---

bed, the infant can manage to fall by moving his or her arms and legs. For example, if the infant in the car seat is placed on the hood of the car while the parent puts shopping bags in the trunk, movement of the infant's arms and legs can cause the car seat to tip and fall off the car. It is important to teach parents about safety from the time they take their baby home from the hospital. Box 6-5 ■ provides areas for client teaching about physical injury and safety.

The baby begins to roll from side to back and can crawl as early as 6 months. It is important to begin the habit of protecting the child from falls at birth. Parents should be taught to use safety gates to prevent the infant from falling down stairs. Particularly when the infant becomes mobile, it is important to secure the gate to the wall following manufacturer's guidelines. Safety in bed may also be a consideration (Box 6-6 ■). Also, in older cribs, the child's head may become trapped between slats because these cribs were not designed to prevent this.

CHOKING.   **Choking** (asphyxiation by a foreign object lodged in the respiratory tract) and suffocation are a particular concern during infancy. Because the baby becomes mobile within a few months and frequently brings hand to mouth, parents must be constantly aware of small objects within the infant's reach and be vigilant to remove them from the baby's environment. The parent should be encouraged to get down on the floor and look for small objects from the infant's perspective. Toys should be inspected to be sure there are no small parts that could come loose and be swallowed by the infant. Any toy labeled "not intended for use by those under 3 years" should be kept out of the infant's reach. Other choking or suffocation hazards include stuffed toys, pacifiers, pillows, and plastic-type materials, including plastic bags and balloons.

The crib should not be close to the drawstring on the curtains or blinds because the infant can get the cord around his or her neck and strangle. Parents should also be aware that hanging mobiles can cause a choking hazard. An

BOX 6-6	CULTURAL PULSE POINTS

Sleeping with Infants in the Same Bed

Consider the family's cultural norms when discussing the risks of parents and children sleeping in the same bed. For example, it is common for Bosnian families to allow children up to age 2 to sleep in the same bed with the parents. Safety teaching about the dangers of the practice must occur, but be sensitive to the client's cultural beliefs.

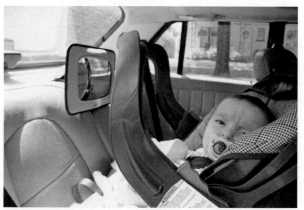

A

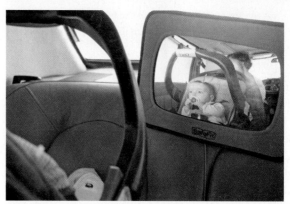

B

infant's crib slats must be close together so he or she cannot get his or her head caught between the slats. Any crib with slats spaced more than 2⅜ inches (6 cm) apart should be discarded. The mattress should fit tightly against the crib rails to prevent body parts from becoming lodged in the crib frame.

CAR SAFETY.   The most common injuries to an infant are caused by automobile crashes, falls, and choking. All infants must be transported in a rear-facing infant car seat. The car seat should be secured according to directions provided by the manufacturer. The safest place for the infant is in the back seat. With the infant in the rear-facing position in the back seat, the parent may have difficulty seeing the infant. Adjustable mirrors are available to allow the driver to see the infant through the car's rear-view mirror (Figure 6-10). The driver should not allow a crying infant to interfere with safe driving practices; he or she should pull off the road and stop before attending to the infant. Information can be obtained from the National Safety Council. Federal Motor Vehicle Safety Standards (American Academy of Pediatrics [AAP], 2006) should be followed regarding use of infant car seats and booster seats. Table 6-4 ■ identifies the recommended use of infant and child car seats. Small or premature infants may not be able to breathe in a sitting position in the car seat. In these cases, they need to use an approved infant car bed until their weight increases. The infant car bed will need to be secured to the automobile's rear seat, and the infant secured into the bed following manufacturer instructions. Infants should never be left alone in a car. In the summer, temperatures inside the car can reach more than 130° F in just a few minutes, subjecting the infant to hyperthermia, brain damage, and even death.

PSYCHOSOCIAL HEALTH

Promoting Self-Esteem

Many child development experts agree that one of the best ways to promote self-esteem in children is to give them a sense of security and to assist them in developing trust. In

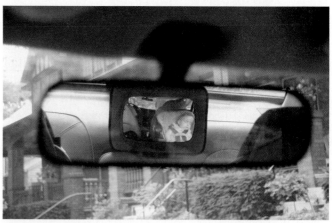

C

Figure 6-10. ■ Adjustable mirrors are available to allow the driver to see the infant through the car rear-view mirror. (**A**) The mirror is positioned next to the infant's car seat. (**B**) *(Facing rear of car)* There is no obstruction between the front seat and the mirror next to the car seat. (**C**) The driver attaches a small mirror to the rear-view mirror in front and slants it so that the infant can be seen from the driver's seat.

infancy, trust is developed as needs are met promptly. Nurses can help parents recognize the infant's cues for hunger, sleep, and nurturing. The nurse should also encourage parents to respond promptly to these cues. This allows

TABLE 6-4	
Use of Infant and Child Car Seats	
CHILD SIZE OR WEIGHT	INSTRUCTIONS
Weight below 20 lb (9 kg)	■ Place infant or convertible seat in back seat of car facing backward. ■ Never place the infant in the front passenger seat. ■ Recline infant at 45 degrees or less (some small infants must be flat in a car bed). ■ Following manufacturer's instructions, fasten seat securely to car using car seat belt. ■ Adjust harnesses to fit snugly at shoulders and legs. ■ Move to a larger seat before the infant's head reaches top of the shell. ■ When using a convertible seat from birth, use one with a 5-point harness.
Birth to 40 lb (18 kg)	■ Use car seat reclined when rear-facing and upright when forward-facing position. ■ Follow manufacturer's instructions for proper position at specified child weights for that product. ■ Move to a high-back child seat or booster when child's ears are above the seat. ■ Always place the seat in the back seat of the vehicle.
Child more than 40 lb (18 kg)	■ Use booster seat for children who have outgrown convertible toddler seat. ■ Follow manufacturer's instruction for installation and for specified child weights for the product. ■ Use booster seat until the vehicle lap and shoulder belts fit correctly. ■ Have all children 12 years and younger ride in the back seat whether or not they are in a car seat.

Note: Air bags can cause serious injury and death when a child is in a car seat in the front passenger seat. Even when not in a car seat, and when the vehicle is not equipped with a passenger side air bag, the back seat is the safest location for all children.

Source: National Safety Council. (2004). *Child passenger safety fact sheet.* Washington, DC: Author.

the infant to learn to trust the parent and will facilitate the process of bonding or attachment.

Promoting Play

Each age group has patterns of play that indicate its level of social development. Many changes occur in the first year of life. Infants rapidly learn about the world around them. Play for the 2- to 3-month-old infant involves learning to grasp and move small lightweight toys. The infant enjoys seeing bright colors and hearing rattling noises coming from the toy. As the infant grows in strength and learns to sit and crawl, play becomes exploring the world. This exploration involves seeing, touching, and tasting the environment.

APPROPRIATE TOYS. Toys for infants should be age appropriate and safe. They should not have small, removable parts or long cords that could be a choking hazard. Rattles are interesting to infants because they make noise and can be easily grasped. Mobiles and baby gyms should be brightly colored or black and white to attract the infant visually. Blocks should have smooth, rounded corners. The older infant is able to stack these successfully. Books with

pictures and few words will interest the infant. Many books are soft sided and easy to grasp.

NUTRITION

Most infants continue to breastfeed or be formula fed during infancy. For more information on these topics, see newborn section in this chapter. Table 6-5 ■ provides information about nutritional needs at different ages. In

TABLE 6-5	
Recommended Caloric Intake by Age Group	
AGE GROUP	RECOMMENDED CALORIC INTAKE
Infant	100–200 kcal/kg/day
Toddler	1,100–1,300 kcal/day
Preschooler	1,300–1,600 kcal/day
School age child	1,600–2,200 kcal/day
Adolescent	2,200–2,800 kcal/day

an effort to prevent childhood obesity, parents should limit infant intake of fruit juices and avoid beverages with high sugar content such as powdered and carbonated drinks. The AAP (2001) suggests that fruit juices never be given to an infant in a bottle but only in a covered cup. This will avoid dental caries and decrease the intake amount.

Solid food is gradually introduced beginning around 6 months. Usually, a thin rice cereal is given once or twice a day. As the infant learns to control his or her tongue and swallow, a thicker consistency of the cereal can be given. Generally pureed vegetables and fruits are then added to the diet, with meats added last. Once teeth erupt, the infant can be given soft finger foods such as crackers, bananas, and cheese. By 12 months, the infant should be encouraged to use a covered cup exclusively for fluid intake.

Infants generally thrive with three set meals and several snacks a day. Placing the infant in a high chair or seat at the table and letting him or her eat only in the kitchen or dining room helps the infant learn social skills associated with meals.

Food allergies or sensitivities (e.g., lactose intolerance) are growing concerns. Parents should be taught to pay attention to any unusual reactions to foods their infants are eating. Some pediatricians recommend avoiding certain foods prior to the age of 2 years, when the child's immune system is more developed. Such foods include eggs, peanut butter, and shellfish. See more about gastrointestinal issues in Chapter 17 ⚭ .

Oral Health

Infants may show signs of teething at 4 months of age. These signs include increased drooling, increased hand-to-mouth activity, attempting to clench hard on objects, disturbed sleep patterns, difficulty in being consoled, and loss of appetite. Teething does not cause gastrointestinal disturbances or fever. Parents should be taught that these symptoms indicate a disease process and that they should consult a health care professional if symptoms do not resolve.

Parents can be taught to apply cold to the infant's gums for relief. Freezing the teething ring or wrapping a piece of ice in a thin towel and applying it to the gums are appropriate methods. The nurse should warn parents not to place a piece of ice in the infant's mouth because this could cause aspiration. Topical anesthetics are available over the counter and can provide temporary relief from the discomfort of teething. If these relief measures are ineffective, systemic analgesics can be used on a short-term basis.

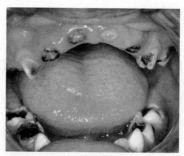

Figure 6-11. ■ Nursing bottle mouth syndrome. This child has had major tooth decay related to sleeping as an infant and toddler while sucking bottles of juice and milk. *Note:* Courtesy of Dr. Lezley McIlveen, Department of Dentistry, Children's National Medical Center, Washington, DC.

Dosing should be discussed with the pediatrician or family practitioner.

Parents should be encouraged to model dental health as soon as teeth begin to erupt. A soft brush or cloth without toothpaste can be used to clean the teeth and gums. The American Academy of Pediatric Dentistry (2003) suggests that children receive fluoride supplementation if the drinking water in the home contains fluoride levels of less than 0.6 ppm.

Infants engage in nonnutritive or recreational sucking. They may suck a pacifier or their thumb, or spend extra time at the breast. There appear to be benefits to this type of sucking, both physically and emotionally. Some parents may be concerned about tooth alignment and forming unwanted habits. The nurse can encourage parents to view this type of sucking during infancy as harmless. However, nurses should teach parents not to allow an infant to suck on a bottle after feeding. This can result in "bottle mouth" (Figure 6-11 ■).

Toddler

HEALTH PROMOTION

Environmental Safety

The toddler is becoming more mobile and inquisitive, so safety becomes more of a challenge. Parents often claim the toddler is "into everything" when he or she is learning to walk and climb. The most common injuries of this age group include automobile injury, falls, burns, poisonings, and drowning. The toddler is not big enough to use car seat belts, but still needs to use a safety seat at all times. The shoulder strap on adult seat belts should not be used because it could cause strangulation. Figure 6-12 ■ illustrates proper use of toddler safety car seats. Again, the safest

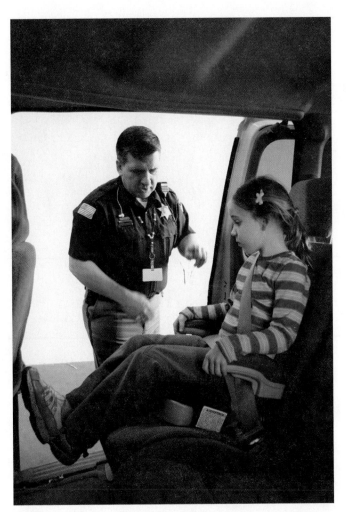

Figure 6-12. ■ It is important to be consistent in use of safety-approved car seats for infants and children. Toddlers and older children can face forward, but still should have the protection of being in the back seat. Front seat air bags can suffocate a child if they inflate, so the general guideline is that children under the age of 12 years should not ride in the front seat of a car.

place for the toddler is in the back seat. The toddler may be able to unfasten the seat belt and may resist being restrained in the seat. However, the parent must insist on safety for all trips, regardless of the distance. Once the car has come to a complete stop with the engine off, the seat belt can be removed.

The toddler must not be left alone in an automobile. Not only can he or she suffer from extreme temperature inside the vehicle, but also the toddler might disengage the brake, put the car in neutral, or start the engine, allowing the car to move and cause an accident.

Inquisitive toddlers often want to explore their environment. As a result, parking lots can be dangerous places. Toddlers are not capable of sensing the hazards of cars as

they pull in and out of parking spaces. Parents must devise a plan for toddler safety when entering or exiting the car. This plan can be complicated by younger children who must be held and by loading groceries or shopping bags. For the overly adventurous toddler, parents may limit outings to times when another trusted adult can accompany them.

Toddlers learn to ride tricycles and other wheeled vehicles. This mobility carries a risk for injury. As toddlers learn to ride these vehicles, they must be taught to wear properly fitting helmets and both knee and elbow pads. Riding in a park where the sidewalks are surrounded by grass is safer than riding on a sidewalk along the street. When riding on a sidewalk, toddlers could ride into the street without being aware of the risk for injury. Therefore, it is important for parents to supervise toddlers who are riding a tricycle outside a fenced area.

Falls are a concern for toddler safety. Body shape changes continually throughout childhood (Figure 6-13 ■). The body shape of a toddler compromises stability. A protuberant abdomen and short legs increase the risk of falls. Toddlers are also learning to climb stairs. At first they go up and down stairs on their knees, but as soon as they are steadier on their feet, they want to walk up and down. They should be taught to use the handrail. Toddlers may be able to move chairs and climb onto the counter. Close supervision is needed at all times. The toddler should be provided with safe climbing toys and be taught acceptable places to climb. Most playgrounds have climbing toys. Parents should be taught to inspect them for poor construction. The ground in and around the toys should be covered with a soft material such as loose bark to decrease injury in the event of a fall.

As toddlers climb onto chairs and counters, medicines, cosmetics, and cleaning supplies become easy to reach. Therefore, all poisonous substances must be kept out of reach or locked away. Childproof lids, electrical outlet covers, and cupboard closures are helpful but not perfect (Figure 6-14 ■). Teaching toddlers to play with toys is an important step in reducing the risk for poisoning. Parents should be aware that many houseplants are poisonous if the child chews the leaves and stems. Poison control center phone numbers and syrup of ipecac should be readily available. Plant reference books are also available with handy guides on plant safety.

Choking remains a hazard for toddlers, even though they do not explore their environment by putting objects in their mouth as infants do. They are eating a greater variety of whole foods, which increases the risk for aspiration. Nuts and meat can be particularly risky for toddlers to swallow. Children should not be given peanuts until they have enough teeth to chew the nut well before

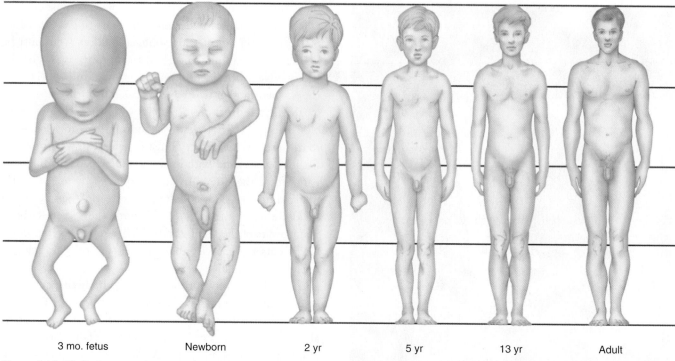

3 mo. fetus   Newborn   2 yr   5 yr   13 yr   Adult

Figure 6-13. ■ Body proportions at various ages.

swallowing. Meat should be cut into small pieces for the toddler. Other foods that could be dangerous are hot dogs, grapes, and hard candy. Parents should insist that children eat in a controlled environment, such as at the dining table, where adult supervision is available. To prevent choking, children should not talk with their mouths full or play while eating.

Injury to the mouth can occur if children are allowed to run or play with things in their mouths. For instance, running or rough play with a popsicle stick, lollipop stick, or

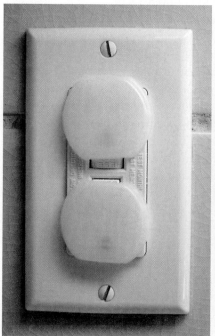

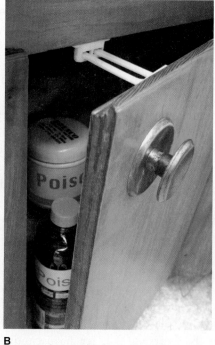

A   **B**   **C**

Figure 6-14. ■ The home needs to be childproofed for safety. (**A**) Safety covers for electrical outlets. (**B**) Childproof locks on drawers and cabinets. (**C**) Mr. Yuk stickers on toxic substances.

toothbrush in the mouth could cause injury to the palate, tongue, gums, or teeth. These objects should be placed out of the toddler's reach.

As toddlers watch routine activities in the kitchen, their curiosity is aroused. They are tall enough to reach the stove and can pull hot pans, spilling contents onto their head, arms, or entire bodies. They can touch the hot burner or open an oven door and turn on stoves with front controls. They can even turn on the burners. Toddlers are fascinated with fire and might reach into a lit fireplace or touch burning candles. They want to mimic adults who are lighting matches and using cigarette lighters. Toddlers should be taught that all heat-producing objects are dangerous and off limits. Parents must not forget that electric cords pose a strangulation hazard to toddlers and also pose a risk for electrical burns or electrocution if they are chewed.

Most toddlers enjoy playing in water. Constant supervision is critical when the toddler is in the bathtub (Figure 6-15A ■). The toddler should be taught to sit and never to stand while in the tub. Nonskid surfaces should be used to prevent falls in the tub. Children might try to play in the toilet water, fish tanks, and mop buckets. The child can fall into these seemingly safe, shallow water sources. Children who fall head first into these tanks do not have the upper body strength to right themselves. Therefore, parents need to protect children from water hazards. Buckets should be emptied when not in use.

Fish tanks should have childproof lids. Toilet seat lids should be down and the bathroom door closed at all times. Swimming pools, hot tubs, ponds, ditches, canals, and rivers are other places in which the toddler might try to play. When possible, fences with locking gates should be used to prevent young children from accessing water hazards. The use of child life jackets near water and on boats is essential. However, flotation devices like arm or doughnut inflatables are not certified life preservers (Figure 6-15B ■). Swimming lessons at an early age might be valuable but cannot guarantee that a child will not drown. Adult supervision is always necessary.

PSYCHOSOCIAL HEALTH

Toilet Training
Children are expected to learn to use the toilet and abandon wearing diapers. This often presents a struggle for the child and for the parent. Parents need to understand how to determine whether the toddler is ready to be toilet trained. They also need assistance in accomplishing this task without bringing shame to the toddler. The nurse can provide this information and teaching to parents. Box 6-7 ■ provides some tips for helping a toddler succeed at toilet training.

Providing Discipline
Toddlers are beginning to develop a measure of independence, even though they are still dependent on the mother

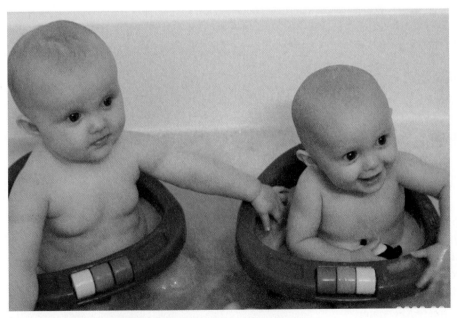
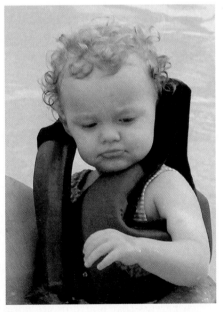

A   B

Figure 6-15. ■ (A) Infants and toddlers can easily lose their balance in a bathtub, and they do not have the muscle strength and coordination to sit themselves back up. These bathing devices allow the parent to bathe both twins at once in the bathtub. (B) Toddlers should not be allowed to play in swimming pools or other deep water without a flotation device. Teach parents to look for life vests that help to support the head above water.

BOX 6-7 CLIENT TEACHING

Hints for Toilet Training

- Create enthusiasm by purchasing the child a proper-sized potty chair. If this is not available, provide a toilet seat insert for the child to sit on, and place a stool in front of the toilet for the child to climb on.
- Establish a routine. Place the child on the toilet seat on rising in the morning, before and after naps, before bathing, before bed, and at regular intervals throughout the day.
- Wipe female children from front to back to model proper technique. Use clean toilet tissue to remove fecal matter.
- Teach hand washing after toileting.
- Transitional diapers may be helpful. They are easier for the child to manipulate and give a better sense of bladder and bowel awareness.
- Develop a reward system, possibly giving the child a small reward when he or she uses the potty chair. Some children are often motivated by "big girl" or "big boy" underwear.
- Create an environment of patience and praise. Do not punish accidents.
- If the child does not cooperate, wait a few weeks and try again.

or caregiver. Consistency in limit-setting is important at this age. Children can begin to learn social expectations (to sit at the table when eating, not to eat food that has fallen on the ground, etc.). The more consistent the parent is in establishing norms, the easier it will be for the child to accept them.

This is the time when children learn to say "NO." When the child performs a negative behavior or refuses to participate in a desired behavior, it is important for the parent to respond in clear and consistent ways. The following steps are generally recommended for toddler discipline:

1. Give the child a warning that the behavior is unacceptable and name the consequence if the child continues.
2. If the toddler continues the behavior, provide the consequence. Usually, "time-out" is a good method for disciplining a toddler (1 minute of time-out per year). The toddler should be removed from the physical situation and placed where there are no toys or other diversions so the time-out is focused on thinking about the behavior.
3. After time-out, direct the child's attention to an activity that is not associated with the previous behavior.

Temper tantrums are also common in this age group. Teach parents that tantrums are normal for toddlers, and that it is most important for them to remain calm and not to give in to the behavior. Time-out may be useful. If tantrums occur in public, it may be necessary to remove the child from the situation or to hold the child firmly until

the tantrum has subsided. Remind parents to reinforce good behavior by praising the child when he or she regains control.

Promoting Play

Toddlers enjoy the company of others, even though they may not play together. This side-by-side play is known as **parallel play** (Figure 6-16 ■). Toddlers imitate the behavior of others, such as talking on the telephone, hammering, or sweeping. The toddler also likes to climb, ride big-wheeled toys, and swing. Fine motor skills are continuing to develop by scribbling with a pen and turning pages in a book.

APPROPRIATE TOYS. Toddlers need toys that provide action. Examples of these types of toys are pull toys, puzzles, shape sorters, dolls, and sports equipment. Toddlers also need toys to improve their creativity. Crayons, washable markers, and musical instruments will spark the toddler's creativity. Toys that challenge a toddler, such as books and blocks, are also good choices. Box 6-8 ■ provides information for teaching parents and caregivers about toy safety.

NUTRITION

Parents are often concerned that the toddler is not eating enough food. As the rate of growth slows, a toddler's body needs decrease. The amount of food consumed over several days is more indicative of adequate intake than the intake meal by meal. The general rule is 1 tablespoon of each food offered per year of age. For the toddler to consume the needed nutrients, a variety of foods should be offered from all food groups in order. The pediatrician or family

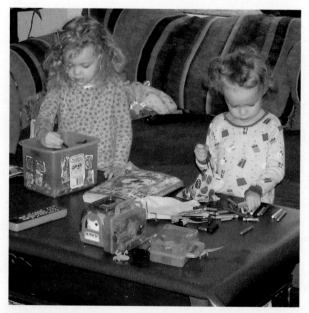

Figure 6-16. ■ In toddler and preschool years, children often participate in parallel play, enjoying each other's presence while having separate playthings.

BOX 6-8	CLIENT TEACHING

Toy Safety

Under Age 3

Children younger than age 3 tend to put everything in their mouths.

- Avoid buying toys with small parts that could create a choking hazard.
- Never let children of any age play with uninflated or broken balloons because of the choking danger.
- Avoid marbles, balls, and games with balls that have a diameter of 1.75 inches or less. These products also pose a choking hazard to young children.

Children at this age pull, prod, and twist toys.

- Look for toys that are well made, with tightly secured eyes, noses, and other parts.
- Avoid toys that have sharp edges and points.

Age 3 to 6 Years

- Avoid toys constructed with thin, brittle plastic that might easily break into small pieces or leave jagged edges.
- Look for household art materials, including crayons and paint sets, marked with the designation "ASTM D-4236." This means the product has been reviewed by a toxicologist and, if necessary, labeled with cautionary information.
- Teach older children to keep their toys away from their younger brothers and sisters.

Age 6 to 12 Years

- For all children, adults should check toys periodically for breakage and potential hazards. Damaged or dangerous toys should be repaired or thrown away.
- If buying a toy gun, be sure the barrel, or the entire gun, is brightly colored so it is not mistaken for a real gun.
- If you buy a bicycle for any age child, also buy a helmet and make sure the child wears it.
- Teach all children to put toys away when they are finished playing so they do not trip or fall on them.

Read the Label . . .

The U.S. Consumer Product Safety Commission (2003) requires toy manufacturers to meet stringent safety standards and to label certain toys that could be a hazard for younger children. Look for labels that give age recommendations and use that information as a guide. Labels on toys that state "not recommended for children under 3 . . . contains small parts" are labeled that way because they may pose a choking hazard to children younger than age 3. Toys should be developmentally appropriate to suit the skills, abilities, and interests of the child.

Shopping for toys during the holidays can be exciting and fun, but it can also be frustrating. There can be thousands of toys to choose from in one store, and it is important to choose the right toy for the right age child. Toys that are meant for older children can be dangerous for younger children.

---

practitioner may recommend a daily multivitamin for the picky eater. Allowing the toddler to choose between healthy options, such as the kind of juice or a choice between two kinds of cereal, will encourage positive eating habits and satisfy the toddler's search for independence.

After 12 months of age, parents may introduce cow's milk into the diet of their child. Prior to 1 year of age, cow's milk is an insufficient source of iron and exclusive use of cow's milk would put the infant at risk for anemia. There is also considerable evidence that many children have an allergy to cow's milk. Parents should observe closely for adverse reactions when they introduce cow's milk into the diet of their toddler.

It is also time to help the toddler learn to use a spoon and fork. At first toddlers may pick the food up in one hand and put the food onto the spoon before putting it into the mouth, or they may hold the utensil backwards (Figure 6-17 ■). With practice, they learn to scoop the food into the spoon with one hand. Using a bowl instead of a plate may help the toddler practice this fine motor skill. It is important to cut the food into small, bite-sized pieces. The toddler has not yet learned how much food to put into his or her mouth at a time. Close supervision will avoid a choking hazard.

Oral Health

As the toddler gains more teeth, caring for the teeth becomes a higher parental priority. This is a good time to take the child to the dentist for the first time. This will help the child get used to going to the dentist at regular intervals. Pediatric dentists are available in many communities, providing a child-friendly environment.

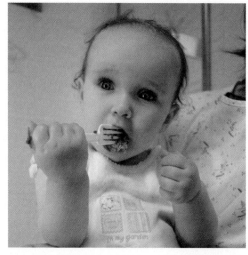

Figure 6-17. ■ Bit by bit, toddlers learn the complicated task of eating with utensils.

Preschooler

HEALTH PROMOTION

Environmental Safety

The preschooler is becoming more independent. The parent may begin to feel comfortable with leaving the preschooler to play by him- or herself for brief periods of time. As the preschooler learns numbers and letters, he or she can be taught to call 9-1-1 to reach emergency help. However, the preschooler does not completely understand cause and effect and needs to be provided with a safe place to play. For example, the preschooler may not understand that climbing on a stool to reach the cookie jar could lead to a fall. Motor vehicle accidents, burns, and drowning remain the leading causes of injury.

The older preschooler can independently get into the car and fasten the seat belt. However, he or she may forget to fasten the seat belt correctly. It is important for the driver to verify that the seat belt is fastened before the car is started. Because the child is growing physically, eventually the booster seat will no longer be needed and the regular car seat belt will be best. The back seat continues to be the best location for the child. It may be tempting to have an older preschooler sit in the front seat, but front and side air bags still pose a danger to the smaller child.

> ### clinical ALERT
>
> Teach parents always to place infants in rear-facing, safety-approved car seats until the infant is at least 1 year old <u>and</u> weighs at least 20 pounds. Car seats should be used until the child reaches the maximum weight for the car seat or until straps do not fit over the shoulders. Children should then use booster seats until a seat belt fits properly over the shoulder and across the hips. This is usually when the child is 4 feet 9 inches tall and between 8 and 12 years of age (AAP, 2006).

Striving for independence, the preschooler may choose to go into a lake or pool unsupervised. The preschooler is not cognizant of the dangers of swimming alone. Running water in ditches and canals also poses a danger. The preschooler likes to watch toy boats, sticks, or other items floating in moving water. He or she might try to reach them and fall into the current. For these reasons, it continues to be important to provide constant supervision in or around water.

Preschoolers have an understanding of "hot" and the hazard of fire but still need to be watched near stoves and fires (Figure 6-18 ■). With reminding, they can blow on hot food before eating. They should be taught not to play with matches and to stop, drop, and roll if their clothes are on fire. They can learn escape routes in case of fire and should practice them on a monthly basis. If a preschooler is

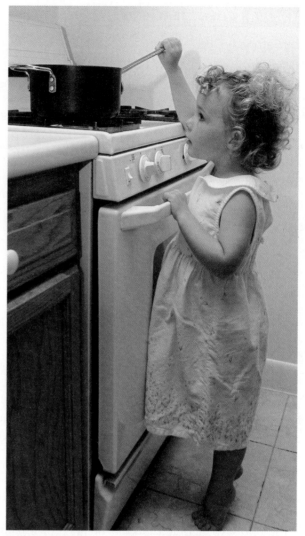

Figure 6-18. ■ Placing hot pots on back burners with handles turned inward is one way to prevent injury to children.

in a daycare facility, basic fire safety may also be taught there. Box 6-9 ■ lists fire safety rules for the home.

TEACHING ABOUT "STRANGERS." It is never too early to talk to children about trusting people they do not know. They should also be taught about appropriate and inappropriate touch. Although parents do not want to scare children unnecessarily, they have to be taught not to get into a car or go anywhere with someone they do not know. A family "password" could be used to identify those individuals whom the child could trust. Children should be taught to close the bathroom door when using the toilet, to dress and undress in private, and to keep their "private parts" covered. The preschooler is old enough to wash themselves with parent supervision, and should be taught to do so, instead of having others wash or touch their breasts or perineum.

Preschoolers should also be taught to tell parents if they believe they have been or are being touched in bad ways.

BOX 6-9   CLIENT TEACHING

Fire Safety for the Home

- Place a fire detector on every floor of the home. Check the batteries regularly.
- Maintain at least two working fire detectors in the home.
- Discuss an exit strategy with children in case of fire. Have rehearsals regularly.
- Store flammable liquids such as gasoline and paint away from heat sources, and do not smoke around these substances.
- Regularly inspect electrical cords and discard any that are frayed.
- Never leave candles unattended.
- Store matches and lighters in locked cabinets.
- Post emergency numbers where the child can easily read them.

Abusers are most often people children already know, so they may not think of them as "strangers."

Health Education

During the preschool years, a child's brain is rapidly developing. This is an optimal time to promote learning that will influence a lifetime of healthy behaviors. Organized learning often begins during this period when the child attends day care, mother's morning out programs, or preschool programs. These settings provide an excellent opportunity to learn about healthy behaviors.

Learning in the school setting can be quite appealing to the child, and it promotes retention of the information. Games and skits that incorporate peers and friends entice the child to listen attentively. Craft activities provide the child with an ongoing reminder of the lessons learned. Many health topics are appropriate for the school environment. These include seat belt use, personal hygiene, disease prevention, importance of daily exercise, and proper nutritional habits.

PSYCHOSOCIAL HEALTH

Providing Discipline

During the preschool years, the goal of discipline is for the child to develop a sense of responsibility for his or her actions. The child is able to understand the cause and effect of most of his or her actions and can choose behavior accordingly. The preschooler also desires to please the adults in his or her life. He or she wants to be obedient and often feels guilty if he or she is not.

One form of discipline found to be effective during the preschool years is the use of isolation or "time-out" for disobedient behavior. After the expected behavior is clearly defined and the child chooses an alternative action, the child can be placed in a safe setting for a defined period of time. This safe setting could be a certain chair in a specific room or an area of a room that is devoid of toys and other forms of entertainment. After the child has been isolated for the defined period of time, he or she should be asked by the caregiver what he or she learned as a result of this discipline. The parent may need to help the child understand the lesson by supplying hints and further teaching.

It is important for all caregivers in the child's life to provide the same type of discipline and expect the same behaviors. This will enhance the child's expected behavior. These caregivers must be careful to communicate to the child that the unwanted behavior is why the discipline is implemented, not because the child is "bad."

Play and Appropriate Toys

Preschoolers begin to socialize and indulge in **associative play** by learning to share and by working together on a project. Associative play occurs when children are engaging in the same activity but without formal organization. The preschooler develops fine motor skills by using scissors, crayons, and glue. They enjoy making art projects with adult supervision. They are learning colors, shapes, numbers, and letters. The preschooler uses dramatic play in acting out the events of daily life. By using dolls, furniture, and clothing, the preschooler not only portrays the events of the world, but can also learn new things. The nurse should use playtime to assess the child's social skills and get clues into the family interaction from the child's point of view. The nurse should also use this time to teach the preschooler about health care issues and upcoming procedures. For more information, see Chapter 8 ⚭.

NUTRITION

The preschooler generally eats three meals and two snacks a day. Mealtime is a social event because the preschooler enjoys participating in conversation. The preschooler also wants to be involved in food preparation. This is a good time to teach about nutritious foods, food preparation, refrigeration, cleanliness, and safety around stoves and other kitchen utensils and appliances. The preschooler can be given routine tasks such as setting the table, clearing away dirty dishes, and putting away leftover food.

A balanced diet, with adequate amounts of fruit, vegetables, protein, grains, and dairy, is desirable for the preschooler. Some fat is necessary to absorb fat-soluble vitamins and to ensure proper metabolism; however, saturated fat must be limited. Unfortunately, foods high in saturated fats, such as hamburgers, French fries, and chicken nuggets, satisfy the preschooler's taste. Parents can be encouraged to serve these foods only on special occasions instead of routinely.

Oral Health

By age 7, children begin to lose their baby teeth. It is not uncommon to have several missing teeth at a time. Soft, easy-to-chew foods may be needed until the permanent teeth come in. Dental care is important to be sure permanent teeth are well cared for and in proper alignment.

School-Age Child

HEALTH PROMOTION

Environmental Safety

School-age children are learning to take responsibility for their own safety. Automobile safety continues to be of concern. Pedestrian and bicycle safety also poses a risk. School-age children may travel to and from school by themselves or in small groups. If they ride a school bus, they must be taught to cross well in front of the bus so the driver can see them. They also need to follow the safety rules of pedestrian travel consistently (Box 6-10 ■). They need to be told to watch for cars because the driver may not see them. School-age children should be taught to cross the street at crosswalks or intersections, being alert for cars making turns at the corner. When sidewalks are not available, they should walk on the side of the road facing traffic. This would allow them to move completely off the roadway if a car is approaching them too closely.

They might ride a bicycle and need to learn safety rules, including how to ride in traffic. School-age children should be taught to ride their bicycles on the side of the road, in the same direction as traffic flows. Wearing a properly fitted helmet is essential, and both elbow and knee pads are recommended (Figure 6-19 ■). In-line skates and skateboards must never be used in traffic. Protective equipment, including a helmet and elbow and knee pads, should be worn at all times.

School-age children can be depended upon more often to follow directions. They are learning cause and effect but may become careless as they "show off" for friends. Injury from fire, drowning, and poison usually occurs as a result of carelessness and experimentation rather than from unknown dangers. It is important for parents to talk frequently with their children about safety and family rules. Parents should know where and with whom their children are at all times.

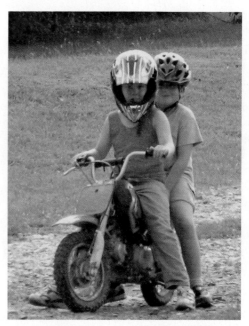

Figure 6-19. ■ Children on motorized bikes are at risk for injury. Helmets are essential. Kneepads and elbow pads can help reduce the risk.

School-age children still need general supervision in order to prevent careless behavior.

School-age children may come home from school to an empty house and may remain unsupervised until parents return from work. The term **latch-key children** has been used to describe these children, who may be as young as 5 years. As a result of spending a large amount of time alone, these children are at greater risk for dangers related to drugs, smoking, crime, behavior problems, and peer pressure. They become lonely or bored and feel more stress than children who are supervised after school. The National Crime Prevention Council (O'Neil, Kelly, & Kirby, 1995) recommends that communities offer afterschool programs to prevent children's involvement in dangerous activities and to encourage academic excellence.

As school-age children become more independent and mobile, they must also be aware of injury from assault. Many children have been taught "not to talk to strangers" and presume a "stranger" to be an evil-looking individual. However, most child molesters seem nice, friendly, and gentle. They use ploys such as "help me find my dog" to lure children into unsafe areas. Many children arrive home from school before parents are home from work and are alone for a short time. They should be taught not to open the door to strangers and should demonstrate that they are responsible before being left alone. Older children should not be expected to care for younger siblings until they are mature enough to handle the responsibility. Community resources, available through the local public health department and

---

BOX 6-10	CLIENT TEACHING

Pedestrian Travel

- Walk on sidewalks.
- Walk at the side of the road when sidewalks are not available.
- Walk facing traffic when sidewalks are not available.
- Cross the street at corners or crosswalks.
- Cross the street when the signal indicates it is safe.
- Check traffic in all directions when crossing without a light.
- Ride bicycles along the side of the road or in the bike lane.
- Ride bicycle in the same direction as traffic flow.

local police department, help parents talk with their children about the danger of assault.

School-age children may begin to experiment with fire, including matches, lighters, and fireworks. Fire dangers include setting themselves on fire, starting a fire resulting in property damage, and causing injury to others trapped in the burning building. Fire safety must be reviewed frequently.

School-age children may have witnessed adults using, caring for, and storing firearms. They may find firearms in their house and want to show them to friends. Even when children have received instruction not to touch a firearm, research shows that most children are fascinated with a gun when they find it. They pick it up (Figure 6-20 ■) and even point it at friends. Firearms must be unloaded, locked with a trigger lock, and stored in a locked cabinet. Some states provide trigger locks free of charge. Ammunition should be kept in a separate locked storage area.

PSYCHOSOCIAL HEALTH

Promoting Self-Esteem

The school-age child is developing his or her sense of self-concept. The ability to make appropriate decisions, to problem solve, and to be successful contributes to his or her self-esteem. The school-age child also begins to address issues of body image and sexuality. The nurse can help parents promote the

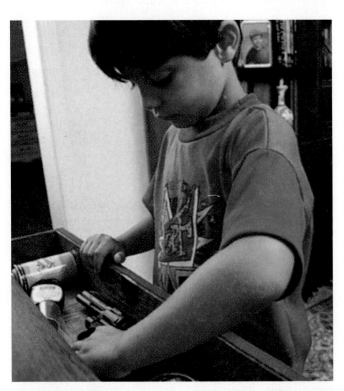

Figure 6-20. ■ Teach children never to touch guns without a parent present. Be sure to teach parents that all ammunition must be removed from guns and kept safely locked away from all weapons. Safety locks should always be in place on weapons.

school-age child's self-esteem by encouraging them to praise the child for successes. When a child experiences a failure, the parents should be encouraged to assist the child in problem solving and should promote a sense of accomplishment in seeking alternative solutions to address the problem.

Promoting Play

The school-age child has learned that everyone has a role and can take part in **cooperative play.** Cooperative play is organized play such as games at school or sports. School-age children understand that games have rules and are eager to follow them. They become frustrated when others do not follow the rules and may act out their frustration. School-age children learn competition and the concepts of winning, losing, teamwork, and doing your best. Children in this age group have an increasing desire to spend time with friends and begin to develop long-term relationships.

Providing Discipline

School-age children like to know the rules, and they generally want to play by the rules. They are gaining an understanding of "fair play" and may complain, "It's not fair," when they see peers getting special favors.

School-age children are learning how to solve problems and regulate their own activities. They can be invited to participate in finding solutions to problems among family or friends. Parents should be encouraged to ask for their children's input while still realizing that their children need their guidance and discipline.

This is often the stage at which hyperactivity, attention deficit, and anxiety disorders are identified. The nurse can provide information and referrals to help the parents set up the care they may need. (See also Chapter 16 ⚭.)

Bullying is also identified in the school-age child. Nurses can teach parents to interrupt bullying behaviors in their own children and to follow up if they hear of bullying in their child's school or play group.

NUTRITION

As children enter school, they begin to eat at least one meal a day away from home. Many school-age children have not been exposed to food outside their home. They may not like or eat the food found at school. Parents should thoroughly assess the child's likes and dislikes when deciding whether to purchase cafeteria food or to pack the child a lunch. Eating in a busy cafeteria may be distracting to 6-year-olds, and they may not have enough time to finish their meal. For this reason, nutritious after-school snacks and a balanced evening meal are essential. Eating at school makes mealtime a social occasion for school-age children. Table manners should be encouraged and reinforced in the home and at school. School-age children are capable of using utensils properly, contributing to conversation, listening when others speak, and assisting in serving food to others. Proper hygiene should also be encouraged.

Toward the end of the school-age period, there might be a period of rapid growth as the child prepares for adolescence. With this period of rapid growth comes an increase in appetite and the need for adequate nutrition.

Oral Health

Loss of primary teeth and the eruption of permanent teeth occur during the school-age period. The nurse can teach parents and the child proper ways of pulling these primary teeth. The nurse can also discourage improper ways of pulling teeth, such as tying a string to the tooth and attaching the other end of the string to a doorknob while the door is closed quickly. This method may cause further injury to the child's mouth, jaw, and head.

As the permanent teeth appear and the jaw line grows, the school-age child may have crooked teeth or a misaligned bite. Parents often consult an orthodontist during this period. If the orthodontist determines that the child will need braces, preliminary measures may be implemented in the school-age period.

Adolescent

HEALTH PROMOTION

Environmental Safety

Adolescents are at increased risk for injury related to their tendency toward risk-taking behavior and the belief that no harm can come to them (see Figure 5-7 ⬤⬤). In fact, though, motor vehicle crashes and suicide are the leading causes of adolescent death. The ability to drive a car gives the adolescent freedom from parental supervision. Although teenagers may have developed the skills to maneuver a car though traffic, they may not be mature enough to handle the responsibility. Conversation, use of cell phones, joking, and loud music are common when teens get together, and they cause distraction for the driver. The use of alcohol clouds judgment, resulting in great risk for accident and injury. The risk is not limited to the automobile. These same dangers and concerns relate to the operation of off-road vehicles, snowmobiles, jet skis, and motorcycles. The use of safety devices such as seat belts and helmets is important. Adult supervision can help only when the adult teaches and enforces safety rules.

Many teens participate in physically challenging sports such as soccer, football, baseball, basketball, track, and swimming. They may overestimate their endurance, competence, and athletic ability, causing them to take more risks. Proper training, supervision, and correct use of protective equipment may prevent unnecessary injuries.

Health Education

Many schools provide a health course for the adolescent. This course provides an opportunity for the educator to present topics related to the health care needs of the adolescent, while also assessing the health behaviors of the class. The nurse is an ideal educator for this type of program.

Topics covered in this class include decision making, **peer pressure** (influencing a person to follow the desire of another person or group), dating, sexuality and sexual intimacy, sexually transmitted diseases, substance abuse, mental health concerns such as depression and anorexia nervosa, and accident prevention. Because some of this content may be uncomfortable to present in a mixed-gender setting, students are often divided into male and female sections.

PSYCHOSOCIAL HEALTH

Promoting Self-Esteem

Teen suicide rates and violence are increasing. Teens face many issues today, including peer pressure to smoke, drink alcohol, take drugs, and participate in premarital sex. Many teens feel ill equipped to handle these issues. Adolescents need an opportunity to express their fears and frustrations. The nurse can provide strategies for managing these stressors.

Teens may seek social support by joining a gang to strike out at those they feel are against them. They may get involved in illegal activities as a result. Some teens turn the anger and violence inward and take their own lives. Parents need to keep the lines of communication open, know what their teen is doing at all times, and encourage nonviolent activities. Community resources are available to help parents faced with raising teens. For more information on issues of teen sexuality, see Chapter 18 ⬤⬤. For more information on substance abuse and psychosocial disorders of the adolescent, see Chapter 16 ⬤⬤.

Types of Play

The adolescent is rapidly making the transition from childhood play to adult play. As a result, team sports, extracurricular activities, and attending movies and concerts often occupy the adolescent's free time.

Peers

The adolescent begins to try out more risky adult activities, including car racing, motorcycle riding, and jet boating. Being with friends and peer groups soon becomes more important than spending time with parents. Teens look to each other for approval (Figure 6-21 ■). By late adolescence, male-female relationships are developing, and sexual encounters might be part of the "play." Unfortunately, other activities such as use of alcohol and illegal drugs might become part of the adolescent's recreational time. Nurses

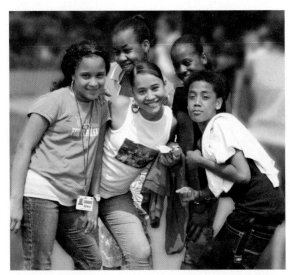

Figure 6-21. ■ Peers are the most important group among teens.

should help parents and teens prepare for the responsibilities and consequences of adult play.

Providing Discipline

Although teenagers are learning the important task of setting their own rules and boundaries, they still need guidance and discipline during this developmental stage. Remind parents of the value of positive feedback at this time. Praise can reinforce desired behaviors, such as keeping up with their studies, helping with tasks at home, and maintaining good hygiene.

This is a time to emphasize a few basic and crucial rules. Emphasize respect, and show respect for the teenager by never belittling the teen in front of peers. Discuss the teen's unacceptable behavior, rather than labeling him or her as a "bad person." Keep rules simple and fair (e.g., "Avoid risky behaviors that could hurt you and others.") Gradually increase the teen's independence as he or she exhibits more responsibility. Irresponsible behavior can be tied to a restriction in freedom. For example, if a teen deliberately stays out past curfew, the parent may restrict the teen from going out the following weekend. Try to discuss rules in terms of how they apply in the adult world. Teens are more likely to cooperate with behaviors that all adults should follow than with limits that seem like power plays by figures in authority.

NUTRITION

Meeting the nutritional needs of the adolescent is a challenge. The rapid growth spurt and increased muscle mass result in a need for 2,000 to 3,000 calories daily. Teens active in sports require an even higher caloric intake. Requirements for iron, calcium, zinc, and vitamins all increase. To meet these requirements, three meals per day, with nutritious snacks between meals, are needed (Abrams,

2001). Figure 6-22 ■ shows an example of a dietary screening survey for adolescents.

Calcium intake has been found to be particularly important during adolescence, and adequate intake has been linked with the prevention of osteoporosis. The deposition of calcium is five times greater prior to menarche than that of adult women. Adequate calcium and vitamin D during early adolescence is effective in enhancing bone mineral composition.

Adolescents can prepare much of their own food and frequently eat with friends. Their diet should contain protein, milk, fresh fruits, and vegetables daily. However, many adolescents choose high-calorie, high-fat, convenience foods. The adolescent should be taught to make healthy food choices. Nutritional teaching and counseling are most effective when conducted in a group setting with the teenager's peers.

Oral Health

During adolescence, individuals are at increased risk for caries. This risk is due to immature enamel, a diet high in refined carbohydrates and acid-containing beverages, and poorly established oral habits. The nurse should assess for and encourage regular dental check-ups, brushing, and flossing.

The adolescent may pierce his or her tongue, lip, cheek, or uvula. These piercings have been found to compromise oral and overall health. If they are done in nonaseptic conditions, disease transmission may occur. Such diseases include hepatitis, tuberculosis, tetanus, and other bacterial or viral infections. Other hazards of oral piercings include hemorrhage, airway obstruction, pain, scarring, tooth damage, speech impediment, and nerve damage. The nurse should assess a client's oral cavity for the presence of these piercings and include the risks and hazards in health promotion teaching.

ADOLESCENT SEXUALITY AND TEENAGE PREGNANCY

More than 50% of adolescent girls and 75% of adolescent boys report engaging in sexual intercourse before the age of 18. This high-risk behavior not only increases the incidence of teenage pregnancy; it also exposes the teens to sexually transmitted infections or diseases (STIs or STDs). Decreasing the incidence of adolescent pregnancy and STIs is an objective of the U.S. Department of Health and Human Services and of many school systems.

Peer pressure can lead the adolescent to experiment in high-risk activities. The combination of peer pressure, feelings of invincibility, and elevated sex hormones and sex drive may lead adolescents to engage in premarital sexual intercourse. Some begin to develop a monogamous relationship, at least for a while. Other teens fail to develop a close relationship with one person and move from partner to partner in a short period of time or have multiple partners at one time. Nearly half of

1. Which of these meals or snacks did you eat yesterday?
   _____ Breakfast
   _____ Morning snack
   _____ Lunch
   _____ Afternoon snack
   _____ Dinner/supper
   _____ Evening snack

2. Do you skip breakfast three or more times a week?
   _____ Yes _____ No

3. Do you skip lunch three or more times a week?
   _____ Yes _____ No

4. Do you skip dinner/supper three or more times a week?
   _____ Yes _____ No

5. Do you eat dinner/supper with your family four or more times a week?
   _____ Yes _____ No

6. Do you fix or buy the food for any of your family's meals?
   _____ Yes _____ No

7. Do you eat or take out a meal from a fast-food restaurant two or more times a week?
   _____ Yes _____ No

8. Are you on a special diet for medical reasons?
   _____ Yes _____ No

9. Are you a vegetarian?
   _____ Yes _____ No

10. Do you have any problems with your appetite, like not feeling hungry, or feeling hungry all the time?
    _____ Yes _____ No

11. Which of the following did you drink last week?
    _____ Regular soft drinks
    _____ Diet soft drinks
    _____ Fruit-flavored drinks
    _____ Whole milk
    _____ Reduced fat (2%) milk
    _____ Low-fat (1%) milk
    _____ Fat-free (skim) milk
    _____ Flavored milk (for example, chocolate, strawberry)
    _____ Coffee/tea
    _____ Tap/bottled water
    _____ Juice
    _____ Sports drinks
    _____ Beer/wine, hard liquor

12. Which of these foods did you eat last week?

Grains
   _____ Bread   _____ Cereal/grits
   _____ Rolls   _____ Popcorn
   _____ Bagels   _____ Noodles/pasta/rice
   _____ Crackers   _____ Tortillas
   _____ Other:_____

Vegetables
   _____ Corn   _____ Greens (collard, spinach)
   _____ Peas   _____ Green salad
   _____ Potatoes   _____ Broccoli
   _____ French fries   _____ Green beans
   _____ Tomatoes   _____ Carrots
   _____ Other:_____

Fruits
   _____ Apples/juice _____ Peaches
   _____ Oranges   _____ Pears
   _____ Grapefruit/juice   _____ Berries
   _____ Grapes/juice _____ Melon
   _____ Bananas
   _____ Other: _____

Milk and Other Dairy Products
   _____ Whole milk _____ Yogurt
   _____ Reduced-fat (2%) milk   _____ Cheese
   _____ Low-fat (1%) milk   _____ Ice cream
   _____ Fat-free (skim) milk _____ Flavored milk
   _____ Other:

Meat and Meat Alternatives
   _____ Beef/hamburger   _____ Sausage/bacon
   _____ Pork   _____ Peanut butter/nuts
   _____ Chicken   _____ Eggs
   _____ Turkey   _____ Dried beans
   _____ Fish   _____ Tofu
   _____ Cold cuts
   _____ Other: _____

Fats and Sweets
   _____ Cake/cupcake   _____ Chips
   _____ Pie   _____ Doughnuts
   _____ Cookies   _____ Candy
   _____ Other: _____

13. Do you have a working stove, oven, and refrigerator where you live?
    _____ Yes _____ No

14. Were there any days last month when your family didn't have enough food to eat or enough money to buy food?
    _____ Yes _____ No

15. Are you concerned about your weight?
    _____ Yes _____ No

16. Are you on a diet now to lose weight or to maintain your weight?
    _____ Yes _____ No

17. In the past year, have you tried to lose weight or control your weight by vomiting, taking diet pills or laxatives, or not eating?
    _____ Yes _____ No

18. Did you participate in physical activity (for example, walking or riding a bike) in the past week? If yes, on how many days and for how long?
    _____ Yes _____ No

19. Do you spend more than 2 hours per day watching television and videotapes or playing computer games? If yes, how man hours per day?
    _____ Yes _____ No

20. Do you take vitamin, mineral, herbal, or other dietary supplements (for example, protein powders)?
    _____ Yes _____ No

21. Do you smoke cigarettes or chew tobacco?
    _____ Yes _____ No

22. Do you ever use any of the following?
    _____ Alcohol/beer/wine
    _____ Steroids (without a doctor's prescription)
    _____ Street drugs (marijuana/speed/crack/heroin)

Figure 6-22. ■ Dietary screening for adolescents. (Reprinted from Story, M., Holt, K., & Sofka, D. (Eds.). (2002). *Bright futures in practice: Nutrition* (2nd ed.). Arlington, VA: National Center for Education in Maternal and Child Health and Georgetown University, Nutrition Tools Appendix. Used with permission.)

high school seniors report having had sexual intercourse. As mentioned, frequent sexual contact with multiple partners increases the exposure to STIs and the likelihood of pregnancy.

Teens in lower socioeconomic levels engage in sexual relations at nearly the same rate as other teens. However, they have a disproportionate number of teen pregnancies. The lower socioeconomic level adolescent may not have the same access to birth control measures as their counterparts in higher socioeconomic levels. They may not feel that higher education and career development are realistic goals. Instead, they may transition into adulthood by engaging in sexual intercourse and becoming parents. In contrast, teens in higher socioeconomic levels often have ready access to various forms of contraception. They may have been raised with the expectation that they will go on to college or a career before parenting. These teens may be more likely to use contraceptive methods or to terminate pregnancy if it occurs.

Unintended Pregnancy

An unfortunate issue that develops from sexual relationships among adolescents is unintended pregnancy. Pregnancy, occurring while the adolescent girl is in a period of rapid growth and physical maturation, puts additional stress on the body and increases the risk to her and the infant. Teen mothers have a higher incidence of complications such as gestational (pregnancy-induced) hypertension, gestational diabetes, and preterm labor. Early and regular prenatal care is essential to their health. However, the teen mother may deny or try to cover up the pregnancy for some time and not seek help.

Once pregnant, the teenage mother and father have some very difficult decisions to make. How should they tell their parents? Should they get married? Should the pregnancy be continued or terminated? Will the child be raised in the family? Will the child be adopted by another family? Some parents provide emotional and financial support when they discover their teen is pregnant. Other parents refuse any form of support, because they believe the teen has committed a "terrible sin."

If there were several sexual partners, the teen may not know the identity of the father. Even if she knows the father, he may or may not accept responsibility and offer support. The teen mother may not have the cognitive and emotional resources to make objective decisions for her own well-being or the well-being of her child.

NURSING CARE

PRIORITIES IN NURSING CARE

When assisting clients and their families with issues related to illness prevention and health promotion, the nurse should focus on recognizing environmental hazards that would place a child's health or safety at risk. The nurse should also teach parents and other caregivers to develop strategies to prevent injury or illness.

ASSESSING

The nurse plays an important role in assisting parents to learn and teach health-promoting behaviors. As children gain cognitive abilities and become increasingly responsible for their own wellness, the nurse can be involved in assessing the degree of ability the child has developed.

DIAGNOSING, PLANNING, AND IMPLEMENTING

Nursing diagnoses for health promotion and illness prevention might include:

- Deficient **K**nowledge related to unidentified or unmanaged environmental safety hazard
- Disturbed **T**hought Process related to deficits in reality orientation and problem-solving abilities due to immature cognitive abilities
- Imbalanced **N**utrition: More than Body Requirements, related to familial pattern of eating dinners and snacks at fast-food restaurants
- Compromised Family **C**oping related to lack of information about successful methods of providing discipline

Some outcomes for these diagnoses are as follows. The client and/or parent will:

- Identify current hazards in or around the home and develop a plan to protect the child and avoid injury
- Demonstrate the ability to make reasonable choices between two or more alternatives
- Exhibit an understanding of good nutrition by identifying the most healthful choices from a fast-food menu
- Explain why discipline helps the child and describe the steps the parent will take in upholding discipline

The nurse's role in providing support to these clients would include the following:

- Assess the child's gag reflex. *A present gag reflex gives an indication of a child's ability to swallow properly although aspiration may still occur.*
- Teach parent to feed an infant in an upright position and maintain this position for 30 minutes after feeding. *Aspiration can be avoided when the child is in an upright position.*
- Teach parent to remove small objects from the infant's or toddler's environment. *Small objects may become lodged in the child's airway.*
- Teach parents to observe for symptoms of aspiration: coughing, choking, excessive drooling. *Response time to aspiration is decreased with prompt symptom recognition.*

- Teach parents to assess the home environment for safety hazards and to prevent the child's access to hazardous areas. *Children are at increased risk for injury in presence of environmental hazards. Parents should be proactive in avoiding injuries. This includes a range of items: safety catches on medicine cabinets, locks on gun cabinets, and separate cupboards for alcoholic beverages.*
- Encourage the use of personal protective equipment. *Seat belts, bike helmets, knee and elbow pads, and so forth, can protect the child from injury. Teens who drive independently should be asked if they routinely use seat belts.*
- Encourage parents to attend a course that teaches life-saving techniques such as the Heimlich maneuver. *All parents and caregivers should know the Heimlich maneuver. The ability to perform the maneuver immediately may mean the difference between life and death.*
- Ask about the child's activities outside school. *The child's activities outside school give a clearer picture of behaviors that are health promoting (e.g., an outside sport) or risk creating (e.g., hours of video games each day).*
- Ask how the child likes school or what is his or her favorite activity at school. *This question can help create discussion about behavior issues or learning difficulties. It may also raise other psychosocial problems, such as low self-esteem.*
- Assess the child's ability to reason and make appropriate safety decisions. Observe the parent's ability to provide adequate care. *Assessment identifies level of ability to provide self-care. If the nurse observes a parent who is endangering the child by poor decisions, the nurse must report the behavior.*
- Teach parent and child the associated risks of behaviors that compromise personal health. Provide information in a nonjudgmental manner. *Knowledge of risks may lead to changed behaviors. A nonjudgmental approach is more easily accepted and leads to greater cooperation.*

EVALUATING

The care plan is revised until expected outcomes are achieved. To evaluate the effectiveness of interventions, the nurse would gather data concerning:

- The parent/client's injury prevention plan
- Identification of environmental hazards
- Avoidance of aspiration
- The client's decisions regarding self-care behaviors.

NURSING PROCESS CARE PLAN
Pediatric Client with Unintentional Poisoning

A parent of a 3-year-old male child calls the poison control center and states that her child had been playing in the neighbor's yard. The child and his friend went into the neighbor's garage, and the child came running out suddenly, crying. The parent noticed a white powdery substance around the child's mouth and a foamy substance in the child's mouth. The parent asks for assistance.

Assessment. The following data should be collected as soon as possible.

- Condition of pupils
- Moderate amount of irritation of the mucous membranes with edema and erythema
- Vital signs: T 98.6° F tympanic, P 96, R 24, BP 90/60
- Parent and child deny nausea, vomiting, or diarrhea
- Pain: child is experiencing mouth and throat pain
- Description of possible toxic substances

Nursing Diagnosis. The following important nursing diagnosis (among others) is established for this client:

- Risk for Injury related to possible poisoning and the presence of toxic substances and physical manifestations

Expected Outcome

- Client will not have complications related to ingestion of toxic substances

Planning and Implementation

- Obtain a specimen of the substance found on the child's face and in his mouth. *Identifying the substance assists in the treatment process.*
- If the poisonous substance is suspected to be corrosive or a hydrocarbon, rinse the mouth with water. *Vomiting should not be induced if there is evidence of mucosal irritation because vomiting would cause further damage.*
- If the poisonous substance is suspected to be medication, induce vomiting. *Vomiting removes the poison from the child's system.*
- Observe for signs of respiratory obstruction and signs of shock. *Various substances may cause respiratory obstruction or shock.*

Evaluation. The client does not experience complications related to poisoning.

Critical Thinking in the Nursing Process

1. What substances, commonly found in a garage, could the child have ingested?
2. What prevention methods would be appropriate for the nurse to discuss with the parent?
3. What is the expected emotional response from the parent following this event?

Note: Discussion of Critical Thinking questions appears in Appendix I.

Note: The reference and resource listings for this and all chapters have been compiled at the back of the book.

Chapter Review

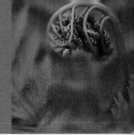

 KEY TERMS by Topic

Use the audio glossary feature of either the CD-ROM or the Companion Website to hear the correct pronunciation of the following key terms.

Illness Prevention
illness prevention, primary prevention, secondary prevention, tertiary prevention

Health Promotion
health promotion, health, spanking

Infant
choking

Toddler
parallel play

Preschooler
associative play

School-Age Child
latch-key children, cooperative play

Adolescent
peer pressure

KEY Points

■ It is important for the nurse to use each contact with the client and family as a time to assess and promote health behaviors and illness prevention.

■ The nurse promotes healthy individuals, families, and communities by role modeling appropriate healthy behavior, providing encouragement to family members, reinforcing the need for change, and recognizing positive efforts.

■ The nurse is involved in three levels of illness prevention: primary, secondary, and tertiary. Primary prevention helps the child avoid illness. Secondary prevention allows for early detection and treatment of illness. Tertiary prevention involves treating illnesses to prevent complications.

■ An essential nursing intervention is health promotion, which includes promoting environmental safety and psychosocial health.

■ Nutritional assessment, teaching, and monitoring of the child's nutritional status are important nursing tasks.

■ Nursing measures to protect the infant include preventing injury from falls and aspiration, promoting the development of trust, and implementing appropriate feeding measures whether formula feeding, breastfeeding, or introducing solid foods.

■ The nurse can be instrumental in protecting the toddler from injuries during play, promoting appropriate toilet training, and discussing methods of discipline with parents.

■ Preschoolers begin to be independent, and the nurse can assist in health promotion by discussing protecting the child from strangers, promoting the use of seat belts, and helping both parent and child to make nutritional food choices.

■ The nurse can help the school-age child take responsibility for his or her own safety by discussing with the child how to stay safe at school, during sporting activities, and after school, especially when home alone.

■ Adolescents frequently compromise their safety by participating in risk-taking activities. The nurse can provide teaching to the adolescent regarding risks associated with certain behaviors such as sexual contact and substance abuse.

 EXPLORE Media Link

Additional interactive resources for this chapter can be found on the Companion Website at www. prenhall. com/ adams.

Click on Chapter 6 and "Begin" to select the activities for this chapter.

For chapter-related NCLEX®-style questions and an audio glossary, access the accompanying CD-ROM in this book.

Animations:

Children and obesity

The importance of physical activity

∞ FOR FURTHER Study

For more information on *Healthy People 2000* and *Healthy People 2010*, see Chapter 1.

See Chapter 5 for additional information on safety and life span issues; see Box 5-5 for some age-specific communication techniques.

For pediatric procedures, see Chapter 8.

See Chapter 10 for more information on childhood diseases and prevention methods.

For more information on psychosocial issues and disorders, see Chapter 16.

See Chapter 17 for more information about gastrointestinal issues.

For more information on issues of teen sexuality, see Chapter 18.

Critical Thinking Care Map

Caring for a Client with Inadequate Nutrition

NCLEX-PN® Focus Area: Physiological Integrity: Basic Care and Comfort

Case Study: An adolescent is being interviewed by the school nurse. She is asked to complete a 24-hour nutrition diary. For breakfast, the teen writes "none." For lunch, the teen writes "chips and cola." For dinner, the teen writes "chicken fingers, fries, and sweet tea." She also states that this is fairly typical for her daily diet.

Nursing Diagnosis: Imbalanced <u>N</u>utrition, Less than Body Requirements

COLLECT DATA

Subjective	Objective
_____	_____
_____	_____
_____	_____
_____	_____
_____	_____
_____	_____

Would you report this? Yes/No

If yes, to: _____

Nursing Care

_____
_____
_____
_____
_____
_____
_____
_____
_____
_____

How would you document this? _____
_____
_____
_____

Compare your documentation to the sample provided in Appendix I.

Data Collected
(use only those that apply)

- Current weight 100 pounds
- T 98.8° F, P 66, R 12, BP 110/60
- Lungs sounds clear bilaterally
- Previous weight 110 pounds
- States typical diet is low in calories
- Skips breakfast
- Deep tendon reflexes (DTR) 2+
- All peripheral pulses present
- Chips and cola for lunch
- Chicken fingers, fries, and sweet tea for dinner

Nursing Interventions
(use only those that apply; list in priority order)

- Present a sample daily meal plan.
- Discuss the hazards of obesity.
- Refer to a dietitian prn.
- Use the food pyramid to discuss essential nutrients.
- Discuss exercise as a method of weight reduction.
- Discuss ways to overcome difficulties related to food preparation and food acquisition.
- Explain importance of nutrition during adolescence.
- Consider hospitalization and feeding tube for nutrition.

NCLEX-PN® Exam Preparation

1 The nurse is preparing to give a hepatitis B vaccine to a newborn. The order reads hepatitis B vaccine 10 mcg IM. The vaccine is supplied in 20 mcg/mL. How many mL will the nurse give? _____ milliliters

2 The registered nurse discusses a teaching plan for primary prevention for a newborn with the LPN. Which of the following interventions would be appropriate?

1. Immunizations
2. Bimonthly visits with the pediatrician
3. Treating diaper rash
4. Changing the formula to a soy product

3 The adolescent admits to being sexually active. Which of the following secondary prevention methods is appropriate for the client?

1. Monthly pregnancy tests
2. Yearly Pap smears
3. Attending an abstinence support group
4. Increasing iron in the diet

4 The toddler has been diagnosed with otitis media. The nurse assists in providing tertiary prevention. Which of the following interventions is a method of tertiary prevention?

1. Hearing screening
2. Administering cephalosporins
3. Keeping the child from interacting with other children for a period of 48 hours
4. Reading books to the child

5 A new mother asks the nurse to suggest appropriate toys for her infant child. Which of the following are appropriate choices?

1. Balloons on ribbons
2. Stuffed animals of any variety
3. Plastic keys on a plastic ring
4. Bright music box attached to the outside of the crib

6 The nurse is assisting the mother of a 6-month-old infant to make appropriate solid food choices. Which of the following could be suggested? Choose all that apply.

1. Rice cereal mixed with breast milk
2. Cheerios
3. Thinly sliced hot dogs
4. Pureed bananas
5. Commercially prepared vegetable puree

7 The nurse has an order to administer *Haemophilus b* conjugate vaccine. He should document all of the following, except:

1. Lot number of the vial used
2. Expiration date of the vial
3. Site of the injection
4. Temperature and blood pressure at time of injection

8 A 17-year-old client states that she smokes and is unwilling to attend smoking cessation classes. Choose the most appropriate nursing intervention.

1. Contact social services to report parental neglect.
2. Discuss reducing the number of cigarettes daily.
3. Obtain a prescription for the nicotine patch.
4. Inform the client that she will have to deal with lung cancer later in life.

9 A 16-year-old female visits the family physician. Height is 5 feet 1 inch. Current weight is 159 pounds. The nurse is concerned about the risk for obesity when the client reveals which of the following?

1. Her single mother works two jobs and is rarely home.
2. Client enjoys smoothies at breakfast and rarely snacks.
3. Client states she is doing well academically.
4. Client has two siblings and lives with her mother and grandmother.

10 The school nurse recognizes pinpoint pupils and drowsiness for several days in a student. Which of the following drugs might the nurse suspect the teen is abusing?

1. Narcotics
2. Amphetamines
3. Depressants
4. Hallucinogens

Answers for NCLEX-PN® Review and Critical Thinking questions appear in Appendix I.

Thinking Strategically About...

You are an LPN/LVN employed by a home health agency. At 0800, you arrive at the office to receive your assignment. You are expected to visit the clients on your assignment and report to the supervising RN by telephone. You can organize your time as you choose. The clients are all within a 3-mile radius from the home health agency office.

The first client, Jenny, is a 3-year-old who suffered a near drowning 6 months ago. She has severe neurologic damage and is in a persistent vegetative state. Her family provides all necessary care in their home with the help of a certified nursing assistant (CNA). A nurse visits on a weekly basis to evaluate the child's condition and make any necessary changes in the care plan.

Your second client is 18-year-old Marie. She delivered her first baby, Jason, 3 days ago. She is not married, has limited financial resources, and has few close friends. She was discharged from the hospital yesterday. She requested a visit from the home health nurse because she has never taken care of a baby and is unsure of herself.

Your third client is Juan, a 13-year-old who received a spinal cord injury in a car crash. Juan is being transferred from the hospital's surgical unit to the rehabilitation unit. The plan is for Juan to go home in approximately 6 weeks. The home health agency where you are employed will be providing home visits at that time. In preparation for Juan's discharge, the house and yard need to be assessed for safety and accommodation for Juan's wheelchair and other equipment necessary for his care. You are to go to Juan's home and complete a home assessment that will be used in a planning session this afternoon with Juan's family, rehabilitation personnel, and the home health supervisor.

CRITICAL THINKING

- What questions should be asked of Marie to add the intellectual standard of depth to your assessment of her coping with being a new mother?
- What questions should be asked of Juan's mother to add the intellectual standard of breadth to your assessment of her house?

- What questions should you ask Jenny's CNA to add the intellectual standard of precision to your assessment of Jenny's nutritional status?

COLLABORATIVE CARE

- What agency should Marie be referred to that will provide support and monitoring of this young family?

MANAGEMENT OF CARE AND PRIORITIES IN NURSING CARE

- In what order will you visit these clients?
- What is your rationale for prioritizing care?

DELEGATING

- When visiting Jenny, how would you determine whether the care delegated to the CNA has been performed appropriately?

COMMUNICATION AND CLIENT TEACHING

- How would you identify what instruction and supervision needs to be provided to the CNA caring for Jenny?
- What follow-up plan would be important in ensuring that Maria has understood the information you have provided regarding infant care?

DOCUMENTING AND REPORTING

- After you have assessed Marie and her baby, if you believe she is at a high risk for neglecting him, what should you do?
- What steps should you take after monitoring the status of Jenny's care?

CULTURAL CARE STRATEGIES

- If Juan is of Hispanic origin, what aspects of his culture should be taken into consideration when planning care for him?

Care of the Ill Child

UNIT II

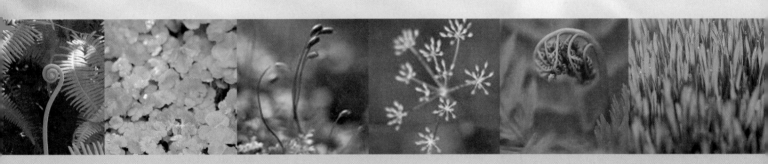

Chapter 7

Care of the Hospitalized or Chronically Ill Child

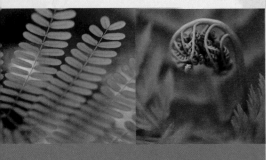

HEALTH PROMOTION ISSUE:
Let's Pretend Hospital

NURSING PROCESS CARE PLAN:
Child Undergoing
Hospitalization for Surgery

NURSING CARE PLAN CHART:
The Child and the Surgical
Experience

CRITICAL THINKING CARE MAP:
Nursing Care of a Child with
Bilateral Hip Splints on a
Rehabilitation Unit

BRIEF Outline

Role of the LPN/LVN
HOSPITALIZED CHILD
Age-Specific Preparation for
Hospitalization
Admission Process
Preparation for Procedures
Care of the Child Before and
After Surgery
Preparation for Discharge

Nursing Care
CHRONICALLY ILL CHILD
Care at Home
Care at School
Rehabilitation
Long-Term Care
Care of the Caregivers
Nursing Care

LEARNING Outcomes

After completing this chapter, you will be able to:
1. Define key terms.
2. Describe how to prepare children for hospitalization.
3. Describe how to prepare parents for their child's hospitalization.
4. Describe the preoperative and postoperative care of children.
5. Describe how to prepare parents and children for discharge.
6. Describe important aspects of care for the chronically ill child and the family.
7. Describe the role of the LPN/LVN in caring for children with acute or chronic disorders.
8. Discuss how to care for children in the home or in long-term care settings.

Community-based nursing practice involves caring for the client and family in any setting. It is generally agreed that the home is the ideal place to care for a child with an **illness** (state of disease or sickness). Illness may be physical or psychological. It may be characterized as **acute** (having rapid onset, severe symptoms, and a short course), **chronic** (long-lasting, slowly progressing), or **terminal** (final, fatal).

Sometimes a child is ill outside the home setting. For example, a child might be healthy when he or she goes to school but become ill during the day. The child might have a chronic condition such as asthma that does not prevent him or her from attending school but that may require care while at school. A child with an acute disorder may require hospitalization. Some children with complex illnesses may not be able to leave home or might be placed in a long-term care setting away from home. The nurse must be prepared to work with other professionals to plan and implement the best care possible for the child and family in any environment.

A child with a minor illness or injury is commonly cared for at home. Parents recall their own upbringing and apply the concepts they learned to care for their own children. For example, if their mother provided them with chicken noodle soup and ginger ale when they had an upset stomach, parents will probably fix these same foods for their children who are ill. If a child has a fever, parents may provide an over-the-counter antipyretic medication, encourage fluid intake, and allow the child to rest.

If the symptoms become worse or do not improve in a reasonable period of time, the parents might seek additional medical attention. The majority of illnesses and injuries will not warrant hospitalization and therefore the child will return home to be cared for by the parents, who will be responsible for administering medication and other prescribed treatments.

When parents have sought medical attention, the nurse should provide detailed instructions about the illness and medical treatment. These instructions generally involve cleanliness, nutrition and fluids, rest, and

medications. Parents can also benefit from teaching about preventing the transmission of the illness to others. Symptoms of complications and follow-up care also need to be discussed.

If the child's illness is serious or acute, it may be necessary to admit him or her to the hospital. Admitting a child to the hospital is a stressful event for the child, as well as for the parents and siblings. The severity of the child's illness might require that the child be admitted for emergency or diagnostic procedures, treatment, surgery, and rehabilitation. The more prepared the child and family are for the hospitalization, the less stress they will experience. This chapter addresses the key issues in caring for the child who is acutely ill or chronically ill in a variety of settings.

Role of the LPN/LVN

The role of the LPN/LVN is to assist in the care of the child. For example, in the office or clinic, the LPN/LVN collects data about the child and family (see Chapter 4 ⬥), assists with diagnostic procedures, and provides instructions for home care or an upcoming hospitalization. At school, the LPN/LVN assists with health screening such as vision or scoliosis detection, administers prescribed medications, cares for the ill child until parents arrive, and provides health teaching, such as hand washing, in the classroom. In the hospital, the LPN provides direct care by assisting with activities of daily living (ADLs) and administers medications within the legal scope of practice. The LPN may use a pediatric admission form to obtain information about the developmental level of the child and can be used to maintain the child's daily patterns and preferences (Figure 7-1 ■). The nurse can help the child through **therapeutic play** (play that allows the individual to deal with fears associated with the health care experience). The nurse can also reinforce rehabilitation therapies and encourage health promotion activities. The LPN/LVN provides verbal and written explanations about plans for discharge.

HOSPITALIZED CHILD

Hospitalization of a child causes stress and anxiety for clients and families. It is the responsibility of the nurse to lessen the stress to the extent possible. When a child is hospitalized, the nursing responsibility seems greater. It is difficult to provide detailed instruction to children who, because of their age, are unable to fully comprehend, or participate in, their care.

Parents might have feelings of fear, guilt, or anger about their child's hospitalization. The two parents may not agree

on treatment. Parents may experience conflict between the need to continue working and the need to be with their child who is ill. Siblings are curious about what is happening to their brother or sister. They might feel responsible for the illness or be fearful that their sibling might die.

Family patterns, structure, culture, and ethnicity (see Chapter 4 ⬥) may affect family functioning when a child is to be hospitalized. Some families may be heavily involved

Infancy (Birth To 1 Year)

Motor / Sensory
- ☐ Follows objects 180°
- ☐ Reaches for objects
- ☐ Smiles / laughs
- ☐ Passes hand to hand
- ☐ Rolls over
- ☐ Sits
- ☐ Crawls
- ☐ Stands
- ☐ Walks

Nutrition
- ☐ Breast-fed
- ☐ Bottle
- ☐ Cup
- ☐ Cereal
- ☐ Baby food
- Frequency of feeding _____
- _____
- ☐ Other _____
- _____

Sleep
- ☐ Crib   ☐ Sleeps alone
- ☐ Bed   ☐ With parent
- ☐ Naps
- ☐ Sleeping pattern _____

Habits
- ☐ Sucks thumb
- ☐ Favorite toy or blanket?

Elimination   Last void _____ Last B.M. _____
Other _____ No of B.M.'s a day? _____
Assessment appropriate for age? ☐ Yes ☐ No
Comments _____

Toddler Through Pre-School (13 Months To 5 Years)

Motor / Sensory
- ☐ Walks
- ☐ Climbs steps
- ☐ Vocalizes
- ☐ Dresses self
- ☐ Bathes self
- ☐ Brushes teeth
- ☐ Combs hair
- ☐ Ties a bow

Nutrition
Does child feed self? ☐ Yes ☐ No
- ☐ Finger foods   ☐ Spoon
- ☐ Fork   ☐ Knife
Does child drink from?
- ☐ Bottle ☐ Cup
- Frequency   ☐ Three meals a day
- ☐ Nap and/or bed time snacks
- Diet   ☐ Regular
- ☐ Other _____
- _____

Play Habits   ☐ Nursery school ☐ Baby-sitter ☐ Home
Favorite games, toys, etc. _____ ☐ Pet
Assessment appropriate for age?   ☐ Yes   ☐ No

Sleep
- ☐ Crib   ☐ Sleeps alone
- ☐ With parent
- ☐ Other _____
- Has child slept away from home?
- ☐ Often
- ☐ Rarely
- ☐ Never
- ☐ Sleeping pattern _____
- _____

Elimination
- ☐ Is child toilet trained?
- ☐ Bowel
- ☐ Bladder
- ☐ Partially
- ☐ Toilet
- ☐ Potty chair
- Last void? _____
- Last B.M.? _____
- Frequency of B.M? _____

Developmental Section
Pediatric Admission Assessment Record

School Age (6 To 11 Years) And Adolescent (12 To 16 Years)

Motor / Sensory
- ☐ Ambulates well
- ☐ Other _____

Sleep
Bedtime? _____
Arise? _____
Bed-wetting? _____
Nightmares? _____

Education
Grade level? _____
Learning disability? _____
_____

Academics
- ☐ Above ☐ Average
- ☐ Below

Habits
- ☐ Smoking   ☐ Thumbsucking
- ☐ Alcohol   ☐ Tantrums
- ☐ Drugs   ☐ Other _____
Socialization Relationship to?
- Parent? ☐ Good   ☐ Poor
- Peers? ☐ Good   ☐ Poor
Hobbies Athletic? ☐ Yes ☐ No
- ☐ Other _____

Assessment appropriate for age?   ☐ Yes   ☐ No

Nutrition
Diet _____
Frequency? _____
Snacks? _____
Likes/dislikes? _____
Dental visits?   ☐ Yes   ☐ No
Condition of teeth?
- ☐ Poor   ☐ Good
- ☐ Appliances
- ☐ Comments _____

Elimination
Last Void? _____
Last B.M.? _____
Frequency? _____
Comments _____

Menses
Age started _____
Last period _____
Problems _____
Vaginal discharge? _____
Sexually active ☐ Yes ☐ No
Oral contraceptives? _____
Exposed to disease? _____
Is there a possibility you could be pregnant? _____

NURSE'S SIGNATURE

DATE

CLIENT IDENTIFICATION

Figure 7-1. ■ Portion of a pediatric admission form showing developmental level and habits of children.

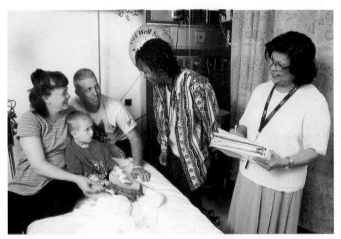

Figure 7-2. ■ Children and their families need to be actively involved in decisions about care when appropriate. Here, the family and staff come together to discuss the child's care in a positive and honest manner.

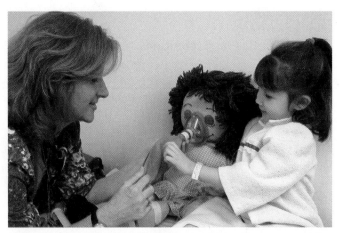

Figure 7-3. ■ A child life specialist works with children, using therapeutic play and helping to familiarize them with the procedures they will undergo. Role-playing is one type of therapeutic play. Putting a mask on a doll gives this child some mastery over an upcoming surgical experience. It is important for children to see and touch medical equipment in order to reduce their fears of the unknown.

in their child's care (Figure 7-2 ■; Box 7-1 ■). Others may prevent siblings from visiting a hospitalized child.

Sensory deficits can increase anxiety for a child who is hospitalized. For example, a child who is deaf may communicate easily at home with their parents, but difficulties arise when caregivers do not know sign language. The hospital may take special measures to provide an interpreter who knows sign language (see sign language in Appendix VII 🔗), but the interpreter is likely to participate only when decisions and plans are being made. Nurses need to be creative to prevent children who are deaf from feeling isolated. Quality nursing care requires that nurses understand the importance of families, cultures, and special needs.

Many larger hospitals have special units designed to care for the pediatric client and the family. These might include special pediatric intensive care units (PICUs);

<table>
<tr><td>BOX 7-1</td><td>CULTURAL PULSE POINTS</td></tr>
</table>

Mexican American Family Support System

The Mexican American family is a strong support system. Although the father is the spokesperson for the family, extended family members may be present during hospitalization. The nurse should include them in explanations about health care.

With every family, it is important for the nurse to try to answer certain questions:

■ Who is the decision maker?

■ Is the family expressive or stoic about their feelings?

■ What kind of physical presence does the family expect or want to have with the hospitalized child?

preoperative and postoperative care units, pediatric oncology, pediatric orthopedics, pediatric burn units, and pediatric rehabilitation units. They may also have overnight facilities (e.g., the Ronald McDonald House) where families can stay during the child's hospitalization. Nurses with expertise in the care of children team with respiratory therapists and physical therapists. A **child life specialist** (trained professional who plans therapeutic activities for the hospitalized child) may be available to plan age-appropriate activities to assist children in working through their feelings about hospitalization, their specific illness, and surgery (Figure 7-3 ■).

Smaller hospitals may not have the luxury of these special units. In small hospitals, children are generally admitted to a private room and cared for by the same nurses and staff as the adult clients. There might be days or weeks when the small hospital has no inpatient pediatric client. Nurses must have adequate resources available to meet the needs of the pediatric client, without interfering with the care of adult clients. If a child life specialist is not available, the LPN/LVN may assist with therapeutic play techniques. Table 7-1 ■ identifies some therapeutic play techniques that might be used.

Age-Specific Preparation for Hospitalization

The reason for hospitalization helps determine guidelines for preparing families for hospitalization activities. If the hospitalization will be for an elective surgery or diagnostic procedure, written and verbal teaching might be coupled with a

TABLE 7-1	
Therapeutic Play Techniques	
TECHNIQUE	**INTERVENTION**
Drawing	■ Use a simple gender-specific picture and have the child draw what he or she thinks is his or her medical problem. ■ Use drawings to explain care, procedures, and surgery. ■ Ask the child, "Tell me about your picture." Be alert for child's emotions such as fear or sadness.
Music	■ Encourage family to bring tapes of favorite music. ■ Use music to relax and reduce stress. ■ If family is unable to visit, have them tape messages to the child. ■ Play time could include musical instruments and singing.
Pets	■ Animals foster relaxation. Safety rules must be followed, and pet must be approved inside the facility.
Puppets	■ Use puppet to ask the child questions. Children may answer puppet instead of person. ■ Perform skits to teach child necessary care.
Role Playing	■ Provide dolls and medical equipment. Help child role-play procedures and/or surgery. ■ Use toys that foster expression of emotions. Dolls with disabilities similar to the child's are available.
Stories	■ Read or make up stories to explain procedure, surgery, or specific illness. ■ Have child make up a story about a picture. ■ Talk about the child's feelings identified in the story.

facility tour. If the hospitalization is for a chronic illness and the client has a history of hospitalizations, the preparation might include a review of past experiences and instruction on any new experiences. In an emergency situation, little time is available, so preparation might be limited to verbal instruction given under stress. In part, the age of the child also determines the method and amount of preparation. The Health Promotion Issue on pages 142 and 143 describes one community's approach to making hospitals feel safe to children.

INFANT

In early infancy, preparation of the child would not be effective and therefore is not necessary. Parents and siblings, however, need instruction and reassurance. It is difficult for them to witness painful procedures (e.g., IV sticks) being performed on the baby. It might be best for only one parent to remain with the infant and the other parent to wait with siblings at this time. The nurse must observe the parents for signs that they might faint (pale, diaphoretic skin and light-headedness) if they are allowed to remain with the infant during these times. A chair should be provided for parents to prevent falls. Following procedures or treatments where restraints are used, the parent should comfort the infant. See Chapter 8 ⚭ for more information regarding assisting with procedures in infants.

The infant needs close supervision while in the hospital. Unless the infant is sleeping, family or trained hospital personnel should be in attendance at all times.

Separation Anxiety

At about 6 months of age and older, the infant is able to identify primary caregivers and develops anxiety when separated from them. This anxiety may also occur in the toddler. **Separation anxiety** is apprehension due to the removal of significant persons or items from the environment. The infant or toddler progresses through three stages of separation: protest, despair, and detachment.

PROTEST STAGE.   When the primary caregiver leaves the child, he or she feels alone and abandoned. The child expresses his or her feelings of being abandoned by loud protests, including screaming and crying. The approach of a nurse or other stranger may result in increased protest. Because of these outbursts, the child may be labeled as "bad."

DESPAIR STAGE.   The crying gradually stops and the child enters the second stage of separation anxiety, despair. The child may fall asleep for a short time. When awake, the child may appear sad and depressed, and lie quietly, not playing with toys. The child may be labeled as "adjusting."

When the parents return, the child may regress to loud protests at the next separation.

DETACHMENT STAGE.   In the third stage, detachment, the child becomes more interested in the environment, and plays and behaves as "usual." He displays disinterest in parents and significant others. The child appears to have adjusted to the separation. However, the nurse must understand that the child is using a defense mechanism to cope with the pain of separation. If the child remains in the detachment stage, long-term and often permanent disruption of parent-child bonding may occur. In this case, professional help is needed to heal the parent-child relationship.

Promoting a Sense of Security

It is important to encourage as much parental involvement as possible. If parents are unable to remain with the child, other familiar adults may help reduce separation anxiety. Leaving the child with a favorite toy or blanket may help ensure a feeling of security. If the parents will be absent for some time, leaving a picture can help the child feel connected to the parents. Parents should be encouraged to talk to the child about leaving them for a short time, indicating that they will return. Even though the child may not understand the situation, honest communication from the parents helps develop trust. Parents should be discouraged from "slipping away when the child is distracted" because this can break the trust bond.

TODDLER

The toddler is beginning to understand that people get sick and that, in a short time, they get better. Toddlers have no understanding of cause and effect and may think that something they said or did caused the illness. The toddler is beginning to identify body parts and can point to "where it hurts."

Remember that toddlers use magical thinking in their mental processing. Seeing other children with tubes, dressings, or IVs, toddlers might think something bad or mysterious has happened to the children and become afraid it will happen to them as well. It is important to tell toddlers that the treatments they (or others) are having will fix their body and "make it better." Instruction needs to be brief and given just prior to the procedure. If the procedure will be painful, toddlers need to be told that it will hurt but that holding still will help. If possible, a parent should be present to support the child emotionally.

Toddlers are very attached to their parents, and separation still causes extreme anxiety. For more information, see the section on Separation Anxiety in this chapter. Parents should be encouraged to be present as much as possible and to participate in care. Besides pictures of parents, it may be helpful to have audiotapes or other reminders left with children when the parents are absent. A favorite toy or blanket may help the toddler feel more comfortable.

Unless they are sleeping, toddlers require one-to-one supervision. This can be provided by the parents, family, volunteers, assistive personnel, or nurses. It is critical for safe care that staffing be provided to allow for this level of supervision.

PRESCHOOLER

The preschooler is learning about safety and daily practices to keep healthy. To the extent possible, following routine practices in the hospital should be encouraged. Preschoolers are beginning to think about cause and effect but may not be correct in the association. Preschoolers might think that something they did caused the illness. For example, if a preschooler did not pick up his toys as his mother instructed and then later vomited, he might think he became sick because he had not obeyed his mother. Preschoolers need reassurance that the illness or injury is not their fault.

Although preschoolers can be away from parents for a brief period of time, they are easily frightened by new people and experiences. Parents should be encouraged to participate in care and reinforce instructions provided by the nurse. Preschoolers may be left unattended for a few minutes but generally should be supervised at all times. Familiar objects (Figure 7-4 ■) continue to provide a sense of security for the preschooler. Rituals and family routines should continue as much as possible.

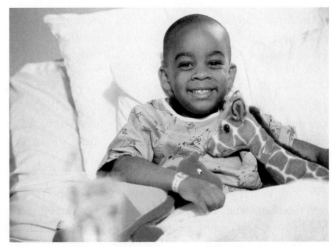

Figure 7-4. ■ This child has brought a favorite toy from home to make the hospital environment feel more secure and familiar. (Getty Images, Inc. Taxi, Ken Chernus.)

HEALTH PROMOTION ISSUE

LET'S PRETEND HOSPITAL

The elementary school nurse contacts the pediatric unit of a local hospital. She has assessed several students exhibiting signs and symptoms of anxiety prior to scheduled surgical procedures. These students have unrealistic expectations about the hospital. They do not have correct information about what will happen to them at the hospital. They seem overly fearful and express dread about going to the hospital. The school nurse has also heard some of the students express negative emotions about nurses and doctors. Although she can manage each student as the need arises, she feels that all children would benefit from instruction about what happens to them at the hospital. The school nurse would like to collaborate with the staff of the pediatric unit to develop a program to familiarize children with the hospital in an effort to decrease their anxiety.

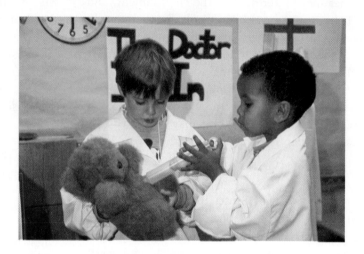

DISCUSSION

Unfamiliar experiences, often perceived as a threat, produce feelings of dread, apprehension, anxiety, and fear in children. Anxiety in its mild form serves as a warning signal, allowing the individual to manage the situation appropriately. However, when anxiety levels rise, the individual may become incapable of coping. Symptoms of anxiety can include but are not limited to tachycardia, tachypnea, increased perspiration, decreased mental acuity, gastrointestinal upset, increased urination, difficulty sleeping, dizziness, restlessness, and headache. The client may also feel helpless or preoccupied with the situation causing the anxiety. They may also demonstrate some type of regressive behavior.

Anxiety may be classified as mild, moderate, or severe. Children and parents can be taught to recognize the symptoms of anxiety and implement anxiety-reducing behaviors before the anxiety levels rises. Removing unnecessary stimuli from the anxious child is a simple method for easing their symptoms.

Recognizing potential anxiety-producing situations and taking steps to prevent the development of anxiety in children is a valuable goal for the health care provider. If a child is oriented to his or her environment and aware of the surroundings, familiarization is increased and comfort is promoted. In a 1984 study, researchers studied the fears of children related to medical events and their medical knowledge. Two groups were studied. One group attended a mock hospital event and the other did not. Children who attended the Let's Pretend Hospital event verbalized fewer fears and greater medical knowledge.

PLANNING AND IMPLEMENTATION

Following several organizational meetings with the school nurse, hospital representatives, and faculty from a school of nursing, a plan is developed to present a "Let's Pretend Hospital" to the community.

Who Presents the Program?

Event organizers should include representatives from a local hospital, the school nurse association, and representatives of a school of nursing to include nursing students, faculty and staff, media relations, campus security, and maintenance.

Who Attends Let's Pretend Hospital?

Students from area elementary school can be invited to attend this field trip offered free of charge. The students should be of a developmental age to appreciate and enjoy the activity. Kindergarteners or first graders would most likely benefit most from the learning activity that engages the imagination.

What Happens at the Event?

Let's Pretend Hospital should most likely be a multiday event in order to accommodate the number of area students who will register. Any area of the hospital that a child may encounter should be represented. The admissions office teaches the child the procedure for getting registered to the hospital. The child and her parent can fill out paperwork, answer questions, and have a hospital identification band applied. In the emergency room, the child explores situations that might bring them to the hospital in an emergency situation. Assessment techniques are described as well as procedures such as stitches and casting. In the lab the child learns about various diagnostic tests. They are allowed to handle blood tubes, agar plates, cotton swabs, and syringes. They can look at bacteria under a microscope. A client room is decorated colorfully and brightly. Students are able to "ride" on the hospital bed, play with hospital food on a hospital tray, and interact with nurses in cartoon character scrubs. The operating room is set up with green drapes, instruments, and staff dressed in scrubs. Children learn about the environment as well as the effects of anesthesia. In the x-ray department students can view broken bones under black lights and strobe lights. Finally, in the discharge area children hear about discharge teaching. Offering a tour of a real ambulance would be both exciting and educational for the children. A safety room can also be offered to teach children fire safety, poison safety, and stranger safety in a fun, interactive environment.

Where is the Event Conducted?

Let's Pretend Hospital should be conducted outside of the "real" hospital setting. Options for settings would include community centers, churches, or a school of nursing.

What are Specific Supplies?

The event is planned with a blend of realism, creativity, and fun. All activities and environments should be nonthreatening. Hospital volunteers can register classrooms and assist in distributing goodie bags. Goodie bags can contain surgical masks and hats, coloring books about going to the hospital, first aid supplies such as Band-Aids or bandages, and pamphlets about becoming a nurse or becoming a physician. Students are greeted as they exit their bus. Brightly colored posters decorate the halls and the rooms. Stuffed animals provide patient models. Use of stickers, balloons, and sidewalk chalk add to the festive atmosphere of the event. Nursing students provide lively entertainment and teaching through role play, songs, and skits.

Who Benefits from this Project?

Sponsoring agencies can benefit from media exposure. Television, radio, newspapers, and websites can promote the event and display photographs of the interactions between the child and the sponsoring agencies. The benefits to the nursing student are plentiful. The experience allows them opportunities to apply principles of growth and development, practice communication techniques, provide community service, provide health teaching, interact with prospective employers, promote their profession, and develop leadership skills.

SELF-REFLECTION

Try to remember an event from your childhood when you were frightened by medical personnel or a medical facility. What were your fears? What were your concerns? What or who made your fears worse? What or who relieved your fears and concerns? How can you adjust your practice to ease the fears of children?

SUGGESTED RESOURCES

For the Nurse

Heamann, D. (1994). Let's Pretend: A hospital teaches children about health care. *Nursing Forum, 29*(4), 5–9.

Elkins, P., & Roberts, M. (1984). A preliminary evaluation of hospital preparation of nonpatient children: Primary prevention in a "let's pretend hospital." *Child Health Care, 13*(1), 31–36.

For the Client

Bourgeois, P. (2000). *Franklin goes to the hospital.* New York: Scholastic Paperbacks.

Karim, R. (2002). *This is a hospital, not a zoo!* Boston: Clarion Books.

Search Internet websites for sponsoring agency reports of their "Let's Pretend Hospital" experiences.

SCHOOL-AGE CHILD

School-age children can participate actively in their care and treatment (Figure 7-5 ■). They can understand written and verbal instructions, ask questions, and be responsible for some aspects of planning and care. They continue to need parental support but generally do not experience extreme anxiety when parents are absent. Bringing a favorite item from home continues to offer comfort. This item may be a book, music, or an electronic game.

If the school-age child will be hospitalized for more than a few days, assignments can be obtained from the school to keep the child from getting behind in their schoolwork. School-age children enjoy a variety of activities and can be left alone for brief periods of time. Computer games, books, and movies can be used to fill time. The nurse should interact frequently with the school-age child but may not be required to remain in the room all the time.

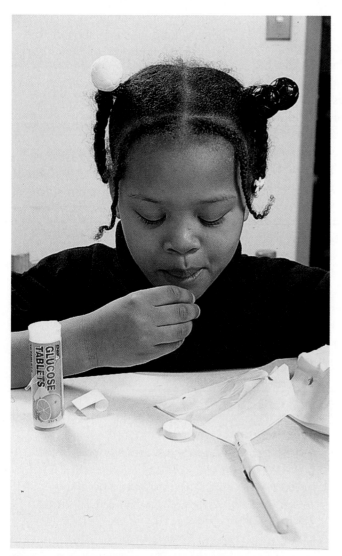

Figure 7-5. ■ This child is old enough to understand the need to take glucose tablets or another form of rapidly absorbed sugar when her blood glucose level is low.

ADOLESCENT

Many adolescents want to be active participants in their care. However, they might be embarrassed, modest, or uncomfortable about their changing bodies. They might have participated in activities that put them at risk for illness or injury without their parent's consent. Adolescents need reassurance that their modesty and privacy will be protected. The nurse needs to provide instructions directly to the adolescent and encourage questions.

Some adolescents want parents present during procedures; others prefer parents to stay in the waiting room. Many adolescents will have frequent visits from their friends. The nurse must maintain control of the environment to ensure that the adolescent has adequate rest and has privacy during treatments. The nurse may request that friends limit their visits to ensure adequate time for nursing care.

Admission Process

The admission process begins the minute a decision for hospitalization is made. The child may or may not have been present at the time the doctor discussed the need for hospitalization with the parents. There may be a few minutes or several days between the decision to hospitalize and the actual admission. Some parents are concerned that the child will be fearful, so they do not tell the child about the hospitalization until the last minute. Although this approach may be appropriate for the young child, the surprise of hospitalization may bring additional stress and fear to the older child. Other parents use a variety of resources to prepare the entire family. Children's books are available that present hospitalization and surgery in a positive light. These stories may be helpful when preparing children for hospitalization (Table 7-2 ■). Drawings that allow children to show their interpretation of the disease or disorder can be useful in discussing treatment with school-age or adolescent children (Figure 7-6 ■).

When the child is brought to the hospital, the nurse must determine the amount and quality of preparation the child and family have received. It is important to establish a positive relationship with the child and family, answer questions, and reduce fear and anxiety as much as possible. Remember that even though parents may have a general understanding of hospital equipment and routines, the experiences will be new for the child. Time must be allowed for adequate explanation, orientation to the environment, and emotional support.

The admission procedure for children is similar to that for adults. The child and family must be oriented to the environment, including the location of the bathroom, use of nurse's call light, and instructions on how to raise and

TABLE 7-2

Books for Hospitalized Children

TITLE AND AUTHOR	READING LEVEL	PUBLISHER AND PUBLICATION DATE	DESCRIPTION
Chemo Girl: Saving the World One Treatment at a Time (Paperback) by Christina Richmond	All ages	Jones & Bartlett; 1st ed., 1996	Describes chemotherapy and cancer treatment through superhero, Chemo Girl
Doctor Maisy (Maisy) (Paperback) by Lucy Cousins	Baby-preschool	Candlewick; 2001	Maisy and Tallulah play hospital; Poor Panda is sick but feels much better with Doctor Maisy in charge; when it's Maisy's turn to need help, Nurse Tallulah comes to the rescue
My Friend the Doctor (Hardcover) by Joanna Cole	Baby-preschool	HarperCollins; 2005	A reassuring, cheery book about going to the doctor
Kevin Goes to the Hospital (The On My Way Books) (Hardcover) by Liesbet Slegers	Baby-preschool	Kane/Miller; 2002	A book that will explain, comfort, and make less scary the experience of going to the hospital
The Hospital (Talk-about-Books No. 15) (Board book) by Debbie Bailey	Baby-preschool	Annick Press; 2000	Explores in a positive and realistic fashion what children can expect if they go to a hospital
How Do Dinosaurs Get Well Soon? (Hardcover) by Jane Yolen	Ages 4–8	Blue Sky Press; 2003	Playful read-aloud verse and wonderfully amusing pictures relieve children's fears about being sick
What Is Cancer Anyway?: Explaining Cancer to Children of All Ages (Paperback) by Karen L. Carney	Ages 4–8	Dragonfly; 1998	This book provides basic, essential information when someone in the family has cancer
Kathy's Hats: A Story of Hope (Hardcover) by Trudy B. Krisher	Ages 4–8	Albert Whitman & Company; reprint ed., 1992	A story about chemotherapy treatments and hair loss
A Day with Dr. Waddle (Paperback) by Center for Basic Cancer Research	Ages 4–8	KSU Center for Basic Cancer Research; 1988	A coloring workbook educates children about cancers, and addresses fears and misconceptions
Why, Charlie Brown, Why?: A Story About What Happens When a Friend Is Very Ill (Hardcover) by Charles M. Schulz	Ages 4–8	Ballantine Books; 2002	*Peanuts* gang faces leukemia in a good friend; a story of a child dealing with great challenges and profound questions
Henry and the White Wolf (Hardcover) by Tim Karu	Ages 4–8	Workman; 2000	Storybook and allegory drawn from teenager's own feelings of being in the hospital
A Night Without Stars (Paperback) by James Howe	Ages 9–12	Aladdin; 1996	Girl about to undergo open heart surgery meets patient who answers questions and becomes a friend
Jamie Drum's Massive Recovery (Paperback) by Paul Davies	Ages 9–12	Element Books Ltd.; 1998	Entertaining, inspirational, and funny book about a 13-year-old boy in the hospital
Let Him Live (One Last Wish) (Paperback) by Lurlene Mcdaniel	Ages 9–12	Laurel Leaf; 1993	17-year-old boy awaiting a liver transplant; his "one last wish" money is used to build a center for terminally ill kids

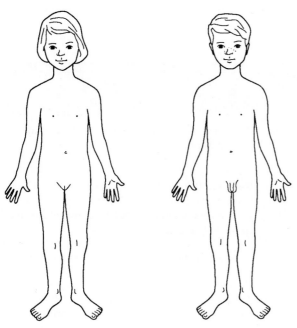

Figure 7-6. ■ The nurse can use a simple gender-specific drawing of a child's body to encourage children to draw what they think about their medical problems. Such drawings reveal the child's interpretation, which the nurse can work with to provide appropriate care.

lower the head of the bed. A toddler or young child may be placed in a crib with a vinyl top to prevent him or her from climbing out (Figure 7-7 ■).

clinical ALERT

For safety, the mattress must fit securely in the crib. The distance between the slats should be no greater than 2³/₈ inches (6 cm). If the child is capable of climbing, a hard bubble top should be secured to the crib.

Hospital routines should be discussed, including meal time, unit security, and visiting hours. The child will be asked to put on hospital attire, and the nurse will complete and document an assessment. Although the focus of the assessment will be the child's presenting medical condition, the nurse should also evaluate the child's level of growth and development. The child's height and weight should be obtained (see procedures in Chapter 8 ⊕). The nurse should observe the child's behavior and question the child and parents to determine if the child has met developmental milestones. The charge nurse will determine client problems and begin the nursing care plan.

Preparation for Procedures

To some extent, preparing the child and family for procedures is not different from preparing an adult for the same procedure. Providing instruction, obtaining informed

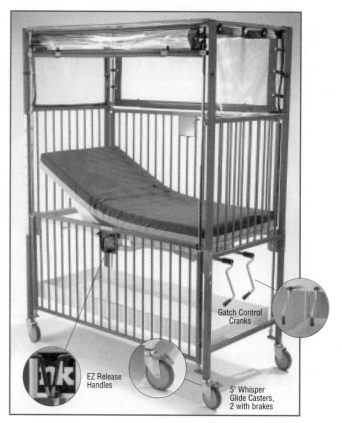

Gatch Control
Cranks

EZ Release
Handles

5" Whisper
Glide Casters,
2 with brakes

Figure 7-7. ■ A vinyl-top crib protects a climbing child from injury. The side bars slide up, and the clear plastic unrolls to connect with it. (Courtesy of nk Medical Products.)

consent, giving medication, assessing health status, and documenting care are the same. However, more time needs to be spent in preparing the child for procedures. Some children will need a brief explanation immediately before the procedure, whereas others will need detailed information several days ahead of time. If too much time is allowed between instruction and the procedure, some children might forget the instructions; in contrast, others might become upset, worrying about what is ahead. Parents are instrumental in preparing the child. See Table 7-2 for some resources that can be used to prepare children for hospitalization and procedures. For more information on nursing procedures in pediatrics, see Chapter 8 ⊕.

Children like to dress up as part of play. Fear of the unknown can be decreased by helping children dress like a doctor or nurse, play with a doll, and use equipment similar to that used in the procedure. This therapeutic play can be used one-to-one with the child, or in small groups of siblings or children experiencing similar procedures.

In most cases, the actual procedure will be the same as for an adult. However, conscious sedation may be used to keep the child calm, provide for the child's safety, and limit the child's memory of the experience. Conscious sedation is discussed later in this chapter.

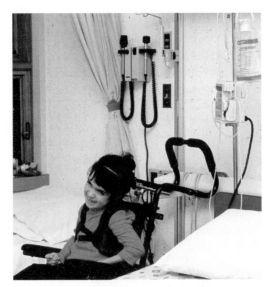

Figure 7-8. ■ This child, who is getting tube feedings or other infusions during the day, can be easily and safely transported in a wheelchair equipped with a safety harness. The tube feeding or infusion on the pole can be rolled with the child from place to place. Pumps can be attached to the pole to regulate infusion rates.

TRANSFER SAFETY

If the child is to be transported to another area of the hospital for the diagnostic exam or treatment, safety is an issue. The child should be transported in a crib with high sides, a youth bed, or a wheelchair with a safety harness, or on a stretcher (Figure 7-8 ■). The child should be lying down with the side rails raised. A safety belt may be fastened across the child's abdomen to prevent the child from falling off the stretcher. Children should not be left unattended.

Care of the Child Before and After Surgery

BEFORE SURGERY

The care of the child before and after surgery is similar to the care of the adult. In all clients, psychological preparation helps relieve fear of the unknown. Children need to be reassured that parents will be able to remain with them as long as possible and will be there shortly after they awaken. They should be introduced to key operating room personnel and be shown surgical attire. For example, the anesthesiologist wearing surgical scrubs and a surgical hat should meet the child and talk briefly about how he or she will observe the child during the surgery. The anesthesiologist should put on a surgical mask in front of the child and explain that everyone in the operating room will be wearing masks. When time allows, the child should have the opportunity to play with anatomically correct dolls, drawings, and surgical attire in order to learn about the surgical experience.

The physical preparation of the child preoperatively is the same as that for adults. A parent or legal guardian must sign the informed consent. Teenage children may also sign a consent form, and in some states, their consent is sufficient to perform certain procedures. See Chapter 3 ⬭ for discussion of legal and ethical issues related to children. The nurse needs to be familiar with legal practices within the state. Preparation includes nothing by mouth (NPO) for several hours, emptying the bladder, initiating an IV infusion, and administering preoperative medication. Local or topical anesthetics may be used for painful procedures such as IV infusions. Figure 7-9 ■ illustrates the application of eutectic (melts easily) mixture of local anesthetics (EMLA) cream.

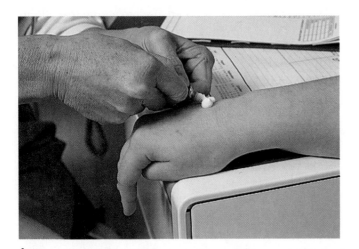

A

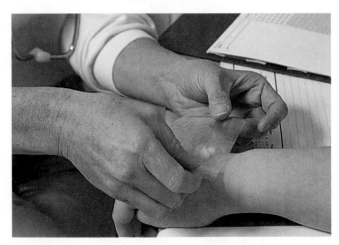

B

Figure 7-9. ■ When painful procedures are planned, use EMLA cream to anesthetize the skin where the painful stick will be made. **(A)** A thick layer of cream is applied over intact skin (½ of a 5-g tube). **(B)** The cream is covered with a transparent adhesive dressing, sealing all the sides. The cream anesthetizes the dermal surface in 45 to 60 minutes.

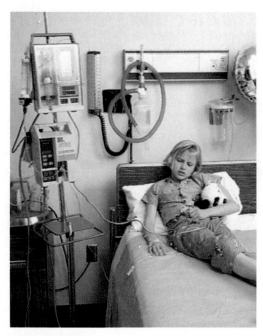

Figure 7-10. ■ The older child is able to regulate a PCA pump.

TABLE 7-3	
Preoperative Checklist	
CHECK WHEN DONE	NURSING ACTIONS
	Consent forms are signed, witnessed, and in chart.
	Child's name band is correct and secure.
	Allergies are noted in chart and highlighted on front cover of chart.
	All prosthetic devices are removed, including orthodontic appliances.
	Loose teeth and tongue piercing are noted in chart.
	Eyeglasses and jewelry are removed.
	Skin preparation and preoperative bath are completed if ordered.
	Clean hospital gown; allow child to wear underwear.
	All ordered tests are completed and reports are on chart.
	Child should void before surgery.
	Keep child NPO (usually 4–6 hours preoperatively).
	Administer prescribed preoperative medication.
	Transport to operating room on stretcher (or in crib).

PCA Pump Instructions

Older children may be trained in use of a patient-controlled analgesia (PCA) device. The **PCA pump** (Figure 7-10 ■) is a device attached to an IV line that allows the client to release pain medication as needed. It is often used as a short-term treatment method after surgery. It is also used in clients who are terminally ill as a way of providing palliative care. After a loading dose of pain medication is administered to initiate pain relief, the client may push a button to obtain more medication as pain intensifies. The pump can be programmed to deliver medication at certain intervals (e.g., during the night) when the client is asleep. It also has a "lockout interval" that prevents too much medication from being administered too quickly.

clinical ALERT

The nurse must ensure that safeguards are in place to protect clients from accidental overdose with PCA pumps:

- The nurse checks the medication order and computes the maximum 24-hour dose to be sure it does not exceed the safe maximum dose for the child (see Procedure 8-38 ⌘).
- The nurse checks the "lockout interval" of the pump to prevent the child from receiving the entire amount of pain medication too quickly.
- The nurse ensures that the pump is locked so changes to the drip rate or amount can only be made by qualified personnel.
- All pump settings are double checked and documented by two licensed nurses.

The PCA pump is useful because it allows the client control over pain relief measures, thus reducing anxiety. There is no significant difference between the amount of analgesic medication used with this and other methods (Smith, 2004).

Preoperative check sheets are used to ensure that all care has been completed. Table 7-3 ■ provides a sample preoperative checklist.

AFTER SURGERY

Following surgery, the child will be taken to a recovery room where routine postoperative care begins. The airway is maintained, level of consciousness is assessed, vital signs are recorded frequently, surgical dressings and drainage tubes are assessed, IV fluids are monitored, and pain control is initiated. (*Note:* The major discussion of pain appears in Chapter 15 ⌘. Also, see Figure 8-12 ⌘ for the Wong-Baker Pain Rating Scale.) In some facilities, parents are allowed to be with the child in the recovery room.

Once the child is stable, he or she might be transferred to the inpatient or ambulatory care room. Routine postoperative care includes monitoring of airway, breathing, and circulation; managing pain; ensuring that elimination occurs; providing fluids and advancing diet as tolerated; monitoring the healing of the surgical incision (see Box 18-1 ⬭); and providing teaching for the client and family as preparation for discharge (see Box 18-5 ⬭). The nurse may teach (or reinforce teaching) about postoperative exercises, such as deep breathing, coughing, and use of the incentive spirometer (IS). Procedure 7-1 ■ describes proper use of the IS.

PROCEDURE 7-1 Teaching Use of the Incentive Spirometer

Purpose
■ To assist lung expansion during the postoperative period

Equipment
■ Incentive spirometer
■ Tissue or paper towel for cleared secretions

Check order ✛ Gather equipment ✛ Introduce yourself ✛ Identify client ✛ Provide privacy ✛ Explain procedure ✛ Hand hygiene ✛ Gloves as needed

Interventions and Rationales

1. Perform preparatory steps (see icon bar above).

2. Explain to parents and child why the spirometer is used. *Lung expansion promotes oxygenation of tissue and clearing of secretions in the airway.*

3. Allow the child to examine the equipment as you describe its use. Point out the elements inside the spirometer tubes (Figure 7-11 ■) and describe how they work. *Having the child handle and feel ownership of the spirometer will encourage compliance.*

4. Indicate the measurements that show how much air the child is inhaling. Tell the child you will mark the highest amount the child can reach. *Having the child focus on the greatest goal possible encourages good results. If there is a presurgical baseline, mark this on the side of the container.*

5. If necessary, show the child how to splint an incision while performing this exercise. *Splinting an abdominal wound will reduce the child's discomfort while performing the exercise.*

6. Instruct the child to exhale as much breath as possible, to close the lips around the mouthpiece of the spirometer, and to inhale slowly. The inside balls or tubes will rise to indicate the amount of air the child is inhaling. Have the child hold the breath for a few seconds and then exhale slowly through pursed lips. *A slow steady breath will fill lungs most completely. Sustained exhalation will concentrate secretions and allow the child to cough them up more easily.*

7. Have the child repeat the procedure two to three times at several points in the day. *This will promote a healthy airway and help in removal of mucus secretions that might otherwise pool in the respiratory tract.*

8. Encourage the child to try to move the balls or tubes higher with each attempt. *Making the exercise into a game encourages repetition and can help promote compliance.*

Note: If an incentive spirometer is not available or is too complicated for the child to use, the child may be given a pinwheel to spin. The child would be encouraged to spin the pinwheel for increasing lengths of time.

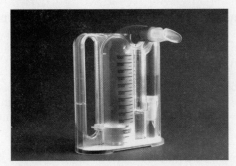

Figure 7-11. ■ The incentive spirometer is an excellent method of promoting lung expansion in school-age and older children. (Pearson Education/PH College)

SAMPLE DOCUMENTATION

(date/time)   IS used every 2 hours with maximum inhalation of two balls. Productive cough of white mucus following IS. J. Seege LPN

The LPN/LVN provides input into the individualized care plan and assists in the implementation and evaluation of care. A postoperative checklist for the nurse is provided in Box 7-2 ■.

CARE OF THE CHILD UNDERGOING CONSCIOUS SEDATION

Conscious sedation is the administration of IV medication to produce an impaired level of consciousness. The child will be able to maintain a patent airway, have protec-

tive reflexes, and respond to physical and verbal stimuli. Conscious sedation is used outside the operating room when sedation is required to perform therapeutic or diagnostic procedures safely. In contrast, **deep sedation** is a controlled state of depressed consciousness or unconsciousness in which the child is unable to maintain protective reflexes. Deep sedation, used during surgical procedures, is administered and maintained by an anesthesiologist or nurse anesthetist.

The medication used for conscious sedation is administered by a skilled RN in an environment where emergency resuscitation equipment and medication are available. Common drugs used for conscious sedation are included in Table 7-4 ■.

Following the procedure, one-to-one observation and care are required until the child has stable vital signs, age-appropriate verbal and physical response, adequate hydration, and a return of orientation at the level prior to sedation. Parents are instructed regarding diet, fluids, home care, and follow-up as appropriate for the specific procedure.

Preparation for Discharge

Preparation for discharge begins at time of admission. Through use of the nursing process, client and family needs for discharge are identified and plans made. An RN is responsible for discharge planning, including establishment of the complete teaching plan, follow-up appointment schedules, home health referrals, and equipment rental. The LPN/LVN helps with routine teaching, making

---

BOX 7-2	NURSING CARE CHECKLIST

Caring for a Child After Surgery

Care of the child after surgery includes both physical and emotional interventions:

☑ Monitor vital signs and compare them to baseline.
☑ Assess for pain.
☑ Provide pain relief and comfort measures.
☑ Support effective airway clearance and monitor for signs of respiratory depression or distress.
☑ Maintain a complete intake and output record, including fluid loss through dressings, tubes, or vomiting.
☑ Check IV status regularly.
☑ Monitor the child's level of consciousness.
☑ Monitor wound site and dressings for signs of complications.
☑ Change dressings as ordered.
☑ Provide or reinforce instructions to family and caregivers.

TABLE 7-4

Pharmacology: Drugs Used for Conscious Sedation

DRUG (GENERIC AND COMMON BRAND NAME)	USUAL ROUTE/DOSE	CLASSIFICATION	SELECTED SIDE EFFECTS	DON'T GIVE IF
diazepam (Valium)	IM/IV less than 5 years, 0.2–0.5 mg slowly every 2–5 minutes up to 5 mg; more than 5 years, 1 mg every 5 minutes up to 10 mg	Anoxiolytic, anti-convulsant	Drowsiness, dizziness, hypotension, respiratory distress	Other drugs are being administered (do not mix)
midazolam (Versed)	IM 0.08 mg/kg IV 0.15 mg/kg followed by 0.05 mg/kg every 2 minutes × one to three doses	Short-acting benzodiazepine anxiolytic, sedative hypnotic	Retrograde amnesia, respiratory distress, hypotension	Severe organic heart disease; caution with renal or hepatic impairment
lorazepam (Ativan)	PO, IV, IM 0.05 mg/kg	Benzodiazepine anxiolytic, sedative hypnotic	Drowsiness, sedation, respiratory distress	Child is younger than 12 years

telephone calls, answering questions, and completing documentation. If the child is going home, all those who will participate in care at home need to be taught proper technique and precautions (see Boxes 18-1 and 18-5 ⊙⊙). If the child will be returning to school, the school nurse, teacher, and office personnel must be made aware of the child's health needs, including medication that needs to be given at school. If the child is going to another care facility, communication with the nursing personnel at that facility is critical for a smooth transition. Documentation should include a detailed description of the condition of the child, the instruction provided to the child and family, and verification that all belongings were sent home with the family.

NURSING CARE

PRIORITIES IN NURSING CARE

Besides meeting the biologic needs of airway, breathing, and circulation, the priority of care for a child who is being hospitalized is to make the child feel safe and secure. Hospitalization can be frightening to the child and family, and care must be taken to alleviate fear to the greatest extent possible.

ASSESSING

Besides normal pre- or postoperative assessments (vital signs, pain, wound drainage, intake and output, etc.), observe the child and family for signs of anxiety and fear:

- Is the child "hiding" behind a parent? Does the child hang on to the parent? *These are signs that the child is scared and seeking the protection of the parent.*
- Does the child talk with parents, family, and nurse (if age appropriate)? *If the child is fearful, he or she may talk only with parents or family but avoid answering the nurse's questions.*
- Is the child crying, screaming, or running away from the nurse? *These are common reactions in the fearful child.*
- Do the parents show any unusual or extreme signs of anxiety, fear, or physical reaction to the situation or procedure? *Parents who are extremely anxious will not be able to adequately support the needs of the child. This observation should be reported to the charge nurse.*

DIAGNOSING, PLANNING, AND IMPLEMENTING

The plan of care is based on the specific medical problem. Because children may not have an accurate understanding of their condition and their environment, hospitalization causes fear of the unknown. One nursing diagnosis for every hospitalized child should be:

- Fear related to hospitalization.

Expected outcomes would include:

- The child will express less fear, either verbally or non-verbally.
- The child will interact appropriately with the nurse.
- The child will rest quietly in bed.

Nursing interventions might include:

- Approach child with a smile and introduce self by first name. Avoid bringing equipment to the bedside during the introductory phase of relationship. *The child is fearful in a new environment. A friendly face can help alleviate fear. Additional equipment will only increase the fear of the unknown.*
- Allow a parent or guardian to remain with child. *Family is reassuring to the child.*
- Allow child to hold a favorite toy or blanket. *The familiarity of a favorite toy or blanket provides security to the frightened child.*
- Provide a tour of the hospital and pediatric unit, including introduction of staff when possible. Allow children to play in the playroom before going to their room (Figure 7-12 ■). *Seeing the environment and staff ahead of time can decrease fear of the unknown.*
- Avoid having the child see other children who are very sick or who have a lot of equipment. *Seeing other children who are very sick or who have a lot of equipment may increase the child's fear. The child's imagination can lead them to believe they will become extremely sick, too.*
- Allow children to see and touch equipment before procedures. Use play therapy when providing instructions. *When a child is allowed to see, touch, and "play" with equipment, procedures and hospital routine are not as frightening.*
- Encourage developmentally appropriate activities when possible. *School-age children may find distraction in books or schoolwork* (Figure 7-13 ■).
- In addition to typical postsurgical care, consider alternative measures that may provide comfort (Box 7-3 ■).
- When possible, assign the same nurses to the child on consecutive days. *The child is able to cope better when familiar staff provides care.*
- Review expected events with parents and answer questions as needed. *Reminders about what is to come can reassure the overwhelmed parent that things are "under control." Providing answers as soon as possible prevents anxiety from building. A calm parent can be more effective in reassuring and calming a child.*
- Encourage parents to provide comfort measures as often as possible (Figure 7-14 ■). *When a child is scared or in pain, the physical presence of the parent can be soothing.*

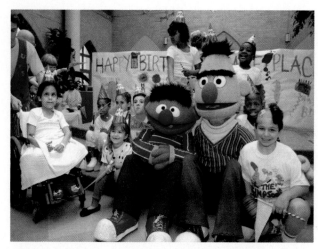

Figure 7-12. ■ Play areas can give the child a welcome diversion from the hospital room. They can also provide space for special events that coincide with hospitalization. (AP Wide World Photo.)

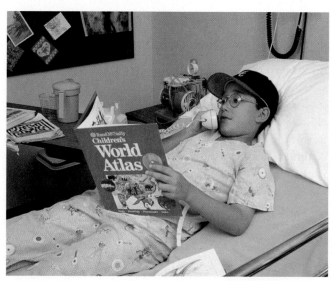

Figure 7-13. ■ It is important that the hospitalized child does not fall behind in schoolwork. As soon as the child is able, schoolwork should be resumed. If the child is unable to get out of bed, all necessary study materials should be brought to the child. The child can consult with teachers or classmates on the phone or via computer.

EVALUATING

The evaluation of the child's level of fear must be made with each interaction. Children need consistency and security in order to rest and heal. Every effort must be made to provide an environment within the hospital that meets this need.

BOX 7-3	COMPLEMENTARY THERAPIES

Postoperative Care

After surgery, the child will need physical and pharmacologic interventions as he or she progresses toward recovery. Along the way, alternative therapies may also be of use. Techniques such as the following may be useful:

■ **Music therapy:** Soft music can be played in the background while a child is resting or sleeping; lively, "happy" music can help draw a child's attention away from pain or worry. A recording of ocean waves or even "white noise" created by a fan can override small background sounds and allow deeper sleep.

■ **Massage:** A gentle hand or foot massage, or gentle stroking of the hair or head, can be done in almost any body position unless contraindicated. Light massage can relieve some pain and can help the child relax. Rocking, if allowed, provides some muscle stimulation, as well as warmth and security. See also Box 1-2 ⬤⬤.

■ **Imaging and relaxation techniques:** A "let's imagine" game or (for older children) a more directed form of guided imagery can help the child focus attention on a place of comfort and happiness. Flexing and releasing portions of the body not affected by surgery (a hand, a foot, etc.) can improve circulation and increase the child's overall comfort.

■ **Hydrotherapy, heat and cold applications:** Hydrotherapy, heat applications, and cold applications may be administered as ordered. However, remember that extra caution is needed with young children, whose skin is thinner than an adult's.

■ **Play therapy:** A variety of play therapy techniques (see Table 7-1) can offer mental relief and diversion to the hospitalized child.

■ **Diversion:** In some hospitals, parents may bring video game units from home and connect them to the television in the hospital room. Children may also bring small electronic devices, such as handheld gaming systems, CD players, or MP3 players. Video and DVD players are available for watching favorite movies.

■ **TENS:** Transelectrical nerve stimulation (TENS) provides low-voltage electrical stimulation to pain areas or areas that innervate a painful area. Cutaneous stimulation provides pain relief to many clients.

Note: Aromatherapy should not be used in the presence of nausea because it could increase nausea and stimulate emesis. Some aromas can also cause respiratory irritation and distress.

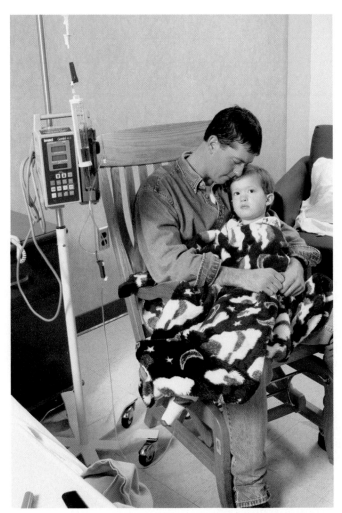

Figure 7-14. ■ The presence of the parent is an important part of pain management.

NURSING PROCESS CARE PLAN
Child Undergoing Hospitalization for Surgery

Five-year-old Timmy is being admitted to the pediatric unit for surgical repair of an umbilical hernia. This is his first hospitalization. His parents told him yesterday of the upcoming surgery.

Assessment

- Timmy appears shy, avoids eye contact, and holds on to his father's hand.
- Timmy answers questions in one or two words in a whisper.
- Timmy's mother rapidly answers all admission questions.
- Timmy's mother asks numerous questions about all the equipment in the room, and about postoperative care.

Nursing Diagnosis. The following important nursing diagnosis (among others) is established for this client:

- Anxiety (Child and Family) related to hospitalization, equipment, and upcoming surgery.

Expected Outcomes

- The child and family will not demonstrate signs and symptoms of anxiety.
- The child and his family will verbalize understanding of equipment and events related to hospitalization and surgical outcome.

Planning and Implementation

- Orient the child and family to the hospital setting. *Familiarity with the environment decreases anxiety.*
- Encourage parents to support the child. *Parents have a better understanding of the hospital environment and routines and can be a valuable support for the child.*
- Ask questions of the parent and child about surgery. *Baseline data direct client and family teaching.*
- Teach about preoperative and postoperative events using age-appropriate techniques such as dolls, drawings, and stories. *Allowing children to play "surgery" with dolls helps identify their understanding of what is happening to them. It also is a good way to identify areas for routine preoperative and postoperative teaching.*
- Reinforce the information the family has about the purpose of surgery. *Reinforcing information helps ensure that family members will remember information accurately for future use.*
- Provide teaching to parents about care of the child after discharge. If hospitalization involved surgery, provide information and teaching for follow-up care (see Boxes 18-1 and 18-5 🔗).

Evaluation. Observe the child and family for signs of decreased anxiety including increased eye contact, normal speech patterns and tone of voice, and relaxed posture. In-depth preoperative teaching should wait until the child and family become comfortable with the hospital environment. See the Nursing Care Plan Chart, Child and the Surgical Experience, on pages 154 and 155. It provides a more in-depth care plan for this child in a format that resembles those used in clinical agencies.

Critical Thinking in the Nursing Process

1. Timmy asks when he can play T ball again. How should the nurse respond?
2. Timmy's parents ask if the umbilical hernia can come back in the future. How should the nurse respond?
3. What would be some indications that surgery should not take place?

Note: Answers for Critical Thinking questions appear in Appendix I.

NURSING CARE PLAN CHART

Child and the Surgical Experience

GOAL	INTERVENTION	RATIONALE	EXPECTED OUTCOME
1. Anxiety, related to preoperative and postoperative events			
The child will demonstrate decreased anxiety behavior	Question the child regarding expectations of hospitalization and previous surgical experiences.	*Previous experiences can influence present anxiety levels*	The child is calm and expresses no other symptoms of anxiety.
	Orient the child to the hospital setting.	*Familiarity with the setting and the people involved in the surgical experience can decrease anxiety by removing fear of the unknown*	
	Explain procedures and prepare the child for what he will experience preoperatively and postoperatively.	*The child is more likely to trust caregivers if they are open, honest and truthful.*	
The child's family will demonstrate reduced anxiety in an effort to adequately support the child through the surgical experience	Encourage the parents to allow the child to ask questions about the surgical experience and to express their feelings related to the experience	*Questioning provides an opportunity to explain the unknown, which decreases anxiety*	Parents are able to deal with their anxious thoughts and behaviors and demonstrate support for their child.
	Encourage parents to demonstrate supportive behaviors to the child such as touch, active listening, providing distraction and reducing environmental stimuli.	*Anxiety-reducing behaviors provided by parents can be effective in assisting the child to manage his or her anxiety*	
2. Ineffective Airway Clearance related to surgical anesthetics and postoperative pain			
The child will maintain adequate ventilation with no respiratory impairment.	Auscultate lungs every 2 hours. Record rate, rhythm, and quality of respiration. Evaluate respiratory rate after administration of analgesics.	*Early identification of respiratory difficulty aids early treatment. Analgesics, especially narcotics, slow the respiratory rate*	The child will have respiratory rate and rhythm WNL and will not demonstrate symptoms of respiratory distress.
	Administer oxygen if ordered.	*Oxygen may facilitate breathing*	
	Encourage the child to turn, cough and deep breathe every 2 hours. Use incentive spirometer, pinwheels, or other appropriate blow toys. Suction airway as needed.	*Repositioning and deep breathing ensures expansion of all lung fields. Coughing facilitates removal or mucus from airways*	
3. Risk for Infection related to surgical procedure and intravenous sites			
The child will not demonstrate symptoms of infection.	Monitor vital signs per hospital routine. Record and report changes from baseline.	*Changes in vital signs, especially increased temperature and pulse, can indicate infection*	The child's vital signs and white blood cell count will be WNL.
	Monitor surgical site, dressings, and drains every hour.	*Excessive drainage may indicate infection*	
	Change or reinforce surgical dressings when saturated with drainage and/or blood.	*Wet dressings can allow organisms to come in contact with the surgical wound*	

(*continued*)

GOAL	INTERVENTION	RATIONALE	EXPECTED OUTCOME
	Check the intravenous site every hour for redness, swelling, pain, or pallor.	*Intravenous lines may become infected or infiltrated*	
4. Risk for Imbalanced Fluid Volume related to intravenous infusion, NPO status, and surgical blood loss			
The child will achieve and maintain proper circulating volume	Monitor vital signs per hospital routine.	*Changes in vital signs, especially pulse and blood pressure, can indicate fluid imbalance*	The child's vital signs, intake and output and hematocrit and hemoglobin will be WNL.
	Record intake and output. Be alert for fluid loss via dressings and watery stools. Evaluate hydration status by skin turgor and mucous membranes.	*Intake and output should be roughly equivalent. Urinary retention may occur as a result of anesthesia. Good skin turgor and moist membranes indicate fluid balance*	
	Monitor laboratory values of hematocrit and hemoglobin.	*Changes in lab values indicate dehydration or overhydration*	
The child will tolerate oral intake when initiated, with no nausea, vomiting, or dehydration present.	Begin oral intake after assessment of bowel sounds. Record vomiting. Administer antiemetics as indicated.	*Vomiting can cause fluid loss*	The child tolerates the progression of oral intake without nausea, vomiting or changes in vitals signs or lab values.

CHRONICALLY ILL CHILD

Some children with chronic illness have a **hereditary condition** (genetic inheritance from a parent or parents). Others have a **congenital condition** (condition present at birth) that results in a chronic disorder. Some of these children, using adaptive equipment, lead a relatively normal life. They attend school, church, and community activities. Some even participate in sports. However, other children have more difficulty adapting and spend their life at home with limited outside activities. Parents need direction and support from nurses in learning to care for these children. Details about specific illnesses are discussed in later chapters of this text.

Care at Home

Caring for a child who is chronically ill at home can be physically, emotionally, and financially draining. Depending on the condition of the child, special equipment might be needed, including beds, ventilators, IV infusion pumps, and wheelchairs (Figure 7-15 ■). Parents either purchase or lease this equipment. The house might need some remodeling to accommodate the equipment. Time and resources are needed for this adjustment. The child might be cared for in a rehabilitation facility or placed in a long-term care facility while the adjustments to the home are being made.

Many children with chronic illnesses need 24-hour care or supervision. For example, if the child's illness involves the respiratory system and requires the child to be on a ventilator, a care provider needs to be present to suction the airway or respond to an emergency. Parents who must work outside the home and care for other children may not be able to provide this 24-hour care. As the child grows, the parent may not be physically able to provide all the care the child needs.

Parents of these children experience varying degrees of emotional trauma. At times, they feel guilt about the condition of their child and their ability (or inability) to provide care. They might blame each other or themselves because they are unable, either physically or financially, to meet the demands the child places on the family. They might be angry with the ill child for "robbing" them of a "normal" family life. Although they love the child, they might entertain wishes that the child would die so the burden of caring for him or her would be lifted.

The nurse has several roles in such situations. To assist the child and family, the nurse not only provides care and uses therapeutic communication to help explore feelings, but also assists the family in finding additional resources. The LPN/LVN can assist with direct care, can provide respite to family members, and can monitor the child's condition.

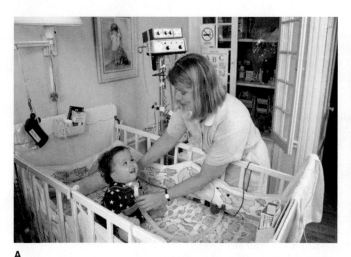

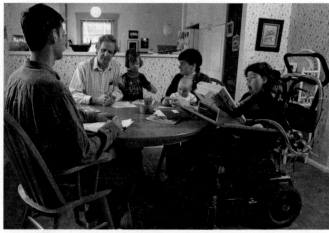

A

B

Figure 7-15. ■ (A) It is often desirable from a family and cost perspective to provide health care in the home, and advances in technology have made this possible. (B) Daily caregiving demands of the child who is medically fragile continue 24 hours a day, 7 days a week. Parents need to identify ways to share the care of the child and other family care management. When the child lives with a single parent, additional health care resources are needed so the parent can sleep.

Care at School

School staff may carry the day-to-day responsibility of providing care for children if they become ill or injured. This responsibility includes care of the child riding to and from school on a bus, care of the child on the playground, and care of the child during field trips and during extracurricular activities. Some school districts are able to have an RN in each school to care for students who are ill or injured (Figure 7-16 ■). In other school districts, an RN must travel between several schools. An LPN/LVN might be hired to assist the RN. In the absence of a licensed nurse, the counselor, teacher, or office personnel will be required to assist a child who is ill or injured until a parent or guardian can be called. It is important to teach the school personnel to care for the child who is ill or injured. Teaching would include basic first aid, cardiopulmonary resuscitation (CPR), and administration of medications.

Most children who become ill at school have a respiratory or gastrointestinal infection. They need to be isolated from contact with other children while waiting for parents or guardians. To prevent spread of infection, anyone caring for these children must wash their hands before having contact with others.

Children at school could also get injured on the playground. These injuries include falls, broken bones, or cuts and scrapes. Basic first aid is needed in most cases. If the injury appears severe, emergency medical personnel should be contacted.

Some common chronic conditions affect children but do not prevent them from attending school. An **individualized education plan (IEP)** is an interdisciplinary plan that pinpoints the special educational needs of a particular student and establishes a plan for meeting them. The IEP may need to be established and may include home tutors, specialized services from speech therapists, transport of the child with disabilities to school, and provisions for specialized medical care as needed. When this is the case, the school nurse works with parents and school personnel to ensure that the health needs of the child are met. Examples of these conditions include asthma, diabetes, cerebral palsy, muscular dystrophy, spinal cord injuries, Down syndrome, and attention deficit disorder.

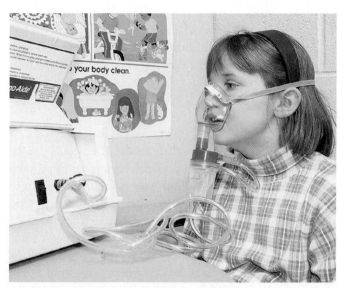

Figure 7-16. ■ This child requires use of a nebulizer during school hours. The nurse or trained school personnel must administer medication on a regular basis.

These children might need assistance with glucose testing, administration of insulin, and diet monitoring. Medication and counseling for children with behavior problems must be provided. Special equipment, such as walkers and wheelchairs, might be needed. Classrooms might need to be altered to make room for this equipment. The child with a spinal cord injury might need respiratory support and airway clearance. The child might need help using the bathroom or eating lunch. Often, an individual is hired to provide this one-to-one care while the child is at school. The nurse should meet with school personnel and parents to assess health needs and to plan, implement, and evaluate care.

Even in the absence of illness or injury, the school nurse is instrumental in collecting health-related data for all school children. Vision testing, hearing testing, and keeping records related to growth and immunizations are but a few examples. Sometimes there might be an outbreak of head lice or infectious disease such as whooping cough. The school nurse must work with other public health department personnel to assess, treat, and evaluate children and to assist in teaching parents.

Rehabilitation

Some children with chronic conditions can benefit from rehabilitation. For example, a child with *Legg-Calvé-Perthes disease* (a disorder characterized by degeneration of the femoral head) will need extensive rehabilitation to learn to walk with leg braces and to regain normal use of the legs once the braces are removed (Figure 7-17 ■). See discussion of musculoskeletal issues in Chapter 20 ⬤⬤. During the rehabilitation process, the child may be admitted to a pediatric rehabilitation unit or a general rehabilitation center. When planning and implementing physical care for the pediatric client, the nurse must also take care to meet the child's growth and development needs (see Figure 7-17B ■). School-age children and adolescents may need a tutor to keep up with school.

Long-Term Care

Some children have chronic conditions that prevent them from attending school or, because of family conditions, prevent them from living at home. These children might be placed in a long-term care facility. Some communities may have a long-term care facility, such as a state school or hospital, that is designed for children with extensive physical and mental disabilities (Figure 7-18 ■). Other communities have only long-term care facilities that have been designed for the elderly. Although placing children with disabilities and clients who are elderly together can promote a special bond, these facilities may not be prepared to deal with the care necessary to stimulate the development of the child. Admitting a child to these facilities poses a challenge for

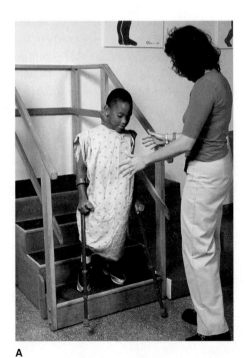

A

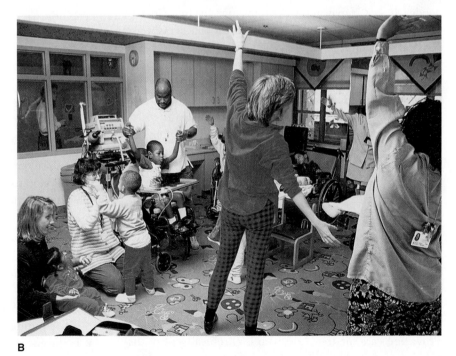

B

Figure 7-17. ■ (**A**) Rehabilitation units provide an opportunity for the child to relearn such tasks as walking and climbing stairs. They provide an important transition from hospital to home and community. (**B**) The nurse can help the child and family accept and adjust to new circumstances. Encouraging a child in a wheelchair to participate in group activities can help build self-esteem, goal attainment, personal satisfaction, and general health.

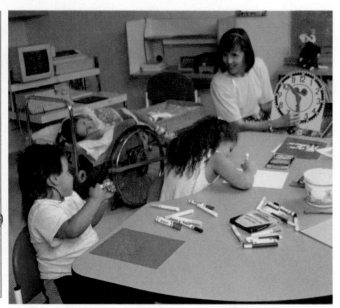

Figure 7-18. ■ Shriner's Hospital in Spokane, Washington, has a special room and teachers for children undergoing lengthy hospital stays, enabling them to remain current with their school work.

the nurses and staff; it also places an emotional and financial drain on the family.

The physical care of the child with chronic disabilities may be similar to that of the dependent adult; however, it has different challenges. With the proper attention, many children with major disabilities can remain stable or progress. Progress may or may not allow them to live independently, but it may allow them to enjoy life in a different way. Activities need to be planned that provide age-specific physical, mental, and occupational therapy. Because progress might be slow, it is important to provide the child with consistent daily therapy for many years.

The nurse needs to work closely with other professionals who have received education specific to the child with a disability in a long-term care facility. Programs of physical therapy, behavioral therapy, and occupational therapy must be designed to meet the needs of each child. Caregivers and therapists must be consistent in their approach to the child. It can be the responsibility of the LPN/LVN to assist in the plan development, supervise unlicensed caregivers, and document changes. Care of these children must be through an interdisciplinary team approach. LPNs and LVNs can be important members of that team.

Care of the Caregivers

Providing care for the child who is chronically ill or disabled on a daily basis is extremely challenging and stressful. The entire family is affected by the amount of attention the child requires. If the child needs close supervision 24 hours a day, parents may take turns monitoring the child

at night while the other parent sleeps. Over time, the caregivers become physically, emotionally, and mentally tired. They can begin to feel trapped. They suffer from burnout. The marriage relationship suffers, and divorce is common.

Siblings in a family with a child who is chronically ill may believe that they must compete for parental attention. They may become jealous of the sibling or angry that the sibling takes so much of their parents' time and financial resources. At school or on the playground, they may be put in a situation of defending their sibling. If they are old enough, they may be asked by the parents to help with the physical care of the child with a disability. These issues place additional stress on family relationships.

It is important for the nurse to address caregiver strain. The nurse can be instrumental in helping the family explore their feelings and develop a plan to prevent burnout. The plan might include a respite support system, taking time for each other and the other members of the family. Sometimes the family needs to discuss obtaining additional help or admitting the child to a long-term care facility. Resources might include extended family, friends, clergy, support groups, and social services.

NURSING CARE
PRIORITIES IN NURSING CARE

The priorities in providing care for the child who is chronically ill or disabled include providing a safe environment for the child. The nurse can also provide activities that promote healing. These activities should also promote growth and development in the child. The nurse must also be attentive to provide caregiver support.

ASSESSING

An assessment of the environment where the child will live and develop must be made in advance of the child's arrival. The environmental assessment must include the following questions:

- What is the functional level of the child?
- What assistive devices are needed for the child?
- Can the child access the bathroom, dining area, and bedroom?
- Are the rooms large enough to accommodate any necessary equipment?
- Is the environment safe for the child?
- Is appropriate care available 24 hours a day?
- Is transportation available for the child to attend school, church, and clinic visits?
- What is the child's current developmental level?

- Are the care activities and household duties shared by members of the family?
- Is a support system available to provide respite for the caregivers?

DIAGNOSING, PLANNING, AND IMPLEMENTING

In addition to nursing diagnoses for the specific disorder, other nursing diagnoses might include:

- **S**elf-care Deficit (specific to the individual child) related to physical impairment
- Delayed **G**rowth and Development related to effects of physical disability
- Interrupted **F**amily Processes related to compromised health status of the child
- Risk for **C**aregiver Role Strain related to inadequate resources to provide care for the disabled child

Expected outcomes for these diagnoses include:

- The child will provide as much self-care as possible in a safe environment.
- The child will maintain or show progress in growth and development.
- The caregivers will verbalize appropriate methods of managing stress

The nurse would perform the following interventions to assist children who are chronically ill and their families:

- Help parents provide a safe environment for the child, taking into account any needed equipment or accommodation. *The home of a child who is chronically ill may need many adjustments in order for a safe environment to exist.*

- Encourage the child to care for self as much as possible. *Self-care aids the child's development and supports self-esteem.*
- Encourage parents to allow child to care for self as much as possible. *The parents may want to do things "for" their child. Remind them that they are showing love when they allow the child to do all he or she can.*
- Teach caregivers to provide necessary care. *All caregivers must receive instruction so safe and adequate care can be provided.*
- Encourage caregivers to verbalize feelings. *Teach caregivers that verbalizing feelings will allow them to look at the situation honestly and work together for solutions.*
- Encourage caregivers to make a plan to minimize stress. *Planning time for self and for activities that minimize stress will allow the caregiver to return refreshed to continue giving care.*
- Provide written referrals for the child and family. *Resources and support groups can help the child and family cope more effectively.*

EVALUATING

Evaluation must be an ongoing process. Once a safe environment has been established, changes will only need to be made if the child's condition changes. The child's growth and development should be evaluated every 3 to 6 months and the plans updated. Caregiver strain should be evaluated with each nursing contact.

Note: The reference and resource listings for this and all chapters have been compiled at the back of the book.

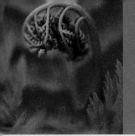

Chapter Review

 KEY TERMS by Topic

Introduction
illness, acute, chronic, terminal

Role of the LPN/LVN
therapeutic play

Hospitalized Child
child life specialist, separation anxiety, PCA pump, conscious sedation, deep sedation

Chronically Ill Child
hereditary condition, congenital condition, individualized education plan (IEP)

KEY Points

- The needs of the individual child and family must be assessed, and an interdisciplinary plan must be developed.

- Teaching must be provided to the child, parents, and members of the community who will be responsible for aspects of care.

- The child's limited understanding of what is occurring produces anxiety over hospitalization and diagnostic and therapeutic procedures.

- It is important for the nurse to help relieve stress by providing age-specific preparation for hospitalization and for every procedure the child will experience.

- The child who is chronically ill or disabled may require care at school, at home, or in a rehabilitation center or long-term care facility. Nurses in these areas must be prepared to meet the child's physical and developmental needs.

- Caregivers need support to prevent fatigue and burnout.

 EXPLORE Media Link

Additional interactive resources for this chapter can be found on the Companion Website at www.prenhall.com/adams.

Click on Chapter 7 and "Begin" to select the activities for this chapter.

For chapter-related NCLEX®-style questions and an audio glossary, access the accompanying CD-ROM in this book.

Animations:

Client pain assessment

FOR FURTHER Study

For additional complementary therapies, see Box 1-2.

See Chapter 3 for discussion of legal and ethical issues related to children.

Information about culture, ethnicity, and family is discussed in Chapter 4.

Procedures for child and Figure 8-12 The Wong-Baker Scale are found in Chapter 8.

The Wong-Baker rating scale is shown in Figure 8-12.

The major discussion of pain is provided in Chapter 15.

For information about monitoring the healing of the surgical incision, see Box 18-1. For postsurgical client teaching before discharge, see Box 18-5.

Musculoskeletal rehabilitation is discussed in Chapter 20.

Details about specific illnesses are discussed in body systems chapters (11 to 22) of this book.

A sign language chart is provided in Appendix VII.

Critical Thinking Care Map

Caring for a Child with Bilateral Hip Splints on a Rehabilitation Unit

NCLEX-PN® Focus Area: Physiologic Integrity

Case Study: Andrew Paulson, a 10-year-old with Legg-Calvé-Perthes disease, has been admitted to the rehabilitation unit of a children's hospital. Andrew's disease has been stabilized, and he has been fitted with bilateral hip splints. He will be on the rehabilitation unit for a minimum of 1 month before he is discharged.

Nursing Diagnosis: Risk for Delayed Development related to prolonged rehabilitation

COLLECT DATA

Subjective	Objective
_____	_____
_____	_____
_____	_____
_____	_____
_____	_____
_____	_____
_____	_____

Would you report this? Yes/No

If yes, to: _____

Nursing Care

_____
_____
_____
_____
_____
_____
_____
_____
_____

How would you document this? _____
_____
_____
_____

Compare your documentation to the sample provided in Appendix I.

Data Collected
(use only those that apply)

- BP 108/62
- Is in fourth grade
- Does not like school
- Weight 89 lb
- Enjoys reading fiction stories
- States pain in both hips
- States he misses playing football
- Good strength in upper extremities

Nursing Interventions
(use only those that apply; list in priority order)

- Tell him he must attend classes to keep up with his schoolwork.
- Limit extra reading until schoolwork is completed.
- Orient to environment and facility routine.
- Insist he participate in physical therapy activities.
- Administer pain medication as ordered.
- Insist he perform ADLs with minimal assistance.
- Contact teacher to obtain information about school assignments.

NCLEX-PN® Exam Preparation

1 A 10-month-old child was admitted to the pediatric unit with newly diagnosed cystic fibrosis. The nurse would expect this child to respond to the staff with which of the following behaviors?

1. outward hostility
2. fear of strangers
3. frequent negativism
4. occasional jealousy

2 A child with cystic fibrosis is to be treated with a mist tent while in bed at home. Before discharge, which of the following is most important for the discharge planner to evaluate?

1. the size of the child's bedroom
2. the child's respiratory rate while sleeping
3. who will provide care for the child at school
4. the relationship of the parents

3 An 8-year-old has been prescribed antibiotic tablets every 6 hours. One dose is due during school hours. The parents should be advised to:

1. keep her home from school until the antibiotics are gone.
2. have her skip the dose while at school.
3. have school personnel administer the dose.
4. have her double the next dose.

4 When caring for a 3-year-old child in the hospital, it is important to keep the routine as close as possible to the _____ environment.

5 A 4-year-old Native American girl has been admitted for surgery tomorrow. Her family requests that the medicine man be allowed to burn incense and dance in the child's room before surgery. The nurse should respond:

1. "Modern medicine will make her better. Those primitive measures are of no use."
2. "I will provide space and privacy for you. Please keep any music or chanting to a low volume to avoid disturbing other clients."
3. "That is not allowed within the hospital environment."
4. "Because of hospital policy, I cannot allow you to burn anything."

6 A pediatric client is severely disabled and is being cared for at home. When the home health nurse arrives, the mother is pale, weak, and tearful. She states she has not slept for several nights because her child has been having diarrhea. The nurse should respond to the mother:

1. "The diarrhea is probably caused by the child's antibiotics."
2. "I will make arrangements for the child to be admitted to the nursing home."
3. "Can you tell me how you are feeling right now?"
4. "I will let the doctor know about the child's diarrhea."

7 When discussing home care for a 5-year-old client who is paraplegic, the nurse should question the family about all of the following. Place them in priority order.

1. plans for the child to attend kindergarten
2. the need to bathe the child quickly after soiling
3. transferring the child from bed to wheelchair
4. evacuation plan in case of fire
5. frequency of changing the child's position

8 How should a 9-month-old infant be transported to surgery?

1. In a crib with the side rails up
2. On a stretcher with the safety belt fastened
3. In his mother's arms
4. On a youth bed with the side rails up

9 A 3-year-old child is being admitted to a nursing home for long-term care following a severe brain injury acquired in a car accident where both parents were killed. In planning care for this child, the nurse should consider which of the following?

1. a private room to allow for the equipment
2. a semiprivate room with an elderly roommate
3. a room away from the nurses' station to avoid disrupting the child's sleep
4. refusing to admit the child because a nursing home is for the elderly

10 A 16-year-old is admitted to the hospital for knee surgery following a football injury. In providing preoperative teaching, the nurse should:

1. Provide brief instruction immediately before surgery to lessen anxiety.
2. Provide detailed instruction to the client with a parent present.
3. Provide instruction only to the parents so they can sign the consent form.
4. Question the client about the use of illicit drugs when the parents are out of the room.

Answers for NCLEX-PN® Review and Critical Thinking questions appear in Appendix I.

Chapter 8

Procedures for the Pediatric Client

BRIEF Outline

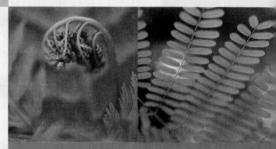

LEARNING Outcomes

After completing this chapter, you will be able to:
1. Define key terms.
2. Describe alterations in data gathering in the care of children.
3. Identify specific adaptations for selected procedures in the care of children.
4. Discuss the role of the LPN/LVN in adapting procedures in the care of children.

Many of the same nursing and medical procedures used in the care of adults are used in the care of children. However, some procedures must be adapted to the size and age of the child. This chapter describes the common adaptations that should be made to provide safe nursing care.

Assessment of the Child

Assessment involves the collection of data and interpretation of the findings in order to make a decision regarding care of the individual. The assessment of the child is organized like assessment of the adult, but the approach is quite different (Table 8-1 ■). The reason for assessment, the environment in which the assessment is done, and the condition of the child all influence the extent of data collected. For example, if the child is brought to the clinic for a well-child check-up, his or her physical and cognitive growth and development and emotional well-being are assessed. If the child is brought to the office because of a minor injury, the physical assessment is focused on that cause. The cognitive assessment might be directed at the cause of the injury so the child can be taught about safety issues. If the child is acutely ill in the hospital, the physical assessment is more in depth. In-depth cognitive assessment is not done because he or she could regress during the illness, and the cognitive and emotional assessment would, therefore, not be accurate.

Although an assessment of an adult is generally conducted from head to toe, it may be better to assess the child in a different order. For example, it is easier to hear heart and lung sounds when a child is quiet. Because touching a child's ears might cause the child to cry, it would be better to take a tympanic temperature after listening to heart and lung sounds.

To begin, the nurse assesses the general condition of the child by answering questions such as the following:

1. What is the child's general appearance? Does the child appear sick or well? Is he or she clean or dirty?
2. What is the child doing? Playing, laughing, or crying? (*Note*: The child may be crying because of the illness.) Is he or she being held by a parent or sitting alone?

Answers to these questions will help guide the nurse in determining the subsequent order of the assessment.

It is important to obtain the cooperation of both the child and the parent (Figure 8-1 ■). At times, much of the assessment can be done while the child is sitting on the parent's lap. This parental contact provides needed security for the small child. Any part of the assessment that might be painful, embarrassing, or frightening should be done last. More detailed assessments of each body system are outlined in Chapters 15 to 28.

TABLE 8-1

Gathering Data from the Pediatric Client

DATA	
SUBJECTIVE	
Demographic data	Full name, contact information, birth date, gender, race, religion
Reason for visit	Statement of the problem in the child's or the parent's words; onset, symptoms, and relieving factors of the problem
Past medical history	Illnesses, hospitalizations, surgeries, accidents (including dates and treatments); current medications (including over-the-counter medications and vitamins); immunization record; known drug, food, and environmental allergies; hazardous substances—alcohol intake, tobacco intake (including smokeless tobacco products), illegal drugs
Family history	Diseases, congenital anomalies, deaths, genogram, review level of support, type of dwelling, source of family income
Review of systems	NOTE: Begin with the system of the presenting problem. Integumentary, head-ears-eyes-nose-throat (HEENT), respiratory, cardiovascular, gastrointestinal including nutritional history, genitourinary, musculoskeletal, neurologic, and endocrine; include psychosocial concerns
OBJECTIVE	
Baseline data	Height, weight, head and chest circumference, vital signs
Physical examination	General appearance, level of consciousness (LOC) NOTE: Begin with the system of the presenting problem. Integumentary, HEENT, respiratory, cardiovascular, gastrointestinal including nutritional history, genitourinary, musculoskeletal, neurologic, and endocrine

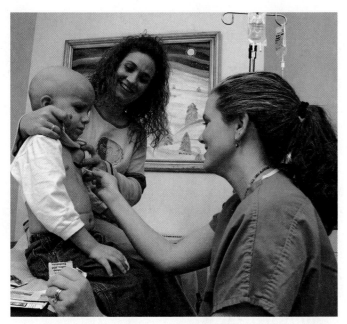

Figure 8-1. ■ Family-centered care policy permits parents to be present during a procedure performed on their child. The parent plays an important role in providing security and comfort to this child who is having his port accessed for an IV infusion treatment.

Discussing Procedures with Children

With the infant and very young child, parents need to be informed about the procedure. The nurse should provide a simple explanation defining the rationale for the procedure, outlining the steps of the procedure, and describing how the parent can assist with the procedure. Allowing the child to touch or play with the equipment may increase the child's sense of security. Parents need an opportunity to ask questions about the procedure. It is best to give them time to ask questions before the procedure begins.

Older children, with greater cognitive ability, need a simple explanation of the procedure. It is often better to time the explanation for immediately before the procedure. This prevents the child from focusing on a painful or invasive procedure and becoming more afraid. The nurse should also allow children ample opportunity to ask questions and discuss fears. Older children and adolescents are curious about their bodies and about the planned procedures. They may even be asked to sign informed consent forms, along with their parents, agreeing to allow the procedures to be done (see more in Chapter 3 ⊕).

Common Procedure Steps

When performing procedures with children, certain basic steps are taken, just as they are with adults. Adaptations of the basic interventions may be made based on age or developmental level. These steps are represented by an icon bar in each procedure in this book:

1. Check the client chart for an appropriate physician's order.
2. Gather all necessary equipment so the procedure can be completed more efficiently, without interruption.
3. Introduce yourself to increase the child's comfort level. When the child is young, fear can be decreased when introductions are made to the parent first. The child can then view the nurse as safe because the parent was comfortable with him or her.
4. Identify the client by checking the identification band or bracelet.
5. Provide privacy. Age and developmental level are important; a young child will want the parent's presence, while an adolescent might not.
6. Explain the procedure. Obtain consent if necessary.
7. Wash hands. Follow standard precautions and facility policy. Often rinse-free hand sanitizers can be used.
8. Don gloves if necessary. Again, follow standard precautions and facility policy.

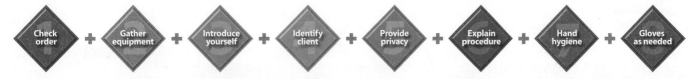

OBTAINING VITAL SIGNS

Temperature

The safety of the child must be taken into consideration in choosing a thermometer and route of measurement. Mercury thermometers have mostly been eliminated from health care facilities due to possible mercury exposure from a broken glass shaft (Box 8-1 ■). Temperature can be recorded in both Celsius and Fahrenheit. Box 8-2 ■ provides a review of conversion formulas.

Electronic thermometers are commonly used. There are a variety of routes for obtaining a temperature with an electronic thermometer. A young child may not be able to follow the directions to keep the mouth closed and not bite the thermometer, so an oral route may not be safe and may not provide an accurate measure. An axillary temperature is safe, but it often takes longer to obtain.

Glass Thermometers

The use of glass thermometers in public health care facilities is rare. Glass thermometers have several disadvantages and hazards, including difficulty reading the temperature, increased time required to obtain the temperature, risk of mercury exposure, and risk for injury related to broken glass. Many parents may still have glass thermometers in their homes. Therefore, the nurse needs to discuss these disadvantages and hazards with the family.

The hazards of mercury exposure are affected by the method of exposure. The amount of mercury contained within most thermometers is very small. If the mercury is swallowed, it is rarely absorbed in the stomach and usually passes through the digestive system. If the mercury is touched, it may cause a skin rash. The greatest risk from mercury occurs with inhalation.

The LPN/LVN can discuss with families the proper methods for handling a mercury spill in the home. Caution the family not to sweep the mercury because this causes it to break into many pieces. Recommend wearing heavy rubber gloves to avoid skin exposure. The mercury may be picked up with an eyedropper, scoop and heavy cardboard, or duct tape. The mercury, and all utensils and clothing exposed to the mercury, must be triple bagged and then sealed in a plastic container. Instruct the client to call the local health department for proper disposal locations. Caution them not to wash material exposed to the mercury in the washing machine because this could contaminate the whole washing machine. The client should ventilate the area for 48 hours.

Note: Sphygmomanometers may also contain mercury.

clinical ALERT

The axillary temperature is one degree *lower* than the oral temperature. Chart the axillary temperature as the numeric value read from the thermometer. Include in your documentation the route of the temperature as "AX."

Some Common Conversions in U.S. and Metric Measurements

1 g = 1 mL (used when weighing diaper to determine fluid output)
1 grain = 60 mg
15 grains = 1 g
1 oz = 30 mL
2.2 lb = 1 kg (used when recording in metric or computing body mass index [BMI])
1 inch = 2.5 cm (used when recording in metric)
39 inches = 1 yd 3 inches = 1 m (used when recording in metric)

A rectal temperature is accurate, but it is not a common procedure because taking a rectal thermometer runs the risk for perforating the anus if the child moves.

clinical ALERT

The rectal temperature is one degree *higher* than the oral temperature. Chart the rectal temperature as the numeric value read from the thermometer. Include in your documentation the route of the temperature as "R."

A tympanic thermometer, which bounces infrared light off the tympanic membrane to measure body temperature, is generally less traumatic for the child and obtains a reading quickly. Measurement of tympanic temperature is described in Procedure 8-1 ■.

Chemically treated tapes that are placed on the child's forehead may also be used to determine temperature. Normal temperature ranges for children are the same as for adults. Table 8-2 ■ shows the normal ranges in vital signs for different ages. Methods for obtaining temperature readings are provided in Procedure 8-1.

Normal Vital Sign Ranges by Age

AGE	TEMPERATURE IN DEGREES CELSIUS/FAHRENHEIT	PULSE (AVERAGE AND RANGE)	RESPIRATIONS (AVERAGE AND RANGE)	BLOOD PRESSURE (mm HG)
Newborns	36.8 (Axillary)/ 98.2	130 (80–180)	35 (30–80)	73/55
1–3 years	37.7 (Rectal)/ 99.9	120 (80–140)	30 (20–40)	90/55
6–8 years	37 (Oral)/ 98.6	100 (75–120)	20 (15–25)	95/57
10 years	37 (Oral)/ 98.6	70 (50–90)	19 (15–25)	102/62
Teen years	37 (Oral)/ 98.6	70 (50–90)	18 (15–20)	120/80
Adult	37 (Oral) 98.6	80 (60–100)	16 (12–20)	120/80
Older adult (older than 70)	36 (Oral) 96.8	80 (60–100)	16 (15–20)	Possible increased diastolic

PROCEDURE 8-1 | Measuring Temperature

Purposes

- To determine a child's body temperature and compare to normal ranges
- To identify variances in normal temperature ranges
- To report abnormal temperatures, in a timely fashion, in an effort to facilitate treatment

Equipment

- Electronic or tympanic thermometer, or thermometer tape
- Disposable probe covers
- Water-soluble lubricant
- Disposable gloves

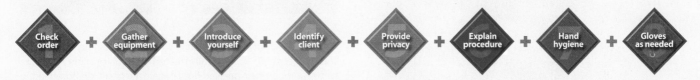

Check order + Gather equipment + Introduce yourself + Identify client + Provide privacy + Explain procedure + Hand hygiene + Gloves as needed

Interventions and Rationales

1. Perform preparatory steps (see icon bar above).
2. Determine client's normal range of temperature by reviewing the chart.
3. Apply a disposable probe to the thermometer shaft. *This prevents transmission of infection.*
4. Position the child in a supine, side-lying, or seated position. *It will be easier for the nurse to manage the child's movements in these positions.*
5. Take the temperature, safely dispose of the probe cover, document the temperature reading and route, and report abnormalities. *Quality care includes safe practice plus timely documentation and reporting.*

TAKING A TYMPANIC TEMPERATURE

6. Position the pinna.
7. For the child younger than 3 years, pull the pinna down and back (Figure 8-2A ■).
8. For the child older than 3 years, pull the pinna up and back (Figure 8-2B ■). *These positions straighten the ear canal.*
9. Place the probe in an anterior position, occluding the outer canal. *The temperature will be more accurate if the probe is positioned toward the tympanic membrane. Occluding the canal will provide core body temperature.*
10. Take the temperature according to manufacturer's recommendations. *In most models, a reading appears on a screen (Figure 8-2C ■).*

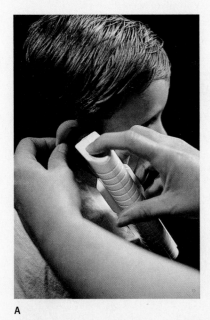

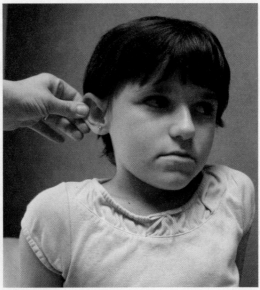

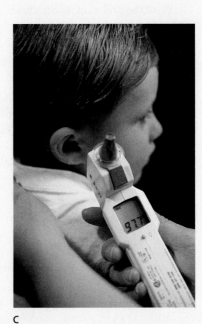

A   B   C

Figure 8-2. ■ Position for inserting thermometer when tympanic route is used. (**A**) Younger than 3 years. (**B**) Older than 3 years. (**C**) Digital readout of temperature appears within 1 minute.

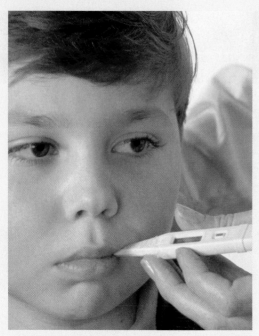

Figure 8-3. ■ Measuring oral temperature. It is important to position the tip of the electronic thermometer under the child's tongue and to make sure the child's lips are closed around the base. (Carolyn A. McKeone/Photo Researchers, Inc.)

11. Return thermometer to the base. *This restores the battery charge.*

TAKING AN ORAL TEMPERATURE

6. Apply a probe cover. *This protects the child from microorganisms on the equipment.*

7. Place the probe under the child's tongue and ask him or her to close the mouth but not clamp down with the teeth (Figure 8-3 ■). *Accurate body temperature is detected when the probe is placed near the large blood vessels in the posterior sublingual pocket.*

8. Leave the thermometer in place according to manufacturer's recommendations. *Most digital and electronic thermometers will signal completion with a beep.*

TAKING ORAL TEMPERATURE WITH PACIFIER THERMOMETERS

6. Although they are not common in health care facilities, the nurse should be aware of thermometers within pacifiers (Figure 8-4A ■). Teach parents to follow manufacturer's directions and to cleanse the thermometer carefully after each use. Teach that the instrument should not be used as a regular pacifier and that it should be discarded if any part becomes cracked or broken. *A pacifier thermometer is unlikely to be used in an institution. Caution parents that misuse or incomplete cleaning could spread infection.*

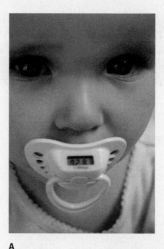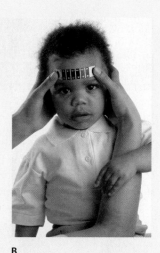

A   B

Figure 8-4. ■ (**A**) Thermometers within pacifiers may be used by some parents. (**B**) A chemically treated tape can provide temperature readings when pressed firmly against a clean, dry forehead. Usually, these temperature-measuring devices are only accurate within 1 or 2 degrees. (B: Dorling Kindersley)

USING A CHEMICAL THERMOMETER

6. Chemical (tape) thermometers may be used in some facilities. Place the tape firmly against a clean, dry forehead (Figure 8-4B ■) and hold it at the ends until one area of the tape becomes lighter. Record the temperature noted under the lightest portion of the tape.

TAKING AN AXILLARY TEMPERATURE

6. Apply probe cover. Place the probe in the child's axilla and secure by holding his or her arm close to the side (Figure 8-5 ■). *Accurate body temperature is detected when the probe is placed near the large blood vessels in the axilla.*

7. Leave the thermometer in place according to manufacturer's recommendations. *Most digital and electronic thermometers will signal completion with a beep.*

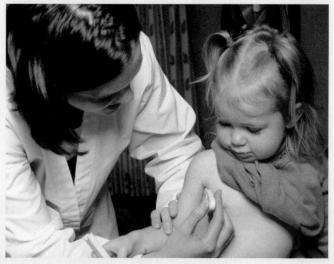

Figure 8-5. ■ Measuring the axillary temperature.

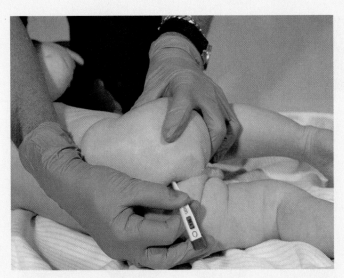

Figure 8-6. ■ Taking a rectal temperature reading from an infant.

TAKING A RECTAL TEMPERATURE (FIGURE 8-6 ■)

6. Apply probe cover. Apply water-soluble lubricant to disposable probe. *Lubricant makes insertion easier and minimizes risk of damaging the anus.*

7. Enlist the assistance of another staff member. *Restraint may be necessary and will decrease the risk of injury.*

8. Retract buttocks and insert the probe no deeper than ½ inch for the infant and 1 inch for the child. *Accurate body temperature is detected when the probe is placed near the large blood vessels in the anus. Risk for injury is minimized by paying attention to the depth of insertion.*

9. Leave the thermometer in place according to manufacturer's recommendations. *Most digital and electronic thermometers will signal completion with a beep.*

SAMPLE DOCUMENTATION

(date) 0800   *(Note: Temperature portion only. This is a focused part of a complete documentation entry.)* Temperature 100.9 °F AX. Reported to Dr. Phillips, orders received. R. Copper LPN

Pulse

Because of fat distribution and small arteries, obtaining an accurate radial, carotid, popliteal, and pedal pulse may be difficult. Generally, an apical pulse, counted for 1 minute, is obtained on a child (Figure 8-7 ■). The pulse rate decreases with age until the normal adult range is reached by age 16 (see Table 8-2). Procedure 8-2 ■ provides more information on obtaining pulse rates in children.

Respiration

Children use the diaphragm as the main muscle of breathing. (See Chapter 12 ⬮⬮ for further information on the anatomy and physiology of respiration in the pediatric client.) Because the diaphragm is used, the nurse can observe or feel the abdominal movement to count the number of respirations in a minute.

clinical ALERT

If the respiratory rate is greater than 60, report this finding immediately to the nurse in charge and/or the doctor. At a respiratory rate of 60 or greater, little oxygen can get to the alveoli for gas exchange.

The respiratory rate decreases with age until the normal adult range is reached by age 16 (see Table 8-2). See Procedure 8-3 ■ for more information on obtaining the respiratory rate in children.

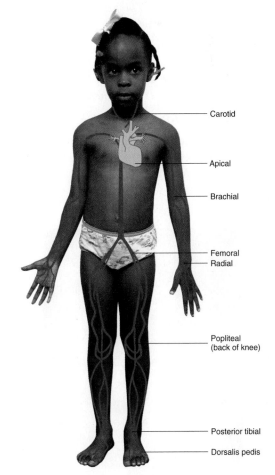

Figure 8-7. ■ The sites used to assess pulses in children.

Carotid
Apical
Brachial
Femoral
Radial
Popliteal (back of knee)
Posterior tibial
Dorsalis pedis

PROCEDURE 8-2 Obtaining Pulse Rate

Purposes

- To determine a child's pulse rate and compare to normal ranges
- To identify variances in normal pulse rate
- To report abnormal pulse rates, in a timely fashion, in an effort to facilitate treatment

Equipment

- Clock or watch with second hand
- Stethoscope

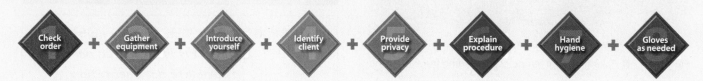

Check order + Gather equipment + Introduce yourself + Identify client + Provide privacy + Explain procedure + Hand hygiene + Gloves as needed

Interventions and Rationales

1. Perform preparatory steps (see icon bar above).

2. Determine client's normal pulse rate by reviewing the chart (see Table 8-2).

3. Position the infant in a supine position and the child in a supine or seated position. *This position allows adequate access for listening to pulse sounds.*

4. Determine the pulse and document rate, rhythm, strength, equality, location and any abnormalities. *Accurate readings provide a baseline for further care, or give information about the client's change in status.*

AUSCULTATING AN APICAL PULSE

5. Choose a time to listen to the heart when the infant or small child is quiet or asleep. *An accurate pulse rate is difficult to assess when a child is crying.*

6. Place the diaphragm of the stethoscope over the apex of the heart (Figure 8-8 ■). Do not attempt to listen through the child's clothing. *The apex or **point of maximal impulse** (PMI) is the site where the heart rate can be best heard. Heart sounds can be muffled if assessed through clothing.*

7. Listen for two distinct heart sounds, lub-dub of rhythm. *The two heart sounds are S1 (closing of the AV valves) and S2 (closing of the semilunar valves). Together they make one heartbeat.*

8. Count the heartbeat for a full minute. *This provides the most accurate assessment of the apical pulse.*

PALPATING A PERIPHERAL PULSE

5. Use the fingertips to locate the child's pulse (Figure 8-9 ■). Peripheral pulse sites are brachial, radial, carotid,

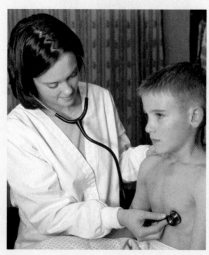

Figure 8-8. ■ Assessing the apical heart rate.

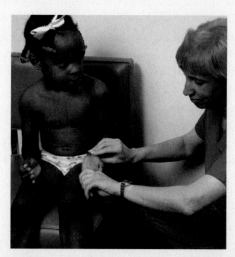

Figure 8-9. ■ Place the fingerpads firmly over each point to evaluate the pulsation.

femoral, popliteal, posterior tibial, and dorsalis pedis. *Fingertips are used instead of the thumb to avoid detecting your own pulse in the thumb.*

6. Assess rhythm and strength of the pulse. (See Chapter 19 ⚭ for more about pulse rhythms.) *Rhythm is assessed by determining the space between the beats and is described as regular or irregular. Strength is assessed by the amount of pressure exerted with each beat. Strength can be documented by using the following scale:*

   0 = Absent

   1+ = Thready or weak

   2+ = Normal

   3+ = Increased

   4+ = Bounding or strong

7. Assess equality of pulse sites by comparing proximal and distal sites. For example, compare the apical pulse to the radial pulse. *This comparison identifies possible alterations in circulation.*

8. Count pulse rate for a full minute. *This makes it easier to notice any irregularities and/or irregular pulse. Once the nurse is experienced at taking pulse rates, the pulse may be counted for 30 seconds and multiplied by 2 to calculate the beats per minute (bpm).*

clinical ALERT

Avoid pressing the carotid pulse, bilaterally, at the same time. This could stop blood flow to the brain.

SAMPLE DOCUMENTATION

(date) 1100   *(Note: Pulse rate portion only. This is a focused part of a complete documentation entry.)*
Radial P 68, 2 + equal bilaterally.
S. Brown LVN

PROCEDURE 8-3   Obtaining Respiratory Rate

Purposes

- To determine a child's respiratory rate and compare to normal ranges
- To identify variances in normal respiratory rates
- To report abnormal respiratory rates, in a timely fashion, in an effort to facilitate treatment

Equipment

- Clock or watch with second hand

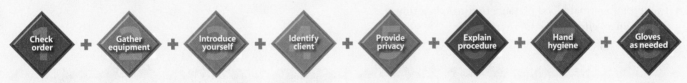

Check order + Gather equipment + Introduce yourself + Identify client + Provide privacy + Explain procedure + Hand hygiene + Gloves as needed

Interventions and Rationales

1. Perform preparatory steps (see icon bar above).

2. Determine client's normal range of respirations by reviewing the chart (see Table 8-2).

3. Position the infant or child in a supine position.

4. Observe the abdomen rise and fall in the infant and young child. Observe the chest rise and fall in the older child and adolescent. The nurse may need to place a hand on the chest or abdomen to feel the rise and fall. *Infants and young children breathe from their diaphragm; thus, the abdomen will rise and fall. Older children breathe more in the chest.*

5. Observe the depth, rhythm, and effort required for respirations.

6. *Depth describes the volume of air exchanged and may be documented as "deep" or "shallow."*

7. *Rhythm refers to the spacing of the respirations and may be described as "regular" or "irregular."*

8. *Effort refers to the energy expended during respirations and may be described as "with effort" or "without effort" or as "labored" or "unlabored."*

9. Count respirations. Document respiratory rate, depth, rhythm, and effort, and report any abnormalities. *One respiration consists of an inspiration (inhalation) and an expiration (exhalation).*

Blood Pressure

The procedure for obtaining a blood pressure is the same as for adults (Procedure 8-4 ■). It is important to explain the procedure to the child using age-appropriate language. Reassure small children that the cuff will not pinch for long. Some clinical agencies require blood pressure to be measured only on older children or on the extremely ill younger child. Blood pressure readings on small children and infants are generally done with Doppler ultrasound equipment.

Although using the upper arm and brachial artery is most common for obtaining blood pressures, using the thigh and popliteal artery or calf and posterior tibial artery is also common in infants and small children. To obtain an accurate measurement, the correct cuff size must be used. The cuff should cover two-thirds of the upper arm, thigh, or calf. If the cuff is too large, the blood pressure will read a false low. If the cuff is too small, the blood pressure will read a false high. The

---

PROCEDURE 8-4 **Measuring Blood Pressure**

Purposes

■ To determine a child's blood pressure and compare to normal ranges
■ To identify variances in normal blood pressure
■ To report abnormal blood pressure findings, in a timely fashion, in an effort to facilitate treatment

Equipment

■ Variety of sizes of blood pressure cuffs (Figure 8-10 ■)
■ Electronic blood pressure monitor, or sphygmomanometer and stethoscope

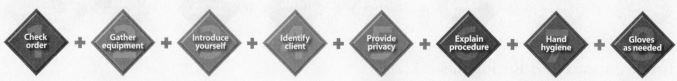

Check order + Gather equipment + Introduce yourself + Identify client + Provide privacy + Explain procedure + Hand hygiene + Gloves as needed

Interventions and Rationales

1. Perform preparatory steps (see icon bar above).
2. Determine client's normal blood pressure range (see Table 8-2).
3. Discuss the fact that the arm will be squeezed tightly for a short period of time. *The client will be more compliant when the procedure is explained beforehand.*

4. Position the client in a seated or recumbent position.
5. Wrap the proper size cuff 1 inch above the antecubital space for an upper arm blood pressure or 1 inch above the popliteal artery for a thigh blood pressure. *If the cuff is too large, the blood pressure equipment will give a false low reading. If the cuff is too small, the blood pressure equipment will give a false high reading.*

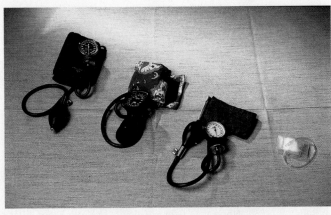

Figure 8-10. ■ Blood pressure cuffs are available in various types and sizes for pediatric clients.

6. Obtain blood pressure and document, reporting any abnormalities.

ELECTRONIC BP ASSESSMENT

7. Turn the power switch on.

8. Position the extremity at the level of the heart. *The blood pressure will be higher than normal if the extremity is lower than the heart.*

9. Press the start button and wait for a reading.

10. Record the digital BP reading.

MANUAL BP ASSESSMENT

7. Close the valve of the sphygmomanometer.

8. Palpate the brachial artery. *This identifies the proper stethoscope placement.*

9. Place the bell or diaphragm of the stethoscope against the artery with the dominant hand (Figure 8-11 ■). With the nondominant hand, inflate the bulb of the sphygmomanometer 30 mm Hg above the client's normal systolic blood pressure. *This provides enough pressure to observe a reading at the first sound.*

10. Slowly release the valve of the bulb of the sphygmomanometer at a rate of 2 to 3 mm Hg/second. Observe the number on the dial corresponding with the presence of the first sound. *This is the systolic pressure.*

11. Continue releasing the air in the bulb at the same rate. Observe the number on the dial corresponding with the disappearance of the pulse. *This is the diastolic pressure.*

clinical ALERT

In children younger than 12 years of age, the diastolic pressure is noted as a muffling of the pulse and not as a disappearance of the sound.

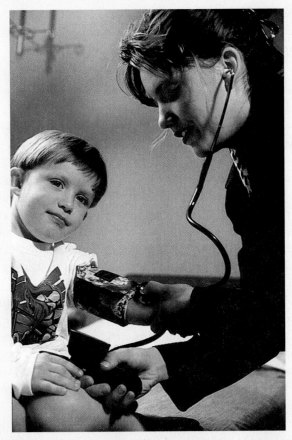

Figure 8-11. ■ With the cuff snugly wrapped around the arm, hold the arm with the cubital fossa at the level of the heart and place the stethoscope against the artery with the dominant hand.

12. Release the remainder of the air in the bulb quickly and remove the cuff.

SAMPLE DOCUMENTATION

(date) 1800   *(NOTE: Blood pressure portion only. This is a focused part of a complete documentation entry.)* BP 112/66 L arm, seated position. F. Darnell LVN

blood pressure in children is lower than in adults and gradually increases until the normal blood pressure ranges are reached by age 16 (see Table 8-2).

Apgar Score

The newborn's adaptation to life outside the uterus is evaluated using an Apgar score (see Procedure 8-5 ■ and Table 8-3 ■). This evaluation is routinely completed at 1 and 5 minutes, but can be used anytime the newborn's condition is in question. Each item—heart rate, respiratory rate, muscle tone, reflex irritability, and color—is assigned a score of 0 to 2, and then totaled. A total score of 8 to 10 requires no additional care. A score of 4 to 7 requires the administration of oxygen and stimulation.

A score of 0 to 3 indicates that the infant needs immediate resuscitation. Figure 12-8 ⬤⬤ will show some of the equipment and techniques used for infant cardiopulmonary resuscitation (CPR). CPR requires special training plus review courses to ensure that the nurse is using up-to-date methods and is following the most current guidelines.

TABLE 8-3			
Apgar Score			
SIGN	SCORE		
	0	1	2
Heart Rate	Absent	Slow — under 100	Over 100
Respiratory Rate	Absent	Slow — irregular	Good crying
Muscle Tone	Flaccid	Some flexing of extremities	Active motion
Reflex Irritability	None	Grimace	Vigorous cry
Color	Pale blue	Body pink, extremities blue	Completely pink (if light skinned); absence of cyanosis (if dark skinned)

Note: Score: 0–4 requires resuscitation efforts; 4–7 requires administration of oxygen and rubbing the back to stimulate breathing; 8–10 requires no special attention

---

PROCEDURE 8-5 Obtaining an Apgar Score

Purposes

- To evaluate the physical condition of the newborn at birth
- To determine the need for resuscitation efforts

Equipment

- Neonatal stethoscope
- Bulb syringe
- Warm towels

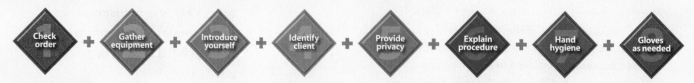

Check order + Gather equipment + Introduce yourself + Identify client + Provide privacy + Explain procedure + Hand hygiene + Gloves as needed

Interventions and Rationales

1. Perform preparatory steps (see icon bar above).

2. Assess the heart rate by auscultation or palpation where the umbilical cord meets the abdomen.

3. Assign a score for heart rate: 0 for absent; 1 for HR less than 100; 2 for HR less than or equal to 100.

4. Assess respiratory effort. Crying indicates good respiratory effort.

5. Assign a score for respiratory effort: 0 for absent; 1 for slow or irregular respirations; 2 for regular respirations or vigorous crying.

6. Assess muscle tone by determining degree of flexion and resistance when straightening the extremity.

7. Assign a score for muscle tone: 0 for flaccidity; 1 for some flexion of extremities; 2 for active motion and good flexion.

8. Assess reflex irritability by physically stimulating the infant during the drying process.

9. Assign a score for reflex irritability: 0 for no response to stimulation; 1 for a notable grimace; 2 for a cry elicited by stimulation.

10. Assess skin color. Observe closely for pallor and cyanosis.

11. Assign a score for skin color: 0 for overall cyanosis and pallor; 1 for acrocyanosis; 2 for pink skin tone over the newborn's entire body.

12. Total the assigned score.

13. Provide appropriate care related to Apgar score. For 8–10: continue with routine newborn care. For 4–7: tactile stimulation and oxygen administration is needed. Scores less than 4: newborn resuscitation is required.

SAMPLE DOCUMENTATION

(date/time)   *(Note: Apgar portion only. This is a focused part of a complete documentation entry.) Caucasian male delivered vaginally. Cord clamped and cut by Dr. L. Hogan. Infant transferred to warmer and dried vigorously. Apgar score 8 @ one minute. W. Brown LVN*

Pain, the Fifth Vital Sign

Pain is considered the fifth vital sign, and the Joint Commission on Accreditation of Healthcare Organizations (JCAHO) requires regular assessment and documentation of it. Pain is subjective; therefore, it exists when the client says it does. The assessment of the pediatric client with regard to pain may be difficult. The infant and small child may not be able to verbalize pain (see Health Promotion box on pages 176 and 177). The difficulty of assessing pain in children contributes to inadequate pain control. Physiologic responses to pain (e.g., tachycardia, tachypnea, pupil dilation, and pallor) may last only a short time. The nurse must look at other indicators of pain, such as restlessness, short attention span, facial grimacing, moaning, crying, posturing or splinting, anorexia, and sleep disturbances (insomnia, drowsiness, or constantly sleeping). The nurse should keep in mind that the child who has had surgery or an injury is likely to be in pain to some degree. Special pain assessment tools have been developed to assist with the evaluation of pain in children (Figure 8-12 ■). Pain assessment is further addressed in Procedure 8-6 ■.

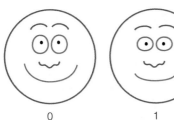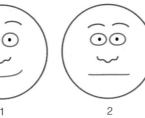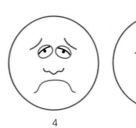

0	1	2	3	4	5

1. Explain to the child that each face is for a person who feels happy because he or she has no pain (hurt, or whatever word the child uses) or feels sad because he or she has some or a lot of pain.

2. Point to the appropriate face and state, "This face..." :
   0—"is very happy because he (or she) doesn't hurt at all."
   1—"hurts just a little bit."
   2—"hurts a little more."
   3—"hurts even more."
   4—"hurts a whole lot."
   5—"hurts as much as you can imagine, although you don't have to be crying to feel this bad."

3. Ask the child to choose the face that best describes how he or she feels. Be specific about which pain (e.g., "shot" or incision) and what time (e.g., Now? Earlier before lunch?)

Figure 8-12. ■ Wong Pain Rating Scale for children 3 to 7 years. (From Hockenberry, M. J. [2005]. *Wong's essentials of pediatric nursing* [7th ed.]. St. Louis, MO: Mosby, p. 1301. Copyright by Mosby Inc. Reprinted with permission.)

HEALTH PROMOTION ISSUE

DEVELOPING A THERAPEUTIC RELATIONSHIP WITH A PEDIATRIC CLIENT

The LPN/LVN working in a pediatrician's office is concerned because her past nursing experience has been with adult clients in an acute-care setting. She states that she has never worked with children before and is having some difficulty relating to them. She is most distressed that the children seem afraid of her. The children will not open up to her and talk to her about issues related to their health care. She is concerned that these factors will affect the type of nursing care she is able to give and ultimately affect the child's health care. She wants some assistance in performing her nursing tasks without scaring the children.

DISCUSSION

For the nurse to assist the child to become healthy, a positive nurse-client relationship must be established. This relationship develops over time, demonstrates respect and confidentiality, is client focused and not nurse focused, and has respect and mutual trust as its basis.

For the relationship between a child and a nurse to be therapeutic, the nurse must display caring behaviors mixed with a professional attitude that conveys competence. Trust develops when children believe that the nurse cares about them and is capable of helping them through a situation. Trust develops as the nurse:

- Listens attentively to what the child says, even if the child is talking about cartoons or toys.
- Displays empathy. Empathy includes recognizing the child's needs, acknowledging the child as real, and showing the child that the nurse is working diligently to meet expressed needs.

- Is honest with the child. Children can see through dishonesty. They need straight, simple responses or an honest "I don't know."
- Is genuine. Caring cannot be contrived. Caring for a child requires knowledge of their developmental levels, of their emotional status, and of their social history. The genuine nurse displays spontaneous behaviors that seek to restore and protect the child.

As the nurse communicates with children, she must recognize that this is accomplished both verbally and nonverbally. Although many people think that spoken words convey our message, in actuality nonverbal communication conveys more than 80% of our message. Nonverbal communication includes our personal appearance. It is said that an opinion of us is formed by other individuals within the first 3 seconds of our first encounter. This opinion is developed before we ever say a word and is largely based on our dress, our posture, our facial expressions, and our gait.

Verbal communication is more than the words we say; it is also how we say them. The nurse can communicate a message effectively by speaking with enthusiasm, energy, and at a pace that indicates interest and not anxiety. Verbal communication should be easy to understand, clear, and as brief as possible.

The timing of verbal communication is also important. The message can go unheard if the child is not ready or willing to listen.

Children learn in different ways. Some must hear the information, whereas others must see it. Still others need to use their hands (e.g., write information or handle a stethoscope) before they can learn.

Developmental levels also influence how a child learns. For instance, a preschooler enjoys learning by trial and error. An adolescent needs to learn independently.

The nurse must consider the child's vocabulary, education, psychomotor abilities, emotional status, societal values, and attention span when developing a teaching plan.

It is also important to choose an appropriate teaching strategy. The nurse can use demonstration to teach a skill and then ask the child to return demonstration. The nurse could also model specific behaviors. Teaching aids may assist the nurse in communicating the proper information. Written materials, posters, anatomic models, games, videos, computers, or dolls may be used in both formal teaching and informal teaching.

PLANNING AND IMPLEMENTATION

Development of a Nurse-Client Relationship

Prior to the child's appointment, the nurse reviews the child's chart, noting any medical or social history that

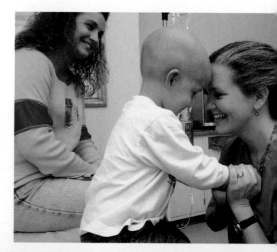

would affect the behavior of the child. The nurse should note the child's age and recall information about the appropriate developmental age. The nurse should practice pronouncing the child's name and note any special likes or dislikes that are noted in the chart. For example, if the child likes a certain cartoon character, the nurse might be able to find a Band-Aid with that character on it or place the child in an exam room decorated with this character. Be sure to include this documentation in the child's chart and update as needed.

Social interaction at the beginning of the appointment is necessary to help ease the child's anxiety and to develop a trusting relationship. The nurse should be at eye level with the child when speaking directly to him or her (see Figure 8-1). Initially, the nurse should avoid touching the child until trust is established.

As the appointment progresses and the nurse seeks to understand the health care needs of the child, listening becomes vital. Active listening requires much energy and is vital in achieving trust. Listening behaviors include eye contact and body language that suggests a willingness to listen (e.g., relaxed body parts, a face-to-face position, a slight leaning toward the child). Listening also requires silence on the nurse's part. As the child speaks, the nurse must actively consider the child's words and not try to develop a wise or witty comeback while the child is speaking. Only after gathering all subjective and objective data can the nurse develop a plan of action. Plans developed before data collection is complete are likely to be ineffective.

Appropriate Communication Techniques

Pediatric nurses often choose bright-colored uniforms that will appeal to children. Hair should be neat. Makeup should look natural, so as not to distract or frighten the child. Posture should be erect but not tense.

Children can read the thoughts of the nurse through the nurse's facial expressions. It is important for nurses to learn to control feelings of disgust, impatience, or boredom. The nurse's face needs to display interest, enthusiasm, and energy. If a child confides that he or she has been abused by an adult, the nurse must not express horror or anger. The nurse's face should convey interest and concern so the child will continue to share information.

When communicating verbally with children, the nurse should speak to them in language and terms that they can understand. The nurse should use open-ended questions when trying to obtain information from a child. Questions such as "Tell me how your tummy feels" or "What happened to your leg?" will elicit more information than a question that can simply be answered with a "yes" or "no."

Appropriate Teaching Methods

The nurse needs to have a variety of teaching aids available in order to conduct formal or informal teaching for the child. A simple drawing of the body can help the nurse describe a disease, procedure, or surgery. Dolls or puppets appeal to preschoolers.

In school settings, videos are often a way of providing information. If videos are used, the dialogue should be appropriate for the age group. Slides or photographs should also be age appropriate. For example, photographs of genitalia should not be shown in a classroom of mixed genders. The nurse should carefully assess readiness to learn and evaluate learning following the teaching session.

With diligence and continued effort, the nurse should be able to relate to the pediatric client and provide effective care.

SELF-REFLECTION

When a child reacts negatively to you, what feelings do you have? If a child has never acted negatively toward you, imagine what the scenario might look like. Be honest about your feelings. When you encounter a strange environment, what factors make you feel more uncomfortable? What factors make you feel more comfortable? What do you need to change in your nursing practice to help develop trust with your clients? To communicate better with your pediatric clients? To be more effective in providing them with teaching as it relates to their health care?

SUGGESTED RESOURCES

For the Nurse

Blackwell, P., & Baker, B. (2002). Estimating communication competence of infants and toddlers. *Journal of Pediatric Health Care, 16*(1), 19–35.

Humphries, J. (2002). The school health nurse and health education in the classroom. *Nursing Standard, 16*(17), 42–45.

Sydnor-Greenberg, N., & Dokken, D. (2001). Communication in healthcare: Thought on the child's perspective. *Journal of Child and Family, 4*(3), 225–230.

| PROCEDURE 8-6 | # Pain Assessment |

Purposes

- To assess the nature of the child's pain to include location and intensity
- To report findings to the appropriate personnel in an effort to assist in the relief of the child's pain

Equipment

- Variety of pain assessment scales that are appropriate for the child's age

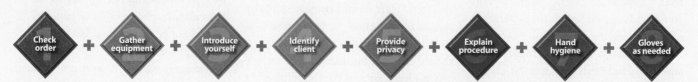

Check order + Gather equipment + Introduce yourself + Identify client + Provide privacy + Explain procedure + Hand hygiene + Gloves as needed

Interventions and Rationales

1. Perform preparatory steps (see icon bar above).
2. Observe the child for manifestations of pain. *Objective data related to pain may be obtained through observation.*
3. If the child is verbal, ask him or her to describe the location and intensity of pain. *The verbal child should be able to assist the nurse by indicating the location and severity of the pain, according to a numeric scale.*
4. If the child is young but able to communicate, the nurse uses the scale to determine a pain level using nonverbal cues. *The child can point to the face that most resembles the pain he or she feels, or to the part of the body that hurts the most.*
5. Document objective and subjective data gathered.

SAMPLE DOCUMENTATION

(date) 2200   *(Note: Pain portion only. This is a focused part of a complete documentation entry.)* 9-year-old boy crying, moaning. States "my head really hurts." Rates headache as 8 on a scale of 10. Shades closed. TV turned off. Cool cloth applied. Report given to charge nurse. E. Gorden LPN

GROWTH MEASUREMENTS

Growth measurements can be taken in U.S. or metric units, depending on facility policy. Box 8-3 ■ provides some commonly needed conversions (inches to centimeters, etc.)

Height

With the infant or child lying supine, use a tape measure, measuring stick, or measurement mat to measure the child's length. Length is assessed from crown to heel. Once the child is able to stand, the height measurement can be obtained with the child standing against the measuring stick. Procedure 8-7 ■ provides more information on measuring height and length.

BOX 8-3

Conversion Formulas

Celsius to Fahrenheit:
From °C **up** to °F:

$$°F = 1.8 \times °C + 32$$

First **multiply** ° by 1.8; then **add** 32.

Fahrenheit to Celsius:
From °F **down** to °C:

$$°C = °F - 32 \text{ divided by } 1.8$$

First **subtract** 32 from °F, then **divide** by 1.8.

PROCEDURE 8-7   Measuring Height and Length

Purposes

- To obtain an accurate measure of the client's height or length
- To report abnormal findings in a timely fashion, in an effort to facilitate treatment; abnormal findings might include lack of growth in height between yearly well-child visits

Equipment

- Tape measure, yard stick, meter stick, or measuring mat
- Stadiometer
- Platform scale with stature-measuring device

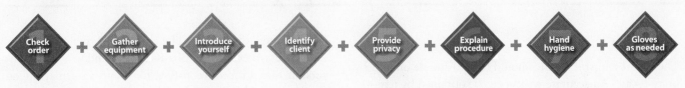

Check order + Gather equipment + Introduce yourself + Identify client + Provide privacy + Explain procedure + Hand hygiene + Gloves as needed

Interventions and Rationales

1. Perform preparatory steps (see icon bar above).

FOR INFANTS

2. Place the infant in a supine position.

3. Place the infant's head against a flat surface. Extend legs until the knee is straight.

4. Use a tape measure, measuring stick, or measuring mat to measure from the crown to the heel (Figure 8-13A ■). Note the length in inches or centimeters.

5. Plot the measurement on a standardized growth chart. *Note:* Appendix II 🔗 shows growth charts from infancy to age 18.

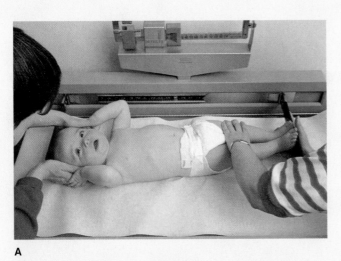

A

Figure 8-13. ■ **(A)** Measure an infant's length carefully from the crown of the head to the heel. **(B)** Standing height measurements are taken routinely at each well-child visit to assess the child's rate of growth. Position the head in an erect and midline position while the shoulders, buttocks, and heels touch the wall. Move the headpiece down to touch the crown. Measure the height reading to the nearest 0.5 cm. or ¼ inch.

Head in midline

Line from eye canthi parallel to stadiometer headpiece

Shoulders touching

Buttocks touching

Heels touching and together

B

FOR CHILD

2. Have the child stand erect, with bare feet and the head level, with the back of the head against the measuring device (Figure 8-13B ■).

3. Place the headpiece onto the child's crown.

4. Note the height in inches or centimeters.

5. Plot the measurement on a standardized growth chart.

Weight

The infant and small child should be laid supine on a calibrated scale. An accurate weight can be obtained by removing the child's clothing. A lightweight absorbent pad can be used to serve as a barrier against cold and moisture. The nurse should hold one hand above the child to guard against injury. If the child is able to stand, weight can be obtained on an upright balance scale. The nurse should seek to weigh the child similarly at each visit. For instance, the child should always be with or without shoes, fully clothed or in underclothing only. The child's privacy and modesty should be protected. See Box 8-2 for pound/kilogram conversion and Procedure 8-8 ■ for more information on obtaining weights.

Body Mass Index

The body mass index (BMI) is used differently in children and adults. The BMI for children is gender and age specific and is called the BMI-for-age. It can be used for children from age 2 through adolescence. The BMI is

---

PROCEDURE 8-8   **Obtaining Weight**

Purposes

■ To obtain an accurate measure of the client's weight
■ To report abnormal findings, in a timely fashion, in an effort to facilitate treatment

Equipment

■ Infant scale, calibrated
■ Floor scale, calibrated

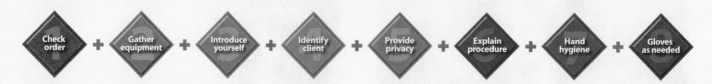

Check order + Gather equipment + Introduce yourself + Identify client + Provide privacy + Explain procedure + Hand hygiene + Gloves as needed

Interventions and Rationales

1. Perform preparatory steps (see icon bar above).

FOR INFANTS

2. Place the infant in seated or supine position on the infant scale (Figure 8-14 ■).

3. Stand close to provide safety for the infant.

4. Read the scale when the infant is still.

5. Plot the weight on a standardized growth chart.

FOR CHILD

2. Ask the child to stand on the scale without shoes.

3. Read the digital scale or balance the weights to obtain a reading.

4. Plot the weight on a standardized growth chart.

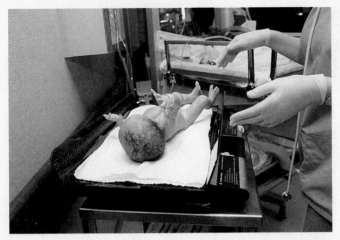

Figure 8-14. ■ Weight. The caregiver's hands are poised near the newborn as a safety measure.

(date) 0900   *(Note: Weight portion only. This is a focused part of a complete documentation entry.)* 11-year-old male, 48 inches, 100 lb. D. Deen LVN

derived by calculating the weight in kilograms divided by height in meters squared (Procedure 8-9 ■). This measurement can indicate whether a child is underweight, overweight, or at risk for becoming overweight. However, it should be remembered that children's body fat changes as they grow and also according to their gender.

Head Circumference

Using a tape measure, the head circumference is measured from slightly above the eyebrow, above the pinna of the ear, and around the occiput (see Procedure 8-10 ■). Head circumference should be obtained on all children younger than 36 months of age and any child with a neurologic defect.

PROCEDURE 8-9   Calculating Body Mass Index

Purpose

■ To determine a child's risk of being underweight or overweight

Equipment

■ BMI-for-age chart

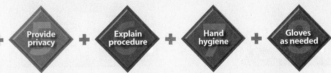

Interventions and Rationales

1. Perform preparatory steps (see icon bar above).
2. Plot the child's weight and height in relation to gender.
3. Obtain BMI. Calculate the BMI by dividing the child's weight in kilograms by the height in meters squared. For example, if a 17-year-old boy weighs 180 lb and is 78 inches tall:

    180 lb divided by 2.2 lb/kg = 81.8 kg

    78 inches divided by 39 inches/m = 2 meters

    81.8 kg divided by 2×2 =

    81.8 kg divided by 4 m² =

    20.45 is BMI

This boy would have a BMI a bit lower than the 50th percentile for his age (Ball & Bindler, 2006).

4. Report findings to appropriate personnel.

(date) 1300   *(Note: BMI portion only. This is a focused part of a complete documentation entry.)* 11-year-old male, 48 in., 100 lb BMI 30.6. Report given to C. Cox CRNP. L. April LPN

PROCEDURE 8-10 **Measuring Head Circumference**

Purpose

- To determine normalcy of the infant's head circumference in relation to chest circumference

Equipment

- Tape measure

Check order + Gather equipment + Introduce yourself + Identify client + Provide privacy + Explain procedure + Hand hygiene + Gloves as needed

Interventions and Rationales

1. Perform preparatory steps (see icon bar above).
2. Position the infant in a supine position.
3. Place the tape measure slightly above the eyebrows, above the pinna of the ear, and around the occiput (Figure 8-15 ■). *This is the largest diameter of the infant's head.*

4. Document the head circumference in inches or centimeters. The nurse may also document the amount of *molding* (shaping of the head during the birth process). *Documentation provides information for later comparison.*
5. Compare to chest circumference. *Head circumference is equal to or 2 cm greater than chest circumference until age 2.*
6. Plot the measurement on a standardized growth chart.

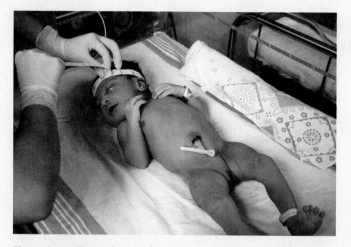

Figure 8-15. ■ Head circumference is usually 33 to 35 centimeters.

SAMPLE DOCUMENTATION

(date) 1500   *(Note: Head circumference portion only. This is a focused part of a complete documentation entry.)* Male infant born vaginally at 1330. Head circumference 33 cm. Chest circumference 33 cm. Moderate amount of molding noted. H. Freida LPN

Torso Circumference

CHEST CIRCUMFERENCE

Using a tape measure, the chest circumference is measured from under the axilla, across the nipples, and around the back (Procedure 8-11 ■). The normal height, weight, and head and chest circumference measurements can be found on growth charts in Appendix II ⚭.

ABDOMINAL CIRCUMFERENCE

Abdominal circumference, or girth, is measured by using a tape measure around the abdomen, at the umbilicus (Procedure 8-12 ■). Although abdominal circumference is not a routine measurement, it may be used when concerned about increasing abdominal distension as in intestinal obstruction.

PROCEDURE 8-11   Measuring Chest Circumference

Purpose
■ To determine normalcy of the infant's chest circumference in relation to head circumference

Equipment
■ Tape measure

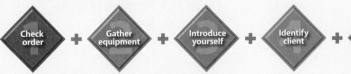

Interventions and Rationales

1. Perform preparatory steps (see icon bar above).
2. Position the infant in a supine position.
3. Encircle the chest with the measuring tape. Place the tape measure against the bare skin of the infant's chest,

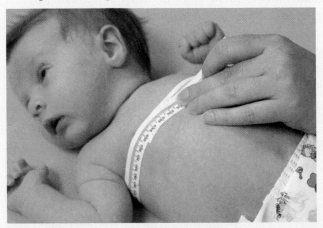

Figure 8-16. ■ Measure chest circumference with the tape flat and at an even distance under the axillae.

at the nipple line, under the axillae (Figure 8-16 ■). *This is the largest diameter of the infant's chest.*

4. Document the chest circumference in inches or centimeters.
5. Compare to head circumference. *Head circumference is equal to or 2 cm greater than chest circumference until age 2.*
6. Plot the measurement on a standardized growth chart.

SAMPLE DOCUMENTATION

(date) 1400   *(Note: Chest-head proportion only. This is a focused part of a complete documentation entry.)* Female infant born at 1349 by cesarean section. Chest circumference 31 cm. Head circumference 32 cm.
B. Smartt LVN

PROCEDURE 8-12   Measuring Abdominal Girth

Purposes
■ To determine normalcy of the infant's or child's abdominal girth
■ To check for abnormal findings such as umbilical and inguinal hernias, bowel obstructions, ascites, constipation, and organ enlargement

Equipment
■ Tape measure

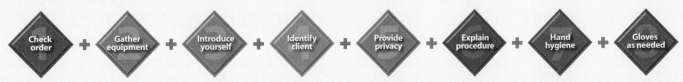

Interventions and Rationales

1. Perform preparatory steps (see icon bar).
2. Position the child in a supine position.
3. Place the tape measure against the bare skin of the child's abdomen, at the umbilicus. *This is the largest diameter of the abdomen.*
4. Document the abdominal circumference in inches or centimeters. *Follow facility policy for unit of measure.*

NEWBORN REFLEXES

Reflexes in newborns are signs of neurologic integrity (Procedure 8-13 ▪ and Figure 8-17 ▪). Some reflexes, like blink, cough, and sneeze, remain intact throughout life. Others disappear by 4 to 6 months. Still others will take 2 years to disappear. Absent or slowed reflexes may indicate prematurity of the infant. They may also result from CNS depressant medications that were transferred to the infant during labor or in breast milk. Reexamination should be done at a later date. Lingering reflexes (those present after the expected time) may indicate neurologic lesions. The child with lingering reflexes should be referred for further evaluation by the primary care provider.

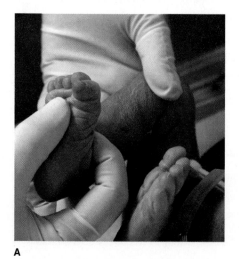
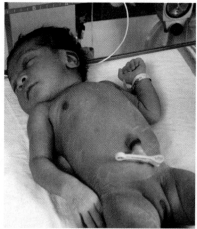
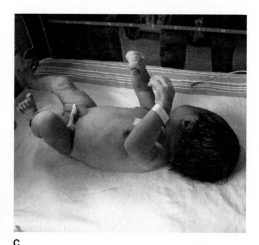

A **B** **C**

Figure 8-17. ▪ **(A)** Newborn exhibiting plantar grasp reflex. **(B)** Newborn exhibiting the tonic neck reflex. **(C)** Newborn exhibiting Moro reflex.

Eliciting Newborn Reflexes

Purpose

- To assess neurologic integrity

Equipment

- Reflex hammer
- Pacifier

Check order + Gather equipment + Introduce yourself + Identify client + Provide privacy + Explain procedure + Hand hygiene + Gloves as needed

Interventions and Rationales

1. Perform preparatory steps (see icon bar above).

2. Elicit the **rooting reflex** by stroking the newborn's cheek. Observe the infant's head turning toward the cheek that was stroked. The infant may also open his or her mouth as if to begin sucking. *The rooting reflex disappears between 3 and 4 months.*

3. Elicit the **sucking reflex** by touching the newborn's lips or placing a gloved finger or pacifier in the newborn's mouth. *The rooting and sucking reflexes are important in feeding. The sucking reflex disappears by 10 months.*

4. Elicit the **palmar grasp reflex** by placing a finger or small object in the newborn's hand. *Newborns grasp the finger tight enough to be lifted from the bed. A weak grasp could indicate cerebral, local nerve, or muscle injury. This reflex lasts 4 months.*

5. Elicit the **plantar grasp reflex** (see Figure 8-17A), by touching the ball of the foot. The toes curl under as if newborns are trying to "grasp" with their feet. *The plantar grasp reflex lasts 8 months, This reflex must disappear before infants are able to walk.*

6. Elicit the **Babinski's reflex** by stroking the lateral side of the foot from heel to toe using either the index finger or the metal end of a reflex hammer. The big toe should dorsiflex and the other toes should flare. *Absence of this reflex could indicate upper motor neuron abnormalities. This reflex disappears before the infant begins to walk.*

7. Elicit the **stepping reflex** by holding the newborn upright with the feet touching the table. Newborns will step as if walking. *Stepping can be observed more frequently 72 hours following birth.*

8. Elicit the **tonic neck reflex** (see Figure 8-17B) by placing the newborn supine on a firm surface. Turn the head to one side, and observe the newborn extend the arm and leg on that side. The opposite arm and leg will flex. This is also called the fencing position.

9. Elicit the **Moro reflex** or **startle reflex** (see Figure 8-17C) by holding the newborn in a sitting position and suddenly lowering the head, by bumping the surface of the crib or clapping loudly near the infant. The newborn will quickly extend (abduct) the arms and clench the fists. The arms will then adduct in an embracing motion. The lower extremities may extend and then flex. A slight tremor may be noted. *This reflex disappears by 6 months of age.*

SAMPLE DOCUMENTATION

(date/time) (Note: Reflexes portion only. This is a focused part of a complete documentation entry.)
Newborn reflexes elicited.
Moro, plantar and palmar grasp, rooting, sucking, stepping, Babinski, and tonic neck reflexes present. H. Stewart LVN

CARE OF THE CHILD DURING DIAGNOSTIC PROCEDURES

Diagnostic procedures are often necessary to determine treatment for the pediatric client. These procedures are often frightening to children. The nurse must be able to communicate in an age-appropriate manner to the child. There are, however, times when a child must be restrained to ensure safety. If possible, the parent should be allowed to accompany the child during procedures.

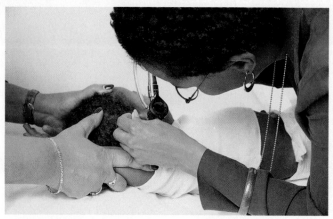

A

Figure 8-18. ■ To restrain an uncooperative child, place the child supine on the examining table. (**A**) Have an assistant hold the child's arms next to the head to restrain the child's head movements. Restrain the child's body movements by lying across the child's body. (**B**) A mummy restraint is an alternative method of restraining all but the head of a child.

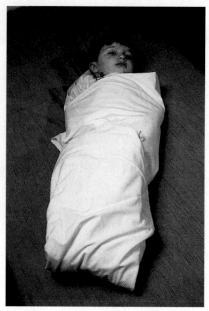

B

clinical ALERT

For procedures in hospital, it is important that the child be taken to an examination room. If painful procedures are performed in the child's room, he or she may become fearful of going to sleep or of being left alone in the room.

Restraining the Child

At times children must be restrained during procedures to protect their safety (Procedure 8-14 ■). Procedures such as medication administration by injection, initiating intravenous access, lumbar puncture, or using an otoscope require some form of restraint. It is important to use the least restrictive type of restraint for the shortest period of time to reach the desired goal. The child's age, size, and condition and the needed procedure are taken into account when deciding on a type of restraint. Parents should be present if possible. However, to prevent feelings of mistrust, avoid requiring the parent to restrain the child.

Often, infants can be restrained by holding them in position (Figure 8-18A ■). Larger children may require a mummy wrap in a sheet (Figure 8-18B ■). Restraint sleeves can be used to keep a young child from bending the arms. This type of restraint is useful to prevent the child from playing with tubes or dressings applied to the arms, head, or chest. Mittens or socks can be put over the hand and pinned to the long sleeve of a shirt to keep the child from grasping and pulling.

PROCEDURE 8-14   Restraining the Child

Purpose

■ To maintain a child's safety during a procedure by restricting movement

Equipment

■ Papoose board
■ Large sheet or blanket, or a mummy board
■ Elbow restraints
■ Tape

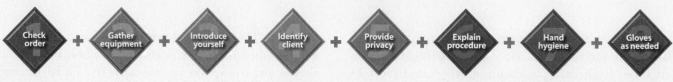

Interventions and Rationales

1. Perform preparatory steps (see icon bar).

2. Obtain an order from the physician to apply restraints. If the child's safety is compromised and restraints must be applied prior to receiving the order, obtain the order within 1 hour. *Legally, the nurse must have a physician's order to apply restraints. The safety of the child is the priority.*

3. Discuss procedure with the child or the parents. *Except for small children, clients will be more compliant when the procedure is explained beforehand.*

4. Solicit the assistance of a coworker. *This will prevent injury to the child.*

APPLYING PAPOOSE RESTRAINTS

5. Place the child in a supine position on a papoose board that has been padded with a towel or blanket.

6. Wrap the fabric around the child according to manufacturer's recommendations (Figure 8-19 ■). Secure with Velcro, paying special attention to securing the joints. *This prevents the child from bending the joint(s) and sustaining injury.*

APPLYING MUMMY RESTRAINTS

For the Infant

5. Place the blanket on a hard surface. Position it in a diamond shape.

6. Fold down the top corner. Lay the infant in a supine position with the neck on the folded edge (Figure 8-20A ■).

7. Wrap the blanket around one arm and under the back (Figure 8-20A).

8. Weave this same part of the blanket under the opposite arm and the back.

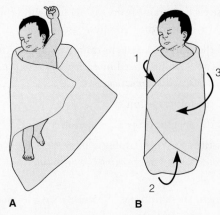

Figure 8-20. ■ Making a mummy restraint.

9. Take the other side of the blanket and bring it over the infant's abdomen and then tuck it under the body (see Figure 8-20B).

10. Fold the remaining corner of the blanket up over the infant's abdomen and tuck (see Figure 8-20B). *These steps ensure a secure hold without injury.*

For the Child

5. Place the blanket on a hard surface. Position it in a diamond shape.

6. Fold down the top corner. Lay the child in a supine position with the shoulders on the folded edge.

7. Wrap one edge of the blanket across the arm, abdomen, and legs, tucking under the opposite arm and under the back.

8. Take the other side of the blanket and bring it over the child's abdomen and then tuck under the back and legs. *These steps ensure a secure hold without injury.*

APPLYING ELBOW RESTRAINTS

5. Place the elbow restraints on the child's arm. Secure the restraint according to manufacturer's recommendations. This may be with pins, ties, or Velcro. Most models are positioned from wrist to axilla (Figure 8-21 ■). *This device will not allow the child to bend the arm and prevents the child from reaching and grabbing.*

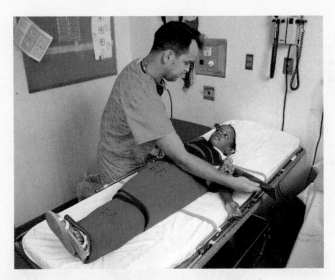

Figure 8-19. ■ Child on a papoose restraint board.

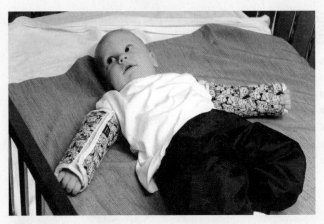

Figure 8-21. ■ Infant with elbow restraints.

6. Release each restraint immediately following the procedure or according to physician's order.

7. Assess the skin where the restraint was applied for redness and compromised integrity. *The skin is the first line of defense against infection.*

8. Assess the joints for injury.

9. Assess the area for proper circulation.

10. Assess the area for neurologic intactness. *These measures determine whether the restraint is constricting nerve conduction.*

11. Document these findings. *Documentation is an essential part of quality nursing care.*

SPECIMEN COLLECTION

Many specimens may need to be obtained for effective treatment of a child. These include blood, urine, stool, wound drainage, sputum, spinal fluid, and throat specimens. Throat cultures are unpleasant for the child and often stimulate the gag reflex, resulting in vomiting. Care must be taken to prevent trauma to the oral pharynx. The head should be held still while the mouth is opened and the pharynx is swabbed.

Collecting urine and stool specimens is a particular challenge with children. Older children may be embarrassed at the thought. Age-specific instruction is essential, and the nurse may obtain assistance from the parent. Stool specimens can be collected directly from the diaper with a tongue blade. To collect a urine specimen from infants and children who are not toilet-trained, a urine collection bag is used. It is important to check the bag frequently for leakage and skin irritation. Methods for collecting specimens are provided in Procedures 8-15 to 8-20 ■.

PROCEDURE 8-15   Obtaining Blood Specimens

Purpose

■ To identify variations in hematologic lab values

Equipment

Capillary test:

■ Lancet
■ Automatic pen to hold lancet, if desired
■ Alcohol swab
■ Collection card
■ Reagent strip
■ Capillary tube
■ Glucometer

Venous and blood cultures:

■ Tourniquet
■ 20- to 27-gauge needle
■ **Vacutainer®** (a hollow, plastic device with a shielded or blunted needle on one end and a sharp needle on the other end that enters the vein (Figure 8-22 ■); it facilitates the collection of blood specimens)
■ Variety of collection tubes or culture media collection bottles
■ Gloves (clean for capillary and venipuncture, sterile for blood culture collection)

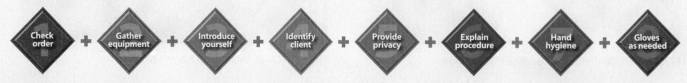

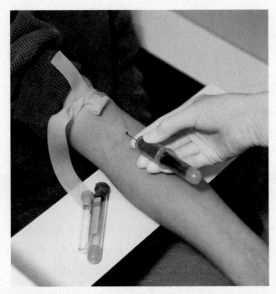

Figure 8-22. ■ Vacutainer® is used in collecting blood specimens. (Getty Images Photodisc)

Interventions and Rationales

Note: ALWAYS work within the nursing practice acts of your state and within facility guidelines.

1. Perform preparatory steps (see icon bar above).

2. Solicit the assistance of a coworker. *This will help prevent injury to the child.*

CAPILLARY SPECIMENS

3. Cleanse site (fingertip or heel) with alcohol or soap and water. *Repeated exposure to alcohol may make the site tough and inappropriate for future collection of specimens.*

4. Puncture the site using the lancet. Obtain at least one drop of blood.

5. Collect specimen onto desired source (collection card, reagent strip, or collection tube).

6. If obtaining a specimen for glucose monitoring, insert reagent into glucometer and proceed according to manufacturer's recommendations.

VENOUS SPECIMENS (FIGURE 8-23A–C ■)

4. Apply a tourniquet proximal to the intended site for venipuncture. *Restricting blood flow to the site allows venous pooling at the site, dilating the vein for easier access.*

5. Determine the appropriate site for specimen collection, using inspection and palpation.

6. Cleanse the site with alcohol or povidone-iodine (according to agency policy). Be sure to verify that the child is not allergic to povidone-iodine. Use firm pressure beginning at the center of the site, creating a circular pattern. *This technique will reduce the likelihood of transferring harmful bacteria to the puncture site* (Figure 8-23B).

7. Steady the site by using the nondominant hand to displace the skin just below the site. Be careful not to touch the previously cleansed site. *This maintains the sterile site and aids insertion of the needle.*

8. Hold the needle with attached Vacutainer, bevel up, at a 15- to 20-degree angle above the previously cleansed site. Insert the needle. Advance until blood return occurs (Figure 8-23C).

9. Insert desired collection tube(s).

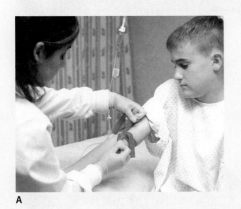
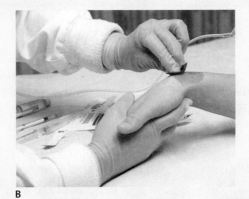
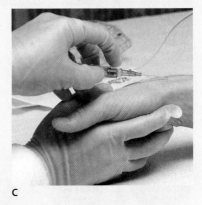

A   B   C

Figure 8-23. ■ Venipuncture procedure. (**A**) The tourniquet is applied to restrict venous blood flow. (**B**) The area for venipuncture is cleaned by the nurse with Betadine and alcohol solutions and dried with a cotton ball. (**C**) The needle is placed with the bevel up and gently inserted into the identified vein.

10. Release tourniquet. *This lessens the pressure, slowing blood flow.*

11. Carefully remove needle and apply pressure to the site. *This ensures that bleeding has ceased.*

12. Cleanse the site and apply a bandage if necessary. Allow the child to select the type of Band-Aid. *Band-Aids often give the child ownership, provide a distraction, and serve as a source of pride for bravery during the procedure.*

13. Label, package, and transport specimen according to agency policy.

BLOOD CULTURES

4. Apply sterile gloves.

5. Proceed as outlined previously for venipuncture, using needle with attached syringe.

6. Withdraw approximately 20 mL of blood.

7. Carefully remove contaminated needle.

8. Discard used needle or syringe and replace with sterile needle using sterile technique.

9. Cleanse top of each collection bottle with an antimicrobial agent.

10. Insert blood specimen in collection bottle. Gently mix. *The blood specimen needs to be mixed with the culture medium to obtain reliable test results.*

11. As ordered, repeat the procedure at desired intervals using another peripheral site and sterile needle for each venipuncture.

12. Apply pressure to site. *This ensures that bleeding has ceased.*

13. Cleanse site and apply bandage if necessary.

14. Label, package, and transport specimen according to agency policy.

15. Document findings.

SAMPLE DOCUMENTATION

(date) 1500 *(Note: Blood specimen collection portion only. This is a focused part of a complete documentation entry.)* 20 mL venous sample obtained from antecubital space using 20-gauge needle and aseptic technique. Pressure bandage applied. Specimen to lab per agency policy for basic metabolic panel.
N. Thomas LVN

PROCEDURE 8-16 Obtaining Urine Specimens

Purposes

- To obtain information concerning chemical composition of the urine sample
- To determine the presence of harmful bacteria or blood in the urine specimen

Equipment

- Infant collection bag or sterile collection container
- Soap, sterile water, and sterile cotton swabs or prepackaged antiseptic wipes
- Alcohol wipes
- Sterile needle with 20-mL syringe (from indwelling catheter only)

Check order + Gather equipment + Introduce yourself + Identify client + Provide privacy + Explain procedure + Hand hygiene + Gloves as needed

Interventions and Rationales

1. Perform preparatory steps (see icon bar above).

USING AN INFANT COLLECTION BAG (FIGURE 8-24 ■)

2. Cleanse the perineum. Wipe with soap, water, and cotton ball from tip of penis to scrotum for males and

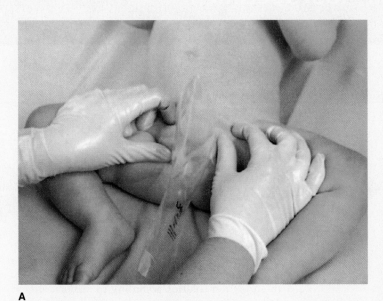 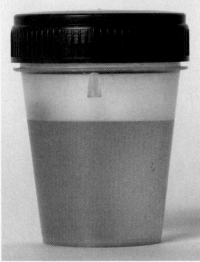

Figure 8-24. ■ **(A)** Attaching the urine collection bag. **(B)** Urine cup. (B: © Dorling Kindersley Media Library.)

clitoris to anus for females. Discard cotton ball. Repeat twice. Rinse with sterile water. *Cleansing removes microorganisms and foreign matter that might alter laboratory results.*

3. Apply urine collection bag with adhesive strips. For males, place over the scrotum and penis. For females, place over entire labia majora (Figure 8-24A).

4. Apply a diaper over the urine collection bag to secure. *The diaper will support the device and prevent the infant from handling the collection bag.*

5. When specimen is obtained, remove gently from the infant's skin.

6. Place entire bag in sterile specimen container.

OBTAINING A CLEAN CATCH SPECIMEN

2. Instruct the child to cleanse the perineum. The LPN may need to assist in this process, using clean gloves, if the child is unable. For a male, use a cleansing swab or soap and water to cleanse the head of the penis in a circular pattern beginning at the tip of the penis and moving outward. *Note:* If a male has foreskin, it should be retracted. For a female, separate the labia and cleanse from the clitoris to the anus. *Note:* Three cleansing swabs should be used. *This technique lessens the likelihood of carrying bacteria toward the urinary meatus. Separate swabs prevent reinfection.*

3. Ask the child to initiate urination.

4. If possible, have the child stop the stream, place the sterile urine container (Figure 8-24B), and begin flow again.

5. Remove container. Instruct child to finish emptying the bladder.

OBTAINING A STERILE URINE SPECIMEN FROM AN INDWELLING CATHETER

2. Clamp the catheter for a few minutes to obtain a specimen.

3. Cleanse the catheter port with an alcohol swab. *This minimizes contamination of specimen with bacteria.*

4. Insert sterile needle with attached syringe into port.

5. Withdraw specimen.

6. Inject specimen into sterile specimen container without touching the sides of the container with the needle or syringe.

7. Unclamp the catheter.

8. Label, package, and transport specimen according to agency policy.

SAMPLE DOCUMENTATION

(date) 1300 *(Note: Urine specimen portion only. This is a focused part of a complete documentation entry.)* Urine collection bag attached to male infant according to agency policy. 30 mL clear, yellow urine obtained. Transferred to sterile specimen container and sent to lab for urinalysis.
B. Brockway LVN

Obtaining a Stool Specimen

Purpose

- To determine the presence of harmful bacteria, parasites, or blood in the stool specimen

Equipment

- Tongue blade or cotton swabs
- Stool specimen container
- Guaiac card and solution for occult blood

Check order + **Gather equipment** + **Introduce yourself** + **Identify client** + **Provide privacy** + **Explain procedure** + **Hand hygiene** + **Gloves as needed**

Interventions and Rationales

1. Perform preparatory steps (see icon bar above).
2. Obtain stool specimen from diaper, bedpan, or commode.
3. Remove amount of specimen needed for particular test with tongue blades or cotton swabs. (Some tests require 2 tsp. Others require the entire specimen.)
4. Place specimen in stool specimen container (Figure 8-25 ■).

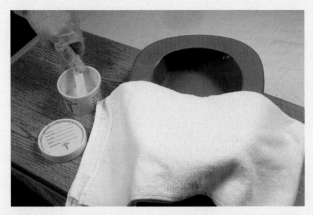

Figure 8-25. ■ Equipment for a stool specimen. In the case of an infant or toddler, the specimen could be collected from a soiled diaper. (Pearson Education/PH College)

TESTING FOR OCCULT BLOOD

5. Smear a thin layer of stool onto the guaiac card.
6. Apply test solution according to manufacturer's instructions.
7. Read results. Document negative or positive findings. Report positive findings.
8. Label, package, and transport specimen according to agency policy.

SAMPLE DOCUMENTATION

(date) 0745   *(Note: Stool specimen portion only. This is a focused part of a complete documentation entry.)* Stool specimen obtained from infant's diaper. Sent to lab for culture. K. David LPN

Obtaining Sample for Wound or Throat Culture

Purpose

- To assist in the detection of harmful bacteria that may be present in wounds, body cavities, or throat

Equipment

- Sterile swab
- Culturette with preserving medium
- Penlight

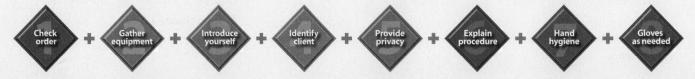

Check order + **Gather equipment** + **Introduce yourself** + **Identify client** + **Provide privacy** + **Explain procedure** + **Hand hygiene** + **Gloves as needed**

Interventions and Rationales

1. Perform preparatory steps (see icon bar above).
2. Gently swab the area to be cultured (Figure 8-26 ■).

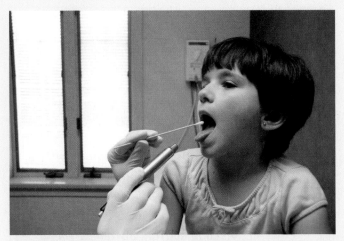

Figure 8-26. ■ A long cotton-tipped applicator can be used as a throat swab or wound swab.

3. Carefully place swab into preserving medium without touching the sides of the tube. *This ensures that bacteria are transferred to the medium and do not adhere to the tube.*
4. Label, package, and transport specimen to lab according to agency policy.

SAMPLE DOCUMENTATION

(date) 1630 *(Note: Wound specimen portion only. This is a focused part of a complete documentation entry.)* Specimen obtained from abdominal incision. Thick, green exudate noted. B. Smartt LPN

PROCEDURE 8-19 # Obtaining a Sputum Specimen

Purpose

■ To assist in the detection of harmful bacteria that may be present in respiratory secretions

Equipment

■ Sterile suction catheter with attached suction trap
■ Sterile saline
■ Sterile specimen container

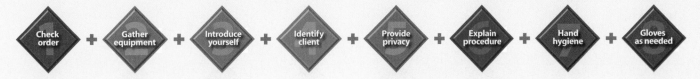

Check order + Gather equipment + Introduce yourself + Identify client + Provide privacy + Explain procedure + Hand hygiene + Gloves as needed

Interventions and Rationales

1. Perform preparatory steps (see icon bar above).

FROM AN INFANT

2. Attach the suction tubing to low suction.

3. Place the catheter in the infant's nose.
4. Clear secretions from tubing with sterile saline (see Procedure 8-27).

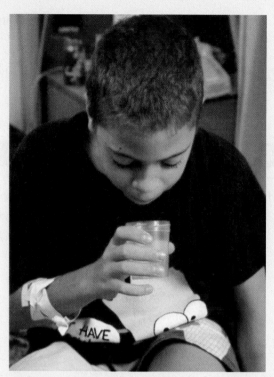

Figure 8-27. ■ Child supplying a sputum specimen.

FROM A CHILD

2. Place the child in a seated position.

3. Instruct the child to take several deep breaths. *This will help cause the client to cough deeply.*

4. Ask the child to spit sputum into the sterile specimen container (Figure 8-27 ■).

5. Label, package, and transport specimen to lab according to agency policy.

SAMPLE DOCUMENTATION

(date) 1000   *(Note: Sputum specimen portion only. This is a focused part of a complete documentation entry.)* Small amount of white, viscous sputum obtained for culture. Specimen to lab.
A. Evans LVN

PROCEDURE 8-20 **Positioning a Child for Lumbar Puncture**

Purposes

■ To provide safety during the lumbar puncture
■ To assist the practitioner in obtaining a spinal fluid specimen

Equipment

■ Clean gloves
■ Light source

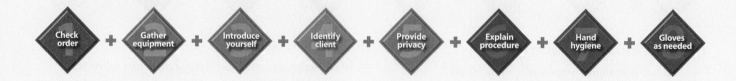

Check order + Gather equipment + Introduce yourself + Identify client + Provide privacy + Explain procedure + Hand hygiene + Gloves as needed

Interventions and Rationales

1. Perform preparatory steps (see icon bar above).

2. Solicit the assistance of a coworker. *This will help prevent injury to the child.*

3. Position the infant in a lateral position (Figure 8-28A ■). Hold infant by placing one hand behind the neck and one hand around the thighs, maintaining a curve in the spine.

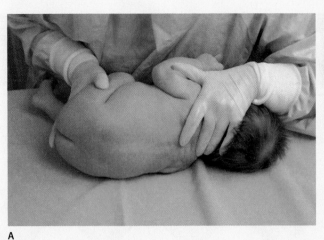 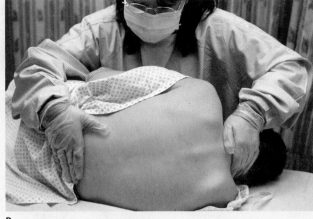

A   B

Figure 8-28. ■ (**A**) Infant positioned for a lumbar puncture. (**B**) Child positioned for a lumbar puncture.

4. Position child in a lateral position (Figure 8-28B ■). Ask him or her to flex both the neck and the knees. Hold the child by placing one hand behind the neck and one hand around the hips.

5. Talk quietly and gently to the child during the procedure. *This serves to lower anxiety levels and increase compliance.*

SAMPLE DOCUMENTATION

(date) 0900   *(Note: Positioning portion only. This is a focused part of a complete documentation entry.)* Assisted child into lateral position, knees and neck flexed. Position secured during lumbar puncture. No complaints voiced following procedure. A. McIntire LPN

ASSISTING WITH NUTRITION

Feeding a Child

There are occasions when the nurse may need to feed a child orally (Procedure 8-21 ■). A child who has had surgery and is in pain may need assistance with nutrition. The visually impaired child may also need help. If increased calories are essential to the child's health, it may be necessary for the nurse to be present at all meals and to encourage increased food intake.

Mealtime should be pleasant and stress-free. Forcing a child to eat puts the child at risk for aspiration because of crying or struggling. Often, giving the child choices will reinforce independence and protect dignity.

Tube Feeding

There are several types of tubes through which a liquid food may be introduced to the client for hydration or nourishment. In gavage feeding, the stomach tube is inserted through the nares, pharynx, and esophagus, and into the stomach. Care must be taken to ensure that the tube is in the stomach before the liquid nourishment is introduced (discussed in Procedures 8-22 ■ and 8-23 ■). After the fluid is instilled or after the tube feeding is finished, the tube is removed. It is reinserted for the next feeding. In some agencies, introduction of the feeding tube in a small infant is not an LPN/LVN function.

PROCEDURE 8-21 Feeding a Child Orally

Purpose

- To encourage the child in obtaining adequate nutritional intake

Equipment

- Child-size utensils
- Straws
- Divided plates to keep food separate

Check order + Gather equipment + Introduce yourself + Identify client + Provide privacy + Explain procedure + Hand hygiene + Gloves as needed

Interventions and Rationales

1. Perform preparatory steps (see icon bar above).

2. Create an environment conducive to eating. Limit distractions. Remove items with strong odors. Consider feeding child in an area other than the hospital room.

3. Cut food into bite-size pieces. *This will help prevent choking.*

4. Offer the child's favorite foods if they are allowable to prescribed diet. *This encourages compliance.*

5. Use straw in a covered drink container. *This will avoid spills.*

6. Use praise only and avoid negative comments. *This will make mealtime pleasant and encourage the child to eat.*

7. Document the percentage of meal eaten.

SAMPLE DOCUMENTATION

(date) 1200 | *(Note: Oral feeding portion only. This is a focused part of a complete documentation entry.)*
80% of regular diet consumed. Assisted child by cutting meat and encouraging bites. Mother present during meal.
L. Gayle LVN

However, gastric suction may be performed by the LPN in most facilities (see Procedure 8-24 ■).

If tube feeding is expected to be a long-term necessity, the physician may insert a gastric tube or jejunostomy tube. Liquid nourishment can then be introduced. The tube remains in place between feedings. Skin care around the tube is important to prevent skin breakdown and infection. At times, the tube needs to be replaced. Once the stoma has healed, the gastric or jejunostomy tube can be replaced by the LPN/LVN according to state board of nursing rules and agency policy.

There are many commercially prepared tube feeding formulas. The specific formula to meet the nutritional needs of the child is ordered by the doctor. All opened containers should be stored in the refrigerator. The liquid nourishment must be administered at room temperature to avoid stomach cramping.

Giving small amounts of tube feeding frequently is safer than introducing large quantities that might distend the stomach and cause vomiting or aspiration. At times, feedings are introduced by an intermittent bolus. At other times, feedings are by slow continuous infusion. It is important to assess the amount of residual tube feeding fluid periodically to determine if the feeding is being digested. **Residual volume** is the amount of the feeding that remains in the client's stomach. It is obtained by aspirating and measuring gastric contents before the feeding is begun. If the residual volume is equal to or greater than the amount of feeding being given per hour, stop the feeding and reevaluate in 1 hour. If the residual volume continues to be high, it is an indication that the child is not digesting the nourishment properly. If this finding is assessed, the supervising nurse and/or physician should be notified. Most facilities have their own protocols for handling tube feedings and residual volumes.

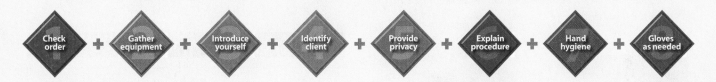

PROCEDURE 8-22   # Inserting and Removing an Orogastric and Nasogastric Tube

Purposes

- To provide nutritional supplementation or medications
- To remove stomach contents

Equipment

- Variety of sizes orogastric or nasogastric tubes
- Suction equipment
- Litmus paper
- Water-soluble lubricant
- 20-mL syringe

Check order ✛ Gather equipment ✛ Introduce yourself ✛ Identify client ✛ Provide privacy ✛ Explain procedure ✛ Hand hygiene ✛ Gloves as needed

Interventions and Rationales

1. Perform preparatory steps (see icon bar above).

2. Solicit the assistance of a coworker. Consider restraints prn. *This helps prevent injury to the child.*

3. Position the child in Fowler's position. *This position utilizes gravity when inserting the tube and helps minimize aspiration of fluid.*

4. To determine the length of the orogastric tube to be inserted, measure the tube from the mouth to the tragus of the ear to the xiphoid process. Mark appropriately.

5. To determine the length of the nasogastric tube to be inserted, measure the tube from the tip of the nose to the tragus of the ear to the xiphoid process (Figure 8-29 ■). Mark appropriately.

6. Apply lubricant to the tip of the tube for easier insertion.

7. For the orogastric tube, insert the tube into the child's mouth with the neck hyperextended and advance it toward back of the throat. Continue advancing until mark is reached.

8. For the nasogastric tube, insert the tube into the child's nares with neck hyperextended and advance it straight. If resistance is met, increase pressure slightly or rotate the tube. Continue advancing until mark is reached.

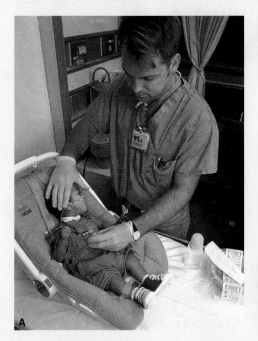

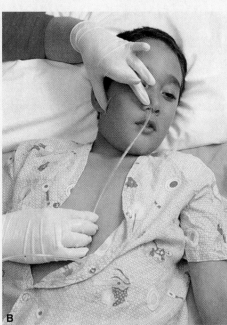

Figure 8-29. ■ Measuring for nasogastric tube placement. (**A**) Infant. (**B**) Child. (A similar technique is used in measuring for orogastric tube insertion.)

clinical ALERT

The child's gag reflex may be elicited when either tube reaches the oropharynx. If this occurs, have the child take small sips of water while you continue to advance the tube.

9. Use the syringe to aspirate a small amount of gastric content. Test the pH of the gastric contents using the litmus paper. *A pH of 3 or less indicates gastric contents and, therefore, proper placement.*

10. Secure the tube with tape or (if available) a manufactured product that holds nasogastric tubes in place (Figure 8-30 ■). *It is important to secure the tube to prevent it from dislodging.*

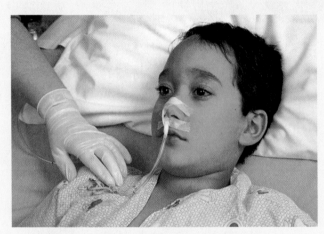

Figure 8-30. ■ Nasogastric tube taped securely in place.

TUBE REMOVAL

11. Position the child in Fowler's position to avoid aspiration if gagging occurs.

12. Cover the child's chest with a towel. *Secretions sometimes drip off the tube when it is removed.*

13. Put 10 to 20 mL of air into the tube to remove secretions in tube.

14. Remove tape, ask the child to hold his or her breath, and to close his or her eyes. Then clamp and gently withdraw the tube. *This prevents secretions from getting in the eyes.*

15. Suction prn.

SAMPLE DOCUMENTATION

(date) 1600   *(Note: Nasogastric tube portion only. This is a focused part of a complete documentation entry.)* NG tube inserted per agency policy. Aspiration of gastric contents reveals pH 2. Low suction attached. No nausea or GI distress noted. J. Baker LPN

PROCEDURE 8-23 # Administering a Gavage/Tube Feeding

Purpose

■ To provide nutritional support when the child is unable to obtain adequate calories orally

Equipment

■ Nutritional supplementation
■ Tap water
■ 20-mL syringe
■ Clean towel

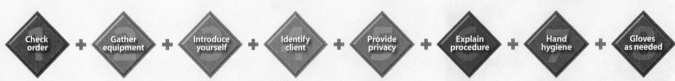

Check order + Gather equipment + Introduce yourself + Identify client + Provide privacy + Explain procedure + Hand hygiene + Gloves as needed

MediaLink ● Gavage Tube

Interventions and Rationales

1. Perform preparatory steps (see icon bar above).

2. Allow nutritional supplement to reach room temperature. *This will prevent cramping.*

3. Position the child in a Fowler's or high Fowler's position. Place a towel across the child's abdomen. *This position prevents aspiration, and the towel helps keep the child's clothing free of soiling.*

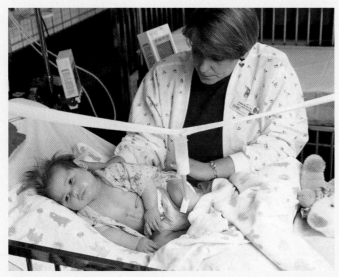

Figure 8-31. ■ Gravity assists the flow of a gavage feeding to this hospitalized infant.

4. Check placement (see Procedure 8-22).

5. Assess residual gastric volume. *The feeding should be withheld if the residual volume is too great because this indicates that digestion may be altered. The agency may designate this volume, and the physician may include the residual volume in the original order.*

6. Flush the tubing with tap water. *This is necessary to clear the tubing of gastric contents.*

7. Clamp the tubing and attach barrel of syringe or primed tubing for continuous feeding.

8. For bolus feeding, raise barrel of syringe no more than 18 inches above the child's abdomen. Fill the syringe

with nutritional supplement. Unclamp the tubing and allow supplement to flow slowly into tube (Figure 8-31 ■).

9. Watch the infusion carefully and do not allow air into the tube. Clamp the tubing. *Air could cause the child to have gas.*

10. Maintain the child in the Fowler's position for 1 to 2 hours. *This will prevent aspiration.*

11. Following the bolus feeding with a flush of tap water. *The amount of the flush will typically be ordered by the physician.*

12. For continuous feeding, label the bag with date and time. Set the rate as prescribed and monitor it closely.

SAMPLE DOCUMENTATION

(date) 0845   *(Note: Gavage/tube feeding portion only. This is a focused part of a complete documentation entry.)* No gastric residual obtained. Orogastric tube flushed with 10 mL tap water. 30 mL Enfamil with iron given bolus via orogastric tube. 30 mL tap water flushed following feeding. HOB at 45 degrees.
A. David LPN

PROCEDURE 8-24 Performing Gastric Suction

Purpose
■ To remove gastric contents for further evaluation or decompression

Equipment
■ Suction equipment
■ Litmus paper

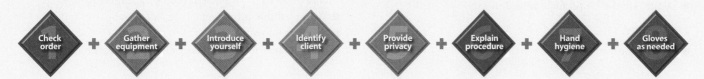

Check order + Gather equipment + Introduce yourself + Identify client + Provide privacy + Explain procedure + Hand hygiene + Gloves as needed

Interventions and Rationales

1. Perform preparatory steps (see icon bar).
2. Check for proper tube placement (see Procedure 8-22).
3. Attach gastric tube to suction equipment.
4. Suction according to physician order.
5. Document color, consistency, and amount of gastric contents suctioned.

ASSISTING WITH ELIMINATION

The nurse can assist in promoting normal elimination patterns by encouraging a diet adequate in fiber and fluids, as well as regular exercise. If the child becomes constipated, oral medication, suppositories, or an enema might be ordered. The administration of a suppository or enema is an invasive procedure, so age-specific instructions are essential. To ensure the child's safety during these procedures, a second nurse may be needed to help restrain the child. Procedures 8-25 ■ and 8-26 ■ offer more information on assisting with elimination.

shift into or out of the cells. A smaller volume of solution, administered with less pressure, is needed for children. The following volumes are given unless other volumes are ordered by the physician:

Infant = 40–100 mL
Toddler = 100–200 mL
Preschooler = 200–300 mL
School age = 300–500 mL
Adolescent = 500–700 mL

Enema

Administer the solution ordered by the physician. Commercially prepared solutions are available in pediatric dosage. The solution should be isotonic to prevent fluid

Urinary Elimination

The nurse can assist in promoting normal urinary elimination by encouraging an adequate fluid intake and regular emptying of the bladder. If the child's bladder

---

PROCEDURE 8-25 **Administering an Enema**

Purposes

- To clear the bowel of feces, relieving constipation
- To prepare the bowel for a procedure

Equipment

- Solution ordered

- Enema container or bag with attached tubing. For the infant, syringe with bulb or size 10 to 12 French rectal tube. For the child, size 14 to 18 French rectal tube (Figure 8-32 ■).
- Water-soluble lubricant
- Waterproof pads
- Bedpan, bedside commode, or accessible bathroom

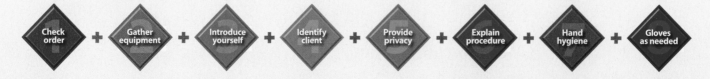

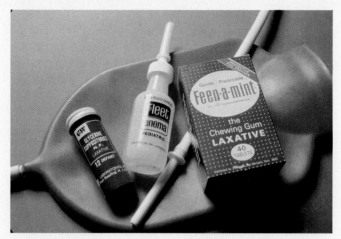

Figure 8-32. ■ Enema equipment, suppositories, and laxatives. (Pearson Education/PH College)

Interventions and Rationales

1. Perform preparatory steps (see icon bar).

2. Solicit the assistance of a coworker. *This will help prevent injury to the child.*

3. Prepare equipment. Prime the tubing. Ensure appropriate temperature.

4. Position the child in a left lateral position, knees flexed. Place waterproof pad underneath the child.

5. Lubricate tip of rectal tube with water-soluble lubricant.

6. Insert the rectal tube. For the infant, 1 to 1.5 inches. For the child, 2 to 3 inches.

7. Raise the container above the child's hips. Avoid raising it higher than 12 to 18 inches. *Raising the container higher*

than the recommended height will cause an increased pressure gradient on the colon. This could cause colon damage.

8. Open the clamp and allow fluid to infuse slowly over 10 to 15 minutes.

9. Gently remove rectal tube, asking the child to hold the fluid for the prescribed amount of time. For the infant, the buttocks are held together.

10. Assist the child onto the bedpan or to the bedside commode or bathroom to expel the contents of the enema.

11. Assist the child with hygiene measures.

SAMPLE DOCUMENTATION

(date) 0630	*(Note: Enema portion only. This is a focused part of a complete documentation entry.)* 100 mL soap suds enema given. M. McCune LPN
(date) 0640	assisted to BR to expel enema. M. McCune LPN
(date) 0655	approximately 100 mL enema expelled. Assisted with perineal and anal hygiene. M. McCune LPN

becomes distended, the nurse should encourage emptying of the bladder by assisting the child to the bathroom, providing privacy, placing the child's hand in warm water, and providing water to drink. If the child is unable to empty the bladder, urinary catheterization may be necessary.

Urinary catheterization may cause anxiety and discomfort for the child. The nurse should thoroughly explain the procedure to both the parent and the child, using a kind, soft tone when communicating with the child. Choosing the smallest size catheter and lubricating the catheter well can reduce discomfort for the child.

PROCEDURE 8-26 — Inserting an Indwelling Catheter

Purpose

■ To provide continuous decompression of the bladder

Equipment

■ Disposable catheterization tray, containing the appropriate size catheter and sterile equipment for cleansing the perineum
■ Tape
■ Light source

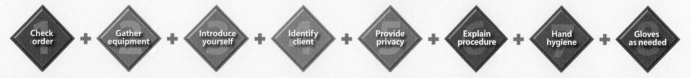

Check order + Gather equipment + Introduce yourself + Identify client + Provide privacy + Explain procedure + Hand hygiene + Gloves as needed

Interventions and Rationales

1. Perform preparatory steps (see icon bar above).

2. Solicit the assistance of a coworker. *This will help prevent injury to the child.*

3. Provide for the child's privacy.

4. Position the child in a supine position with knees flexed and abducted.

5. Apply sterile gloves.

6. Prepare the equipment: Pour antiseptic solution in reservoir; test the bulb for patency by injecting the syringe filled with sterile water (leaving this syringe attached to the tubing); lubricate the tip of the catheter.

7. Drape the perineum with the provided drape.

8. With the dominant hand, dredge cotton balls in antiseptic solution by holding them with forceps.

9. For the female child, separate the labia with the nondominant hand. Clean the perineum, from front to back, laterally. Discard cotton ball. Repeat on other side. Wipe midline, from urethral meatus to anus. Discard.

10. For the male child, with the nondominant hand, retracting the foreskin if necessary, grasp the penis, separate meatus with thumb and forefinger. With the dominant hand, use a circular motion to clean from the meatus outward. Discard cotton ball and repeat until head of penis has been cleansed entirely. Recommended practice is three times.

11. Use the dominant hand to pick up the lubricated catheter.

12. Insert catheter into the meatus until urine is returned or seen in tubing.
    - For the female: 2 to 3 inches plus 1 inch following presence of urine
    - For the male: 4 to 5 inches plus 1 inch following presence of urine

clinical ALERT

Do not advance the catheter using force if resistance is felt. Encourage the child to relax the perineal muscles by taking deep breaths in through the nose and out through the mouth. If this is unsuccessful, remove the catheter and obtain a size smaller. Attempt catheterization again.

13. Hold the catheter with the nondominant hand. Use the dominant hand to inflate the bulb with the attached sterile water-filled syringe.

14. Pull back gently on the catheter until resistance is met. *This verifies proper placement of the bulb in the bladder.*

15. Secure the catheter by taping tubing to the child's leg.

16. Perform hygiene to remove antiseptic solution. *Antiseptic solution may cause irritation.*

SAMPLE DOCUMENTATION

(date) 1245   *(Note: Catheter portion only. This is a focused part of a complete documentation entry.)* Urinary catheter #10 inserted per sterile technique with return of clear, yellow urine. Tubing secured to leg with tape. No complaints voiced. L. Lynn LVN

RESPIRATORY PROCEDURES

Airway Clearance

Maintaining a patent airway is the nurse's highest priority in client care. The nurse must be familiar with various types of suctioning equipment and be able to use them properly. A bulb syringe may be used to remove secretions from the nose and mouth of an infant. This piece of equipment has the advantage of being small and portable.

Compress the bulb and insert the tip into the mouth. Releasing the bulb will draw secretions into the bulb tip. Empty the bulb syringe by covering the tip with a tissue

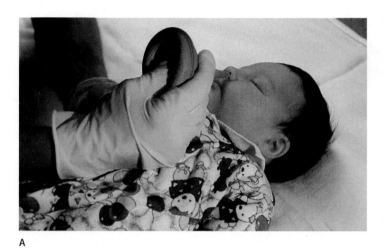
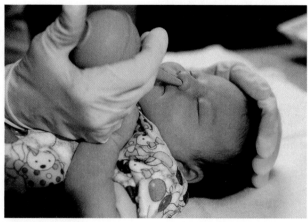

A   B

Figure 8-33. ■ **(A)** Insertion of a deflated tube bulb syringe. **(B)** Removal of a reinflated bulb syringe.

or cloth and then squeezing bulb again, forcing the secretions from the tip. After suctioning the infant's mouth, suction the nares in the same manner as described here (Figure 8-33 ■). Rinse the bulb syringe with water when done.

Suctioning the airway of an infant or child is the same as for adults except that a smaller size suction catheter is used. Because of the small air passages in the nose, it may be difficult to insert a suction catheter. The suction catheter can be introduced into the mouth and advanced into the pharynx. Suction is then applied to remove secretions. However, when suction is applied, air is pulled out of the lungs. For this reason, preoxygenation is important and the *maximum* amount of time suction is applied is 5 to 10 seconds. Table 8-4 ■ lists suggested endotracheal tube and suction catheter sizes.

An infant or child may have an endotracheal or tracheostomy tube for airway maintenance. Suctioning through these devices requires care and practice. The nurse, if authorized, can insert a suction catheter through the endotracheal or tracheostomy tube to remove secretions (Figure 8-34 ■). At times the oral/pharyngeal catheter is advanced into the trachea. Follow facility policy regarding tracheal suction by an LPN/LVN. Procedure 8-27 ■ describes steps for several types of suctioning.

TABLE 8-4		
Suggested Endotracheal Tube and Suction Catheter Size for Children		
AGE	ENDOTRACHEAL TUBE SIZE (mm)	SUCTION CATHETER SIZE (FRENCH)
Premature newborn	2.0–2.5	5
Newborn	3.0–3.5	6–8
6 months	3.5	8
12–18 months	4.0	8
3 years	4.5	8
5 years	5.0	10
6 years	5.5	10
8 years	6.0	10
12 years	6.5	10
16 years	7.0–8.0	12

Source: Adapted from Dieckman, R., Brownstein, D., & Gaushe-Hill, M. (eds.) (2nd ed.), (2006). *Pediatric education for prehospital professionals.* American Academy of Pediatrics. Sudbury, MA: Jones and Bartlett Publishers.

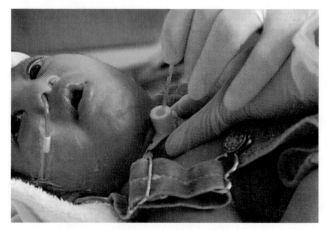

Figure 8-34. ■ Tracheostomy tube suctioning.

PROCEDURE 8-27 Suctioning a Child

Purposes

- To remove respiratory secretions to assist ventilation
- To obtain a specimen in order to detect harmful bacteria

Equipment

- Bulb syringe
- Normal saline
- Suction catheter, variety of sizes
- Oxygen source, resuscitation bag and mask
- Tracheostomy tubes

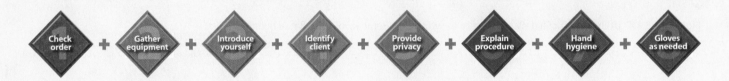

Check order + Gather equipment + Introduce yourself + Identify client + Provide privacy + Explain procedure + Hand hygiene + Gloves as needed

Interventions and Rationales

1. Perform preparatory steps (see icon bar above).
2. Solicit the assistance of a coworker. *This will help prevent injury to the child.*
3. Prior to the procedure, assess the child's breath sounds, respiratory rate and effort, and patency of airway. *This provides data for evaluating the effectiveness of the procedure.*
4. After suctioning, assess respiratory status.

USING THE BULB SYRINGE

5. Position the infant in a supine position. The older child may be in a seated position.
6. Clean the oral cavity by depressing the bulb and inserting the tip of the syringe into the left buccal cavity of the child's mouth. Repeat in the right buccal cavity. *Placing the syringe into the buccal cavity avoids eliciting the gag reflex.*
7. Depress the bulb into a tissue or towel to clear the bulb syringe.
8. Depress the bulb and place the tip of the syringe into the nares. *If the bulb is not depressed prior to insertion, air could force the secretions into the nasopharynx.*
9. Release the bulb and withdraw secretions.
10. Wipe tip of bulb to remove debris.
11. Rinse the bulb syringe by depressing it into a cup of water and flushing it out. Repeat until clean.

SUCTIONING A CONSCIOUS CHILD

5. Place child in a semi-Fowler's position with neck hyperextended.
6. Attach suction tubing to source of suction. See Table 8-4 for selecting the size of the suction catheter and the

endotracheal tube. Use settings as ordered by physician or according to agency policy.

7. Apply sterile gloves. *This prevents exposure to and spread of microorganisms.*
8. Insert the suction catheter into the naris. Close the suction port with the thumb to initiate suction. Limit suctioning to 5 to 10 seconds. Repeat in other naris.
9. Suction the mouth in the same manner.

SUCTIONING A CHILD WITH DECREASED LEVEL OF CONSCIOUSNESS

5. Administer oxygen by face mask. *Preoxygenating the child avoids hypoxia during suctioning.*
6. Position the child in a lateral position. *The lateral position can prevent aspiration because it prevents the tongue from falling back and blocking the oropharynx. It allows gravity to assist in the drainage of secretions.*
7. Apply sterile gloves.
8. Moisten the catheter with water and insert the suction catheter into the naris. *Moistening the catheter eases insertion.*
9. Close suction port with thumb to initiate suction. Limit suctioning to 5 to 10 seconds.
10. Apply oxygen mask. *This improves oxygenation.*
11. Repeat in other naris.
12. Apply oxygen mask.
13. Suction the mouth in the same manner.
14. Apply oxygen mask.
15. To remove secretions beyond the hypopharynx and trachea, advance the catheter further. Apply suction by occluding the suction port. Rotate gently on withdrawal.

This removes secretions attached to the walls of the trachea. Rotation also prevents suction equipment from adhering to one spot.

SUCTIONING THE TRACHEOSTOMY TUBE

5. Inform the child that suctioning may cause coughing and dyspnea.

6. Position the child in a supine position with the head of bed raised 30 degrees to prevent aspiration.

7. Attach oxygen source to resuscitation bag.

8. Apply sterile gloves.

9. Using the nondominant hand, remove the humidity source from tracheostomy tube.

10. Preoxygenate the child as ordered.

11. With the dominant hand, insert suction catheter into the tube without suction. Advance the catheter no farther than 0.5 cm below the opening of the tracheostomy tube (see Figure 8-34).

12. Apply intermittent suction, rotating the catheter during withdrawal to remove the maximum amount of secretions. Do not suction for longer than 5 to 10 seconds.

13. Withdraw the catheter completely and apply oxygen. *Suction removes both oxygen and secretions.*

SUCTIONING THE ENDOTRACHEAL TUBE

5. Position the child in a supine position with head of bed raised 30 degrees to prevent aspiration.

6. Attach oxygen source to resuscitation bag.

7. Apply sterile gloves.

8. Have assistant disconnect the ventilator.

9. Preoxygenate the child as ordered. *This prevents hypoxia.*

10. With the dominant hand, insert the suction catheter into the tube without suction. Advance the catheter no farther than 0.5 cm below the opening of the ET tube.

11. Apply intermittent suction, rotating the catheter during withdrawal. Do not suction for longer than 5 to 10 seconds. *Rotation ensures greater removal of secretions. It also prevents suction from adhering to one spot.*

12. Withdraw the catheter completely and apply oxygen.

13. Reconnect ventilator.

14. Repeat prn.

15. Clear the suction catheter using sterile saline.

SAMPLE DOCUMENTATION

(date) 0845 *(Note: Suctioning portion only. This is a focused part of a complete documentation entry.)* R 32, uneven and labored. Cough ineffective. Rhonchi auscultated bilaterally. Sterile oral/pharyngeal suctioning performed according to policy. Moderate amount of thick, white secretions obtained. Breathing less labored, R 22. J. Edward LPN

Oxygen Administration

Oxygen can be administered to an infant or child by cannula, catheter, mask, hood, or tent (Figure 8-35 ■; Procedures 8-28–8-30 ■). The method of administration is determined by the amount of oxygen required and the client's tolerance. High concentrations of oxygen given over a long period of time can be damaging to some body tissues. Retinal damage and lung disorders from oxygen administration are discussed in Chapter 18 ⚭ of this text. Frequent assessment of blood oxygen concentration is essential to prevent tissue damage (Procedure 8-29). Arterial blood gas analysis is most accurate, but measuring blood oxygen tension through the skin via pulse oximetry is an acceptable noninvasive method of assessment. The recording should be obtained as close to the child's head as possible.

Oxygen is a dry gas and may need to be humidified prior to administration. Humidifier reservoirs can be a host for growth of microorganisms and a source of infection. Facility policy should be followed regarding the use and cleaning of humidifiers and humidifying equipment.

clinical ALERT

All safety measures used for administration of oxygen to an adult should be followed with children as well. These include placing "No Smoking; Oxygen in Use" signs on doors; removal of static-causing materials, including wool or nylon blankets and toys; and instructing clients and visitors about oxygen precautions.

Often, the best method of administering humidified oxygen to children is by tent. The tent is usually set up by the respiratory therapy department, but the nurse must be

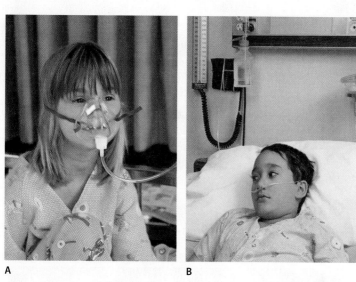

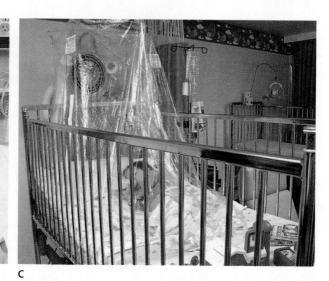

A   **B**   **C**

Figure 8-35. ■ **(A)** Simple face mask. **(B)** Nasal cannula. **(C)** Oxygen tent.

able to set up and monitor the equipment's functioning. Follow facility policy and manufacturer's recommendations on use of the equipment.

Generally, the tent consists of a frame that is suspended over the bed or crib (see Figure 8-35C). Plastic "roof and walls" are draped over the frame and tucked under the mattress. Humidified oxygen is forced into the tent by a pump. Gauges are used to determine the oxygen concentration inside the tent. The amount of oxygen is adjusted to maintain the desired concentration. Opening the tent lowers the oxygen concentration. Therefore, it is important to plan

and implement care to decrease the amount of time the tent is open.

The high humidity level inside the tent causes condensation on everything inside the tent. The cool, moist air can cause the child to chill. The bed linen and client clothing should be changed to keep the child warm and dry. Nonabsorbent toys should be placed in the tent to entertain the child. The nurse can help decrease the child's anxiety about being inside the tent by reassuring him or her that the tent will make it easier to breathe and that the nurse will always be available.

PROCEDURE 8-28   # Administering Oxygen to Children

Purpose

■ To provide the prescribed concentration of oxygen to the child

Equipment

■ Oxygen supply, including a flowmeter
■ Device to humidify the oxygen
■ Nasal cannula, face masks, or oxygen tent
■ Oxygen tubing

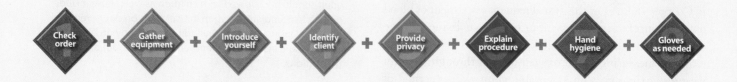

Check order ➕ Gather equipment ➕ Introduce yourself ➕ Identify client ➕ Provide privacy ➕ Explain procedure ➕ Hand hygiene ➕ Gloves as needed

Interventions and Rationales

1. Perform preparatory steps (see icon bar).

2. Set up oxygen delivery method, including humidification.

3. Turn on oxygen to prescribed flow rate.

4. Place the face mask over the bridge of the child's nose to the cleft of the chin (see Figure 8-35). OR
   Place the nasal cannula into the anterior naris and put an elastic band around the child's head. OR
      Surround the child in the hospital bed with the oxygen tent. Secure the edges of the tent to deliver prescribed oxygen dosage and prevent escape of oxygen.

SAMPLE DOCUMENTATION

(date) 0700   *(Note: Oxygenation portion only. This is a focused part of a complete documentation entry.)* O_2 *per nasal cannula at 2L/ minute applied. Band secured around head. K. Coffey LPN*

PROCEDURE 8-29 # Monitoring Oxygen Status

Purposes

- The pulse oximetry is used to measure oxygen saturation of the blood.
- The apnea monitor is used to measure breathing patterns.
- The peak expiratory flow rate (PEFR) meter is used to measure pulmonary function in the child.

Equipment

- Pulse oximeter, variety of sizes
- Apnea monitor, electrodes, alcohol swabs
- PEFR meter

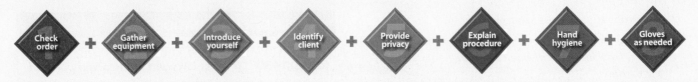

Check order + Gather equipment + Introduce yourself + Identify client + Provide privacy + Explain procedure + Hand hygiene + Gloves as needed

Interventions and Rationales

1. Perform preparatory steps (see icon bar above).

PULSE OXIMETRY

2. If continuous pulse oximetry is ordered, set alarms at prescribed parameters.

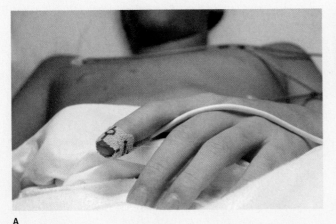

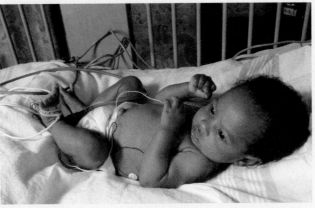

A   B

Figure 8-36. ■ **(A)** Pulse oximeter on finger. **(B)** Pulse oximeter on infant's foot.

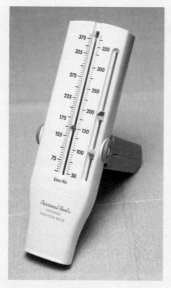
A

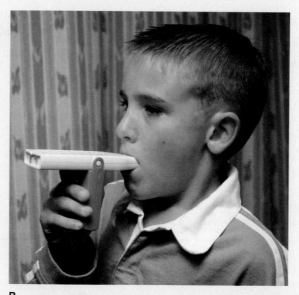
B

Figure 8-37. ■ (**A**) Peak expiratory flow rate (PEFR) meter. (**B**) Child using PEFR device.

3. Apply the sensor to the index finger, the large toe, or the earlobe (Figure 8-36 ■). If using the finger or toe, ensure sensor is positioned on the nail. If possible, have the probe at the level of the child's heart.

4. Obtain readings.

5. Assess skin at site every 2 hours.

APNEA MONITOR

2. Set alarms at prescribed parameters.

3. Apply alcohol to electrode sites. Allow to dry. *This removes body oils and will ensure more effective attachment of electrodes.*

4. Apply electrodes in the following pattern: one on the right side, one on the left side, and one on the lateral side of the abdomen.

5. Assess respiratory rate and pulse if alarm sounds.

PEFR MONITOR

2. Set the PEFR monitor (Figure 8-37A ■) according to the child's previous scores.

3. Instruct the child to put the mouthpiece in the mouth (Figure 8-37B ■). The child should then take a deep breath and blow as hard as possible into the meter.

4. Observe the score shown on the meter.

5. Repeat two to three times. Average the scores.

6. Compare the scores with previous scores.

7. Administer prescribed treatment, prn.

SAMPLE DOCUMENTATION

(date) 1430 *(Note: Oxygen monitoring portion only. This is a focused part of a complete documentation entry.)* R 77. Pulse oximetry applied to infant's earlobe. 88%. O_2 applied via face mask at 4 L/minute per order. S. Locke LVN

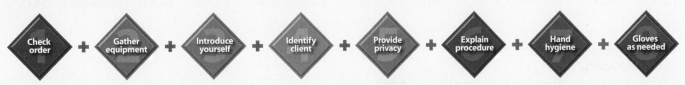

PROCEDURE 8-30   # Assisting with Airway Insertion

Purpose

- To assist the practitioner in inserting an artificial airway in an effort to maintain an airway of the conscious or unconscious child
- Suction equipment, including resuscitation bag
- Water-soluble lubricant

Equipment

- Oropharyngeal airways, variety of sizes
- Nasopharyngeal airways, variety of sizes
- Endotracheal tubes, variety of sizes, including stylet
- Tape
- Laryngoscope, variety of blade sizes

Check order + Gather equipment + Introduce yourself + Identify client + Provide privacy + Explain procedure + Hand hygiene + Gloves as needed

Interventions and Rationales

1. Perform preparatory steps (see icon bar above).

OROPHARYNGEAL

2. Assist in the selection of the proper size tube (see Table 8-4). The front flange should be at the level of the central incisors, and the distal end should reach to the angle of the jaw (Figure 8-38A ■).

3. Hold the child's head midline. Avoid flexion or extension. *This position ensures proper alignment of the trachea.*

NASOPHARYNGEAL

2. Assist in the selection of the proper size tube. Measure from the tip of the nose to the tragus of the ear (Figure 8-38B ■).

3. Lubricate airway with water-soluble lubricant.

4. Position the child in a supine position with HOB elevated.

ENDOTRACHEAL TUBE

2. Assist in the selection of the proper size tube (see Table 8-4). For a child older than 2 years, add 16 to the age in years and divide by 4. This sum will yield the size of ET tube necessary. Also, compare the diameter of the child's fifth finger to the diameter of the ET tube to select the proper size.

3. Position the child in a supine position and hyperflex the neck.

4. Secure the tube with tape after insertion. Assess the child's respiratory status.

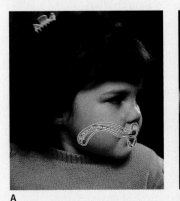 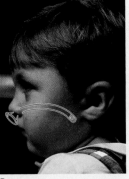

A   B

Figure 8-38. ■ (**A**) Estimating the size of an oropharyngeal airway. (**B**) Estimating the size of a nasopharyngeal airway.

SAMPLE DOCUMENTATION

(date) 0815   *(Note: Airway insertion portion only. This is a focused part of a complete documentation entry.)* Nasopharyngeal airway inserted. Tube taped in place. Positioned child in left lateral position. R 32 and even. H. Payne LPN

PHARMACOLOGY AND MEDICATION ADMINISTRATION TO CHILDREN

The administration of medications to children carries great responsibility. Extensive research must be conducted on the use, long-term effects, and dosage of medications for children. Absorption, metabolism, and excretion of drugs in adults differ from those actions in children because children's body systems may be immature (Table 8-5 ■). Allergic reactions, toxic effects, or other adverse reactions may be dramatic and more severe in children. Drug literature must be read carefully and followed for client safety.

All dosage calculations and measurements must be checked for accuracy. Some facilities require dosages of certain drugs to be checked by two nurses. Some examples are Lanoxin, insulin, heparin, and chemotherapy agents. In some facilities, the LPN/LVN is not permitted to calculate

TABLE 8-5

Effects of Medications on Children Versus Adults

BODY COMPONENT OR SYSTEM	VARIATION	ABSORPTION RATE VARIABLES	NURSING IMPLICATIONS
Muscle Mass Infant 10–11 years Adult	25% 40% 50%	Decrease in absorption due to erratic blood flow to muscle tissue	Less muscle tissue available in children for injections
Body Fat Infant 1 year 4 years 10–11 years Adult	16% 22–24% 12% 18–20% 15%	Some drugs are dependent on the amount of fat tissue	Blood levels increase with fat saturation effects Different variable in percentage of fat may lead to different milligram per kilogram dosage to achieve therapeutic blood levels
Body fluid Infant 1 year 4 years 10–11 years Adult	70–80% 58–60% 60% 60% 50–60%	Dehydrated state can alter the needed dosage and response to medication	Greater milligram-per-kilogram dosage of water-soluble drugs is needed in young children
Skin Children Adult	Thin dermis and epidermis Relatively inactive sebaceous glands before puberty Larger surface	Affects the absorption of topical medication	Prone to skin irritations and allergies
Gastrointestinal system Infant 2 years	Gastric emptying time: 6–8 hours Peristalsis is irregular in infants Gastric emptying time: 2 hours Gastrointestinal tract long in proportion to body size	Erratic absorption of oral medication, especially in newborns and infants Infant and young child's pH level affects acidic drugs; basic drugs are more readily absorbed	Infant having a lower gastric pH level will not metabolize medications effectively

(continued)

BODY COMPONENT OR SYSTEM	VARIATION	ABSORPTION RATE VARIABLES	NURSING IMPLICATIONS
Liver	Less developed in infants and young children Lower levels of liver enzymes	Maternal hormones, free and fatty acids compete with the neonate plasma protein-binding sites. They decrease the biotransformation rates, causing toxic effects of some drugs to be reached more readily	Drugs that bind to plasma proteins are needed in smaller doses Monitor the infant's and young child's blood levels. Monitor for side effects
Cardiovascular system	Infants have a poorly developed peripheral circulation	May cause intramuscular and subcutaneous injections to absorb erratically	
Endocrine system	Increased levels of sex steroids in adolescents Sexual maturity Genetic makeup Male adolescents	May compete for enzymes necessary for drug metabolism May affect the rate of elimination May influence the metabolism and elimination of certain drugs May increase binding in certain drugs	
Neurologic system	Blood-brain barrier is not mature in children younger than age 2	Central nervous system stimulants and depressants often cause unpredictable results	
Renal system Infant Children and Adults	Glomerular filtration rate 30–50% that of an adult Mature rates are reached within 6 months Lower tubular secretions Urinary pH (more acidic) Higher tubular secretion at night	Longer half-life in infants for drugs excreted by glomerular filtration and by tubular secretion Increased reabsorption of acidic drugs	Can lead to an increase in dehydration and overhydration Observe closely for drug toxicity
Immune system	Immature	Allergies are more common, especially in skin and respiratory systems	Carefully record any drug reaction
Respiratory system Infant Children	Alveoli are immature and not fully functional Breathe almost totally through the nose Proportionally smaller lungs and shorter and narrower upper and lower respiratory passages than adults have	They have a higher metabolic rate	Respiratory rate is higher

BOX 8-4

Pharmacology: Dosage Problems

1. Calculate the dosage for the following medication orders.
   The recommended dosage of Ceclor is 20 mg/kg/day in three divided doses. How many mg should a child weighing 20 kg receive per day?

   ANSWER: Multiply 20 mg by 20 kg. This equals 400 mg/day, which is the recommended dosage of Ceclor per day for a child weighing 20 kg.

2. The physician orders Demerol 0.5 mg/lb IM. A child weighs 27 lb. How many mg should the child receive? You have a syringe of Demerol 50 mg/1 ml. How many ml should the child receive?

   ANSWER: Multiply 0.5 mg by 27 lb. This equals 13.5 mg and is the ordered dosage of Demerol. The next step is to work the problem using the formula D/H $\times$ Q. In this scenario you would use 13.5/50 $\times$ 1 = 0.27 mL. The nurse would draw 0.27 mL of Demerol into the syringe and administer the medication intramuscularly.

3. The doctor orders 35 mg of Demerol every 3 hours prn for pain. The child weighs 10 kg. The package insert states that the recommended dosage for pain relief in children is 0.5 mg/lb to 0.8 mg/lb. Is it safe to give the 35 mg ordered?

   ANSWER: Convert kg to pounds. Multiply 10 kg by 2.2. This equals 22 lb. Next multiply the lower end of the range and the upper end of the range by the child's weight in pounds. 0.5 $\times$ 22 = 11 mg and 0.8 $\times$ 22 = 17.6 mg. Therefore, a child weighing 22 lb should receive a dose of Demerol between 11 and 17.6 mg. This dose is too high for this child. The medication should not be given, and the physician should be contacted.

fractional dosages. State Board of Nursing regulations and facility policy must be followed. Box 8-4 ■ provides some dosage problems.

Pediatric doses are smaller than adult doses. Orders are usually written for milligrams of the drug per body weight of the child per 24 hours, as well as the number of doses the child is to receive per day. The nurse must calculate the number of milligrams per dose the child is to receive. Before administering medication to a child, the nurse should verify that the dose is within the recommended amount allowed for the size of the child. If a dose is questionable, the physician, pharmacist, or nurse supervisor should be consulted.

Oral Administration

The oral route of administration of medication may be preferred in children because it is less invasive and has a slower absorption rate (Procedure 8-31 ■). However, at times it is a challenge to get the infant or small child to swallow the oral medication. Children younger than 5 years of age may have difficulty swallowing pills or capsules. Medication may have a bitter taste and should be mixed in a pleasant-tasting medium. Mixing medication in common foods such as orange juice, applesauce, or pudding may cause the child to develop a dislike for those foods. Consult the pharmacist before opening capsules or crushing tablets to ensure that

PROCEDURE 8-31   Administering Oral Medications

Purpose

■ To provide medication that has been ordered to a child who requires treatment of a medical condition

Equipment

■ Measuring device: medicine cup, eye dropper, syringe, spoon
■ Mortar and pestle
■ Prescribed medication
■ Food or beverage of the child's choice

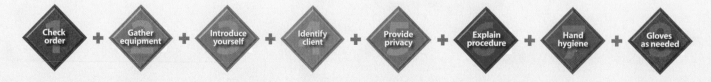

Check order + Gather equipment + Introduce yourself + Identify client + Provide privacy + Explain procedure + Hand hygiene + Gloves as needed

Interventions and Rationales

1. Perform preparatory steps (see icon bar above).

2. Prepare medication appropriately. Crush medications if permitted. Do not crush enteric-coated medications, time-release capsules, or other capsules.

3. Mix crushed medication in food or beverage of the child's choice. Be sure it is not the child's favorite food. *If the favorite food is used and the medication flavor is unpleasant to the child, the child may develop a dislike for the food as well.*

4. Measure carefully. *Pediatric doses must be extremely accurate.*

5. For the infant, place in a supine position. Use an eyedropper. Squeeze a small amount in the buccal area of the infant's mouth. Allow the infant to swallow, and repeat until medication is consumed. *This method should be used to prevent aspiration.*

6. For the child, place in a semi-Fowler's position. Children can sit if conditions permit. Administer the medication, small portions at a time, with a syringe or medicine cup.

7. Avoid administering oral medications while the child is crying. *This will prevent aspiration.*

SAMPLE DOCUMENTATION

(date) 1545   *(Note: Oral medication administration portion only. This is a focused part of a complete documentation entry.)* 40 mg acetaminophen given PO as ordered. Medication crushed and mixed with strawberry gelatin.
H. Hurley LVN

the action of the drug will not be altered. Generally, enteric-coated tablets and time-release capsules cannot be crushed.

Liquid medication must be measured accurately in a medicine cup, oral syringe, or medicine dropper. Medication may be given directly from the syringe or dropper into the buccal pocket of the mouth. Give small amounts at a time to avoid choking. Older children may drink the liquid from the medicine cup. The nurse may need to restrain the child to administer the proper dosage. A crying, struggling child may spill or aspirate medication.

Ear, Eye, or Nose Drops

When administering medications in the eye (Procedure 8-32 ■), ear (Procedure 8-33 ■), or nose (Procedure 8-34 ■), the child may need to be restrained for the procedure. This will help prevent injury to the child. To administer medications in the ear in children younger than 3 years, it is important to pull the pinna of a child down and back (see Figure 8-2A). For the child older than 3 years, pull the pinna up and back (see Figure 8-2B). This will straighten the ear canal and allow the medication to be administered properly. Table 8-6 ■ discusses routes of medication administration in children.

PROCEDURE 8-32   ## Administering Ophthalmic Medications

Purposes

■ To provide prescribed medications to the eye safely
■ To remove debris from the eye

Equipment

■ Prescribed medication, drops, or ointment
■ Sterile gloves
■ Tissues
■ For irrigation: prescribed irrigation solution and tubing or syringe, basin, towels

Check order + Gather equipment + Introduce yourself + Identify client + Provide privacy + Explain procedure + Hand hygiene + Gloves as needed

Interventions and Rationales

1. Perform preparatory steps (see icon bar).

2. Solicit the assistance of a coworker. *This will help prevent injury to the child.*

3. Position the child in a supine position with head extended.

4. With gloved hand, pull down the lower lid, exposing the conjunctival sac (Figure 8-39 ■).

5. Place the prescribed drops or ointment in the center of the conjunctival sac. *This will prevent placement of medication directly onto the cornea.*

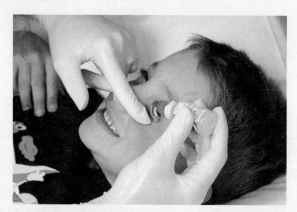

Figure 8-39. ■ Administering an ophthalmic medication. The child is instructed to close his eye and pretend to look up toward his head. The nurse then gently retracts the lower lid and inserts the medication.

6. Have the child close the eyes for 30 seconds and keep the head midline. *This will prevent the medication from running out of the eyes and promotes absorption.*

FOR EYE IRRIGATION

7. Turn the child's head slightly, with the affected eye down. *This will prevent contamination of the unaffected eye.*

8. Place towel under the child's head.

9. If using tubing, prime the line first.

10. Gently separate the upper and lower eyelids with thumb and forefinger of dominant hand.

11. Open the clamp on the tubing and allow fluid to flood the eye. Turn the flow off periodically to allow the child to close the eye.

SAMPLE DOCUMENTATION

(date) 0725 *(Note: Ophthalmic medication administration portion only. This is a focused part of a complete documentation entry.)* 0.2 in. ribbon of Illytocin applied to both eyes. No redness or exudate noted. M. Martin LPN

PROCEDURE 8-33 # Administering Otic Medications

Purposes

■ To provide prescribed medications safely to the ear
■ To remove debris from the ear

Equipment

■ Prescribed otic medication equipped with dropper
■ Cotton ball
■ For irrigation: prescribed solution, otoscope, syringe with tubing, emesis basin, towels

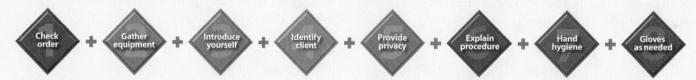

Check order + Gather equipment + Introduce yourself + Identify client + Provide privacy + Explain procedure + Hand hygiene + Gloves as needed

Interventions and Rationales

1. Perform preparatory steps (see icon bar above).

2. Solicit the assistance of a coworker. *This will help prevent injury to the child.*

3. Correctly identify the child with the identification band.

4. Position the child in a supine position with head turned to the side and the affected ear up (Figure 8-40 ■).

5. Pull the pinna in the appropriate direction according to the child's age (see Figures 8-2A and B).

6. Hold the dropper above the ear and instill prescribed number of drops. Never occlude the ear canal completely. *Occlusion can create a pressure change and damage the eardrum.*

7. Place a cotton ball loosely in the opening of the ear.

8. Have the child lie in this position for 5 to 10 minutes. *This will give the medication time to be absorbed.*

ASSISTING WITH IRRIGATION OF THE EAR CANAL

9. Warm prescribed solution to body temperature. *Solution below body temperature may cause nausea and vertigo.*

10. Hand the practitioner the otoscope. *The tympanic membrane should be seen as intact with the otoscope to avoid further damage.*

11. Position the child in a supine position with the head turned and the affected ear up.

12. Place the emesis basin under the affected ear. Place a towel over the child's neck and shoulders. *This will prevent clothing from becoming saturated.*

13. Draw up 20 mL of solution in syringe with attached tubing.

14. Repeat as necessary.

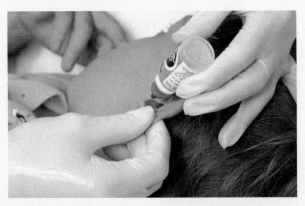

Figure 8-40. ■ Administering an otic medication.

SAMPLE DOCUMENTATION

(date) 0945   *(Note: Otic portion only. This is a focused part of a complete documentation entry.)* Left ear irrigated with 40 mL of normal saline. Return of 40 mL yellow-tinged fluid. R. Love LVN

PROCEDURE 8-34   Administering Nasal and Inhaled Medications

Purpose
■ To provide prescribed medications to the nasal cavity safely

Equipment
■ Prescribed medication, drops, or aerosol
■ Delivery device, dropper for nasal and nebulizer for aerosol medications

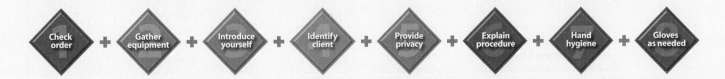

Check order + Gather equipment + Introduce yourself + Identify client + Provide privacy + Explain procedure + Hand hygiene + Gloves as needed

Interventions and Rationales

1. Perform preparatory steps (see icon bar above).

2. Solicit the assistance of a coworker. *This will help prevent injury to the child.*

NASAL MEDICATIONS

3. Position the child in a supine position with the head hyperextended.

4. Administer medication into nares as ordered.

5. Have the child maintain the position for 5 minutes. *This will give the medication time to absorb.*

AEROSOL MEDICATIONS

See Chapter 12 ⬯ for further discussion on the use of aerosol medications in the treatment of asthma.

3. Position the child in a semi-Fowler's position. *This position enables easier lung expansion than the supine position.*

4. Instruct child to place the tubing in the mouth and breathe deeply for approximately 10 minutes. Observe the child to be sure that he or she understands the instructions.

SAMPLE DOCUMENTATION

(date) 1130 *(Note: Nasal/inhaled medication administration portion only. This is a focused part of a complete documentation entry.)* 0.05% naphazoline hydrochloride, 2 sprays, administered in both nostrils. C. Wellman LPN

Rectal Suppositories

Rectal suppositories are a common route of administration for pediatric drugs when the child is unable to take oral medications (Procedure 8-35 ■ Figure 8-41 ■). The child may need to be restrained for the procedure. Insert the suppository into the anus. Using the small finger, push the suppository into the rectum approximately 1 inch (½ inch for the infant).

Medications by Injection

Medications administered by the parenteral route include intramuscular (Procedure 8-36 ■), subcutaneous (Procedure 8-37 ■), intradermal (Procedure 8-38 ■), and intravenous routes (Figure 8-42 ■). These sites are used when it is important that drugs be metabolized quickly. Also, an injection may be preferred when drugs would have a high

TABLE 8-6

Routes of Drug Administration by Age in Children

AGE	ORAL LIQUID	SUBLINGUAL	INTRAMUSCULAR INJECTION OR SUBCUTANEOUS INJECTION	INTRAVENOUS
Infant	Preferred route; may be administered by dropper into buccal sac	Generally avoided because of their inability to keep pill under tongue	Vastus lateralis used. Many sites are not well developed enough for IM injection	Veins are very small. Scalp, wrist, or ankle veins may be used for IV administration. Armboard and restraints required to maintain site
Toddler and preschooler	Preferred route of administration. Administered by syringe or cup. Greater predictability of the drug action by this route	Carefully assess the child's ability to swallow	Few possible sites because of low muscle mass. Gluteus maximus used as site after toddler has been walking for 1 year	Access difficult because of vein size; armboard and restraints required to maintain site. Greater predictability of the drug action by this route
School-age child	Preferred route of administration. Administered by syringe or cup. Greater predictability of the drug action by this route	Carefully assess the child's ability to swallow	Sites as for adult	Greater predictability of the drug action by this route
Adolescent	Preferred route of administration. Administered as liquid, tablet, or capsule. Greater predictability of the drug action by this route	Same as for adult	Sites as for adult	Greater predictability of the drug action by this route

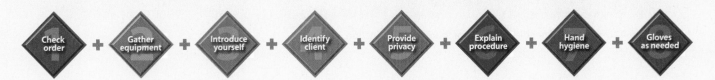

PROCEDURE 8-35   Administering Rectal Suppositories

Purpose

- To provide prescribed medications in the rectal canal safely

Equipment

- Prescribed medication, stored in the refrigerator
- Water-soluble lubricant
- Nonsterile gloves

Check order + Gather equipment + Introduce yourself + Identify client + Provide privacy + Explain procedure + Hand hygiene + Gloves as needed

Interventions and Rationales

1. Perform preparatory steps (see icon bar above).
2. Solicit the assistance of a coworker. *This will help prevent injury to the child.*
3. Correctly identify the child with the identification band.
4. Place the child in the left lateral position.
5. Lubricate the suppository with water-soluble lubricant. *This allows for easier insertion.*
6. For infants and toddlers, the nurse uses the little finger and carefully inserts the suppository just beyond the internal sphincter (about ½ inch or 1.25 cm) (see Figure 8-41).
7. For the older child, use the index finger and carefully insert the suppository just beyond the internal sphincter (about 1 inch or 2.5 cm).
8. Have the child maintain this position for 5 to 10 minutes. The nurse may also need to hold the buttocks together for about 1 minute. *This will facilitate absorption of the medication and prevent the medication from being expelled.*

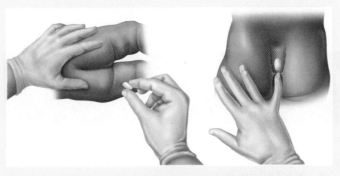

Figure 8-41. ■ The suppository is inserted gently just past the internal sphincter (about 1 inch or 2.5 cm in children; about ½ inch or 1.25 cm in infants). In infants, the little finger may be used instead of the index finger to insert the suppository.

SAMPLE DOCUMENTATION

(date) 0900   *(Note: Rectal medication administration portion only. This is a focused part of a complete documentation entry.)* T 101.9; 325 mg acetaminophen given rectally. R. Ress LPN

(date) 1000   Temp 99.9 degrees F. resting without complaint. R. Ress LPN

---

probability of irritating the child's stomach if given by mouth. Several sites are used when administering medication by injection. Intradermal medications can be given on the ventral surface of the forearm or the scapula. Subcutaneous injections can be given in the deltoid, abdomen, lower back, scapula, and thigh. Intramuscular injections are given to the infant in the vastus lateralis muscle. For the child who has walked for 1 year, injections are given in the ventrogluteal muscle. For the child who has appropriate muscle mass, and when small amounts of medication are to be given, the deltoid site can also be used (Figure 8-43 A–C ■).

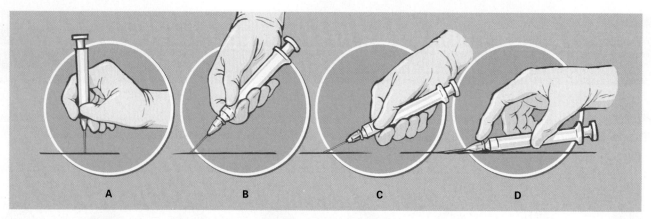

Figure 8-42. ■ Angle of needle insertion for four types of injection.

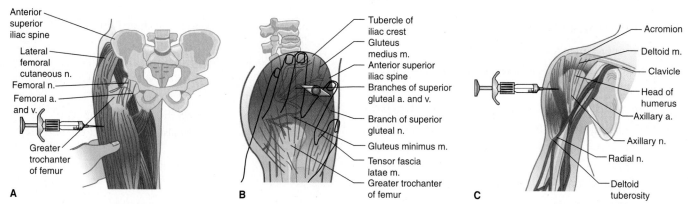

Figure 8-43. ■ Intramuscular injection sites. (**A**) Vastus lateralis. (**B**) Ventrogluteal. (**C**) Deltoid. (Adapted from Bindler, R., & Howry, L. (1997). *Pediatric drugs and nursing implications* (2nd ed.). Stamford, CT: Appleton & Lange, pp. 39–42.)

PROCEDURE 8-36 Administering Intramuscular (IM) Injection

Purpose

■ To provide prescribed medications intramuscularly in a safe manner

Equipment

■ Prescribed medication
■ 21- to 25-gauge needle with lengths 0.5 to 1 inch
■ 1- to 3-mL syringe
■ Alcohol swab
■ Adhesive bandage

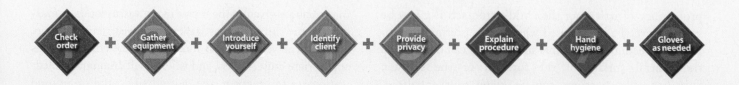

Check order ✛ Gather equipment ✛ Introduce yourself ✛ Identify client ✛ Provide privacy ✛ Explain procedure ✛ Hand hygiene ✛ Gloves as needed

Interventions and Rationales

1. Perform preparatory steps (see icon bar).

2. Solicit the assistance of a coworker. *This will help prevent injury to the child.*

3. Correctly identify the child with the identification band.

4. Ensure that the amount of medication is appropriate for the child's age and the muscle chosen as the site (Table 8-7 ■).

5. Choose the correct site for administering a medication intramuscularly. *For the infant, the vastus lateralis (Figure 8-43A) is used. For the toddler who has been walking for 1 year or more, the ventrogluteal (Figure 8-43B) can be used, but is still not preferred until the child has been walking for several years.*

6. Choose the correct size needle. *A smaller gauge needle should be used for injections into the smaller muscles such as the deltoid. The child's muscle mass and body weight should also be taken into consideration.*

7. Position the child according to the site chosen (Figure 8-43C). *For the deltoid site, place the child in the lateral position. This restrains one arm on the surface under the child so the arm receiving the injection can be restrained by the nurse. To use the vastus lateralis site, place the child in the supine position or seated on an adult's lap with the adult restraining the arms (Figure 8-44 ■). To use the ventrogluteal site, place the child in the prone position.*

8. Cleanse the site with alcohol from the center outward.

9. Insert the needle quickly at a 90-degree angle with the dominant hand.

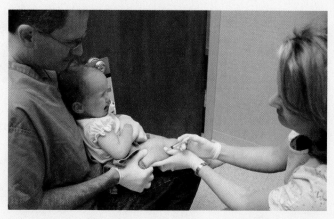

Figure 8-44. ■ The child is restrained by an adult while an injection is being administered. The vastus lateralis is the appropriate site for a child of this age.

10. Using the nondominant hand, pull back on the plunger slightly, observing for the return of blood. Be careful not to move the needle because this can cause additional discomfort.

11. If there is no blood, inject the medication slowly, remove the needle, and massage the site.

12. If there is blood in the syringe, withdraw the needle without injecting the medication. *Blood indicates that the needle is in a blood vessel. Injecting the medication at this point would mean that the medication will be administered intravascularly.*

13. Needles cannot be recapped. Dispose of needle and syringe in the proper container. *The equipment used for an intramuscular injection is considered to be contaminated and poses the threat of transmitting harmful substances.*

TABLE 8-7

Appropriate Volumes for IM Administration by Age

AGE	MAXIMUM AMOUNTS
Infant	Aoid volumes greater than 0.5 mL.
Toddler	Avoid volumes greater than 1 mL.
Older child and adolescent	Deltoid: Avoid volumes greater than 1 mL. Vastus lateralis: Avoid volumes greater than 2 mL. Gluteal: Avoid volumes greater than 3 mL.

SAMPLE DOCUMENTATION

(date) 1500 *(Note: Intramuscular injection portion only. This is a focused part of a complete documentation entry.)* 1 mg dexamethasone administered IM in right vastus lateralis. Band-Aid applied. Weaver LVN

| PROCEDURE 8-37 | Administering Subcutaneous (SQ) Injection |

Purpose

- To administer prescribed medications subcutaneously in a safe manner

Equipment

- Prescribed medication
- 25- to 26-gauge needle with lengths 3/8 to 5/8 inch
- 1- to 3-mL syringe
- Alcohol swab
- Adhesive bandage

Check order + Gather equipment + Introduce yourself + Identify client + Provide privacy + Explain procedure + Hand hygiene + Gloves as needed

Interventions and Rationales

1. Perform preparatory steps (see icon bar above).

2. Solicit the assistance of a coworker. *This will help prevent injury to the child.*

3. Choose the correct site for administering a medication subcutaneously. *Sites available for subcutaneous injections include the deltoid, the abdomen, the thighs, the lower back, and the scapula.*

4. Position the child according to the site chosen. *For the deltoid site, place the child in the lateral position. This restrains one arm on the surface under the child so the arm receiving the injection can be restrained by the nurse. To use the abdominal site, place the child in the supine position. To use the lower back or scapular site, position the child in the prone position.*

5. Cleanse the site with alcohol from the center outward.

6. Insert the needle quickly at a 45-degree angle with the dominant hand (see Figure 8-42).

7. Using the nondominant hand, pull back on the plunger slightly, observing for the return of blood. Be careful not to move the needle because this can cause additional discomfort.

8. If there is no blood, inject the medication slowly, remove the needle, and massage the site, unless administering heparin or insulin. *The effect of these two medications may be altered if massage occurs after injection.*

9. If there is blood in the syringe, withdraw the needle without injecting the medication. *Blood indicates that the needle is in a blood vessel. Injecting the medication at this point would mean that the medication will be administered intravascularly.*

10. Never recap a needle. Dispose of needle and syringe in the proper container. *The equipment used for a subcutaneous injection is considered to be contaminated and poses the threat of transmitting harmful substances.*

SAMPLE DOCUMENTATION

(date) 0730   *(Note: Subcutaneous injection portion only. This is a focused part of a complete documentation entry.)* Two units regular insulin administered SQ in RUQ. A. Page LVN

Intravenous (IV) Administration

The intravenous route is routinely used to administer pediatric medications (Procedures 8-39 ■ and 8-40 ■). It is generally less traumatic to the child than intramuscular injection every few hours. Care must be taken to ensure proper dilution of the medication. Infusion pumps are predominantly used to regulate the rate of administration. The site must be assessed for infiltration and patency before administration of each dose of medication. Many drugs are irritating to tissues and if infiltration occurs, the physician must be notified. In some areas, the administration of pediatric medications by the intravenous route is not an LPN/LVN function, and state board of nursing regulation and facility policy must be followed.

PROCEDURE 8-38   # Administering Intradermal (ID) Injection

Purpose

- To inject prescribed medication intradermally in a safe manner
- 1-mL syringe
- Alcohol swab

Equipment

- Prescribed medication
- 27-gauge needle with lengths ¼ to ⅜ inch
- Adhesive bandage

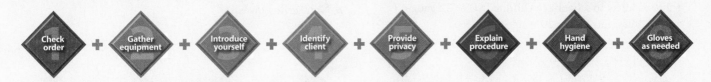

Interventions and Rationales

1. Perform preparatory steps (see icon bar above).

2. Solicit the assistance of a coworker. *This will help prevent injury to the child.*

3. Choose the correct site for administering a medication subcutaneously. *Sites available for intradermal injections include the ventral surface of the forearm and the scapula.*

4. Position the child according to the site chosen. *To use the forearm site, place the child in a semi-Fowler's position. The older child who is able to understand the importance of holding still may be seated for this injection. To use the scapular site, position the child in the prone position.*

5. Cleanse the site with alcohol from the center outward.

6. Insert the needle quickly at a 15-degree angle with the dominant hand (see Figure 8-42).

7. Do not aspirate.

8. Inject the medication slowly, creating a wheal or blister. *This verifies placement of the medication in the dermis.*

9. Withdraw needle and do not massage. *It is important for the medication to stay at the site.*

10. Mark the site with a permanent marker for future assessment.

11. Needles cannot be recapped. Dispose of needle and syringe in the proper container. *The equipment used for an intradermal injection is considered to be contaminated and poses the threat of transmitting harmful substances.*

SAMPLE DOCUMENTATION

(date) 1430   *(Note: Intradermal injection portion only. This is a focused part of a complete documentation entry.)* 0.1 mL purified protein derivative antigen given ID in right ventral forearm. Wheal marked with permanent marker. Parent instructed to return to clinic in 48 hours. _____
T. Thomas LPN

Initiating Intravenous Access to Administer Intravenous Fluid

Purposes

- To initiate intravenous access properly
- To infuse prescribed intravenous fluid in a safe manner

Equipment

- Tourniquet or rubber band if accessing a scalp vein
- Antiseptic solution, alcohol, or povidone-iodine
- IV catheter:
  - For infants, 24 gauge
  - For toddlers to school-age children, 20 to 22 gauge
  - For adolescents, 18 to 20 gauge
  - Butterfly needles, which are 22 to 25 gauge, can be used in temporary situations

- T connector, flushed
- Saline-filled and/or heparin-filled syringe
- Prescribed IV solution
- Appropriate tubing
- Armboard, variety of sizes
- Tape
- For saline or heparin lock, needleless catheter cap
- Rate-controlling device such as a pump, Buretrol (Figure 8-45 ■), Soluset, or Metriset
- Nonsterile gloves

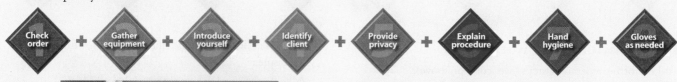

Check order + Gather equipment + Introduce yourself + Identify client + Provide privacy + Explain procedure + Hand hygiene + Gloves as needed

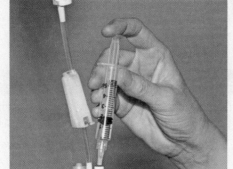

A

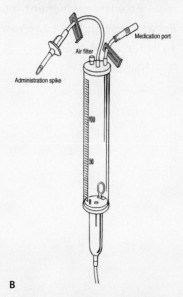

Medication port
Air filter
Administration spike
100
50

B

Figure 8-45. ■ Buretrol device. (**A**) Adding medication to the volume-control device. (**B**) Parts of the volume-control infusion set.

Interventions and Rationales

1. Perform preparatory steps (see icon bar above).
2. Solicit the assistance of a coworker. *This will help prevent injury to the child.*
3. Attach the tubing to the IV bag and prime.
4. If using a rate-controlling chamber device, attach to the IV bag. Fill chamber with 50 mL of IV fluid.
5. Position the child in a supine position. Restrain as necessary.
6. Apply tourniquet.
7. Use inspection and palpation to locate an appropriate vein (see Figure 11-8 ⊂⊃ for pediatric venous access sites).
8. Release tourniquet.
9. Apply armboard to location chosen (Figure 8-46 ■).
10. Reapply tourniquet.

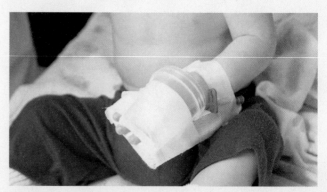

Figure 8-46. ■ This intravenous site on a hand has been placed on an armboard, securely wrapped, and covered with part of a plastic cup to prevent the child from disrupting the line.

11. Cleanse the site with antiseptic solution as outlined in facility policy. Use a circular pattern, beginning at the desired puncture site and moving outward. *This pattern of cleansing the site moves bacteria away from the injection site.*

12. Carefully insert the catheter at a 15-degree angle, bevel up. As blood appears in the catheter, carefully advance the catheter. Remove needle. Apply pressure at the end of the catheter and release tourniquet.

13. Quickly attach T connector and flush with saline-filled syringe.

14. Attach prescribed IV solution and set to infuse at the prescribed rate per pump or by gravity.

15. Tape the catheter securely.

CONVERTING IV TO SALINE OR HEPARIN LOCK

16. Prime needleless cap with the saline- or heparin-filled syringe.

17. Clamp the T connecter. *This prevents loss of blood through the catheter.*

18. Discontinue IV tubing from the catheter hub and quickly insert the needleless cap.

19. Open the clamp. Attach and inject the saline or heparin slowly to flush the needleless cap. *Heparin keeps the site patent by preventing clots at the site.*

20. Remove the syringe and clamp the T connector.

21. Secure the site according to agency policy.

SAMPLE DOCUMENTATION

(date) 1330   *(Note: Initiating IV portion only. This is a focused part of a complete documentation entry.)* IV of 250 mL D51/2 NS started with 22-gauge catheter into R antecubital space after cleansing with antiseptic solution. Rate set per pump at 50 mL/hour. K. Adams LPN

PROCEDURE 8-40   Administration of Intravenous (IV) Medications

Purpose

■ To infuse prescribed medication intravenously in a safe manner

Equipment

■ Prescribed medication
■ Syringe and needle or needleless system
■ Appropriate tubing
■ Alcohol swabs
■ Nonsterile gloves

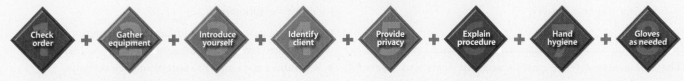

Check order + Gather equipment + Introduce yourself + Identify client + Provide privacy + Explain procedure + Hand hygiene + Gloves as needed

Interventions and Rationales

1. Perform preparatory steps (see icon bar above).

BOLUS ADMINISTRATION

2. Prepare prescribed amount of medication for bolus.

3. Assess the IV line for patency. *Line must be clear and open for medication to infuse properly.*

4. Cleanse the access port with alcohol.

5. Insert needle or needleless syringe into the cleansed port.

6. Inject medication slowly, observing closely for changes in the child's condition. *IV medications go directly into the bloodstream and so take effect quickly.*

7. Increase the intravenous fluid rate for several minutes to flush the medication from the tubing. *This ensures that all medication is delivered to the client.*

INITIATING A SECONDARY INFUSION

2. Obtain the prescribed medication from the pharmacy in either a 50-mL or a 250-mL bag of fluid or a prefilled syringe (5 mL or 60 mL).

3. Attach secondary tubing.

4. Cleanse port on primary line and attach secondary tubing.

5. Hang the secondary bag on the IV pole, lower than the primary line, or set the pump accordingly. *The bag that is highest will infuse first.*

6. For the prefilled syringe, insert into infuser and set to infuse according to manufacturer's instructions.

7. When medication is infused, discontinue secondary line and resume primary infusion.

SAMPLE DOCUMENTATION

(date) 0730 *(Note: Administering IV medication portion only. This is a focused part of a complete documentation entry.)* 363 mg ampicillin in 150 mL D$_5$W IVPB hung to infuse rapidly. D. Day LPN

Storage of Medication

Safe storage of medicines is essential. In an acute- or long-term care facility, medications are kept locked in storage cupboards or drawers for safety. Medication cannot be left at the bedside. Intravenous infusion pumps must be locked so the rate of administration cannot be adjusted by clients or visitors. In the home, medication should be safely stored out of reach of the child.

NURSING CARE

PRIORITIES IN NURSING CARE

When caring for children before, during, and after procedures, the nurse must remember that the child is typically in a foreign environment, among strangers, and exposed to frightening instruments and situations. There is often pain associated with procedures, which only increases the child's fear. Adequate preparation for the procedure, as well as a kind, comforting, and gentle manner, can assist the child in overcoming fear and anxiety.

ASSESSING

The nurse assesses the child's anxiety, fear, and stress before, during, and after procedures. Subjective statements related to the child's anxiety should be documented. The speaker (parent or child) should be identified. Younger children with verbal skills are likely to admit fear or anxiety before, during, or after the procedure. Older children and adolescents may want to project a brave attitude and often deny fear. Irritability, preoccupation, lack of eye contact, restlessness, trembling, GI distress, urinary frequency, confusion, and increased pulse, blood pressure, and respirations may all be objective signs of fear, anxiety, and stress related to procedures.

DIAGNOSING, PLANNING, AND IMPLEMENTING

Nursing diagnoses for a child who is required to have a procedure are as follows:

- **A**nxiety related to the situational crises of a procedure
- **F**ear related to threat of physical harm caused by the procedure
- **F**ear related to a lack of knowledge about the procedure
- **I**neffective **C**oping related to the threat created by the procedure

Some outcomes for a child who is required to have a procedure might include:

- The child will not demonstrate negative behaviors related to anxiety.
- The child will be able to manage fearful thoughts.
- The child will seek and express understanding of accurate information about the procedure.
- The child will take part in some forms of diversion, relaxation, or play.

The nurse's role in providing support to these clients includes the following:

- Teach the parent and child factual information about the procedure. *Increased knowledge helps reduce anxiety and fear.*
- Encourage the child to express anxiety verbally. *Expressing concerns relieves the child and allows the nurse to address the concerns.*
- Provide verbal and nonverbal support before, during, and after the procedure. The appropriateness of touch as a method of giving nonverbal support may vary among cultures (Box 8-5 ■). *The child should understand that the nurse respects feelings. Respect builds trust in the nurse-child relationship.*
- Arrange for the care of the child to be consistent. *Continuity of care builds trust and increases the child's comfort.*
- Allow the child to have a comfort item or parent present during the procedure. *Familiar items or family members increase the child's comfort level.*

BOX 8-5   CULTURAL PULSE POINTS

Use of Touch as Nonverbal Support

Most procedures require the nurse to use touch. Personal space and cultural norms must be taken into consideration when implementing procedures. Casual touch should be avoided in children of Asian or Native American descent. European cultures are more comfortable with casual touch. Permission should be obtained from the child and his or her family, regardless of culture, prior to the procedure. However, this is especially important when the child is uncomfortable with casual touch.

- Give the child some choices in the procedure whenever possible. These choices could include which arm to start the IV, going to the procedure room or staying in the hospital room for the procedure, or what type of bandage they receive. *Choices allow the child to have ownership in the procedure and may help reduce fear.*
- Decrease the child's environmental stimulation before, during, and after the procedure. Lower the lights, turn off the TV, and close the door. *A quiet, calm environment is more comforting to the child.*

EVALUATING

Evaluating a child with anxiety or fear related to a procedure includes continually observing for manifestations of fear, anxiety, and inability to cope. The nurse should document these and report them appropriately. Remember to document interventions aimed at reducing anxiety and fear prior to using restraints during procedures.

NURSING PROCESS CARE PLAN
Client with Fractured Arm

Keri is 3 years old. She sustained a broken left arm and facial cuts in an automobile accident. Her fractured arm required an open reduction and internal fixation. The facial lacerations required sutures. Keri's dad is at her bedside, but her mother was injured in the accident and is currently in surgery. Upon return from surgery, Keri is grimacing and crying softly. Her vital signs are T 98.6 °F, P 144, R 35, and BP 100/60.

Assessment

- Grimacing, crying softly
- Elevated pulse, respiration, and blood pressure
- Facial wounds with sutures
- Left arm post open reduction and internal fixation

Nursing Diagnosis.   The following important nursing diagnosis (among others) is established for this client:

- Acute **P**ain related to surgical and facial wounds

Expected Outcomes.   Expected outcomes for this client are:

- Will be able to express pain verbally or nonverbally using an appropriate pain scale.
- Will experience reduced pain.

Planning and Implementation

- Administer medication as ordered. *Medications relieve pain and pain perception.*
- Teach child signs and symptoms of pain, especially nonverbal signs. Use a pain scale with facial expressions to assist a child with limited vocabulary. *Children need instruction in recognizing pain and reporting it promptly in order to initiate pain relief methods quickly.*
- Teach parent signs and symptoms of pain, especially nonverbal signs. Use a pain scale with facial expressions to assist parents in recognizing pain. *Parents need instruction in recognizing pain and reporting it promptly in order to initiate pain relief methods quickly.*
- Allow the child to "assist" in medication administration. For example, give the child a clean empty syringe (no needle, no medication) to play with while the nurse is administering the medication. *This gives the child a feeling of control and provides a method of distraction as well.*
- Implement nonpharmacologic pain relief methods such as positioning, use of cold or heat application, or playing soothing music to relax the child between medication administrations. *Nonpharmacologic pain relief methods complement pharmacologic methods and may extend their effectiveness. These nonpharmacologic methods (see Box 7-3 ■) may also allow the client to be weaned sooner from the use of pharmacologic methods of relieving pain.*
- Monitor medication effectiveness. *Adequate assessment of medication effectiveness allows the nurse to respond quickly when the medication is ineffective.*

Evaluation.   Prompt evaluation of pain management provides the nurse with an avenue to provide client-specific pain relief measures.

Critical Thinking in the Nursing Process

1. What distraction activities would be appropriate for this child?
2. What response should the nurse give the girl when she asks where her Mommy is?
3. Based on this girl's age, how might she express pain?

Note: Discussion of Critical Thinking questions appears in Appendix I.

Note: The reference and resource listings for this and all chapters have been compiled at the back of the book.

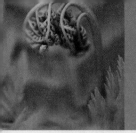

Chapter Review

 KEY TERMS by Topic

Use the audio glossary feature of either the CD-ROM or the Companion Website to hear the correct pronunciation of the following key terms.

Obtaining Vital Signs
point of maximal impulse

Newborn Reflexes
rooting reflex, sucking reflex, palmar grasp reflex, plantar grasp reflex, Babinski's reflex, stepping reflex, tonic neck reflex, Moro reflex, startle reflex

Specimen Collection
Vacutainer®

Feeding a Child
residual volume

KEY Points

- The order of assessment in children is often organized so the least comfortable or most invasive parts are done last. This allows more successful and accurate measurement of pulse and respiratory rate.

- Children are generally fearful of procedures, especially those of an invasive nature. The nurse provides appropriate teaching and emotional support to the child to alleviate this fear.

- Older children and adolescents will generally cooperate better if they are informed about a procedure ahead of time and understand its purpose.

- Small children may cooperate less if informed ahead of time about painful procedures. Inform parents of small children ahead of time, and give limited information to the small child directly before performing the procedure.

- Parents or caregivers need the reason for the procedure, the steps in the procedure, the results expected, any risks associated with the procedure, and follow-up measures required after the procedure.

- The scope of practice varies from state to state and facility to facility. Common sense coupled with nursing judgment should guide decisions when adjustment to any procedure is needed.

- The child's safety during procedures is the nurse's primary responsibility. This is accomplished by performing the procedure correctly, restraining the child when necessary, and observing his or her well-being following the procedure.

- Correct documentation should include the date and time the procedure was performed, objective information about the procedure results, and condition of the child following the procedure. The nurse must also record any further nursing measures that were necessary related to the procedure, including any reports given.

- The use of appropriate equipment is important for procedures involving pediatric clients. For example, blood pressure is altered when cuff size is incorrect. Needle sizes must also be chosen based on the child's weight and age.

- Children younger than 3 years should have intramuscular injections in the vastus lateralis because gluteal muscles have not developed adequately.

- Fluid overload is a significant complication for pediatric clients receiving intravenous infusion. The nurse must be vigilant in assessing rate of infusion, the condition of the IV site, and systemic effects of the intravenous infusion.

- The nurse must be constantly aware of the child's airway and oxygenation. Aspiration is avoided by proper positioning and feeding methods. Upright positioning will assist respiratory effort of the child with breathing difficulties. The nurse is responsible for correctly administering oxygen by nasal cannula, face mask, or oxygen hood.

 EXPLORE MediaLink

Additional interactive resources for this chapter can be found on the Companion Website at www.prenhall.com/adams.

Click on Chapter 8 and "Begin" to select the activities for this chapter.

For chapter-related NCLEX®-style questions and an audio glossary, access the accompanying CD-ROM in this book.

Animations

Child physical assessment	Applying a mummy wrap
Blood pressure	Gavage tube
Capillary pressure	Ostomy care
Client pain assessment	Proper use of a metered dose inhaler
Pulse oximeter	
Throat culture	Adolescent ear
Tracheostomy	Lung sounds
Metered dose inhaler	Evaluating deep tendon reflexes

FOR FURTHER Study

Discussion of informed consent forms and other legal forms is in Chapter 3.

For an illustration of pediatric venous access sites, see Figure 11-8.

For further discussion on the use of aerosol medications in the treatment of asthma, see Chapter 12. Figure 12-8 shows some of the equipment and techniques used for infant cardiopulmonary resuscitation (CPR).

For more about heart sounds, see Chapter 13.

For standardized growth charts, see Appendix II.

Critical Thinking Care Map

Caring for a Child Requiring Restraints
NCLEX-PN® Focus Area: Safe and Effective Care Environment

Case Study: Casey, an 18-month-old male, needs to have a nasogastric tube inserted for persistent vomiting. Casey is crying and kicking as the nurse takes him to the procedure room. He is yelling, "No, no, no." The nurse decides that in order to do the procedure safely she needs assistance from a colleague and will need to restrain Casey during the procedure.

Nursing Diagnosis: Risk for Injury, related to nasogastric tube insertion

COLLECT DATA

Subjective	Objective
_____	_____
_____	_____
_____	_____
_____	_____
_____	_____
_____	_____
_____	_____

Would you report this? Yes/No

If yes, to: _____

Nursing Care

_____
_____
_____
_____
_____
_____
_____
_____
_____
_____
_____
_____

How would you document this? _____
_____
_____
_____

Data Collected
(use only those that apply)

- Crying
- Kicking and screaming
- Yelling "no, no, no"
- Face red
- Carotid pulse 120 bpm
- 50 mL green vomitus
- 100 mL yellow urine
- Phenergan 12.5 mg, rectal suppository inserted

Nursing Interventions
(use only those that apply; list in priority order)

- Administer Phenergan 12.5 mg, rectally.
- Measure urine output every shift.
- Obtain physician's order for mummy restraints.
- Provide emotional care during and after procedure.
- Enlist assistance of a colleague during procedure.
- Remove restraints immediately after procedure.
- Assess restraints every 15 minutes.

Compare your documentation to the sample provided in Appendix I.

NCLEX-PN® Exam Preparation

1 For which of the following children would it be appropriate for the nurse to measure head circumference? Select all that apply.

  1. 6 months
  2. 1 year
  3. 6 years
  4. 2 years
  5. 3 years
  6. 5 years

2 What is the best method the nurse can use to measure urine output in the infant?

  1. Inserting an indwelling catheter
  2. Weighing the diapers
  3. Applying an external collection bag
  4. Weighing the infant after each voiding.

3 The most appropriate nursing intervention for a child in an oxygen tent is:

  1. Changing linens frequently.
  2. Allowing the child to enter and exit the tent at will.
  3. Providing several stuffed animals for the child to play with.
  4. Providing the child with a fan to assist with lowering the temperature.

4 The nurse needs to give an infant an intramuscular injection of hepatitis B vaccine. Where should the injection be given?

  1. Deltoid
  2. Dorsogluteal
  3. Rectus femoris
  4. Vastus lateralis

5 An infant, shortly after birth, is coughing, and the nurse hears a moist sound on inspiration. Which of the following nursing interventions is most appropriate?

  1. Suction the mouth, then the nose.
  2. Insert an endotracheal tube and attach to continuous suction.
  3. Insert a feeding tube and attach to continuous suction.
  4. Suction the nose, and then the mouth.

6 In which of the following situations can the nurse apply restraints? Select all that apply.

  1. on all children in the hospital
  2. only when other methods of restraint fail
  3. as the first choice of restraint
  4. to keep the arm immobilized during injections
  5. to prevent the child from pulling the bandage

7 The nurse needs to insert a rectal suppository in a 6-month-old infant. Choose the appropriate method(s):

  1. Insert using the index or little finger.
  2. Insert $1/2$ inch into the rectum.
  3. Both 1 and 2.
  4. Never given.

8 Which of the following vital signs, obtained from a 2-year-old male, would require the nurse to report the findings?

  1. P 150, R 50
  2. P 120, R 35
  3. P 125, R 38
  4. P 140, R 40

9 Which of the following vital signs, obtained from a 15-year-old female, would require the nurse to report the findings?

  1. P 100, BP 130/90
  2. P 70, BP 119/80
  3. P 60, BP 110/78
  4. P 90, BP 115/70

10 When choosing an assessment method, which of the following is appropriate for a child experiencing pain?

  1. Assess head to toe so no areas are forgotten.
  2. Assess only physical symptoms.
  3. Put the child on a bed or table.
  4. Assess areas that are painful last.

Answers for NCLEX-PN® Review and Critical Thinking questions appear in Appendix I.

Chapter 9

Care of the Family with a Dying Child

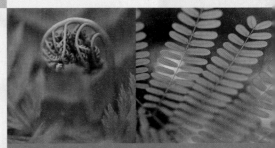

BRIEF Outline

Grief Process

Anticipated Loss

Family of the Dying Child

Nurses' Grief

Culture and Grief

Caring for the Dying Child

Legalities Related to Death

Nursing Care

Signs of Impending Death

Care After Death

Death-Related Religious
and Cultural Practices

LEARNING Outcomes

After completing this chapter, you will be able to:

1. Define key terms.
2. Describe the stages of grief.
3. Describe the role of the LPN/LVN in caring for dying children and their families.
4. Describe the signs of impending death.
5. Discuss the process of organ donation.

HEALTH PROMOTION ISSUE:
Pediatric Organ Donation

NURSING PROCESS CARE PLAN:
Care of a Child Dying at Home

NURSING PROCESS CARE PLAN
CHART:
Comforting the Dying Client
and Family

CRITICAL THINKING CARE MAP:
Care of Mother Who Is Grieving

Threats to a child's life may be expected—as in a chronic illness or a progressively disabling condition—or be unexpected—as in a premature birth or accident. How the child, parents, and siblings cope with the threat will depend on the circumstances surrounding the event and the child's condition. If the child dies from a chronic, terminal disease such as muscular dystrophy, the child and family have time to adjust to the impending death. The parents and siblings who become involved in the care of the terminally ill child can feel that they have contributed to making the dying child as comfortable as possible. However, when an acute illness or unexpected injury threatens the life of a child, the parents and siblings are thrust into the unfamiliar environment of an emergency room or intensive care unit. The parents and siblings, unable to assist with care, may be totally unprepared to cope with the loss.

Nursing care of children with chronic disorders is discussed in Chapter 7 . This chapter will focus on helping the family through the grief process, making preparation for the death, and providing care after death.

Grief Process

Much research has been done since the mid-1960s about the grief process. Five stages of loss or grief have been identified (Kübler-Ross, 1969) and described in detail in many nursing textbooks. These stages will be reviewed and applied to the real or anticipated loss of a child.

Loss, either real or perceived, is experienced when something is removed from the body or the environment. The loss could be tangible, such as the amputation of a limb, the death of a pet, or misplacing a favorite toy. The loss could be intangible, such as the loss one's job, health, or respect. **Grief** is a feeling of extreme sadness resulting from a loss. At times, circumstances are such that we anticipate the loss before it occurs. In these cases, the stages of grief will be experienced twice: once when the loss is initially anticipated, and again when the loss actually happens. It is important to note that individuals move through the stages of grief at different rates, but all stages. The five stages are shown in Figure 9-1 ■.

Stages of Grief	
Shock	No! I don't believe it!
Anger	**It's not fair! I don't deserve this!**
Bargaining	If you just make me better, I promise I'll …
Depression	*Leave me alone.*
Acceptance	I am ready now.

Figure 9-1. ■ Five stages of grief have been identified, but clients do not always experience all five stages. They may only experience some of the stages, or they may move back and forth from one stage to another.

STAGE 1 SHOCK AND DISBELIEF

The initial reaction to a loss is one of shock and disbelief. The conscious mind is trying to process what is happening. Sensory perceptions may be altered. Time seems to stand still. It may take several minutes for the parent to understand what is being said. It may be several hours or days before the complete impact of the situation has "sunk in." Often parents describe their feelings during this time as being disconnected, in a daze, or "out of it." For most parents, the period of intense shock passes in about 24 hours. During this time, they grope for answers and explanations. They may think the situation is just a bad dream and they will wake up. They may make statements like, "This can't be happening," or, "This isn't real." Because of their emotional state, information may need to be repeated several times. The nurse must be gentle in explaining and reinforcing the reality of the situation (Figure 9-2 ■).

Parents display a wide range of behaviors on hearing bad news. The parent may scream, cry, or collapse to the floor. They may remain in control, they may strike out at the nearest object, or they may try to run away. They may yell at the person who is telling them the news. The nurse must anticipate any of these reactions and be ready to provide support. Parents should not be alone at this time. If they try to run away, it is important for someone to go with them. Running away in an extreme emotional state puts the parent at risk for injury to themselves and to others.

STAGE 2 ANGER

As the reality of the situation begins to penetrate the conscious mind, anger begins to surface. The parents may direct the anger at themselves in the form of guilt, or they

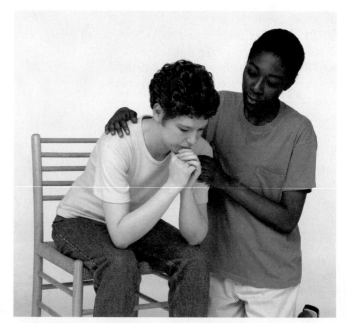

Figure 9-2. ■ In the stage of shock, therapeutic touch and presence of the nurse can support the family. (Dorling Kindersley Media Library.)

may direct it toward the spouse, health care providers, other children, others involved in the situation, or God. In their anger, parents frequently make accusing or threatening comments. They may physically try to assault the person they believe is responsible for the child's death. It is important for the nurse to maintain objectivity, to help defuse the situation, and to help the grieving parent work through the anger in a positive manner.

STAGE 3 BARGAINING

To bargain means to make a deal (if I do something for you, then you do something for me). The bargaining stage of grief has this type of thinking. In anticipation of the death of their child, parents may bargain with doctors, nurses, or God. Comments such as "I'll do anything, just save my child's life" indicate the parent is bargaining to prevent the loss. When death has occurred, parents may say, "I would do anything just to have one more day with my child." The nurse must understand these comments and support the parents as they come to the realization that there is nothing that can be done to change the inevitability of death.

STAGE 4 DEPRESSION

Depression is a state of persistent sadness. When grieving a loss, depressed individuals lack energy and enthusiasm to perform all daily activities. They may experience persistent hopelessness, tearfulness, and a sense of worthlessness. The times of sadness seem to come in waves. They are interspersed with times of relative calm as they remember happy experiences. Although this depressed state may last for up to a year, they should begin to have longer periods of happiness and shorter periods of extreme sadness. If depression prevents them from performing daily activities and interacting socially, professional help may be needed. The nurse can be instrumental in helping parents explore and understand their feelings. Because of the seriousness of depressed states, early recognition and referral is important.

STAGE 5 ACCEPTANCE

The loss of a child is the most difficult experience a parent endures. When the birth of a child is expected, parents begin to dream and plan for the future. When the child dies or has a life-threatening illness or injury, the parents not only lose the child, but they also lose the dream. Over time the parent comes to accept the loss. They are able to make new dreams and plans for the future. To keep the memory of the lost child alive, parents need to be encouraged to reminisce about the happy times, keep some pictures around the house, or keep in contact with the child's friends. Serving as a resource to other grieving families may help the parents to find some good out of their loss.

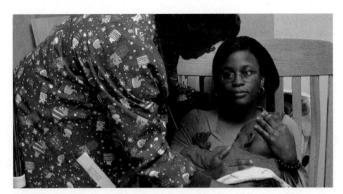

Figure 9-3. ■ This 3½-year-old's condition has deteriorated rapidly, and death is expected within 2 to 3 days. The nurse's role now is to keep the child as comfortable as possible and to support the family.

Anticipated Loss

Anticipated loss occurs during a life-threatening illness or injury. Anticipated loss begins when the parent first hears the diagnosis of the life-threatening illness (Figure 9-3 ■). If parents are present at the time of injury, they begin to make judgments about the extent of injury and possible prognosis. If they are not present at the time of injury, the anticipated loss begins the moment they are notified of the injury. When the child's condition is uncertain, the parents begin to anticipate death, permanent damage, or disfigurement. They imagine how their life will be changed if the child does not recover fully. They experience sadness at the thought of losing the lifestyle they have known, and the hardships ahead.

If the child's condition stabilizes and improves, the parents adjust and make plans for transfer or discharge. If the child's condition is terminal, parents remain in the emotional turmoil of grief. If the child's illness involves periods of remission and exacerbation, the parents will have periods of calm acceptance and periods of emotional stress. As the child's condition deteriorates, the parents will need to make plans for terminal care. Following the death, the parents will again move through the grief process.

Family of the Dying Child

DYING CHILD'S CONCEPT OF DEATH

Care of the dying child is one of the most challenging experiences of nursing, requiring great sensitivity and compassion for the child and for the entire family. The age and developmental stage of the ill child influence his or her reaction to impending death. Table 9-1 ■ identifies children's understanding of and reaction to death at each stage of development.

The infant has no concept of illness or death, but will develop separation anxiety when the parents or primary

TABLE 9-1		
Children's Understanding of Death		
CHILD'S AGE	**CONCEPT OF DEATH**	**BEHAVIOR**
Infant	Has no concept of death. May react to caregiver stress.	Crying, fussy, eats less. May sleep more than usual.
Toddler	Has no true concept of death. Aware someone is missing, but unable to tell temporary separation from permanent loss.	Separation anxiety, clinging to parents. Biting, hitting, and refusing to eat or sleep.
Preschooler	May have beginning understanding of death of pets. Believes death is temporary, and believes magic can cause death or return life.	Shows aggression, throws things, hits, is hyperactive. Fears going to sleep due to nightmares. Asks a lot of questions about death.
School-Age	Understands that death is permanent. Understands that death will happen to everyone.	Tries to act "grown-up" and not cry. Tries to help with household chores. May develop stomachache or headache.
Adolescent	Understands death is associated with illness and trauma. Fear of death conflicts with feeling invincible. Recognizes effects of death on parents and others.	May develop severe depression including suicide attempts. May exhibit risk-taking behaviors.

care provider are out of sight. The toddler responds to the anxiety of the parent. In a strange environment, they fear body mutilation and the possibility of pain. Even 5-year-olds can tell the seriousness of illness. They are aware of death but may not have a concept of its permanence. Young children can see their body deteriorate and feel the effects of toxic chemicals as the disease progresses. They may realize they are dying based on their own body changes and seeing other children who are undergoing treatment. Although the young child may not be able to express anxiety over death, they do express fear of body mutilation. Even when not told they are dying, children know their condition is worsening.

Children often keep their fears of dying to themselves. They are aware of the stress their family is undergoing, and they do not want to contribute to it. They fear the family will abandon them if they express anger over their illness and impending death. Because of their own fears and feelings of hopelessness, parents may not recognize the child's emotional needs and fears

Adolescents are old enough to understand death and what is happening to them. However, because of their stage of development, adolescents have additional challenges. Adolescents struggle for independence and their own identity. They are preoccupied with their body image at a time when terminal illness may result in disfigurement. Dying teens may feel isolated from their friends at a time when peers are an important part of their development. As death

nears, adolescents should be allowed as much control over events as their condition allows.

The nurse must be diligent in providing care to the terminally ill child, while promoting a normal growth and development pattern and supporting the family and peers. Whether in the hospital or at home, helping the ill child maintain contact with peers will reduce the feeling of isolation (Figure 9-4 ■).

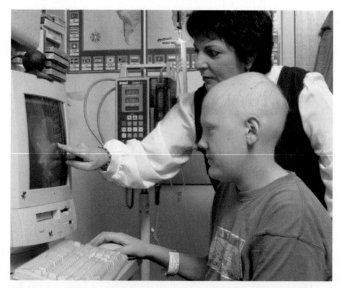

Figure 9-4. ■ This teenager and his mother are exploring computer chat rooms of terminally ill children receiving palliative care.

The biggest challenges to nursing care come not from the physical needs but from the emotional needs. The nurse must be sensitive to the verbal as well as the nonverbal communication. By providing opportunities for fantasy play, storytelling, and art projects, the nurse encourages the child to express feelings for which they may not have words. Box 9-1 ■ identifies strategies for communicating with the dying child.

At times, the parents request that the child not be told about the prognosis. This can put the nurse in an emotional conflict if the child asks about the condition. Table 9-2 ■ identifies questions commonly asked by terminally ill children. In such a situation, the nurse should tell the parents about the child's questions. Parents may feel unprepared to talk with the child and answer questions about dying. The nurse can anticipate the child's questions and give the parent developmentally appropriate words to use in discussing death. The family may benefit from a referral to a professional who has experience in bereavement and in counseling children and families.

PARENTS OF THE DYING CHILD

The death of a child is the most painful experience a parent will have to endure. When the death is sudden and unexpected, such as following an accident, the parent has little time to adjust to the shock. At times, due to resuscitation efforts, the parents may not be able to stay with the child. A private room should be provided for them. If possible, one spokesperson from the medical team should keep the

TABLE 9-2

Answering Children's Questions About Death

QUESTION	ANSWER
What will death be like?	"I think it will be peaceful. What do you think?"
What will happen to me when I die?	"What have your parents told you about what will happen to you?"
Will I be punished for the bad things I have done?	"Do you think you will be punished?"
When will I be with (person closest to child) again?	"I think (person) will be with you when they die."
Will my parents be all right?	"Your parents will miss you because they love you, but they will be all right."
Will I experience pain?	"We will try to keep the pain away. Let us know if you hurt, OK?"

family informed of the child's condition. When death appears inevitable, the spokesperson should provide time for the parents to absorb information of the child's worsening condition.

Federal regulations require the family to be given the option of donating the child's organs for research or transplant. Nurses with special education in organ procurement should be called to talk with the family and obtain informed consent. If organ donation is being considered, the physician should be notified immediately because the decision may alter use of some life support medications. The Health Promotion Issue on pages 234 and 235 discusses organ donation.

Family, friends, and clergy should be called at the parents' request. Avoid giving news of death over the telephone. Instead, notify the family that the child has been seriously injured in an accident. Ask them to come to the hospital immediately. Bad news should be given in a private area. Assure parents and family that everything possible was done for the child. Prepare the child's body before allowing the parents to view their child.

When the child is dying of a chronic illness, the parents have more time to prepare for the loss. In most cases of chronic terminal illness, the child gradually deteriorates over a few hours or days. Parents usually have enough time to call family and friends to be with them. After months or years of watching their child struggle for life, parents may wish for the child's death. Parents will grieve, but they will also experience relief that the child is finally at peace.

BOX 9-1   NURSING CARE CHECKLIST

Communicating with Dying Child

☑ Be flexible.

☑ Recognize that some children communicate best through nonverbal means (i.e., art and music). The child may be willing to talk through a puppet or a stuffed animal.

☑ Respect the child's need to be alone and the desire to share. Allow communication, but do not force it.

☑ Be receptive when children initiate conversation.

☑ Be specific and literal in explaining death.

☑ Acknowledge that a child's life can be complete, even if it is brief. Let dying children know they will always be loved and remembered. Help children find a sense of accomplishment and purpose in the lives they have led.

☑ Empower children as much as possible in circumstances concerning their deaths. Reassure them of continued love and physical closeness.

Source: Used with permission from Faulkner, K. W. (1997). Talking about death with a dying child. *American Journal of Nursing, 97*(6), 67–69.

HEALTH PROMOTION ISSUE

Pediatric Organ Donation

Delores and Juan Reyes rushed to the emergency room when their 2-year-old daughter Sandra climbed onto a porch railing and fell on her head onto a concrete patio below. Sandra had been taken to the emergency department by ambulance. Upon arrival at the hospital, Sandra was comatose, her breathing was very slow and shallow, and her pulse was irregular. Within minutes her pupils became fixed and dilated. The toddler did not regain consciousness. The child remained on life support while the doctor talked with the parents in a separate room. Both parents were distraught and stated they "cannot believe their baby is gone." The charge nurse who was staying with or near the parents has the responsibility of discussing the possibility of organ donation with them. The nurse needs knowledge and compassion to discuss this topic with emotionally distraught parents. However, this discussion is not only a legal requirement, but it must take place in a timely manner to ensure the organs are preserved for successful transplantation.

DISCUSSION

In recent years organ transplantation has become an acceptable treatment for clients with organ failure. The primary problem facing organ transplant teams is not the advanced technology required for successful transplantation, but a lack of donor organs, especially for pediatric populations. Annually more than 2,000 children under the age of 17 are on a waiting list for donor organs. Sadly, 30% to 50% of children under 2 years of age will die while

waiting for various organs. Three reasons for this shortage have been identified. Families are not being asked about organ donation. Health care professionals do not pursue potential donors. Families fail to give consent for organ donation.

The process of obtaining donor organs usually begins with health care professionals who treat critically ill children. Any person with severe head trauma should be considered a candidate to donate organs. Most donors have suffered spontaneous intracranial bleeding, gunshot to the head, brain tumors, cerebral anoxia, or drug overdose.

Once a possible donor has been identified, signs of brain death must be recognized and evaluated. In the early 1980s physicians were reluctant to apply brain death criteria to young children. Following years of research and dialogue, it is now agreed that standard brain death criteria can be applied to all

children with the exception of the premature infant.

Whereas medical personnel understand the diagnosis of brain death, families and the general public are often confused by it. This is especially true when the brain-dead individual is a child. Often parents, in shock from grief, may not fully understand that their child will not recover. Parents may deny that their child is dead. They may not accept that all life support measures can and will be discontinued whether they give permission for organ donation or not. Organs cannot be removed until the client is declared brain dead and the parents or legal guardians give consent.

In 1998, the Health Care Financing Administration (HCFA) instituted a requirement that all hospitals notify the Organ Procurement Organization (OPO) of any death or impending death. This requirement is further supported by the federal law titled "Required Request."

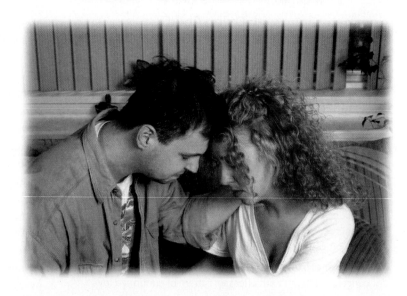

Federal policies require any hospital receiving Medicare and Medicaid reimbursements to establish a program for organ donation. The Joint Commission for the Accreditation of Healthcare Organizations (JCAHO) has a similar requirement.

The OPO evaluates the potential donor's medical and social history for any issue that would rule out organ donation. If the OPO supports the organ donation, the next step is to discuss the idea with the family. This is a very delicate subject to discuss at a very emotional time. Many feel the physician who determines the child to be brain dead should be the person to discuss organ donation with parents. Some physicians, however, feel this could be viewed as conflict of interest and suggest someone else would be better suited. As part of the plan required by the 1998 HCFA recommendations, hospitals have designated trained individuals, who work in collaboration with OPO, to meet with the family.

Timing of the discussion with the family is critical. The family must be given time to understand fully the meaning of "brain dead," to move past the shock and disbelief of their loss, and to have their questions answered. Then the topic of organ donation can be discussed. Many families are grateful for the opportunity to donate their child's organs and to know that "something good will come out of this tragedy." Other parents express discomfort with the discussion before having time to adjust to their loss.

Some families feel the discussion is hasty and callous. When families are treated with respect and compassion, they will be more open to organ donation discussion.

Donor families rely on health care professionals for comfort, support, and accurate information. Donor families should understand that the cost of organ donation is the responsibility of OPO and not of the donor families. Funeral ceremonies usually are not delayed or altered because of organ donation.

It takes time for recipients to be identified and contacted and for transplant teams to be prepared. Recovering or harvesting donated organs is a highly technical and specialized surgical procedure. Specially trained surgeons, anesthesiologists, nurses, and technicians may need to travel to the donor. During this time, the child's stability and organ function must be maintained. This includes maintaining normal cardiac output and tissue perfusion, ensuring adequate ventilation, preventing infection, maintaining adequate urinary output, maintaining fluid and electrolyte balance, and regulating body temperature. OPO personnel coordinate these activities.

PLANNING AND IMPLEMENTATION

All children in critical condition with a brain injury or disease should be assessed by health care professionals for the possibility of becoming an organ donor. The function of all body systems must be assessed frequently. Signs of decreased function should be reported promptly and intervention begun to stabilize the child's conditions.

Initially the child's condition may not warrant a call to OPO, or talking with the family. However, the nurse must anticipate that if the child's condition deteriorates, organ donation may become an issue. The nurse must be knowledgeable of the requirement of discussing organ donation and be aware of facility policy. The nurse needs to remember that whatever the family's decision, it will be a good one if they have been given information in a caring manner.

Emphasis needs to be placed on public awareness of organ donation. Families should talk about donation and share their decision with other family members and their primary health care provider. The nurse has the role of discussing the option of organ donation with families, including their own.

SELF-REFLECTION

What are your own thoughts about organ donation at death? Do you have any religious or cultural opposition to the idea? Are you in favor of the idea? What effect could your own opinion have when you are dealing with parents who must make this decision for their child?

SUGGESTED RESOURCES

For the Nurse

This website provides articles from the Northeast Florida Medicine Journal including the September 98 article *Issues in pediatric organ donation* by

Carman Koch D'Agostino. National Organ Procurement and Transplantation Network. *UNOS Update.* Spring 1998.

Being happy for the death of their child may bring feelings of guilt. At this time parents need to be encouraged to talk about their feelings. They should be told that it is okay to let go of the child and be relieved that the suffering is over.

Over time, parents will work through the grief process and come to accept the loss of their child. However, there will continue to be times when an event, birthday, or anniversary will stimulate the grief process again. These new periods of sadness may last only a few hours or they may last for days. They are likely to become less frequent over time, but will probably be with the parents forever.

SIBLINGS OF THE DYING CHILD

The reaction of siblings to the terminal illness and death of a child is as individual as the reaction of adults. Many factors, including age, development, birth order, and length of the illness, can influence the reaction of siblings. As stated earlier, very young children do not have an understanding of death, so they may not know why their brother or sister is no longer present. Very young children, reacting to the stress of their parents and other family members, may realize that the ill child is no longer present, but they may forget once they are gone for some time. If the dying child is the eldest, the younger siblings may feel that when they "grow up," they, too, will die. Siblings may feel that the loss of a sister or brother is punishment for something they have done, or that somehow the death was their fault. Some children may be jealous of the attention the ill child has received and then feel guilty once the child dies. Many children have difficulty sleeping for fear they will not wake up.

Siblings need support and compassion. The nurse needs to explain what is happening in age-appropriate language (Figure 9-5 ■). If the child is dying from a chronic illness, the siblings should be allowed to participate in care as much as possible. Encouraging and helping the siblings to make cards, posters, or gifts will help them as well as the ill child. When death does happen, the nurse should make statements like: "His heart stopped beating and it will never start again." "She will never be in pain again." Such statements help the siblings understand the finality of death. Siblings need to understand that their parents are grieving and may not be able to respond to their needs as usual. Friends and family members are invaluable to assist with routine household chores and to provide as much stability in the home as possible.

GRANDPARENTS OF THE DYING CHILD

The grief of grandparents is unique. When a parent becomes a grandparent, a special bond develops with the grandchild. Grandparents develop a feeling of pride in their own children, and fulfillment that their family heritage

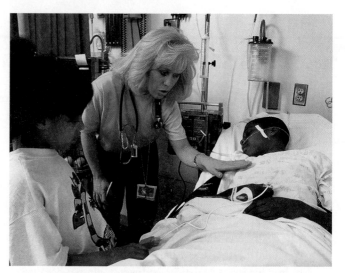

Figure 9-5. ■ When siblings visit the dying child, be prepared to answer questions honestly and in a manner that they can understand.

will continue. When a child dies, a part of that family heritage dies, too. The grandparent grieves over the loss. When a child dies, the grandparents also feel intense pain for their own child's loss. Having to watch their adult child in pain, and being unable to relieve it, the grandparents experience helplessness and guilt. As they try to be strong for their child, the grandparents may find that their own needs go unrecognized and unmet.

The nurse can offer support by encouraging the grandparents to express their feelings. By acknowledging the grandparents' loss and feelings of helplessness, the nurse communicates empathy for them. This opens a therapeutic relationship with the nurse that allows the grandparents to feel comfortable talking about their loss.

Nurses' Grief

Nurses grieve over the loss of their clients. Most enter the nursing profession to be of help to others. When a client dies, nurses may feel as though they failed to provide quality care. When the client is a child, the nurse may feel she has failed the client, the parents, and the family.

When caring for a terminally ill child, the nurse develops a close relationship with the child and the family. In order to remain objective and professional, many nurses begin to withdraw from the relationship prior to the death. When the nurse has children or grandchildren the same age as the dying child, the nurse may have more difficulty maintaining a professional relationship. The nurse may have difficulty identifying the child's and family's needs because of her own defenses against the feeling of hopelessness and helplessness. When nurses realize the inevitability of a child's death, they experience feelings of

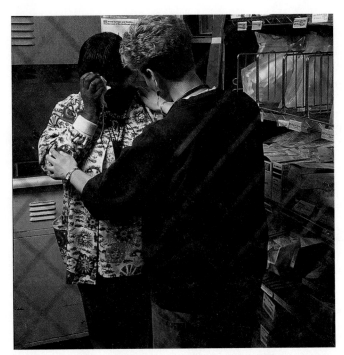

Figure 9-6. ■ Nurses who work with the dying need to express their own grief in a supportive environment after a child's death. Nurses who do not share their sadness and grief with colleagues may be unable to continue to provide supportive care to the next families who need compassionate care.

anger, frustration, sadness, and powerlessness. These feelings can interfere with the nurse's decision making and good judgment.

It is important for nurses in these circumstances to share their grief with other health care professionals (Figure 9-6 ■). Nurses who work frequently with dying children and their families must learn to cope with grief while maintaining their objectivity, empathy, and compassion. The employing agency must acknowledge the nurse's stress. Employee support groups and debriefing sessions with mental health professionals help nurses to manage their feelings.

The nurse must also remember that he or she is human, and humans grieve. The family wants a nurse who provides care with compassion. If the nurse sheds a tear at times, the family will not see the nurse as weak and unprofessional, but as a person who cares about them and their child. This sharing of human emotion speaks more than words.

Culture and Grief

The nurse should work closely with the family of a dying child. In order to be most helpful, the nurse must understand the family's culture. There are many culturally influenced rites and rituals surrounding death. Table 9-3 ■ identifies some common cultural traditions regarding mourning and after-death care.

A nurse may sometimes work with a family whose culture is not familiar. In this situation, the nurse must ask the family questions. Statements like "What are your traditions when a child dies?" can be helpful. Box 9-2 ■ provides some insight into cultural approaches to illness. The most important aspect of care for the child and family is to provide care with compassion and understanding of the extreme stress the family is undergoing. Many times, a gentle touch or sitting quietly with the family is the best intervention at the time.

COMPLICATED (OR DYSFUNCTIONAL) GRIEF

Complicated grief (dysfunctional grief) occurs when an individual is unable to accept what has happened and move on with life. "Forgetting" the lost child is never a goal. However, being able to work through the pain and continue with other activities is a sign of healthy grieving. The individual who is unable to continue with activities of daily living needs professional assistance. Signs of dysfunctional grieving might include:

- Continuous crying.
- Sleep disturbances, including being unable to sleep or wanting to sleep all the time.
- Eating disturbances, including overeating or undereating.
- Being unable to manage household activities, or an obsession with household activities to the point that other things are omitted.

BOX 9-2	CULTURAL PULSE POINTS

Respecting Cultural Practices Related to Illness and Death

At death, cultural practices and patterns generally surface, even if people have drifted from many cultural habits in daily life. Problems may arise if a health care team does not understand behavior that is normal or expected within a culture. For example, a Southeast Asian may use "coining" (rubbing coins) as a way to try to heal a sick person. A person from the Caribbean might look to a witch or *shaman* (medicine man) to help regain health. After death, some American Indians cleanse the body, drum, and then open the window to release the person's spirit. These behaviors might seem bizarre to a nurse who does not understand them or who feels they somehow "break the rules."

When a family presents an idea that is foreign, the nurse should ask questions and try to understand what the practice means to the family in the context of their culture. If possible, a "cultural translator" should be asked to participate, to explain the meaning of the behavior and customs, and to help the staff accommodate these rituals as much as they can.

Source: Adapted from Eby, Linda. (2005). *Mental health nursing care.* Upper Saddle River, NJ: Prentice Hall, p. 133, Box 8-7.

TABLE 9-3

Cultural Traditions in Mourning and After-Death Rites

RELIGIOUS GROUP	POSSIBLE RITUALS	ORGAN DONATION OR AUTOPSY BELIEFS
Native Americans	Beliefs and practices vary widely. Navajo do not touch the deceased or their belongings. Mourning is done in private.	Varies among tribes.
Baha'i	No embalming or cremation; must be buried within an hour's travel distance of place of death. Body washed and wrapped in shroud. Prayer for the Dead recited.	Decision left to individual.
Buddhism	Last-rite chanting at bedside. Cremation common. Prayers weekly for 49 days to help soul in its transformation and possible rebirth.	Organ donation considered act of mercy, autopsy individual choice.
Catholicism	Sacrament of the sick. Obligated to take ordinary but not extraordinary means to prolong life. Burial preferred (in Catholic cemeteries). Cremation allowed, but remains must be interred, not scattered.	Autopsy, organ donation acceptable.
Christian Science	Unlikely to seek medical help to prolong life. Disposal of body and parts decided by family.	Individual decides about organ donation.
Hinduism	No restrictions to right-to-die issue. Religious prayers chanted before and after death. Body washed, wrapped in white cloth, laid in coffin. Cremation common. Men and women display outward grief, do not take part in any rituals for length of mourning period. Thread tied around wrist signifies a blessing; do not remove. No embalming.	Autopsy, organ donation acceptable.
Islam	Attempts to shorten life prohibited. Body is washed only by Muslims of same gender, wrapped in a plain cloth (kafan). Only burial is permitted by Islamic law (Shari'ah). Prayer for forgiveness recited.	Organ donation acceptable. Autopsy only for medical or legal reasons.
Jehovah's Witness	Use of extraordinary means to prolong life is individual choice. Burial determined by family preference.	Autopsy if required by law. Organ donation forbidden.
Judaism	If death is inevitable, no new procedure needed, but must continue those ongoing. Body ritually washed. Burial as soon as possible, all body parts must be buried together. Seven-day mourning period.	Autopsy permitted in certain circumstances; organ donation is a complex issue.
Mennonite	Do not believe life must be continued at all cost.	Autopsy, organ donation acceptable.
Mormonism	If death inevitable, promote a peaceful and dignified death. Burial in temple clothes. Burial preferred to cremation ("dust to dust").	Autopsy permitted with permission of next of kin. Organ donation is permitted.
Protestantism	Burial or cremation is individual decision.	Autopsy, organ donation are individual decisions.
Seventh-Day Adventist	Follow ethic of prolonging life. Disposal of body and burial are individual decisions.	Autopsy, organ donation acceptable.

Source: Data from Spector, R. E. (2000). *Cultural diversity in health and illness* (5th ed., pp. 137–138, 144–149). Upper Saddle River, NJ: Prentice Hall Health; Death and dying. *(1997). Hinduism today.* Published by Hindu Press International; Funeral rites and customs. (2000). Microsoft Encarta Encyclopedia.

- Being unable to work or participate in social activities within 3 to 6 months of the death.
- Being unable to dispose of any of the child's belongings.
- Being unable to show signs of sadness (no crying, no emotional response).

The LPN/LVN who sees these signs should inform the RN or physician. A referral to a counselor and antidepressant medication may be needed.

Caring for the Dying Child

PALLIATIVE CARE

As the child's condition deteriorates, decisions about palliative care must be made. The term **palliative care** or **palliative management** involves a shift in treatment goals from curative toward providing relief from suffering. Relief of suffering in dying clients goes beyond identifying and treating physical symptoms. The emotional, spiritual, and existential components of suffering and pain must also be addressed. It is important to note that palliative management can occur even in a hospital setting. The following are the major principles of palliative care.

- The overall goal of treatment is to optimize quality of life; that is, the hopes and desires of the dying person are fulfilled as much as possible.
- Death is regarded as a natural process, to be neither hastened nor prolonged.
- Diagnostic tests and other invasive procedures are minimized, unless they are likely to alleviate symptoms.
- Use of "heroic" treatment measures is discouraged.
- When using narcotic analgesics, the right dose is the dose that provides pain relief without unacceptable side effects.
- The client is the "expert" on whether pain and symptoms have been adequately relieved.
- Clients eat if they are hungry, drink if they are thirsty; feeding and fluids are not forced.
- Care is individualized and based on the goals of the client and family.

HOSPICE CARE

Once the decision has been made for palliative care, the family may be referred to hospice services. **Hospice care** is based on the holistic concepts of palliative care, which emphasizes quality of life rather than cure. The hospice movement was founded by the physician Cecily Saunders in London, England, in 1967 and was later extended to the United States. It grew rapidly after the enactment of the Medicare Hospice Benefit in 1983. The Medicare Benefit systematically outlines who can provide care, at what time, and in what way. Another facet of the Medicare program is

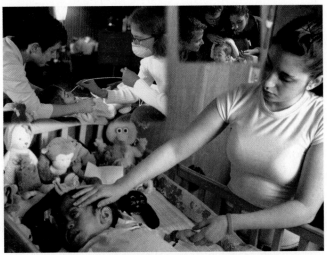

Figure 9-7. ■ Hospice care programs such as Pathways KIDS work with the client and family to provide quality of life for the dying child. Comfort measures and attention to emotional, psychological, and spiritual concerns are the priorities. (Photos courtesy of Sophia's Garden Foundation. © 2002–2005 Karen Schreiber.)

to provide the client with durable medical equipment, such as oxygen and a hospital bed. As with palliative care, the principles of hospice care can be carried out in a variety of settings. However, the most common settings are the client's home or extended care facilities. Autonomous hospice and hospital-based palliative care units are also becoming more available.

Hospice services can range from comprehensive to a focus on selected specialties such as symptom control and pain management services (Figure 9-7 ■). Hospice care is always delivered by a team of health care professionals, regardless of the setting, in order to ensure a holistic approach to care. The team members generally consist of the dying one, family and caregivers, physicians, nurses, aides, chaplains, social workers, and volunteers.

Entrance or admission into a hospice program requires a physician referral that can occur several ways. The referral may be initiated by the physician who finds at some point that curative treatment is no longer an option. The Medicare guideline governing admission is a prognosis of 6 months or less of life expectancy. Obviously, this has to be an educated guess, and clients should not be denied claims if they live longer than 6 months. Typically, the referring physician discusses the referral with the client and family and either contacts the hospice team or contacts the discharge planner or social worker to assist with the transition.

COMFORT MEASURES

Comfort measures are important for the dying child and for the family. By assisting with providing comfort, family

MediaLink

Hospice and Palliative Nursing

BOX 9-3	COMPLEMENTARY THERAPIES

Comfort for a Dying Child

Providing comfort is a primary concern for the dying child. Pain management is an important nursing intervention. When medical interventions cannot control pain, the nurse looks to alternative methods to reduce or remove pain. The following are some methods of addressing pain relief:

Biofeedback
With biofeedback, a client uses special machines to learn how to control such body functions as heart rate, blood pressure, and muscle tension. Biofeedback is sometimes used with people who have cancer to help them cope with pain and reduce anxiety.

Distraction
Distraction means turning your attention to something other than the pain. Distraction may actually work better than medicine when pain is sudden and intense or brief (lasting 5 to 45 minutes). It can be useful while waiting for pain medicine to start working. Distraction may be all that a person needs if pain is mild. It can even be a powerful way of relieving even the most intense pain temporarily. Some people think that a person who can be distracted from pain does not have severe pain. This is not necessarily true.

Skin Stimulation
Skin stimulation is the use of sensations (pressure, friction, temperature change, or chemicals) to excite the nerve endings in the skin. By providing a strong sensation that is not pain, we are able to lessen or block the pain sensation. Skin stimulation also alters

the flow of blood to the affected area, which can reduce or remove pain. **Note:** Skin stimulation should not be used on areas of skin receiving radiation therapy, because it may increase trauma to the skin.

Pressure
Pressure is a method of relieving pain in some instances. Pressure can be applied with the entire hand, the heel of the hand, the fingertips, knuckles, the ball of the thumb, or with both hands. Pressure can be applied for about 10 seconds to 1 minute over or near the pain. Pressure is usually most effective if it is applied as firmly as possible without causing pain.

Vibration
Vibration over or near the area of pain may bring temporary relief. The scalp attachment of a handheld vibrator often relieves a headache. A vibrator placed at the small of the back may help low back pain.

Cold or Heat
Heat often relieves sore muscles; cold lessens pain sensations by numbing the affected area. Preference for heat or cold may be very individual.

Menthol Preparations
Menthol preparations for pain are available in creams, lotions, liniments, or gels. When rubbed into the skin, they increase blood circulation to the affected area and produce a soothing feeling that lasts for several hours.

---

members feel useful because they are contributing to their child's care. Comfort measures include:

- Frequent position changes. *Weak children may be unable to turn themselves. Frequent position changes relieve pressure on bony prominences, facilitate drainage of respiratory secretions, and ease breathing.*
- Frequent oral care, including swabbing mucous membranes with applicators and water and applying ointment to lips. *Mouth breathing dries mucous membranes and lips. If a child is unable to swallow, oral fluids should not be given.*
- Liquid tears. *Liquid tears may be needed if the child does not blink often enough to prevent drying of the cornea.*
- Pain medication as ordered. *Pain medication is frequently ordered "as needed." Pain medication should be administered to the dying child to maintain the blood level.*
- Provide alternative methods of reducing pain whenever possible (Box 9-3 ■). *Alternative methods such as distraction and biofeedback can be helpful in coping with pain.*

Legalities Related to Death

The nurse's roles in legal issues related to death are determined by the laws of the region and the policies of the health care institution. For example, in some states a nasogastric

feeding tube cannot be removed from a person in a persistent vegetative state without a prior directive from the client. In other states, the removal is allowed at the family's request or a physician's order. Many of these legal issues stimulate strong ethical concerns. The nurse may need support from other team members in understanding and providing appropriate care to clients facing death.

ADVANCE DIRECTIVES
The Patient Self-Determination Act, implemented in 1991, requires all health care facilities receiving Medicare and Medicaid reimbursement to do the following:

- Recognize advance directives.
- Ask clients whether they have advance directives.
- Provide educational materials advising clients of their rights to declare their personal wishes regarding treatment decisions, including the right to refuse medical treatment.

There are two types of advance medical directives: the living will and the *health care proxy* or surrogate. The living will provides specific instructions about what medical treatment the client chooses to omit or refuse (e.g., cardiopulmonary resuscitation [CPR], intubation, ventilatory support) in the event that the client is unable to make those decisions.

The health care proxy, also referred to as *durable power of attorney for health care*, is a written statement appointing someone else (e.g., a relative or trusted friend) to manage health care treatment decisions when the client is unable to do so. For example, it is often used for specific clients who are in a coma, are having life-sustaining procedures, or are receiving artificial nutrition or hydration.

In most cases, parents are the decision makers for their children. However, in some states children as young as 15 years may sign informed consent forms. They may also determine whether they wish to be organ donors and whether they wish to terminate life-sustaining treatment. (See more on legal and ethical nursing issues in Chapter 3 ⬭.)

Nurses should learn the law regarding client self-determination for the state in which they practice. They are also responsible for knowing the policy and procedures for implementation in the institutions where they work. The legally binding nature and specific requirements of advance medical directives are determined by individual state legislation (Springhouse, 1996, pp. 156–177).

In most states, advance directives must be witnessed by two people but do not require review by an attorney or notarization. Some states do not permit relatives, heirs, or physicians to witness advance directives. Again, it is important for LPNs/LVNs to be informed of their state and institutional policies and procedures.

DO-NOT-RESUSCITATE ORDERS

Physicians may order "no code" or do not resuscitate (DNR) for clients who are in a stage of terminal, irreversible illness or expected death. A DNR order is generally written when the client or surrogate has expressed the wish for no resuscitation in the event of a respiratory or cardiac arrest. Many physicians are reluctant to write such an order if there is any conflict between the client and family members. A "**comfort measures only**" order is written to indicate that the goal of treatment is a comfortable, dignified death and that further life-sustaining measures are not indicated. Many states permit clients living at home to arrange special orders so that emergency technicians called to the home in the event of a cardiopulmonary arrest will respect the client's wish not to be resuscitated. LPNs/LVNs should be familiar with the federal and state or provincial laws and the policies of their institution concerning withholding life-sustaining measures.

EUTHANASIA

Euthanasia is the act of compassionately putting to death a person suffering from incurable or distressing disease. It is sometimes referred to as "mercy killing." Regardless of compassion, good intentions or moral convictions, euthanasia is illegal in both Canada and the United States. It can lead to criminal charges of homicide or to a civil lawsuit for withholding treatment or providing an unacceptable standard of care.

Voluntary euthanasia, or **assisted suicide**, refers to situations in which the dying individual desires some control over the time and manner of death. Assisted suicide is illegal except in Oregon, where a physician-assisted suicide statute was passed in 1994. That statute permits physicians to prescribe lethal doses of medications to clients who request them and meet certain criteria. Since Oregon's action, several other states have proposed similar laws. Legal challenges and ethical debates continue.

NURSING CARE

PRIORITIES IN NURSING CARE

When death cannot be avoided, the priorities of care for the child and the family include:

- Assistance with comfort measures for the child.
- Preparation of the child and the family by encouraging a plan for after-death activities (notifying family and friends, funeral arrangements, etc.).
- Providing emotional support.

Psychosocial issues will have greater impact in this situation than in other acute situations (such as care of a broken leg). Cultural competency will be important, because pivotal decisions about life events (mourning and burial or cremation, organ donation or not) will need to be made. The nurse will need to encourage expression of grief.

ASSESSING

Because everyone progresses through the grief process individually, the **LPN/LVN** must observe each member of the family to determine the degree of coping and need for support. The child's needs are the priority, especially pain relief, comfort measures, and listening. Therapeutic listening is an important aspect of nursing care for the dying child and the family.

DIAGNOSING, PLANNING, AND IMPLEMENTING

Nursing diagnoses related to the dying child often include:

- Ineffective Coping
- Anticipatory Grieving
- Complicated Grieving

Anticipated outcomes for these nursing diagnoses might be:

- Parents request presence of religious minister.
- Parents express need to seek support of other parents who have lost children.

- Child expresses anger that he/she is dying.
- Father accepts appointment with grief counselor.

The role of the LPN/LVN in providing care for the terminally ill child and the family is one of an assistant. Many times the physical care of the child is routine, including hygiene, nutrition, elimination, and special treatment of the specific disease. Providing this care is generally in the scope of practice of the practical nurse. Techniques of therapeutic communication are important when working with the child and the family. The nurse can help the child express feelings through drawings and play therapy (see Table 7-1 ⬥⬥). When the LPN/LVN identifies signs that children or members of the family are having difficulty expressing their loss, either anticipated or actual, the registered nurse should be contacted.

The plan of care for a dying child and his or her family should include the following nursing interventions:

- Provide measures to keep the child as comfortable as possible. *Comfort measures help relieve the child's suffering and at the same time provide psychological comfort to family.*
- Encourage each member of the family to express his or her feelings. *Talking about loss helps individuals to move through the stages of grief toward acceptance. When they express their feelings, the nurse can determine if they are grieving in the usual manner, or if they are becoming dysfunctional in their grief.*
- Adapt interventions to the age and developmental stage of the individual. (See Chapter 5 ⬥⬥ .) *By adapting interventions to the developmental stage of the individual, the nurse allows the child to express his or her feelings and understanding of the events taking place. The nurse can also help the child to understand the situation better.*
- Identify resources available to the family and assist in accessing support systems. *It is helpful to understand that others have had similar experiences and have come to acceptance. Families and individuals who exhibit signs of dysfunction will need professional help.*
- Attend professional support groups designed to help the nurse through the grief process. *In this kind of situation, nurses can only be therapeutic when their own emotional needs are met.*

EVALUATING

In evaluating the dying child, family and care providers it is important for them to verbalize their feelings. Grief takes a minimum of a year for the family to resolve, so they should be evaluated several times. Besides listening closely to their comments, the evaluator should also observe their behavior including dress, grooming, and crying. This data will be important to determine if the individual is moving through the process or is stuck in one of the stages.

NURSING PROCESS CARE PLAN
Care of a Child Dying at Home

Timmy, a 4-year-old in the end stage of a malignant brain tumor, is dying at home. Besides his parents, his 6-year-old brother, 2½-year-old sister, and maternal grandparents are with him.

Assessment.   Vital signs: T 99.8 (O) P 92, R 28. Timmy's respirations are irregular with moist breath sounds. Timmy sleeps most of the time. He is oriented when he is awake. He moans when turned. Timmy's mother and grandmother sit at his bedside constantly. Timmy's mother is crying. His father and grandfather have left the house to run errands. His brother and sister are playing around the house.

Nursing Diagnosis.   The following important nursing diagnosis (among others) has been established for this client:

- **P**ain related to brain tumor and death process

The following important nursing diagnosis (among others) has been established for the client's mother:

- **G**rieving related to upcoming death of child

Expected Outcomes.   The following expected outcomes have been identified:

- Timmy is resting comfortably.
- Timmy's mother will verbalize her feelings.

Planning and Implementation

- Medicate for pain as ordered. *Keeping the child comfortable will decrease suffering.*
- Turn and massage bony prominences every 1 to 2 hours. *Turning and massage increase circulation to skin and muscles and decrease discomfort.*
- Play soft music, and light aromatic candles. *Soft music and pleasant aromas induce relaxation.*
- Provide emotional support to mother and grandmother through touch, hugs, and encouraging verbalization. *At this time, the mother should be allowed and encouraged to grieve.*

Evaluation.   Be alert for nonverbal cues of discomfort. Respirations may decrease with pain medication. This should be documented, but because it is expected during the dying process, there is no need to notify the RN or physician. Timmy's mother and grandmother should express feelings.

Critical Thinking in the Nursing Process

1. Should Timmy be medicated for pain if his respirations slow to 12, and he continues to moan?

2. Timmy's mother asks, "How much longer will this go on?" How should the nurse reply?
3. What support should Timmy's grandmother receive?

Note: Discussion of Critical Thinking questions appears in Appendix I.

Signs of Impending Death

Although the exact time of death cannot be predicted, physical changes in the child can indicate that death is approaching. If death occurs rapidly, as in a cardiac arrest from an allergic reaction, the signs may not be present. If death occurs slowly from a terminal illness, the signs will probably be present. The changes may take place over a few hours to a few days.

As a terminal illness progresses, the heart becomes less efficient in pumping blood. Initially the pulse increases as the heart tries to meet the body's need for oxygen and nutrients. The heart muscle, receiving its oxygen between beats, becomes hypoxic when there is only a few hundredths of a second between beats. The hypoxic heart becomes irregular and eventually slows. In response to the failing heart, peripheral blood vessels constrict in order to shunt the blood to the vital organs; brain, heart, lungs, liver, and kidneys. The blood pressure drops, the skin becomes **mottled** (a bluish or purplish marbled appearance), and brain function slows. The child may become less responsive and slip into a coma. Reflexes such as cough and blink become absent. The kidneys, sensitive to the low blood pressure, slow and then stop production of urine. Peristalsis slows. Because of the slowing of circulation, blood pools in the pulmonary blood vessels resulting in pulmonary edema, and very moist noisy respirations at times referred to as a "death rattle." The respirations are usually through the mouth and become **Cheyne-Stokes respiration** (a period of progressive depth of breathing followed by a period of apnea) The periods of apnea become longer until respirations cease and the heart stops. The Nursing Care Plan Chart below describes aspects of care for a dying client and family.

Nursing Care Plan Chart

Comforting the Dying Client and Family

GOAL	INTERVENTION	RATIONALE	EXPECTED OUTCOME
1. Ineffective Airway Clearance related to excessive respiratory secretions as evidenced by gurgling sound, "death rattle"			
Client's breathing will be quiet and unlabored.	Place client in semi-Fowler's position	*Keeping the head elevated allows fluid to accumulate in lung bases, easing respirations.*	Client's respiration is less labored.
	Suction the airway prn.	*Suctioning the back of the throat and upper airways may be necessary to clear airway.*	
	Administer low-dose morphine, hyoscyamine, or scopolamine as ordered.	*Anticholinergic medications and morphine are frequently ordered to dry secretions and ease breathing.*	
2. Disturbed Sensory Perception related to changes in neurologic function			
Client will be treated with respect even when perceptions are questionable.	Reassure family that confusion is common.	*Families will be less anxious if they understand what is happening.*	Client and family verbalize what is happening.
	Encourage client and family to talk about what is happening.		Client is treated with respect.
	Tell family that hearing is the last sense to go.	*Family members may not realize the client can hear even when response is absent.*	Family members talk to the client.
	Encourage family to talk to client.	*Family members need reminding to talk to the client.*	*(continued)*

GOAL	INTERVENTION	RATIONALE	EXPECTED OUTCOME
	When providing care, always speak to the client, explaining what you are doing.	*This models good communication for the family.*	
	Keep dim light on at all times	*Being able to see helps client reorient if he or she awakens at night.*	
3. Anticipatory Grieving related to impending death			
Client and family will be able to communicate their feelings to each other openly.	A health care provider (RN, LPN, CNA) should be present.	*Clients and family fear being alone at time of death.*	The client and family communicates openly with each other.
	Provide a clean, quiet environment where people can say "goodbye" in a way reflecting their culture and values. Provide tissues and waste disposal.	*Saying "goodbye" is very a difficult, emotional, and personal time. A clean, quiet environment fosters communication. These interactions will provide lasting memories that help with the grief process.*	
	Ask about the family's culture and religious beliefs. Contact the minister or religious counselor of family's choice.	*A minister has special training to help the client and family. Talking about an afterlife can provide comfort.*	
	Show concern for client and family through touch, sitting quietly with them, and respecting their cultural or religious practices.	*Providing culturally sensitive care, reduces the family's anxiety and gives them more control over the situation.*	

Care After Death

The LPN/LVN can provide postmortem care including making the necessary phone calls and completing documentation. Facility policy will determine whether the LPN/LVN can pronounce the child's death.

PROVIDING POSTMORTEM CARE

After death, some characteristic physical changes occur. **Rigor mortis** is the stiffening of the body that occurs about 2 to 4 hours after death. It results from a lack of adenosine triphosphate (ATP), which is not synthesized because of a lack of glycogen in the body. ATP is necessary for muscle fiber relaxation. Its lack causes the muscles to contract, which in turn immobilizes the joints. Rigor mortis starts in the involuntary muscles (heart, bladder, etc.), then progresses to the head, neck, and trunk, and finally reaches the extremities. Rigor mortis usually leaves the body about 96 hours after death.

Algor mortis is the gradual decrease of the body's temperature after death. When blood circulation terminates and the hypothalamus ceases to function, body temperature falls about 1 °C (1.8 °F) per hour until it reaches room temperature. Simultaneously, the skin loses its elasticity and

can easily be broken when removing dressings and adhesive tape.

After blood circulation has ceased, the red blood cells break down, releasing hemoglobin, which discolors the surrounding tissues. This discoloration, referred to as **livor mortis**, appears in the lowermost or dependent areas of the body.

Tissues after death become soft and eventually liquefied by bacterial fermentation. The hotter the temperature, the more rapid the change. Therefore, bodies are often stored in cool places to delay this process. Embalming prevents the process through injection of chemicals into the body to destroy the bacteria.

After-death (*postmortem*) care may vary somewhat from area to area and culture to culture. However, there are some general principles that can be used as a guide.

CERTIFICATION OF DEATH

The formal determination, or *pronouncement*, of death must be performed by a physician, a coroner, or a nurse. In some areas, police officers or paramedics are also permitted to pronounce death. Again, the granting of the authority to nurses to pronounce death is regulated by the state or province. It may be limited to nurses in long-term care,

---

BOX 9-4

Brain Death Criteria

Clinical Signs
- Irreversible condition
- Apnea with arterial CO_2 level (PCO_2) of at least 60 mm Hg
- No response to deep stimuli
- No spontaneous movement (some spinal cord reflexes may be present)
- No gag or corneal reflex
- No oculocephalic or oculovestibular reflex
- Absence of toxic or metabolic disorders

Confirmatory Tests
- Cerebral blood flow study
- Electroencephalogram

Source: LeMone, P. & Burke, K. (2004). *Medical surgical nursing: Critical thinking in client care* (3rd ed.) Upper Saddle River, NJ: Pearson Education, Box 6-1, p. 145.

---

home health, and hospice agencies, or to advanced practice nurses. By law, a death certificate must be made out when a person dies. It is usually signed by the attending physician and filed with a local health or other government office. The family is usually given a copy to use for legal matters, such as insurance claims. (Box 9-4 ■ lists criteria for diagnosing brain death.)

CARE OF THE BODY

Nursing personnel may be responsible for care of a body after death. Postmortem care should be carried out according to the policy of the institution. Because care of the body may be influenced by religious law, the nurse should check the client's religion and make every attempt to comply with the family's wishes.

If the deceased's family or friends wish to view the body, it is important to make the environment as clean and pleasant as possible and to make the body appear natural and comfortable. All equipment, soiled linen, and supplies should be removed from the bedside. Some institutions require that all tubes in the body remain in place; in other institutions, tubes may be cut to within 1 inch (2.5 cm) of the skin and taped in place; in others, all tubes may be removed. The nurse should be familiar with the institutional policies and procedures.

Normally the body is placed in a supine position with the arms either at the sides, palms down, or across the abdomen. One or two pillows are placed under the head and shoulders, or the head of the bed is elevated 30 degrees, to prevent blood from discoloring the face by settling in it. The eyelids are closed and held in place for a few seconds. Often, the eyes and mouth do not remain closed and require a mortician's intervention.

Soiled areas of the body are washed. However, a complete bath is not necessary, because the body will be washed by the *mortician* (also referred to as an undertaker or funeral director), a person trained in care of the dead. Absorbent pads are placed under the buttocks to capture any feces and urine released because of relaxation of the sphincter muscles. A clean gown is placed on the client, and the hair is brushed and combed. All jewelry is removed. The top bed linens are adjusted neatly to cover the client to the shoulders. Soft lighting and chairs should be provided for the family to make the surroundings as peaceful as possible.

LABELING OF THE DECEASED

Nurses have a duty to handle the deceased with dignity and respect and to label the body appropriately. Mishandling can cause emotional distress to survivors. Mislabeling can also create legal problems if the body is inappropriately identified and prepared incorrectly for funeral services. In the hospital, the deceased's wrist identification tag is left on, and another tag is tied to the client's ankle or toe, in case one of the tags becomes detached. A third tag is attached to the shroud. All identification tags should include the client's name, hospital number, and physician's name, which in most hospitals is provided via the addressograph plate or hospital card that has the appropriate information already on it.

VIEWING BY PARENTS

If the parents were not present at the time of death, as is common in the emergency department, they should be allowed to be with the child. It is important to make the child's body presentable before the parents' viewing. When the parents see the lifeless body of their child, the reality of the death comes as a great shock. The nurse should stay with the parents to provide support.

CALLING THE MORTUARY

The nurse is responsible for notifying the mortuary selected by the parents. Mortuary staff will come either to the bedside or to the facility morgue to remove the body. All required paperwork must be completed before the child's body is removed. Personal belongings can either be given to the parents or sent with the body, but documentation must be made about their disposition.

AUTOPSY

An **autopsy** or **postmortem examination** is an examination of the body after death to determine more details about the cause of death, to learn more about a disease, or to assist in the accumulation of statistical data. It is performed only in certain cases. The law and the institutional policies and procedures describe under what circumstances an autopsy must be performed, such as when death is sudden and unexpected or occurs within 48 hours of admission to a hospital.

It is the responsibility of the physician or, in some instances, of a designated person in the hospital to obtain consent for autopsy. Consent must be given by the individual in a legal document before death or by the next of kin. Laws in many states and provinces prioritize the family members who can provide consent as follows: surviving spouse, adult children, parents, siblings. After autopsy, hospitals cannot retain any tissues or organs without the permission of the person who consented to the autopsy.

INQUEST

An *inquest* is a legal inquiry into the cause or manner of a death. When a death is the result of an accident, for example, an inquest is held into the circumstances of the accident to determine if there is any blame. The inquest is conducted under the jurisdiction of a coroner or medical examiner. A *coroner* is a public official, not necessarily a physician, appointed or elected to inquire into the causes of death, when appropriate. A *medical examiner* is a physician and usually has advanced education in pathology or forensic medicine. Agency or institutional policy dictates who is responsible for reporting deaths to the coroner or medical examiner.

Death-Related Religious and Cultural Practices

The various cultural and religious traditions and practices associated with death, dying, and the grieving process help people cope with these experiences and give comfort to survivors. Nurses are often present through the dying process and at the moment of death. Knowledge of the client's religious and cultural beliefs helps nurses provide individualized care to clients and their families, even though they may not participate in their rituals associated with death.

Beliefs about preparation of the body, autopsy, organ donation, cremation, and prolonging life can be related to the person's religion. Autopsy, for example, may be prohibited, opposed, or discouraged by Eastern Orthodox religions, Muslims, Jehovah's Witnesses, and Orthodox Jews. Some religions prohibit the removal of body parts and dictate that all body parts be given appropriate burial. Organ donation is prohibited by Jehovah's Witnesses. In contrast to this, Buddhists in America consider it an act of mercy and encourage it. Cremation is discouraged, opposed, or prohibited by the Mormon, Eastern Orthodox, Islamic, and Jewish faiths. Hindus, in contrast, prefer cremation and cast the ashes in a holy river. Prolongation of life is generally encouraged; however, some religions, such as Christian Science, are unlikely to use medical means to prolong life, and the Jewish faith generally opposes prolonging life after irreversible brain damage. In hopeless illness, Buddhists may permit euthanasia.

Nurses also need to be knowledgeable about the client's death-related rituals, such as last rites, administration of Holy Communion, chanting at the bedside, and other rituals, such as special procedures for washing, dressing, positioning, and shrouding the dead. For example, certain immigrants may wish to retain their native customs, in which family members of the same sex wash and prepare the body for burial and cremation. Muslims also customarily turn the body toward Mecca. Nurses need to ask family members about their preferences and verify who will carry out these activities. The nurse must ensure that any ritual items present in the institution be given to the family or to the funeral home at the time of death to prevent lost items.

Note: The reference and resource listings for this and all chapters have been compiled at the back of the book.

Chapter Review

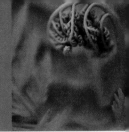

 KEY TERMS by Topic

Use the audio glossary feature of either the CD-ROM or the Companion Website to hear the correct pronunciation of the following key terms.

Grief Process
loss, grief

Culture and Grief
complicated grief, dysfunctional grief

Caring for the Dying Child
palliative care, palliative management, hospice care

Legalities Related to Death
comfort measures only, euthanasia, assisted suicide

Signs of Impending Death
mottled, Cheyne-Stokes respiration

Care After Death
rigor mortis, algor mortis, livor mortis, autopsy, postmortem examination

KEY Points

- Five stages of grief have been identified with any major loss. Not all people go through all stages, and some people experience a stage more than once. It is helpful for the nurse to know the stages in order to communicate well with the client.

- The nurse must provide emotional support or resources for emotional support to the dying child as well as every member of the family.

- The nurse, caring for a dying child, must take time to regain his or her own emotional stability.

- As the child deteriorates, the plan should change from curative care to palliative care.

- The older child and parents should be encouraged to communicate their wishes about advanced directives and do-not-resuscitate orders.

- Facility policy must be followed in providing postmortem care, including providing the death certificate, notifying family, and the mortuary.

- In the case of unexpected death, the family should receive the option of organ donation.

- Family religious and cultural practices related to death should be asked about and honored.

 EXPLORE Media Link

Additional interactive resources for this chapter can be found on the Companion Website at www. prenhall. com/adams.

Click on Chapter 9 and "Begin" to select the activities for this chapter.

For chapter-related NCLEX®-style questions and an audio glossary, access the accompanying CD-ROM in this book.

FOR FURTHER Study

See Chapter 3 for information about legalities in the care of children.

Stages of development are discussed in depth in Chapter 5.

Nursing care of children with specific chronic disorders is discussed in Chapter 7. Table 7-1 lists some forms of therapeutic play.

Critical Thinking Care Map

Care of Mother Who Is Grieving
NCLEX-PN® Focus Area: Psychosocial Integrity

Case Study: Teresa, age 4, has been fighting a leukemia for more than a year. She is now terminal. Her doctor has told the family it is just a matter of time before she will die. The family has decided to have her death take place in the home. Teresa is comatose, her breathing is irregular, and she is beginning to show mottling in her legs. Teresa's mother is at the bedside. An LPN/LVN has been assigned to remain in the home with Teresa and her family.

Nursing Diagnosis: Grieving of mother related to impending death of child

COLLECT DATA

Subjective	Objective
_____	_____
_____	_____
_____	_____
_____	_____
_____	_____

Would you report this? Yes/No

If yes, to: _____

Nursing Care

_____
_____
_____
_____
_____

How would you document this?_____
_____
_____
_____
_____
_____

Compare your documentation to the sample provided in Appendix I.

Data Collected
(use only those that apply)

- Crying quietly
- Telling Teresa they will go to the beach next week
- States Teresa will recover from leukemia
- States she will be relieved when Teresa is gone
- Asking every 10 minutes "how much longer?"
- Identifies signs of impending death
- Stating Teresa will not die

Nursing Interventions
(use only those that apply;
list in priority order)

- Ask mother to help turn Teresa.
- Ask mother to leave during Teresa's routine care.
- Ask mother if other family should be called.
- Ask mother if clergy should be called.
- Agree with mother that Teresa will get better.
- Tell mother not to cry.
- Encourage mother to express feelings.
- Tell mother it will probably be several more days.

1 Which of the following concepts should the nurse be aware of when interacting with parents of a child who died suddenly?

1. The parents had time to engage in anticipatory grief.
2. The parents may feel guilty for not engaging in special activities with the deceased child.
3. The parents feel immediate detachment.
4. The parents may experience an uncomplicated grief response.

2 A 5-year-old with leukemia asks the nurse, "Am I going to die?" The nurse should respond:

1. "Everyone will die sometime."
2. "Of course not, only old people die."
3. "Have you asked your parents that question?"
4. "We can ask the doctor when he comes."

3 The terminally ill adolescent states to the nurse, "I'm just not ready to go." The most appropriate response by the nurse would be:

1. "Tell me more about what you mean when you say that you are not ready."
2. "You're not ready to go where?"
3. "Dying is a natural process, you have nothing to fear."
4. "Yes, I know. Most people don't want to die."

4 In providing support for parents following the death of their child, the nurse needs to be aware that grieving is:

1. Best carried out alone.
2. Socially unacceptable in today's American culture.
3. Essential for good mental health after a loss.
4. Detrimental to emotional health.

5 A 14-year-old girl is having her leg amputated tomorrow due to bone cancer. She has been grieving for the past week, since she was told about the amputation. Which of the following best describes the grief she is experiencing?

1. Complicated grief
2. Perceived grief
3. Bereavement
4. Anticipatory grief

6 In which age group does the child first have a concept that death is permanent?

1. 4–5 years
2. 8–9 years
3. 11–12 years
4. 14–15 years

7 A 17-year-old is terminal with muscular dystrophy. He states, "When my time comes, I do not want any heroic measures." The nurse informs him that a living will:

1. Allows health care workers to withhold fluids and medication.
2. Allows the individual to express his or her wishes regarding care.
3. Is legally binding in all 50 states.
4. Allows the courts to decide when care can be given.

8 Common symptoms of approaching death are: (select all that apply)

1. Loss of control of bowel and bladder.
2. Increased secretions in the throat.
3. Increase in blood pressure.
4. Increased awareness in surroundings.
5. Rapid respirations with periods of apnea.
6. Mottling.

9 After a woman has delivered a 35-week stillborn baby, the nurse should tell the parents:

1. "Just go home and get on with your life."
2. "Hold the baby as long as you wish. I will get hair samples, hand- and footprints for your baby book later."
3. "You are young and can have other children."
4. "Can you make your wife stop crying while I get the room cleaned up?"

10 An 8-year-old has just died at home following a long illness. Place the following interventions in priority order:

1. Call the mortician.
2. Clean the body for viewing.
3. Complete the charting.
4. Call the nursing supervisor and physician.
5. Hold the parents and allow them to cry.

Answers for NCLEX-PN® Review and Critical Thinking questions appear in Appendix I.

Chapter 10

Care of the Child with Communicable Diseases

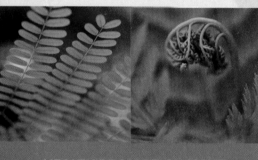

HEALTH PROMOTION ISSUE:
Avian Flu (Planning for the Management of Pandemic Influenza)

NURSING PROCESS CARE PLAN:
Child with Chickenpox

NURSING CARE PLAN CHART:
Child with Influenza

CRITICAL THINKING CARE MAP:
Caring for a Client Requiring Droplet Precautions

BRIEF Outline

Chain of Infection

Risk Factors for Communicable Diseases in Children

Immunizations

Client Teaching to Parents and Children

Common Infections

Infectious Diseases Transmitted by Insects or Animals

Sexually Transmitted Infections

Nursing Care

LEARNING Outcomes

After completing this chapter, you will be able to:
1. Define key terms.
2. Discuss the chain of infection.
3. Explain the specific risk factors for communicable diseases in children.
4. Describe methods of communicable disease prevention in children.
5. Discuss clinical manifestations, diagnostic procedures, and medical management related to childhood communicable diseases.
6. Explain appropriate nursing interventions for children with childhood communicable diseases.

Because children play in close proximity, transferring respiratory secretions and having skin-to-skin contact, diseases spread frequently and easily. **Communicable diseases** are diseases that are transmitted from one person to another by way of direct contact with body fluids (e.g., kissing) or indirectly through contact with contaminated objects (e.g., used tissues).

The nurse has an important role in recognizing these diseases and assisting the family in obtaining appropriate care. Communicable diseases can be prevented in many cases. Another important nursing role is client and family teaching regarding methods of disease prevention.

Chain of Infection

To transmit harmful organisms or **pathogens** from one child to another, there must be a reservoir, portal of exit, portal of entry, and susceptible host (Figure 10-1 ■). The **reservoir** is the site where harmful organisms grow and reproduce. Examples of reservoirs are humans, animals, insects, or soil. A **portal of exit** is the method by which the harmful organism leaves the reservoir. This could be through contact with infected body fluids such as blood or saliva. **Transmission** is the means by which the infectious agent travels from the portal of exit to the portal of entry. The **portal of entry** is the method by which the harmful organism enters a new host. This could be through the gastrointestinal tract, the integumentary system, or the respiratory system. The **susceptible host** is an individual who is at risk for contracting the disease caused by the harmful organism. Young children are more susceptible to harmful organisms because of their immature immune system. The child who is ill, especially the child who is immunocompromised, will have a more difficult time fighting harmful organisms as well.

Harmful organisms are transmitted by direct and indirect methods. Direct methods of transmission of harmful organisms are methods in which there is direct contact with body fluids, skin, or mucous membranes. The indirect method of transmission of harmful organisms can also be called the **droplet method**. In this route of transmission, infected body fluids are released from the mouth or nose via sneezing, coughing, kissing, or just breathing and talking. Droplets can contact the susceptible host immediately, attach themselves to dust particles that are touched later by the host, or actually become suspended in the air. A type of indirect transmission called **airborne transmission** occurs when harmful organisms become suspended in the air. **Fomites** are inanimate objects that transmit harmful bacteria indirectly. Examples of these inanimate objects include personal hygiene items such as combs and hairbrushes, clothing, linens, eating utensils, food, water, or soil.

STAGES OF INFECTIOUS PROCESS

When children become ill with a communicable disease, there are four stages of the infectious process: the incubation period, the prodromal period, illness, and the convalescent period.

The time frame associated with the **incubation period** varies according to the specific disease. The incubation period is the time between the entry of the pathogen into the reservoir and the onset of any clinical signs and symptoms. The pathogen multiplies in number during the incubation period.

The **prodromal period** occurs just prior to the onset of the clinical symptoms. During the prodromal period, the child may have nonspecific symptoms such as a low-grade temperature and lethargy. Children are contagious during this period, and because a specific disease is unrecognizable, they may come in contact with many individuals and pass the disease along.

Illness is the stage in which specific clinical symptoms related to the disease appear. Children can now be diagnosed with the specific disease. The **convalescent period** is the time frame between the beginning of the resolution of symptoms and the restoration of wellness.

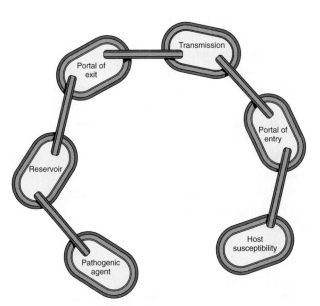

Figure 10-1. ■ Chain of infection. An effective chain of transmission for infection requires a suitable habitat, or reservoir, for the pathogen. A reservoir may be living or nonliving. Transmission may be direct or indirect. Direct transmission involves physical contact between the source of the infection and the new host. Indirect transmission occurs when pathogens survive outside humans before causing infection and disease. To achieve infection control, one of the links in the chain must be broken.

Risk Factors for Communicable Diseases in Children

A healthy person with a functioning immune system is able to avoid many infections before he or she becomes acutely ill. When the organism enters the body, it is recognized by the body as a foreign protein or antigen. With a healthy immune system, the body reacts rapidly by producing a specific antibody to stop or slow the growth of the antigen until white blood cells can destroy the organism. Once antibodies are produced, memory B cells and T cells remember how to identify the antigen and reactivate with the future exposure to the antigen. This process is called **active immunity**. Active immunity provides long-term protection from the harmful organism. **Passive immunity** is the passing of antibodies from the person where the antibody was produced to another person. Passive immunity lasts only a short time. Antibodies are passed from mother to infant through the placenta or through breastfeeding, but in order for the infant to develop long-term immunity he or she must actively produce the antibodies. Passive immunity can also occur as a result of intravenous infusion of immune globulin. As the child interacts with others in society, he or she will be exposed to various communicable diseases and develop antibodies against them.

The child is particularly susceptible to communicable diseases because of many factors. The child's immune system is immature. By age 1, the child will have adult levels of immunoglobulin M antibodies. The child has fewer neutrophils, the white blood cells that assist in the destruction of bacteria. See Chapter 22 ⚭ for more information on the child's immune system.

The child is also exposed to many varieties of harmful bacteria. Parents bring bacteria home from work, and siblings bring bacteria home from school. The developmental level of the child can also play a significant role in the child's risk of infection. A school-age child and adolescent have the cognitive ability to understand the dangers of passing bacteria from the hand to the mouth. These children can therefore make a decision to wash their hands after toileting, avoiding transmission of bacteria. The infant, toddler, and preschooler, however, do not have this cognitive ability.

Children in day care, mother's morning out programs, and church nurseries are exposed to a variety of pathogens. They can also be exposed at family gatherings. The incidence of illness increases as children participate in these activities. Children share toys and food. They are exposed to infected droplets as other children sneeze on them and talk closely in their face.

The child who is hospitalized is at risk for contracting a **nosocomial infection** (infection acquired in a health care setting). These infections increase the cost of hospital stays, make the child uncomfortable, and cause disability or even death. All children are susceptible, but those who are younger than 2 years and are immunocompromised or in a weakened state are at greater risk. The longer a child stays in the hospital, the greater the risk of contracting a nosocomial infection.

Children who travel with their parents to different parts of the world can be exposed to a variety of different diseases. For instance, malaria is prevalent in Southeast Asian countries, Central America, and South America. Children who travel to these areas must be protected from mosquito bites, the route of transmission of malaria. African sleeping sickness is prevalent in the tropical regions of Africa. It is transmitted through the bite of the tsetse fly. The tsetse fly is not susceptible to insect repellent and can bite through lightweight clothing. It is important for parents to avoid taking children into areas inhabited by the tsetse fly. Mosquito netting placed over sleeping areas may help protect the child from these insects.

Children can also be exposed to infectious diseases that are carried into the geographic area in which they live. The Health Promotion Issue on pages 254 and 255 discusses concerns about such a possibility, namely, the transmission of avian flu.

Certain harmful organisms may be used as a weapon in an act of **bioterrorism** (release of deadly infectious agents for the purpose of causing chaos and fear). Common organisms that may be used include *Bacillus anthracis* (anthrax), *Clostridium botulinum* (botulism), *Yersinia pestis* (plague), variola major virus (smallpox), and *Francisella tularensis* (tularemia). These agents can be transmitted by breathing the aerosolized organism or by direct contact.

PRECAUTIONS AND SAFEGUARDS FOR CHILDREN

The most effective way to prevent the spread of communicable diseases is through consistent hand washing. Children may not always wash their hands after using the toilet, blowing their noses, eating, or sneezing. Children put their hands and toys in their mouths, touch their noses and eyes, and thus spread infections. Teaching children how to wash their hands and insisting they do so after using the toilet, before meals, and as often as feasible will help decrease the spread of communicable diseases. Making hand washing fun will often help children wash for the time required to destroy germs. For example, having children sing the "Happy Birthday" song two times while washing hands will ensure that they wash for at least 30 seconds. The nurse must insist parents wash their hands after using the bathroom or changing diapers and before preparing food. Often, a gentle reminder with information about the spread of infection is all that is necessary for parents.

In health care and hospital settings, procedures and precautions need to be implemented to control the spread of infection. Medical asepsis is a basic element of all procedures. The nurse uses health promotion strategies to reduce the number of harmful organisms (e.g., hand washing) and to prevent their spread (e.g., implementing precautions to isolate harmful bacteria to a specific area).

Universal precautions (UP) are defined by the Centers for Disease Control and Prevention (CDC) as a set of precautions designed to prevent transmission of HIV, hepatitis

B virus (HBV), and other blood-borne pathogens when providing first aid or health care. Under universal precautions, blood and body fluids, including cerebrospinal fluid, wound drainage, and oral secretions, of *all* clients are considered to be *potentially* infected with HIV, HBV, and other blood-borne pathogens. Universal precautions include the use of protective barriers such as gloves, gowns, aprons, masks, or protective eyewear. In addition, universal precautions recommend precautions to prevent injuries caused by needles, scalpels, and other sharp instruments or devices.

Standard precautions combine universal precautions and body substance isolation techniques and apply to all clients in the hospital. Standard precautions include:

- Hand washing with plain soap and water before and after client contact.
- Wearing gloves when in contact with blood, body fluids, secretions, excretions, and other contaminated items. (Change gloves when they are contaminated and wash hands before reapplying gloves.)
- Wearing a mask, eye protection, or a face shield when there is a possibility of contacting body fluids during certain procedures.
- Wearing a clean, nonsterile gown to protect skin and prevent soiling of the uniform by contact with body fluids. (Remove the gown promptly, and wash hands thoroughly.)
- Having designated client care equipment such as stethoscope, thermometer, and sphygmomanometer for clients with diseases that can be transmitted to others.
- Ensuring that employees who handle soiled equipment and linen are properly protected from exposure to infected body fluids.
- Handling sharp instruments properly to avoid exposure. (Do not recap used needles. Dispose of these items in proper receptacles.)
- Avoiding mouth-to-mouth resuscitation. Use mouthpieces, resuscitation bags, or other ventilation devices.
- Arranging for a private room for children who can transmit harmful bacteria via airborne or droplet transfer.

Transmission-based precautions include standard precautions plus airborne precautions, droplet precautions, or contact precautions. **Airborne precautions** protect others from diseases such as chickenpox and measles that can be transmitted by the airborne route. The child with these diseases needs to be in a private room that has negative air pressure. The door of the room should be kept closed. Everyone entering the room should wear a high-efficiency particulate air filter respirator mask. If the client leaves the room for any reason, he or she must wear the same type of protective mask.

Droplet precautions are implemented to prevent the spread of infection by the droplet route. A private room is necessary. The door may remain open. Individuals coming within 3 feet of the child must wear a surgical mask. If the client leaves the room for any reason, he or she must wear a surgical mask.

Contact precautions protect individuals from direct contact with the skin or indirect contact with inanimate objects that are infected with harmful organisms. Children requiring contact precautions should be in a private room. Gloves should be worn when entering the room and when providing care that would require contact with infected body fluids. Gowns must also be worn if there is a risk of contacting body fluids with the uniform and removed before leaving the client's room.

Reverse isolation can be used for the child who is immunocompromised. This form of precaution protects the child from harmful organisms that may be brought into the room by hospital personnel or family members. This form of precaution includes requiring every person who enters the child's room to wear a gown, gloves, and a mask. Also, all equipment brought into the room needs to be carefully disinfected. Children who have recently had an organ transplant are often placed on reverse isolation. For more information about organ transplantation, see Chapter 22 ∞. (See Appendix V ∞ for a review of precautions.)

Immunizations

Immunization is the process of inducing resistance to communicable diseases. Immunization is accomplished by the use of **vaccines**, products containing killed, live, recombinant, or conjugated microorganisms administered parenterally to induce immunity. A **toxoid** is also considered a vaccine. Toxoids are toxins that have been treated to destroy the toxic effects while maintaining their capability of forming antibodies against the toxin. The types of vaccines are listed in Table 10-1 ∎. Refer to Chapter 8 ∞ for an in-depth discussion about giving immunizations.

The Advisory Committee on Immunization Practices of the CDC, the American Academy of Pediatrics (AAP), and the American Academy of Family Practitioners collaborate to develop the recommended immunization schedule for children. See Figure 6-3 ∞ for the U.S. recommended immunization schedule from the CDC. Table 10-2 ∎ lists nursing considerations for common pediatric immunizations. For additional information about immunizations, see Chapter 7 ∞.

New vaccines are always in development. For example, each year vaccines are developed for the coming year to guard young children and individuals who are immunocompromised from the effects of influenza. Box 10-1 ∎ provides information about some new pediatric vaccines that are in development.

AVIAN FLU (PLANNING FOR THE MANAGEMENT OF PANDEMIC INFLUENZA)

Because of its geographic proximity, Honolulu is considered the gateway to the Americas by many Asian nations. Outside downtown Honolulu's Chinatown, the nurse works in a 24-hour free-standing medical clinic. On a daily basis, the clinic sees about 60 pediatric clients and 25 adult clients. More than 50% of these clients are tourists, and most of them are from Japan or China. The clinic is staffed by two family care physicians, a family nurse practitioner, two registered nurses, three LPNs, a laboratory technician, a receptionist, and a bookkeeper.

One glance at the clinic's population gives the staff concern that influenza will be brought to America from these Asian countries. Even the children who are now American citizens travel back to their homelands to visit relatives, or the relatives visit America on occasion. The Centers for Disease Control and Prevention (CDC) website shows that Cambodia, Vietnam, China, and Indonesia have the highest number of cases of avian flu and the highest number of deaths resulting from this strain of influenza in 2006.

Concerned about the avian flu and the impact it would have on this community, the staff at the medical clinic decide to be proactive and develop a plan before they have a real problem on their hands. Their initial step in developing the plan was to visit the CDC website for assistance.

DISCUSSION

Prior to discussing the situation, the team learns more about the avian flu. General definitions aid their work:

- The **seasonal flu**, also called the common flu, is a respiratory illness that can be transmitted from person to person. Generally, seasonal flu is caused by influenza A or B. Most people have some immunity to these strains. There is a vaccine available for the seasonal flu. See the Nursing Care Plan Chart on page 274.
- The **avian flu**, also called the bird flu or H5N1, is caused by influenza viruses

that occur naturally among wild birds. H5N1 is deadly to domestic birds. It can be transmitted from birds to humans. Currently, there is no human immunity and no vaccine available.

- **Pandemic flu** is a virulent human flu that causes a global outbreak of serious illness, or pandemic. Because there is little natural immunity, the disease can spread easily from person to person. Currently, there is no pandemic flu. Previous influenza pandemics include the Spanish flu of 1918, the Asian flu of 1957, and the Hong Kong flu of 1968.

This H5N1 virus that now mainly affects birds can become dangerous to humans through two processes: the antigenic drift and the antigenic shift. The **antigenic drift** is the minor genetic changes that occur to the virus as it replicates within the host cells. The **antigenic shift** is an abrupt change or a major change in the virus. The antigenic shift makes the virus capable of infecting humans.

Allen (2006) describes the only known case of person-to-person transmission of the H5N1 virus. The transmission occurred in Thailand when an 11-year-child became ill after handling chickens that were dying. She was hospitalized with symptoms of the avian flu and was cared for by her mother, who did not have any contact with the chickens. The child died of respiratory failure and shock. Her mother developed symptoms 3 days later and died of respiratory complications.

The incubation period of avian flu appears to be 2 to 10 days. Initial symptoms are flulike: chills, fever of 100 °F to 103 °F, persistent malaise, myalgia, headache, eye pain, photophobia, substernal burning sensation, nonproductive cough, sore throat, rhinitis, shortness of breath, and diarrhea (Sheff, 2006). Other possible symptoms include vomiting, abdominal pain, pleuritic

pain, bleeding from the nose and gums, and conjunctivitis. Complications of the avian flu include pneumonia, acute respiratory distress, acute encephalitis, organ failure, and death.

Laboratory results include lymphocytopenia and decreased platelet counts. Radiologic findings include the presence of infiltrates and pneumonia. There are lab tests for the specific H5N1 virus. Respiratory specimens can be tested using virus culturing, antigen tests, or polymerase chain reaction assays.

Treatment for the avian flu is primarily supportive. Clinicians should attempt to prevent the worsening of symptoms. Most clients require admission to intensive care units to monitor fluid and electrolyte balance, oxygenation, circulatory status, and respiratory effort. Oxygen administration, endotracheal intubation, and mechanical ventilation may be necessary. Medication administration may include neuroaminidase inhibitors such as Tamiflu or Relenza, antibiotics to prevent secondary infections, and corticosteroids. Tamiflu can be given prophylactically to children who are 13 years of age or older. It can also be given to children 1 year of age or older with flu symptoms. Relenza can be given to children 7 years of age or

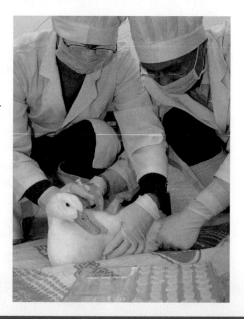

older with flu symptoms. Both Tamiflu and Relenza need to be given within the first 48 hours following the onset of symptoms to have a positive effect.

Clients hospitalized with avian flu should be placed in a private room with standard and contact precautions. Staff members should have the proper equipment to protect themselves, including specially fitted respiratory masks, gloves, gown, and eye protection. Health care equipment such as stethoscope, thermometer, and sphygmomanometer should be dedicated to the client and left in the client's room.

Currently, there is no vaccine available against the avian flu, but several companies are beginning efforts to produce sufficient antibodies to prevent infection.

PLANNING AND IMPLEMENTATION

Using the CDC's *Medical Offices and Clinics Pandemic Influenza Planning Checklist*, the staff of the medical clinic developed an action plan to ensure a proper response to an outbreak of the avian flu. Their first step was to develop a planning committee consisting of an administrator, a physician, a nurse, a receptionist, and a laboratory technician.

They assigned a committee member to monitor any health advisories regarding the avian flu both at the local and state level as well as the federal level. Regular reports were given in the monthly committee meetings, and a mechanism was put in place to give urgent reports when necessary. For instance, this committee member would submit an urgent report when the influenza pandemic is in the United States, when it is in Hawaii, or when it is in Honolulu.

Data collection of influenza cases that present to their clinic was initiated. Analyzing these data allowed the committee to understand their needs for staffing and supplies if the number of cases greatly increased, as they would with a pandemic situation. Reporting cases of pandemic influenza to local and state health departments will be essential. Therefore, one person from the committee was assigned to be the spokesperson for the clinic and manage this task. Contact information (including name, title, agency, telephone number, facsimile number, and e-mail) was obtained and placed in an easily identified location.

Education about the avian flu became the next task. The entire staff, full-time, part-time, and temporary, needed to understand the transmission of the virus, the recognizable symptoms, the treatment plan, and the prevention methods related to the avian flu. Their clients also needed to be educated regarding these same issues. A teaching curriculum was developed, including client handouts. Attention was given to the language and reading level of these materials. The CDC website provided many client education materials already translated into other languages including Spanish, Chinese, and Vietnamese.

It was also necessary to develop a plan for managing the barrage of telephone calls expected during a pandemic. A prioritization plan was developed for handling the clients who were most ill first. This included temporarily canceling physical exams and follow-up appointments to be able to handle the case load. The committee discussed designating separate days for influenza clients in order to decrease the risk of transmission to others. The waiting room situation had to be assessed because this could be a ready

location for transmission. Signs were made that directed clients with influenza symptoms to notify staff members immediately, sit in a designated area, use tissues to cover their cough, dispose of used tissues in designated receptacles, and use no-rinse hand sanitizer frequently.

Staffing was the next issue to be assessed. Priority was placed on administering influenza vaccine or antiviral prophylaxis, if necessary, to all personnel having client contact. The sick leave policy was also reviewed. What would happen if a staff member developed symptoms of the flu at work? What if staff members were needed to care for family members in their home who had symptoms of the flu? Were there enough temporary staff members available if they were needed?

Finally, the planning committee reviewed supplies that would be required during a pandemic outbreak. Supplies of masks, gloves, no-rinse hand sanitizer, syringes, alcohol swabs, and bandages were inventoried. A 2-week reserve inventory of these supplies was obtained. Suppliers of these items were contacted to determine how quickly the items could be acquired in an emergency situation.

This planning took time and energy. However, when the committee gave its final report to the entire staff, a sense of security was experienced by all. With the proper education, supplies, personnel, implementation plan, and support persons identified, the medical clinic staff knew they were prepared to handle an avian flu outbreak in their community.

SELF-REFLECTION

What steps are you taking to personally protect yourself from the flu? Do you receive a flu shot annually? If you answered no, why not?

SUGGESTED RESOURCES

For the Nurse

Allen, P. (2006). Avian influenza pandemic: Not if, but when. *Pediatric Nursing, 32*(1), 76–81.

Ray, M., & Walker-Jenkins, A. (2006). Confronting bird flu: Will pandemic avian flu be the next public health threat? *Lifelines, 10*(1), 21–29.

Sheff, B. (2006). Avian influenza: Poised to launch a pandemic? *Nursing2006, 36*(1), 51–53.

For the Client

Aultshuler, L. (2006). *The Bird-flu primer: The guide to being prepared and surviving an avian flu pandemic.* San Francisco: Sterling & Ross.

TABLE 10-1

Types of Vaccine

TYPE OF VACCINE	DEFINITION	EXAMPLE
Killed	Contains a microorganism that is killed yet capable of causing the body to produce antibodies	Polio vaccine
Live	Contains a microorganism that is live yet altered to be weakened; also called attenuated	Measles, mumps, rubella (MMR) vaccine
Recombinant	Contains a genetically altered microorganism	Hepatitis B (HB) vaccine
Conjugated	Contains an altered organism that is paired with another substance	*Haemophilus influenzae* type B (Hib)
Toxoid	A toxin that has been treated with heat or chemical to weaken the toxic effects while still retaining the ability to produce antibodies	Tetanus toxoid

TABLE 10-2

Nursing Considerations for Common Pediatric Immunizations

IMMUNIZATION TYPE	SIDE EFFECTS	NURSING CONSIDERATIONS
Diphtheria and pertussis vaccines and tetanus toxoid (DTaP) *Route*: Intramuscular *Dosage*: 0.5 mL May give at same time as all other vaccines in a separate site.	*Common*: Redness, pain, swelling, nodule at injection site; temperature up to 101 °F (38.3 °C); drowsiness, irritability, fussiness; anorexia within 2 days of injection. Increase in frequency and magnitude of local reactions with doses 4 and 5 (e.g., entire limb swelling). *Serious*: Allergic reaction, anaphylaxis; shock, fever above 102 °F (38.8 °C); febrile seizure; persistent inconsolable crying; coma or permanent brain damage.	Use same brand for all doses where feasible. Prior to immunization, ask about previous reaction to immunization. DTaP may coincide with or hasten the recognition of a seizure disorder. In children with a history of seizures with or without fever, give acetaminophen at the time of vaccine and then every 4 hours for 24 hours. Shake vaccine before withdrawing. Solution will be cloudy. If it contains clumps that cannot be resuspended, do not use. Inform parents of the chance of increased reaction to doses 4 and 5. Defer the vaccine if the child has a progressive neurologic problem until the child is stable. The series does not need to be restarted, regardless of when the previous dose was given.
Poliovirus vaccine (IPV) *Route*: Subcutaneous or intramuscular, depending on vaccine used *Dosage*: 0.5 mL May give at same time as all other vaccines in a separate site.	*Common*: Swelling and tenderness, irritability, tiredness. *Serious*: Allergic reaction or anaphylaxis.	Prior to immunization, ask if the child has an allergy to neomycin, streptomycin, or polymyxin B (whichever of these antibiotics the specific vaccine to be used contains). Clear, colorless suspension. Do not use if it contains particulate matter, becomes cloudy, or changes color. All doses must be separated by at least 4 weeks. The series does not need to be restarted, regardless of when the previous dose was given.
Measles, mumps, rubella (MMR) vaccine *Route*: Subcutaneous *Dosage*: 0.5 mL	*Common*: Elevated temperature 1–2 weeks after immunization; redness or pain at injection site; noncontagious rash; joint pain.	Prior to immunization, ask if child has allergy to neomycin or gelatin. Observe the child with an egg allergy for 90 minutes after injection. Inquire about immunosuppression.

(continued)

TABLE 10-2

Nursing Considerations for Common Pediatric Immunizations

IMMUNIZATION TYPE	SIDE EFFECTS	NURSING CONSIDERATIONS
May give at same time as all other vaccines in a separate site.	*Serious*: Allergic reaction, febrile seizure; meningitis (usually mild); encephalopathy; thrombocytopenia purpura; rare cases of coma and permanent brain damage.	Instruct adolescent girls of childbearing age to avoid pregnancy for 3 months after immunization. Give tuberculosis test at same time as MMR or 4–6 weeks later. If MMR and Varivax are not given on the same day, space them at least 28 days apart. Reconstituted vaccine is a clear, yellow solution. Give entire contents of reconstituted vial even if more than 0.5 mL. As college students are at greater risk because of decreasing immunity, make sure they have received a second MMR dose.
Hepatitis B (HB) vaccine *Route:* Intramuscular *Dosage:* Engerix-B: 10 mcg or Recombivax HB: 5 mcg May give at same time as all other vaccines in a separate site.	*Common*: Pain or redness at injection site; headache; photophobia; altered liver enzymes. *Serious*: Allergic reaction or anaphylaxis; fever.	Prior to immunization, check status of mother's hepatitis B test and presence of other liver disease. *Note*: If mother has HbsAg+, vaccine must be given to infant within 12 hours of birth along with hepatitis B immune globulin at the same time in another site with a new needle and syringe. Shake vaccine before withdrawing. Solution will appear cloudy. Minimum spacing for children and teens is 4 weeks between doses 1 and 2, and 8 weeks between doses 2 and 3. The last dose in an infant series should not be given before 6 months of age. Vaccine brands can be interchanged for three-dose series. The series does not need to be restarted, regardless of when the previous dose was given.
Haemophilus influenzae type B (Hib) *Route*: Intramuscular *Dosage*: 0.5 mL May give at same time as all other vaccines in a separate site.	*Common*: Pain, redness, or swelling at site. *Serious*: Allergic reaction of anaphylaxis (extremely rare); fever.	Prior to immunizations, ask if child is immunosuppressed. Solution is clear and colorless. If the first dose is given between 7 and 11 months of age, three doses are needed. If the first dose was given at 12–14 months of age, give a booster dose in 8 weeks. If the first dose is given when the child is older than 15 months or younger than 5 years, only one dose is needed. Second and third doses can be given 4–8 weeks after the first. Use the same vaccine preparation for all doses of the primary series if possible. The series does not need to be restarted, regardless of when the previous dose was given.
Heptavalent pneumococcal conjugate vaccine (PCV) *Route*: Intramuscular *Dosage*: 0.5 mL	*Common*: Soreness, swelling, redness at injection site; mild to moderate fever; irritability, drowsiness, restless sleep, decreased appetite, vomiting and diarrhea, rash or hives. *Severe*: Allergic reaction or anaphylaxis	Clear, colorless, or slightly opalescent liquid. In addition to infants, this vaccine is a priority for children ages 2–5 years with sickle cell disease, asplenia, or HIV infection, or in those who are immunocompromised. The vaccine is also a priority for Native American and Native Alaskan children ages 2–5 years because of their increased risk for pneumococcal disease. The series does not need to be restarted, regardless of when the previous dose was given.
Varicella virus vaccine *Route*: Subcutaneous *Dosage*: 0.5 mL	*Common*: Pain or redness at injection site; fever up to 102 °F (38.8 °C) in children. Less commonly a mild vaccine-related rash may occur during first month after the injection. *Severe*: Allergic reaction or anaphylaxis; thrombocytopenia; febrile seizure; central nervous system manifestations.	Prior to immunization, ask if child is immunodeficient, on immunosuppression treatment, or has an allergy to neomycin or gelatin. Determine if a family member is immunocompromised. Clear, colorless to pale yellow liquid when reconstituted. Give the entire contents of the vial even if more than 0.5 mL. Instruct adolescent girls of childbearing age to avoid pregnancy for 3 months after immunization.

(continued)

TABLE 10-2		
Nursing Considerations for Common Pediatric Immunizations (continued)		
IMMUNIZATION TYPE	**SIDE EFFECTS**	**NURSING CONSIDERATIONS**
Hepatitis A *Route*: Intramuscular *Dosage*: 0.5 mL, 1 mL over 17 years for Vaqta, 1 mL over 18 years for Havrix May give at same time as all other vaccines in a separate site	Rare reports of anaphylaxis reaction.	Shake well, slightly opaque white suspension. Can be given for postexposure prophylaxis against hepatitis A. Immune globulin and vaccine can be given at same time in different sites. Vaccine brands can be interchanged.
Influenza *Route*: Intramuscular (all ages), intranasal (5 years and older) *Dosage*: 0.25 mL in infants 6–35 months, 0.5 mL beginning at 3 years May give at same time as all other vaccines in a separate site.	*Common after injection*: May have soreness or swelling at injection site, fever, aches. Life-threatening allergic reactions are rare. *Common after intranasal vaccine*: Runny nose or nasal congestion, fever, headache or muscle aches, abdominal pain, and occasional vomiting.	Thawed intranasal vaccine is pale yellow, clear to slightly cloudy. Administered annually in autumn. Children with no history of influenza illness or vaccine need two doses 1 month apart. Intranasal dose is split (0.25 mL) with a dose divider clip. Administer in each nostril while child is sitting in an upright position. Insert the tip of the sprayer inside the nose and depress the plunger to spray. Children 8 years of age or younger who are receiving the influenza vaccine for the first time should get two doses separated by at least 4 weeks (injectable) and 6 weeks (intranasal). Must be reimmunized each year as immunity wanes.

Source: Data from American Academy of Pediatrics. (2003). *Red Book: Report of the Committee on Infectious Disease* (26th ed.). Elk Grove Village, IL: Author; Immunization Action Coalition. (2004). *Mosby's drug consult 2004*. St. Louis, MO: Mosby; Bindler, R. M., & Howry, L. B. (1997). *Pediatric drugs and nursing implications* (2nd ed.). Stamford, CT: Appleton & Lange.

Immunotherapy is the prevention and treatment of disease using the administration of allergens, immunostimulants, immunosuppressants, interferon, and immune globulin. Many communicable diseases can be treated by immune globulin to diminish the effects of the disease or prevent transmission of the disease. See further discussion of immune therapy in Chapter 22 ⚭.

Client Teaching to Parents and Children

There are many ways in which families can reduce the transmission of communicable diseases among family members. Tissues used to blow the nose should be discarded in a trash receptacle immediately. All family members should wash their hands with soap and water or antibacterial gel after contact with body fluids and excrement. Hand washing should always follow toileting. If a child sneezes or coughs into the hands, the child should immediately wash them. However, recent thinking is that children should be taught to sneeze or cough into the elbow instead of the hands to prevent disease transmission.

Toys and personal linens such as blankets can be a reservoir for harmful organisms such as *Staphylococcus aureus*, *Staphylococcus epidermidis*, and *Clostridium difficile* (Fleming & Randle, 2006). Absorbent toys or linens that become heavily soiled must be discarded or removed from the health care facility by the parent. Soft toys may be cleaned in hot water with detergent containing bleach. Toys should be washed with disinfectant regularly per hospital policy. During periods of communicability, children should not share toys because this increases the likelihood of transmission.

Some practices increase the risk of transmission of certain pathogens. These practices include nail biting, thumb sucking, sharing drinks and eating utensils, and putting items found on the floor or ground into the mouth. The older child can understand the hazards of these practices. However, the younger child's behavior will need to be monitored to prevent the transmission of harmful organisms in these ways.

BOX 10-1

New Vaccines on the Horizon

Human Papillomavirus
In 2006, the FDA approved and recommended the human papillomavirus vaccine in an effort to prevent cervical cancer in women. This inactivate, recombinant vaccine is to be given to 11- to 12-year-old girls in a three-dose series. The series interval is initial injection, dose two in 2 months, and dose three in 6 months. For more information on this vaccine, see Chapter 18 ⬤⬤.

Otitis Media
Alhough still not approved by the U.S. Food and Drug Administration (FDA), a combination *Streptococcus pneumoniae* and *Haemophilus influenzae* vaccine studied in the Czech Republic and Slovakia was found to reduce the incidence of otitis media by 33% (Prymula, 2006).

Rotavirus
The FDA recently approved a vaccine against rotavirus, the most common cause of diarrhea in children. The CDC advises that children be given the three-dose series at 2 months, 4 months, and again at 6 months (Peck, 2006).

Meningitis
Recent outbreaks of meningitis on college campuses have led to the FDA approval of a single-dose vaccine for adolescents age 11 or 12. If unvaccinated, children should receive the vaccine on entering high school or at age 15. Also, college students who will be living in dormitories and who have not been recently vaccinated should be immunized (Rosenfeld, 2006).

REYE'S SYNDROME
Nurses must also teach parents about the risks that exist once children acquire a communicable disease. One serious possible result is Reye's syndrome. Reye's syndrome is an acute *encephalopathy* (a disorder characterized by inflammation of the brain). Untreated, the syndrome is often fatal. Symptoms of Reye's syndrome usually follow a viral illness and may be linked to the intake of aspirin. Because of this association, parents are taught to use acetaminophen or other fever reducers, not aspirin, to reduce fever in a child with a communicable disease.

Initial symptoms include nausea, vomiting, and lethargy but may progress quickly to marked changes in the level of consciousness. The child may become combative, use inappropriate language, have hyperreflexia, develop seizures, and become comatose.

Diagnosis of Reye's syndrome is based on history plus elevated liver enzymes and ammonia levels, decreased blood glucose levels, and prolonged prothrombin time. The ill child is admitted to the pediatric intensive care unit for supportive treatment and close observation. Respiratory ventilation may be necessary. Monitoring for increased intracranial pressure is essential. Intravenous fluids assist in treating hypoglycemia.

TEACHING EMERGENCY PREPAREDNESS
The nurse can assist families in preparing for emergencies such as bioterrorism. The American Academy of Pediatrics recommends that all families have a specified disaster plan. This organization suggests that children be involved in this planning. Children should also be encouraged to assist in creating a disaster kit. This kit should include several days' supply of food and water, pet supplies, warm clothing, rain gear, blankets, toiletries, battery-powered radio and flashlight with extra batteries, a credit card and supply of cash, a first aid kit, and copies of important documents. If a family member has a medical condition, extra medication and supplies need to be included in the kit. If there is an infant in the family and the mother is not breastfeeding, extra infant formula is a necessary element of the disaster kit. For a complete list of items for the disaster kit, contact the American Academy of Pediatrics or visit their website. Nursing care related to traumatic life events is discussed in Chapter 16 ⬤⬤. Also see Box 16-6, Effects of Disasters on Children ⬤⬤.

Common Infections
Communicable diseases are considered to be acute illnesses. They typically have a limited duration and can be considered treatable in most cases. However, depending on the child's state of health, these diseases may prove to be complicated and severe.

It is important for the nurse to understand the route of transmission of these diseases and the incubation period.

Manifestations
Recognizing the clinical manifestations of these diseases can allow for prompt medical management. Many communicable diseases have a distinctive appearance. Figure 10-2 ■ shows clinical manifestations of several common communicable diseases.

Diagnosis and Treatment
Diagnosis is often by clinical manifestations. There may be a history of exposure to another child or children with the disease (particularly with school-age children). Treatment depends on the infectious agent but is generally supportive. Specific information about common pediatric communicable diseases, including transmission and incubation, manifestations, diagnostic tests, and nursing considerations, is

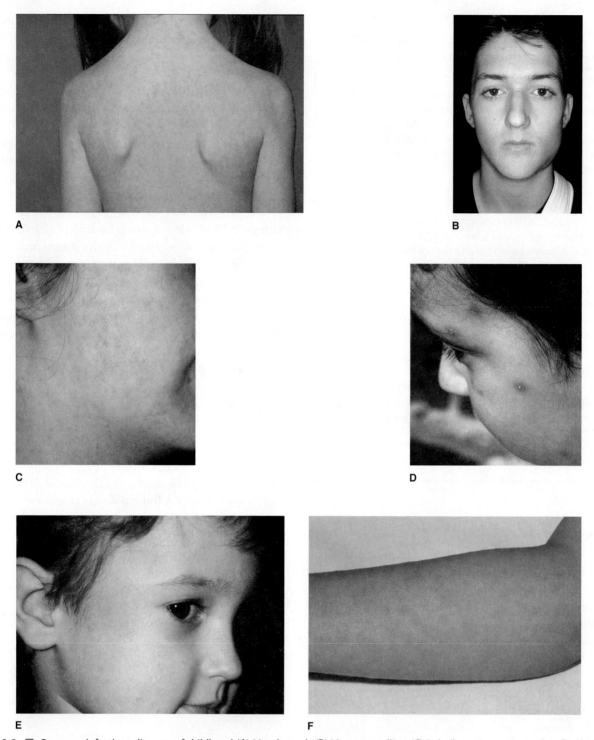

Figure 10-2. ■ Common infectious diseases of childhood. (**A**) Measles rash. (**B**) Mumps swelling. (**C**) Rubella or German measles. (**D**) Chickenpox lesions. (**E**) Fifth disease or erythema infectiosum. (**F**) Scarlet fever (**A** and **C**: NMSB-Custom Medical Stock Photo, Inc. **B**: Phototake NYC. **D**: © Patrick Watson. **E** and **F**: PhotoResearchers, Inc.)

provided in Table 10-3 ■. An important role for the nurse is teaching parents and the public how to prevent these childhood illnesses. The nurse must be prepared to assist the physician in providing medical treatment, with the goal of restoring health to the child.

(Text continues on page 269.)

TABLE 10-3

Common Communicable Diseases of Childhood

DISEASE AND CAUSATIVE ORGANISM	TRANSMISSION AND INCUBATION PERIOD	CLINICAL MANIFESTATIONS	DIAGNOSTIC TESTS AND MEDICAL TREATMENT	NURSING CONSIDERATIONS
Hepatitis B is caused by the hepatitis B virus (HBV).	Transmission: Exposure to body fluids, organ transplants, sexual contact, intravenous drug use and sharing of needles, transplacental, during birth or during breastfeeding. Incubation period: 1–6 months, with an average of 50 days. Children infected with HBV may become a carrier of the virus for life.	Fever, anorexia, nausea, vomiting, rash, arthralgia, pruritus, jaundice, right upper quadrant pain, darkening of the urine, clay-colored stools, hepatosplenomegaly	Diagnostic: Serologic testing to detect the presence of antigens and antibodies to HBV Preventative measures: Routine screening of pregnant women, three-dose series of immunizations against HBV Medical treatment: Bed rest, hydration, well-balanced diet, hepatitis B immune globulin (HBIG) for one-time exposure and infants born to infected mothers	■ Prevent the spread of the virus by good hand washing and other standard precautions. ■ Assist the child and family in planning a high-protein, high-carbohydrate, low-fat diet. ■ Assist the child with activities of daily living and quiet activities to promote rest. ■ Assess carefully for toxic effects of medications because drug metabolism can be altered with liver disorders.
Diphtheria is caused by *Corynebacterium diphtheriae*	Transmission: Direct contact with mucous membranes, skin, or lesions of an infected period or a carrier. Transmission has also occurred indirectly by contact with contaminated surfaces. The bacteria may also reside in unpasteurized milk. Incubation period: 2–7 days or longer. Disease can be transmitted for a period of 2–4 weeks.	Low-grade fever, anorexia, malaise, foul-smelling rhinorrhea, sore throat with hoarseness, stridor or noisy breathing, cervical lymphadenitis. Children with diphtheria have a thick, bluish-white to grayish-black patchy, membranous lesion that can cover the soft or hard palate, the tongue, and the pharynx.	Diagnostic: Cultures of the lesion Preventative measures: Five-dose series of immunizations against diphtheria. The most common immunization against diphtheria is given in conjunction with tetanus and pertussis. Medical treatment: Administration of antibiotics and antitoxins after the child has been tested for sensitivity to horse serum. Observe carefully for airway obstruction.	■ Isolate the child to prevent transmission. ■ Observe carefully for airway obstruction. Keep oral airway and oxygen readily available at all times. ■ Suction prn. ■ Oral liquids may be a choking hazard. Give cautiously. ■ Provide oral hygiene frequently. ■ Assist the child with activities of daily living and quiet activities to promote rest.
Tetanus (lockjaw) is caused by *Clostridium tetani*, also called tetanus bacillus.	Transmission: Indirect contact with contaminated soil, manure, or tools through breaks in the skin or wound. The newborn can become infected if the umbilical cord is cut with a contaminated utensil. Not transmitted from person to person. Incubation period: 3 days to 3 weeks, with an average of 8 days.	Neck and jaw stiffness, difficulty chewing, difficulty swallowing, muscle spasms stimulated by noise or touch, spasms may progress to laryngospasm and compromise respiratory effort, abdominal rigidity progressing to **opisthotonos** (rigid hyperextension of the entire body). The newborn has difficulty sucking, irritability, and nuchal rigidity.	Preventative measures: Five-dose series of immunizations against tetanus. The most common immunization against tetanus is given in conjunction with diphtheria and pertussis. A booster injection is necessary every 10 years for life. Medical treatment: Wound debridement, administration of antibiotics, muscle relaxants for spasms, tetanus immune globulin, nutritional support through enteral methods or total parenteral nutrition; mechanical ventilation is required.	■ Provide a quiet environment, reduce stimulation. ■ Provide wound care. ■ Provide skin care. ■ Observe closely for laryngospasm. Keep oral airway and oxygen readily available at all times. ■ Suction prn. ■ Maintain strict intake and output. ■ Monitor fluid and electrolyte balance.

(continued)

TABLE 10-3

Common Communicable Diseases of Childhood (continued)

DISEASE AND CAUSATIVE ORGANISM	TRANSMISSION AND INCUBATION PERIOD	CLINICAL MANIFESTATIONS	DIAGNOSTIC TESTS AND MEDICAL TREATMENT	NURSING CONSIDERATIONS
Pertussis (whooping cough) is caused by *Bordetella pertussis*.	Transmission: Direct and indirect contact with infected respiratory secretions. Risk for transmission is greatest in the catarrhal stage but may last 4 weeks into the paroxysmal stage. Incubation period: 5–21 days, with an average of 7–10 days	Catarrhal stage: Low-grade fever, rhinitis (coryza), sneezing, lacrimation (tearing), nonproductive cough. Symptoms may last 1–2 weeks. Paroxysmal stage: In children older than 6 months, the cough becomes worse at night. The child produces a "whooping" sound that is a high-pitched crowing sound. The loud cough is the child's effort to expel a thick mucous plug and is due to a narrowed glottis. The coughing episodes are very tiring for the child, and he or she may become cyanotic or red faced. Vomiting may even occur. The infant younger than 6 months will have periods of apnea instead of the characteristic cough. Symptoms may last 1–6 weeks. Convalescent stage: The cough resolves gradually and may return to the cough characteristic of the catarrhal stage.	Diagnostic: Culture and polymerase chain reaction testing. Preventative measures: Five-dose series of immunization against pertussis. The most common immunization against pertussis is given in conjunction with diphtheria and tetanus. Medical treatment: Administration of pertussis immune serum globulin, antibiotics, and corticosteroids; bed rest; removal of environmental factors that aggravate coughing; humidification of the environment, especially where the child sleeps; nutritional support; droplet precautions; oxygen administration	■ Assist the child with activities of daily living and quiet activities to promote rest. ■ Provide adequate ventilation and humidification of the child's room. ■ Suction gently prn. ■ Observe closely for airway obstruction. Keep oral airway and oxygen readily available at all times. ■ Monitor oxygen saturation levels, especially in the infant younger than 6 months. ■ Initiate droplet precautions. ■ Maintain strict intake and output. ■ Monitor fluid and electrolyte balance.
Haemophilus influenzae type B+ (Hib) is caused by coccobacillus *H. influenzae* type B. See Chapter 15 🔗 for more information on meningitis, a common manifestation of this bacterial infection.	Transmission: By direct contact or droplet inhalation. The child may transmit the bacteria during the 3 days following onset of symptoms. Incubation period: Unknown	Manifestations include: Meningitis—sudden onset of headache, stiff neck, irritability, nausea, vomiting, fever Epiglottitis—fever, sore throat, stridor, cough, swollen epiglottis Pneumonia—gradual onset of fever, chills, productive cough, pleuritic chest pain Septic arthritis—joint inflammation, stiffness, joint pain and tenderness	Diagnostic: Evaluation of cerebrospinal fluid (CSF) from a lumbar puncture Preventative measures: Four-dose series of immunizations against Hib Medical treatment: Administration of antibiotics for infected child and other members of the household who have not been vaccinated	■ Initiate droplet precautions. ■ Monitor temperature closely and implement fever-reducing strategies. ■ Provide comfort measures specific to the condition.

Cause	Transmission	Clinical Manifestations	Diagnostic/Medical Treatment	Nursing Interventions
		Cellulitis—localized heat, redness, pain and swelling, fever, chills, headache Sinusitis—swelling and drainage of the mucous membranes, sinus pressure, tenderness and pain, headache Otitis media—ear tenderness, pain and drainage, diminished hearing Bronchitis—productive cough, fever, back pain Pericarditis—fever, substernal chest pain, dyspnea, nonproductive cough		■ Initiate droplet precautions. ■ Observe closely for respiratory distress. Keep oral airway and oxygen readily available at all times. ■ Assist the child with activities of daily living and quiet activities to promote rest. ■ Administer pharmacologic and non-pharmacologic pain relief measures. ■ Implement measures to promote good body mechanics such as proper body alignment when in the bed and performing passive or active range-of-motion exercises.
Poliomyelitis is caused by poliovirus.	Transmission: Direct contact via the fecal-oral and respiratory route. Virus may be transmitted just before and just after onset of symptoms, although the virus may be shed in the feces and respiratory system for 1–6 weeks. Incubation period: 3–36 days, with an average of 7–10 days	Fever, headache, nausea, vomiting, abdominal pain, neck and back pain. These symptoms, in some cases, progress to tremors of the extremities, positive Kernig's and Brudzinski's signs (see Chapter 22 🔗 for more information), hyperactivity (DTR), paralysis, and respiratory distress. The child may develop progressive permanent paralysis, muscle atrophy, and/or severe arthritis.	Diagnostic: Stool or throat cell culture and evaluation of CSF from a lumbar puncture Preventative measures: Four-dose series of immunization against polio Medical treatment: Bed rest, pain management, respiratory support if necessary, physical therapy with the goal of restoring mobility	
Measles (rubeola) is caused by Morbillivirus	Transmission: Direct or indirect with airborne droplets. Incubation period: 8–20 days. The child can transmit measles from the 4th day of the incubation period to 4 days after the rash appears.	High-grade fever, enlarged lymph nodes, malaise, coryza, cough, photophobia, conjunctivitis, Koplik's spots (small, irregular red spots with a bluish-white center appearing on the buccal mucosa). Two to 4 days after the onset of these symptoms, the child develops	Diagnostic: Serologic test for immunoglobulin (Ig)M measles antibody Preventative measures: Two-dose series of immunizations against measles. The most common immunization against measles, MMR, is given in conjunction with mumps	■ Initiate droplet precautions. ■ Assist the child with activities of daily living and quiet activities to promote rest. ■ Assess lung sounds. ■ Suction prn. ■ With high fever, implement seizure precautions.

(continued)

TABLE 10-3

Common Communicable Diseases of Childhood (continued)

DISEASE AND CAUSATIVE ORGANISM	TRANSMISSION AND INCUBATION PERIOD	CLINICAL MANIFESTATIONS	DIAGNOSTIC TESTS AND MEDICAL TREATMENT	NURSING CONSIDERATIONS
		a red maculopapular, pruritic rash that spreads from the face to the trunk and extremities. The rash changes to brown in color, and eventually sloughing (**desquamation**) occurs.	and rubella. A booster injection is now recommended for the adolescent. Medical treatment: Immune globulin may be given to susceptible person up to 6 days after exposure. Bed rest. Administration of antipyretics, anitpruritics, cough suppressants, and antibiotics for secondary infections.	■ Provide skin care, especially when sloughing occurs. ■ Provide frequent oral care. ■ Limit excessive environmental lighting. Some children are sensitive to television.
Mumps (*parotitis*) is caused by *Rubulavirus*.	Transmission: Direct or indirect spread of respiratory secretions. The child may transmit the virus several days before and after the onset of parotitis. Children should not return to school until 9 days after parotitis occurs. Incubation period: 12 to 25 days	Low-grade fever, headache, malaise. An earache soon develops accompanied by unilateral or bilateral swelling of the parotid gland. The male child may develop **orchitis** (unilateral or bilateral inflammation of the testes accompanied by pain).	Diagnostic: Viral culture; serum mumps immunoglobulin (Ig) G antibody titer Preventative measures: Two-dose series of immunizations against mumps. The most common immunization against mumps, MMR, is given in conjunction with measles and rubella. A booster injection is now recommended for the adolescent. Medical treatment: Administration of analgesics and antipyretics. Corticosteroids may be used.	■ Initiate droplet precautions. ■ Administer pharmacologic and non-pharmacologic pain relief measures. ■ Assist child with nutritional intake. Foods should be liquid or soft. Avoid sour foods, which intensify pain. ■ Maintain intake and output. ■ Monitor fluid and electrolyte balance.
Rubella (German measles or 3-day measles) is caused by an RNA virus.	Transmission: Direct or indirect via exposure to respiratory secretions, feces, or urine. The child may transmit the virus 7 days before to 5 days after the onset of the rash. Children should not return to school or day care until 7 days after the onset of the rash. Incubation period: 14–21 days with an average of 16–18 days.	Low-grade fever, headache, malaise, coryza, enlarged lymph nodes. **Forschheimer spots** (erythematous pinpoint lesions of the soft palate) may also occur. After 1–5 days of these prodromal symptoms, a pink, maculopapular rash begins on the face and spreads down the trunk. It disappears in the same order. The fetus exposed to the rubella virus during pregnancy may be born with congenital rubella syndrome. This syndrome is	Diagnostic: Nasal cell culture; serum immunoglobulin (Ig) G or M antibody titer Preventative measures: Two-dose series of immunizations against rubella. The most common immunization against rubella, MMR, is given in conjunction with measles and mumps. A booster injection is now recommended for the adolescent. Medical treatment: administration of antipyretics.	■ Initiate droplet precautions for the hospitalized child. Prevent contact with rubella nonimmune pregnant women. ■ Implement comfort measures.

Disease	Transmission/Incubation	Manifestations	Diagnostic/Treatment	Nursing Care
		characterized by intrauterine growth retardation (IUGR), hepatosplenomegaly, thrombocytopenia, and dark purplish skin lesions.		
Varicella (chickenpox) is caused by varicella-zoster virus.	Transmission: Direct or indirect contact with airborne respiratory secretions, eye secretions, or vesicles. The infected child may transmit the virus up to 5 days before the onset of vesicles and is considered contagious until 6 days following this outbreak, when all vesicles have crusted over. Incubation period: 10–21 days	Low-grade fever, malaise, headache, mild abdominal pain and irritability. 24 hours later the child experiences an outbreak of pruritic macules that progress from papules to fluid-filled vesicles. Lesions begin on the trunk, scalp, and face, spreading to the remainder of the body, including the mouth, eyes, and perineum. Scarring can develop. The fetus exposed to the varicella virus during pregnancy may be born with congenital varicella syndrome. This syndrome is characterized by IUGR, skin scarring, limb hypoplasia (underdevelopment), eye defects, brain defects, and death.	Diagnostic: Tissue culture of vesicle Preventative measures: Varicella immunization any time after 12 months of age Medical treatment: Administration of antipyretics, antihistamines, and acyclovir to reduce the number of lesions for immunocompromised children. Varicella-zoster immune globulin many also be given to immunocompromised children.	■ If the child is hospitalized, implement droplet and contact precautions. Prevent contact with varicella nonimmune pregnant women. ■ Provide skin care. Soothing baths of oatmeal can be suggested. ■ Keep the child's fingernails short to discourage secondary infections from scratching. ■ Avoid the use of products containing aspirin because Reye's syndrome has been associated with the use of aspirin during a varicella outbreak.
Pneumococcal infection is caused by Streptococcus pneumoniae.	Transmission: Direct and indirect spread of respiratory secretions Incubation period: 1–3 days	Manifestations include: Meningitis—sudden onset of headache, stiff neck, irritability, nausea, vomiting, fever Pneumonia—gradual onset of fever, chills, productive cough, pleuritic chest pain Otitis media—ear tenderness, pain and drainage, diminished hearing Bacteremia—fever of unknown origin	Preventative measures: Four-dose series of immunizations against pneumococcal infection Medical treatment: Administration of antibiotics, primarily penicillin and antipyretics.	■ Monitor intake and output. ■ Encourage fluid intake. ■ Monitor for signs and symptoms of respiratory distress.

(continued)

TABLE 10-3

Common Communicable Diseases of Childhood (continued)

DISEASE AND CAUSATIVE ORGANISM	TRANSMISSION AND INCUBATION PERIOD	CLINICAL MANIFESTATIONS	DIAGNOSTIC TESTS AND MEDICAL TREATMENT	NURSING CONSIDERATIONS
Influenza is caused by Orthomyxoviridae.	Transmission: Direct and indirect contact with respiratory secretions Incubation period: 1–4 days	Abrupt onset of fever, chills, cough, malaise, muscle aches, headache, anorexia, nausea, vomiting, diarrhea	Diagnostic: Rapid influenza test using a nasal or throat specimen; viral culture Preventative measures: Annual immunization against influenza Medical treatment: Administration of nonaspirin antipyretics and antivirals	■ Initiate droplet and contact precautions. ■ Encourage fluids to prevent dehydration. ■ Assist the child with activities of daily living and quiet activities to promote rest.
Hepatitis A is caused by the hepatitis A virus (HAV)	Transmission: Exposure to contaminated stool, typically the fecal-oral route Incubation period: 4 weeks with an average of 10–50 days	Fever, anorexia, nausea, vomiting, rash, arthralgia, pruritus, jaundice (in less than 5% of cases)	Diagnostic: Serologic testing to detect the presence of antigens and antibodies to HAV Preventative measures: Two-dose series of immunization against hepatitis A. The first dose can be given at 12 months and the second dose at least 6 months later. Good hand washing, especially following diaper changes. Proper cleaning of changing surfaces and disposal of soiled diapers. Medical treatment: Bed rest, hydration, well-balanced diet, hepatitis A immune globulin for one-time exposure	See previous measures for hepatitis B.
Erythema infectiosum (fifth disease) is caused by human parvovirus B-19.	Transmission: Direct and indirect contact with respiratory secretions and blood Incubation period: 6–14 days	Stage 1—fever, chills, headache, malaise, body aches Stage 2—1 week later, a rash appears on the child's face. It is bright red and looks as if the child has been slapped. Circumoral pallor is also present. One to 4 days later, a lacy, erythematous, maculopapular rash appears on the trunk and limbs, progressing proximal to distal. Stage 3—rash begins to fade but can reappear if the skin is irritated as by the sun.	Diagnosis: Serologic testing to detect the presence of parvovirus B-19-specific immunoglobulin (Ig) M antibodies Preventative measures: Avoid contact with infected children. Medical treatment: Administration of antipyretics and analgesics.	■ Provide skin care. Soothing baths of oatmeal can be suggested. ■ Protect child from exposure to sunlight.

	Transmission / Incubation	Clinical Manifestations	Diagnostic / Medical Treatment	Nursing Care
Exanthem subitum (sixth disease or roseola) is caused by herpesvirus type 6.	Transmission: Unknown; respiratory secretions suspected Incubation period: 5–20 days, with an average of 10 days	If the fetus is exposed to the virus during pregnancy, fetal death may occur. Sudden onset of high-grade fever. The child may play normally and have a good appetite during the 3–4 days of high fever. The fever disappears abruptly and a pale, pink, maculopapular rash appears on the trunk and spreads to the face, neck, and extremities. The rash lasts 1–2 days. Exanthem subitum occurs mainly in children ages 6–36 months.	Medical treatment: Hospitalization is rarely necessary; administer antipyretics.	■ Observe closely for febrile seizures. ■ Teach signs and symptoms to parents. ■ Encourage oral intake of fluids.
Mononucleosis is caused by the Epstein-Barr virus (EBV). Also called *infectious mononucleosis*, glandular fever, or the kissing disease	Transmission: Direct and indirect contact with respiratory secretions, and genital tract secretions, also blood transfusions. *Note:* The virus can be shed for up to 18 months following the clinical disease. Incubation period: 10–50 days	High-grade fever that can last 3–6 days, chills, headache, anorexia, malaise, abdominal pain, left shoulder pain, sore throat, lymphadenopathy, hepatosplenomegaly, weakness, and lethargy, which can last several months.	Diagnostic: Serologic monospot test; testing EBV antibodies by immunofluorescence. Preventative measures: Avoid contact with those who are known to have the disease. Medical treatment: Bed rest, administer corticosteroids for tonsillar swelling, antipyretics for fever, and analgesics for pain.	■ Assist the child with activities of daily living and quiet activities to promote rest. ■ Because of the risk of liver and spleen rupture, teach the child and parents the importance of avoiding contact sports or rough play for approximately 4 weeks or until hepatosplenomegaly has subsided. ■ Encourage the child to maintain adequate hydration. ■ Older adolescents should be told to avoid kissing until several days after the fever has subsided.
Streptococcus A (strep throat) is caused by group A streptococci (GAS). This organism also causes impetigo, scarlet fever, scarlatina, and rheumatic fever. For more information on impetigo, see Chapter 21, and for acute rheumatic fever, see Chapter 13 🔗.	Transmission: Direct contact Incubation period: 2–5 days	High-grade fever and chills with sudden onset, sore throat, dysphagia, malaise, headache, abdominal pain, anorexia, vomiting. Upon inspection, the pharynx appears bright red with white exudates. Cervical lymph nodes are tender. In toddlers, there may be a moderate temperature, rhinitis,	Diagnostic: Secretions of the pharynx and tonsils are tested for the streptococcus, either by a rapid test or culture. Preventative measures: Avoid contact with those known to be infected. Medical treatment: Administer analgesics, antipyretics, antibiotics—penicillin is the drug of	■ If hospitalized, implement droplet precautions. ■ Provide a soft diet. ■ Offer saltwater gargles. ■ Encourage the child and the parents to take the entire prescribed antibiotic regime.

(continued)

TABLE 10-3

Common Communicable Diseases of Childhood (continued)

DISEASE AND CAUSATIVE ORGANISM	TRANSMISSION AND INCUBATION PERIOD	CLINICAL MANIFESTATIONS	DIAGNOSTIC TESTS AND MEDICAL TREATMENT	NURSING CONSIDERATIONS
		irritability, and anorexia, not accompanied by sore throat. Scarlet fever: 12–48 hours following the onset of symptoms, a fine erythematous rash begins on the neck and spreads to the trunk and extremities. In 3–5 days, the rash begins to fade while the tips of the fingers and toes begin to peel. The tongue develops palatal petechiae. This is said to look like a strawberry and therefore is given the name "strawberry tongue."	choice. If the child is allergic to penicillin, erythromycin is given.	■ Encourage the child to replace toothbrush because the organism may be residing there.
Streptococcus B is caused by group B or beta streptococci (GBS).	Transmission: Direct contact with body fluids; intrauterine to the fetus Incubation Period: less than 7 days	Newborn symptoms include: Early onset: Usually occurs within the first 24 hours of life. The newborn has respiratory distress, apnea, and signs of shock. Meconium-stained fluid may be seen at birth. Late onset: Between 1 and 4 weeks, the newborn may develop lethargy, fever, anorexia, and bulging fontanelles. Later effects include blindness, deafness, mental retardation, learning disabilities, and death.	Diagnostic: Complete blood count, chest x-ray, culture of body fluids Preventative measures: Screening of pregnant women for GBS at 35–37 weeks. Intrapartum administration of ampicillin is indicated if the mother tests positive to reduce the risk of newborn infection. Medical treatment: Administration of antibiotics, particularly ampicillin and gentamicin.	■ Observe closely for symptoms of respiratory distress. ■ Keep the infant warm and free from drafts. Chilling increases the risk of respiratory distress. ■ Closely monitor intake and output.

Infectious Diseases Transmitted by Insects or Animals

Many infections are transmitted from human to human. However, some infections may be transmitted to humans from animals or from insects.

LYME DISEASE

Lyme disease (caused by *Borrelia burgdorferi*) can be transmitted through a tick bite. The incubation period is 3 to 32 days following the tick bite. Lyme disease is characterized by three stages. In stage 1, the child may have **erythema migrans** (Figure 10-3 ■; a red rash with a bull's-eye appearance at the site of the bite). The rash will resolve spontaneously in 4 weeks. Other symptoms in stage 1 include malaise, headache, stiff neck, low-grade fever, and muscle or joint aches. Stage 2 is characterized by pain and swelling of the joints, facial palsy, meningitis, and atrioventricular (AV) block occurring 1 to 4 months after the bite. In stage 3, the child has advanced musculoskeletal pain, deafness, and encephalopathy.

clinical ALERT

Parents should be taught the proper method of removing a tick. The nurse can teach the parents to use tweezers to grasp the tick where it has attached to the child's body and to pull gently. Discourage them from squeezing the body of the tick. Teach them to inspect the tick to determine whether the entire tick was removed. (Disease transmission depends on the length of time the tick is attached [some say 24 hours]. If the body of the tick is removed but the head remains embedded in the skin, the disease can still be transmitted.)

Depending on geographic location, a client who presents with possible Lyme disease may need to be tested for babesiosis and possibly ehrlichiosis. *Babesiosis* is a rare parasitic disease found mainly in coastal areas in the northeastern United States. *Ehrlichiosis* is a bacterial disease that is spread by infected ticks. It can usually be treated by antibiotics. Some emergency rooms routinely screen for these diseases. A client who is not improving with antibiotics should be suspected of having a second blood-borne parasite.

Diagnosis and Treatment

Diagnosis of Lyme disease is determined by enzyme-linked immunoabsorbent assay (ELISA) or Western blot tests. Clinical management of the child with Lyme disease includes administering antibiotics, assisting the child in avoiding fatigue by encouraging rest and avoiding strenuous physical activity, and providing pharmacologic and nonpharmacologic pain relief measures.

ROCKY MOUNTAIN SPOTTED FEVER

Rocky Mountain spotted fever, also called *tickborne typhus fever* or *Sao Paulo typhus*, is caused by *Rickettsia rickettsii*. It is transmitted through a tick bite. The incubation period is 2 to 12 days, with an average of 7 days, after a tick bite. The child with Rocky Mountain spotted fever may experience moderate to high fever, which lasts 2 to 3 weeks, malaise, abdominal and muscle pain, nausea and vomiting, a severe headache that is unrelieved, and conjunctival infection. A maculopapular rash that blanches begins on days 3 to 5 (Figure 10-4 ■). It is first found on the extremities and spreads to the trunk. It progresses from maculopapular in nature to petechial (see examples in Figure 21-3 ⊘). The disease carries a risk of gastrointestinal bleeding, disseminated intravascular coagulation (DIC), pulmonary complications, encephalitis, neurologic dysfunction, and cardiac and renal complications.

Diagnosis and Treatment

Indirect immunofluorescent antibody assay, enzyme immunoassay, or indirect hemagglutination test may be used to diagnose Rocky Mountain spotted fever. Clinical management of children with Rocky Mountain spotted fever

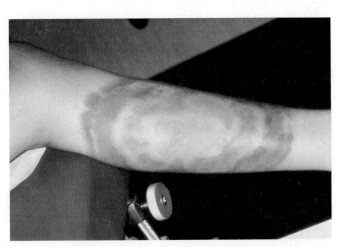

Figure 10-3. ■ Erythema migrans ("target" sign in Lyme disease). (Peter Arnold, Inc.)

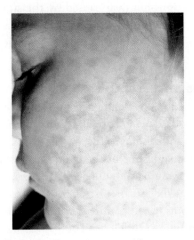

Figure 10-4. ■ Rocky Mountain spotted fever.

includes the administration of antibiotics. The drug of choice is doxycycline. Children should be observed carefully for abnormal bleeding. Emergency equipment should be available in case the child goes into shock. The nurse can help the child avoid fatigue by encouraging rest and discouraging strenuous physical activity. The nurse can also administer pharmacologic and nonpharmacologic pain relief measures.

PROTECTION AGAINST TICK BITES

For children living in tick-prone areas, the nurse may assist the family in implementing preventative measures. These include a three-dose vaccination, LYMErix, to protect against *B. burgdorferi*. LYMErix is recommended for adolescents aged 15 years and older. Children should learn to recognize and avoid tick-infested areas. When walking or playing in these areas, children should wear protective clothing. After being outdoors, the child and parents should examine carefully for ticks and remove them promptly. Insect repellents containing DEET are effective in preventing tick bites. Parents should only apply this chemical when the child is in a high-risk area because there are associated side effects with this product. These side effects include changes in facial skin color; skin rash, hives, and/or pruritis; dyspnea or tachypnea; confusion; seizures; loss of consciousness; muscle cramping; periorbital edema; bradycardia; insomnia; and unusual tiredness or weakness. The insect repellent should not be used on the face, hands, or anywhere the child has a skin irritation. It should be washed off carefully with soap and water.

RABIES

Rabies is caused by *Rhabdoviridae*. Transmission of this harmful organism occurs due to a bite from an animal infected with rabies. The incubation period for *Rhabdoviridae* is 1 to 7 weeks, with an average of 6 weeks. The child is commonly asymptomatic during the incubation period. Initial symptoms include pain at the site of the bite, headache, fever, anorexia, and malaise. Half of the children develop **hydrophobia** (fear caused by the sight of liquid, accompanied by painful contractures in the muscles used for swallowing). Hallucinations, disorientations, manic episodes, seizures, stupor, coma, and death may occur.

Diagnosis and Treatment

Diagnosis of rabies is confirmed by fluorescent antibody staining of the dead animal's brain tissue. Therefore, it is vital to confine the animal, if possible, once it has bitten a child.

Clinical management of the child with rabies includes irrigating and washing the animal bite thoroughly as quickly as possible after the bite occurs. The wound may need suturing. It is important to administer human rabies immune globulin and human diploid cell rabies vaccine (HDCV) as soon as possible after the bite occurs. HDCV is given intramuscularly in five doses on days 0, 3, 7, 14, and 28. If the

---

BOX 10-2   CLIENT TEACHING

Recognizing a Rabid Animal

For an unvaccinated animal to become infected with rabies, it must suffer a bite from an infected animal. Early signs of rabies in an animal are behavioral changes, fever, slow eye reflexes, and chewing at the bite site. After several days, the animal will be irritable, restless, and aggressive; bark frequently; viciously attack inanimate objects; and appear disoriented. Finally, the animal will develop paralysis, starting with the limb that was bitten. As the throat and face become paralyzed, the bark changes, a foamy drool develops, and the jaw drops. Death usually occurs from respiratory paralysis.

animal is found to be rabies free, the series may be stopped. For the child who is diagnosed with rabies, hospitalization is necessary, and contact precautions need to be implemented. The nurse should observe for side effects of the vaccine, which include irritation at the site, pruritis, headache, muscle aches, nausea, and dizziness. The nurse should keep the child with hydrophobia away from liquids.

Providing emotional support to children and their parents prior to confirmation of rabies is an important nursing intervention. Children can be combative in the latter stages of the disease process and may need sedation to avoid exhaustion.

Preventative measures related to rabies include vaccination of all domestic animals against rabies. Children should be taught the dangers of interacting with stray or dead animals. Box 10-2 ■ provides information on how to recognize a rabid animal.

Sexually Transmitted Infections

Several sexually transmitted infections (STIs) may be acquired prenatally or at birth. These diseases include herpes, HIV, gonorrhea, and chlamydia. HIV is discussed more fully in Chapter 22 ⚭. Other STIs are discussed more fully in Chapter 18 ⚭.

There are numerous ways in which children and adolescents can become infected with STIs. These include sexual experimentation, sexual play, molestation, and sexual abuse. Sexual abuse must be considered when a child presents to the health care provider with STIs such as syphilis and gonorrhea. See Chapter 16 ⚭ for more discussion of sexual abuse.

NURSING CARE

PRIORITIES IN NURSING CARE

When caring for children with communicable diseases, the nurse should focus on determining symptoms and the degree of severity of the symptoms. Priority care of these children includes managing fever, preventing respiratory distress, promoting skin integrity, ensuring comfort, and preventing the spread of the infection. The nurse uses skills in communication to teach the child and his or her parents how to manage the care at home and how to prevent the spread of infection.

ASSESSING

The nurse is responsible for collecting data about symptoms of hyperthermia such as flushed skin, increased body and skin temperature, and increased heart and respiratory rates. Children with fevers should be observed for fluid loss and seizure activity. Observe the child for other signs of infection, including a change in activity level, a change in appetite, nausea, vomiting, and diarrhea.

Accurate assessment of the child's respiratory status is important. Besides the respiratory rate, collect data on the depth and rhythm of respirations. Listen to breath sounds anteriorly and posteriorly. Characterize the child's cough. Evaluate the color and consistency of sputum. Look for restlessness, difficulty with speech, orthopnea, and cyanosis.

Ask the verbal child for a report of his or her discomfort and pain. Use pain scales appropriate to the child's age. Observe closely for nonverbal expressions of pain and discomfort such as grimacing, limited attention span, and withdrawal. See Chapter 15 ⟳ for more discussion of the physiology of pain. See Chapter 8 ⟳ for more discussion on pain scales and assessing pain in children.

Collect data on a child's rashes and lesions, including distribution, shape, color, size, and consistency. Determine the presence of prurititis and the degree of discomfort it is causing the child.

Note: Some Eastern cultures may practice traditional medicine that could raise suspicion of abuse. Box 10-3 ■ describes the practices of cupping and coining. Figure 10-5 ■ illustrates these practices.

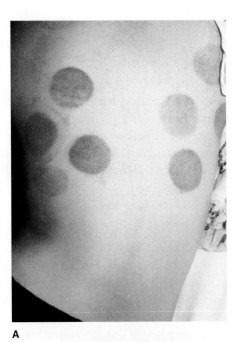

A

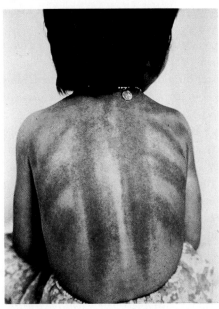

B

Figure 10-5. ■ Cupping (**A**) and coining (**B**) are non-Western healing practices of some cultural groups that must be distinguished from child abuse. (Used with permission of the American Academy of Pediatrics, Visual Diagnosis of Child Physical Abuse Slide Kit. Photographs copyright © AAP/Kempe.)

BOX 10-3   **CULTURAL PULSE POINTS**

Nontraditional Care of Communicable Disease

During periods of illness, alternative medical practices called *coining* and *cupping* may be practiced to relieve pruritus and symptoms of influenza such as muscle aches. This practice may be found among some people of Southeast Asian origin and also among Russian immigrants and Mexican American families.

In coining, a practitioner trained in the practice massages the client's chest, back, and shoulders with medicated ointment. A copper coin or silver spoon is then used to rub down the body parts in a linear fashion. Dark marks are left on the body for several days.

The practice of cupping is done by coating a small jar with alcohol. The jar is then held upside down, and a lighted match burns off the oxygen and creates a vacuum. The jar is then quickly placed on the skin. The vacuum draws the jar, creating a bruiselike mark. Such marks may appear at first glance to be physical child abuse. It is important to explore whether the child was treated with this culturally accepted practice.

DIAGNOSING, PLANNING, AND IMPLEMENTING

Nursing diagnoses for children with communicable diseases might include:

- Hyperthermia related to the infectious process
- Airway Clearance, Ineffective related to airway spasm, excessive or retained secretions
- Pain, Acute related to skin lesions, pharyngitis, cough, chest congestion, etc.
- Skin Integrity, Impaired related to rash, pox, and swelling of the parotid gland.

Outcomes for children with communicable diseases might include that the child will:

- Maintain body temperature within normal limits.
- Have a patent airway.
- Communicate lack of pain or reduced discomfort.
- Be free of complications related to rash, lesions, and blisters (e.g., no purulent drainage, no bleeding of the lesions, no scarring).

The nurse's role in providing support to these children would include the following:

- Avoid the use of aspirin to relieve fever. Use acetaminophen or ibuprofen. *Aspirin increases the risk of Reye's syndrome.* (Reye's syndrome also appears Chapter 15 ⬤ .)
- Implement other methods of cooling the child, such as removing excess clothing, applying cool washcloths, using a circulating fan, or using a cooling blanket. *These methods supplement the use of antipyretics and help to bring down fever.*
- Encourage adequate intake of oral fluids. *This prevents dehydration.*
- Administer humidified oxygen as ordered. *Humidified oxygen loosens secretions and assists in the maintenance of oxygenation.*
- Encourage ambulation if there are no contraindications. If the child cannot ambulate, turn him or her from side to side every 2 hours. *This will promote movement of secretions.*
- Suction the nasopharynx or oropharynx. *This removes secretions blocking the airway.*
- Provide distractions and diversions such as board games, video games, movies, and puzzles. *Distractions promote physical and emotional comfort.*
- Control environmental aspects such as soiled linens, bright lights, warm room temperature, and loud verbal conversations. *These aspects might contribute to the child's discomfort. For instance, a warm room increases the incidence of itching.*
- Provide antihistamines as ordered. Teach parents alternative forms of soothing pruritus for use at home (Box 10-4 ■).

BOX 10-4   COMPLEMENTARY THERAPIES

Methods for Soothing Itchy Skin

Chickenpox (see Figure 10-2) can cause extreme pruritus in children. Several natural remedies are available using common household products.

- Parents can mix ½ cup of vinegar into the bathwater.
- Oatmeal has also been found to relieve the discomfort caused by the virus. Parents can cook 2 cups of oatmeal according to manufacturer's directions. This mixture should be placed into a small cotton bag and secured at the top. The bag is then floated in a warm bath. As the water becomes milky, the solution should be splashed onto the lesions.
- A mixture of baking soda and water can be sponged onto the child's skin and allowed to dry thoroughly.

Antihistamines and alternative therapies assist in the control of itching.

- Keep fingernails clean and short. If necessary, apply mittens to prevent scratching. *This decreases the risk of additional trauma to the skin and secondary infections.*
- Keep skin dry and clean. *Wet, dirty skin could aggravate itching.*

EVALUATING

Changes in vital signs, respiratory status, intake and output, and comfort levels need to be documented and reported to the supervising nurse. Changes in skin lesions need to be documented according to distribution, shape, color, size, and accompanying drainage. The effectiveness of analgesics, antipyretics, antibiotics, and antihistamines should be documented.

NURSING PROCESS CARE PLAN
Child with Chickenpox

Mrs. Word calls the family practice clinic because her 4-year-old daughter, Molly, has chickenpox. Molly's sister had them last week. Mrs. Word is concerned because Molly is scratching her skin. Mrs. Word asks the nurse for suggestions to keep Molly from scratching. She is very concerned that scarring will occur, especially on Molly's face.

Assessment.   The following data should be collected as soon as possible:

- History of present illness
- Risk factors that would contribute to impaired skin integrity such as bowel and bladder control, poor

nutritional status, preexisting skin conditions, impaired cognitive ability, and impaired circulation
- Other possible irritants such as restrictive clothing and harsh body soaps or laundry detergents
- Thorough skin assessment (see Chapter 21 ⬯)
- Current stage of the lesions, including color, distribution, skin temperature, moisture, erythema, and size of the lesion.

Nursing Diagnosis. The following important nursing diagnosis (among others) is established for this client:

- Skin Integrity, risk for impaired related to frequent scratching

Expected Outcomes

- Skin will show no evidence of scratching.
- There will be no complications related to scratching such as irritation, infection cellulitis, or scarring.

Planning and Implementation

- Encourage Mrs. Word to use a mild soap to keep Molly's skin clean and as free of bacteria as possible.
- If Molly still wears a diaper to bed, Mrs. Word needs to be taught that this can irritate her skin and increase irritation. Encourage Mrs. Word to awaken Molly and take her to the toilet once during the night.
- Cut Molly's fingernails short so they do not cut her skin. This could also provide a diversion activity if Mrs. Word chooses to give Molly a "manicure."

- Encourage Mrs. Word to keep Molly's hands busy during the day. She could color, paint, dress her dolls, play with modeling clay, or work puzzles.
- Suggest that Mrs. Word give Molly Benadryl (diphenhydramine hydrochloride) to prevent scratching when Molly is particularly uncomfortable.
- Suggest topical agents such as calamine lotion, oatmeal baths, or baking soda baths to make Molly more comfortable.
- Teach Mrs. Word how to recognize skin irritation, infection, and cellulitis.

Evaluation. Mrs. Word reports that Molly is enjoying her new easel and paints. She is administering Benadryl after lunch and giving her a nightly bath in baking soda. Many of the lesions are beginning to crust over.

Critical Thinking in the Nursing Process

1. Molly's Aunt Betty is 16 weeks pregnant. Aunt Betty is unsure whether she has had chickenpox. What information would you give Mrs. Word concerning Aunt Betty's risk of contracting chickenpox?
2. What is the proper response to a parent who says he or she decided to tie the child's hands to the bed to keep them from scratching?
3. What information would the nurse give to parents to help them recognize symptoms of infection or cellulitis?

Note: Discussion of Critical Thinking questions appears in Appendix I.

NURSING CARE PLAN CHART

Child with Influenza

GOAL	INTERVENTION	RATIONALE	EXCEPTED OUTCOME
1. Hyperthermia related to infectious process			
The child will experience body temperature within normal limits	Encourage the intake of oral fluids	*Adequate hydration assists in the resolution of hyperthermia*	The child experiences normal body temperature.
	Remove excess clothing and linens	*Clothing and linens can complicate hyperthermia*	
	Provide cooling methods including cool washcloths to the axilla, groin, forehead and neck; electric fans; and cooling blankets	*These methods cool the skin and will in turn promote a decrease in core temperature*	
The family will demonstrate appropriate methods of managing hyperthermia	Teach parents to recognize symptoms of hyperthermia and report promptly to include dry skin, headache, tachycardia, increased body temperature, irritability, weakness	*Prompt recognition of symptoms results in prompt treatment*	Family reports symptoms to health care provider. Family will report successful implementation of cooling methods.
	Teach parents to implement cooling methods and to provide antipyretics (not aspirin)	*These methods cool the skin and will in turn promote a decrease in core temperature*	
2. Acute Pain related to infectious process			
The child will have reduced physical and emotional pain	Implement nonpharmacologic pain relief measures to include: position changes, back massage, relaxation and breathing techniques, distraction techniques, patient hygiene, linen change, application of cold or heat, comfortable room temperature, noise reduction, and soothing music.	*Nonpharmacological pain relief measures assist the child in dealing with the emotional aspects of pain and can in turn provide physical pain relief*	The child will report reduced physical and emotional pain.
	Implement pharmacologic pain relief measures as ordered	*Pharmacologic pain agents can reduce or eliminate pain*	
	Use an appropriate pain rating scale to assess pain initially and following implementation of relief measures	*An adequate initial assessment of pain allows the nurse to appropriately manage the child's pain and follow-up assessments allow for a change in the plan of care if necessary*	
The family will demonstrate appropriate methods of managing the child's pain	Teach the family how to recognize pain behaviors	*Prompt recognition of pain will result in prompt implementation of pain relief measures*	Family provides appropriate methods of pain relief.
	Provide instruction to the family about implementing nonpharmacologic and pharmacologic pain relief measures	*Treating both the emotional and physical aspects of pain will result in appropriate management of the child's pain*	

Note: The reference and resource listings for this and all chapters have been compiled at the back of the book.

Chapter Review

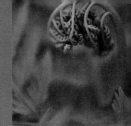

 KEY TERMS by Topic

Use the audio glossary feature of either the CD-ROM or the Companion Website to hear the correct pronunciation of the following key terms.

Introduction
communicable diseases

Chain of Infection
pathogens, reservoir, portal of exit, transmission, portal of entry, susceptible host, droplet method, airborne transmission, fomites, incubation period, prodromal period, illness, convalescent period

Risk Factors for Communicable Diseases in Children
active immunity, passive immunity, nosocomial infection, seasonal flu, avian flu, pandemic flu, antigenic drift, antigenic shift, bioterrorism, universal precautions, standard precautions, transmission-based precautions, airborne precautions, droplet precautions, contact precautions, reverse isolation

Immunizations
immunization, vaccines, toxoid, immunotherapy

Common Infections
opisthotonos, Koplik's spots, desquamation, orchitis, Forschheimer spots

Infectious Diseases Transmitted by Insects or Animals
erythema migrans, hydrophobia

KEY Points

- The nurse has an important role in recognizing communicable diseases and assisting the family in obtaining appropriate care. Another important nursing role is client and family teaching regarding methods of disease prevention.

- For a disease to be transmitted from person to person, there must be a pathogen, reservoir, portal of exit, portal of entry, and susceptible host.

- Stages of the infectious process include the incubation period, the prodromal period, illness or the stage where clinical symptoms appear, and the convalescent period.

- The single most effective way to prevent the spread of communicable diseases is through hand washing.

- Nursing care for children with communicable diseases includes a variety of standards and precautions designed to prevent transmission of the disease or protect the child from additional harmful bacteria. The nurse must be able to implement the following precautions: universal, standard, airborne, droplet, contact, and reverse isolation.

- Immunizations are an essential tool to protect children against communicable diseases.

- Children living in tick-prone areas need added protection from tick bites, which may cause Lyme disease and Rocky Mountain spotted fever. This protection includes insect repellent, long-sleeved shirts, long pants, and a hat when in tick-prone areas and vaccination with LYMErix for older children.

- Comfort measures for children with communicable diseases include pain relief measures and measures to relieve pruritus.

 EXPLORE Media Link

Additional interactive resources for this chapter can be found on the Companion Website at www.prenhall.com/adams.

Click on Chapter 10 and "Begin" to select the activities for this chapter.

For chapter-related NCLEX®-style questions and an audio glossary, access the accompanying CD-ROM in this book.

Animations:
Throat culture

FOR FURTHER Study

Chapter 8 provides procedural steps for giving immunizations.

Acute rheumatic fever is discussed in Chapter 13.

For more information on meningitis and Reye's syndrome, see Chapter 15.

See Chapter 16 for more about effects of disasters on children and sexual abuse.

For additional discussion about STIs, see Chapter 18.

For review of skin assessment and disorders, see Chapter 21.

For more information on HIV, the child's immune system, and organ transplantation, see Chapter 22.

See Appendix II for the U.S. recommended immunization schedule from the CDC.

See Appendix V for a brief review of precautions for infection control.

Critical Thinking Care Map

Caring for a Client Requiring Droplet Precautions
NCLEX-PN® Focus Area: Safety and Infection Control

Case Study: Wendy, a 2-year-old, is admitted to the pediatric unit with a diagnosis of diphtheria. She was recently adopted from an orphanage in Kiev, Russia. Because of her condition, she is placed on droplet precautions and is given a private room. Wendy's adoptive parents decide to stay overnight with her. However, the first time the nurse walks into the room with a mask on, Wendy begins to scream loudly and cry inconsolably.

Nursing Diagnosis: Fear related to unfamiliar environment and people

COLLECT DATA

Subjective	Objective
_____	_____
_____	_____
_____	_____
_____	_____
_____	_____
_____	_____

Would you report this? Yes/No
If yes, to: _____

Nursing Care

_____
_____
_____
_____
_____
_____
_____
_____
_____
_____

How would you document this? _____
_____
_____
_____

Data Collected
(use only those that apply)

- Screaming loudly
- Crying inconsolably
- Harsh cough
- Clenched fists
- Resting with eyes closed in adoptive mother's arms
- Clutching toy stuffed frog while sobbing loudly
- T 99.6
- R 12 and labored
- Rhinorrhea
- Tightened jaw
- Immediately hides head in mother's lap when nurse with mask approaches

Nursing Interventions
(use only those that apply; list in priority order)

- Monitor closely for signs of increasing respiratory distress.
- Keep oral airway, suction equipment, and Ambu bag close at hand.
- Provide Wendy with a mask to put on her frog.
- Stand farther than 3 feet away from Wendy, remove the mask, and greet Wendy pleasantly each time the nurse enters the room. Replace mask. Repeat several times prior to moving close to Wendy.
- Administer oxygen as ordered.
- Suction prn.
- Avoid approaching Wendy or touching her unless she is being held by her adoptive mother or father.
- Administer antibiotics as ordered.
- Provide Wendy with age-appropriate diversional activities such as blocks.
- Give the child a surgical mask to try on.

Compare your documentation to the sample provided in Appendix I.

TEST-TAKING TIP Make a copy of Table 10-3, Common Communicable Diseases of Childhood. With a bright marker, highlight any serious or life-threatening complications. Memorize these facts first. This will help when asked to identify a disease that has a potential complication.

1 The nurse has just completed instruction about active and passive immunity to a couple who is expecting their first child and realizes additional instruction is needed when the wife states:

1. "My child will be protected for life from many diseases through passive immunity."
2. "My child will develop active immunity by producing antibodies to specific organisms."
3. "Through active immunity, my child will develop long-term protection against organisms."
4. "Passive immunity is what my child gets from me and is short-term protection."

2 The mother of an 11-month-old is upset because her child seems to be sick frequently. From the knowledge the nurse has about communicable diseases and susceptibility of children that age, the nurse is able to share some educational points with the mother. The nurse tells the mother that:

1. by age 1, the child will have adult levels of immunoglobulin M antibodies.
2. the child has higher neutrophil levels so should be able to ward off disease.
3. the child's immune system is fully mature at birth.
4. the child must wear gloves when playing with others to prevent disease transmission.

3 The nurse is going to be caring for an infant who was exposed to the varicella virus before birth and has been diagnosed with congenital varicella syndrome. The nurse knows that this is characterized by certain symptoms, which are:

1. asthma, rash, and otitis media.
2. eye and brain defects and underdeveloped arms and legs.
3. polydactyly, pneumocephalus, and rhinitis.
4. urticaria, seborrhea, and psoriasis.

4 The nurse administers a DTaP immunization to a 6-month-old child at the physician's office. The mother calls the office the next day and tells the nurse that the area around the injection site is red and swollen. The nurse instructs the mother to:

1. ignore the redness and swelling.
2. rush the child to the nearest hospital.
3. apply vinegar to the site.
4. place a covered ice pack on the injection site.

5 The nurse is preparing an injection of measles, mumps, rubella vaccine and notices that the child is allergic to neomycin. The nurse plans to:

1. administer the immunization.
2. administer a smaller dose of the immunization.
3. not give the immunization.
4. give the immunization at a later date.

6 A child with roseola is brought into a clinic. While the nurse is providing instructions about care, the mother tells the nurse that she is worried that all of her children will contract roseola. The nurse tells the mother that:

1. the disease is transmitted through uncooked foods.
2. the disease is transmitted through contact with bodily fluids.
3. the cause of the disease is unknown.
4. the disease is transmitted through unpasteurized milk.

7 The nurse is providing home instructions to the parents of a child diagnosed with infectious mononucleosis. The nurse instructs the parents:

1. to allow the child to return to school.
2. to notify the physician if the child develops a fever of greater than 99.9 °F.
3. to keep the child supine for 1 week.
4. to notify the physician if the child develops abdominal pain or left shoulder pain.

8 The nurse has listened to the news about the avian flu, its possibility of transmission, and its threat to humans. The parents of a child are in the clinic for a well-child visit and ask the nurse about the avian flu. The nurse responds:

1. "The avian flu cannot be transmitted to humans."
2. "There is a vaccine available for the avian flu for children older than 3 years."
3. "The avian flu is transmitted through eating the meat of infected pigs."
4. "There is no human immunity or vaccine available for the avian flu."

9 Select the statements about universal precautions that the nurse would use to explain this term. Choose all that apply.

1. It is designed to prevent transmission of HIV.
2. It is designed to prevent transmission of HBV.
3. It is designed to prevent transmission of disease-producing microorganisms transmitted by means of blood, tissue, and body fluids containing blood.
4. It is a standard to follow when providing health care to clients.
5. It is the same as transmission-based precautions.

10 Choose which statements describe standard precautions. Select all that apply.

1. Use mouthpieces, resuscitation bags, or other ventilation devices for mouth-to-mouth resuscitation.
2. Handle sharp instruments properly to avoid exposure.
3. Wear a clean, nonsterile gown to protect skin and prevent soiling of the uniform by contact with body fluids.
4. Immunize with the HBV vaccine.
5. Wear masks, eye protection, or a face shield when there is a possibility of contacting body fluids during certain procedures.
6. Hand wash with plain soap and water before and after client contact.

Answers for NCLEX-PN® Review and Critical Thinking questions appear in Appendix I.

Thinking Strategically About...

Shelby is a 16-year-old who was diagnosed with acute myelogenous leukemia (AML) when she was 12 years old. In the past 4 years, Shelby and her family have become familiar faces on the pediatric unit where you work. Each admission has been different. Sometimes she was anemic and needed transfusions. Other times she was admitted following chemotherapy with nausea and weight loss. At other times she was in need of IV antibiotics because of upper respiratory infections.

As the years have progressed, Shelby's condition has become more and more brittle. She no longer goes into remission, and the search for a suitable donor for bone marrow transplant has not been successful.

Yesterday, Shelby was admitted to the hospital with fatigue, nausea, and symptoms of an upper respiratory tract infection. Vital signs are: T 101.4 °F; BP 102/68; P 66, weak and thready; R 18. Labs reveal: WBC—12.5 (normal values at your institution are 4.4–10.2); hematocrit—27.6 (normal values at your institution are 33.0–46.2); hemoglobin—9.2 (normal values at your institution are 10.7–15.7).

Shelby's parents have requested a private meeting with her physician to discuss her current prognosis. They have asked you to be present at the meeting.

CRITICAL THINKING

Describe your role as an LPN/LVN in the meeting.

COLLABORATIVE CARE

During the meeting, Shelby's physician tells her parents that he believes Shelby is critically ill and may not respond well to treatment. Shelby's mother sobs loudly and cries out that surely no parent on earth feels this level of pain. What type of referrals may be appropriate for Shelby's parents?

DELEGATING

You are working with a certified nursing assistant. Which tasks related to Shelby's care could be delegated to the CNA?

MANAGEMENT OF CARE

List comfort measures that would be appropriate for Shelby in the terminal phase of her disease.

COMMUNICATION AND CLIENT TEACHING

Shelby's mother wants to know what her daughter will feel like as she is dying. How do you respond?

TIME MANAGEMENT AND PRIORITIES IN NURSING CARE

Shelby is not your only client. But, as she declines, her parents state they are afraid to be left alone. How do you manage their request?

DOCUMENTING AND REPORTING

What changes in Shelby's condition would indicate a decline in her condition? How and to whom would you report them?

SPIRITUAL/CULTURAL CARE STRATEGIES

Shelby's parents request that their minister come to the hospital, but he is currently unavailable. What strategy could be incorporated to assist them with their spiritual need?

Pediatric Disorders

UNIT III

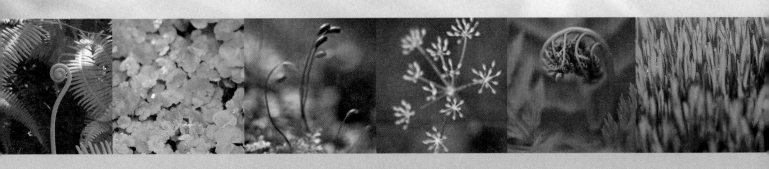

Chapter 11

Care of the Child with Fluid, Electrolyte, and Acid-Base Disorders

NURSING PROCESS CARE PLAN:
Client with Diarrhea

HEALTH PROMOTION ISSUE:
Self-Asphyxiation as a Game

NURSING CARE PLAN CHART:
Child with Respiratory
Alkalosis

CRITICAL THINKING CARE MAP:
Caring for a Client with Fluid
Volume Excess

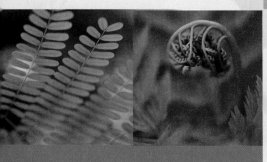

BRIEF Outline

LEARNING Outcomes

After completing this chapter, you will be able to:
1. Define key terms.
2. Discuss fluid and electrolyte balance in children.
3. Discuss acid-base balance in children.
4. Identify alterations in fluid and electrolyte and acid-base balance in children.
5. Describe appropriate assessment and interventions related to fluid and electrolyte and acid-base imbalances.

A finer line exists between fluid balance and imbalance in children than in adults. The percent of water in the body varies with age (Figure 11-1 ■). In adults, the percentage of water ranges from 50% (females) to 55% (males). Approximately 50% of a child's weight consists of water. In infants, water comprises 60% of body weight. In the newborn, 75% of the weight is water. Because of this high percentage of water, fluid and electrolyte imbalances are much more dangerous in pediatric clients than in adults.

Principles Related to Fluids and Electrolytes

To provide the best nursing care to children with fluid and electrolyte disorders, the nurse must recall foundational principles related to the body's fluids and electrolytes. Health is maintained when fluids and electrolytes are balanced within the body. This state of balance is called **homeostasis**.

FLUIDS

The largest component of the body is water. Body fluids are distributed in two distinct compartments: intracellular and extracellular. Intracellular fluid is found within the body cells. Extracellular fluid is found outside the body cells. Extracellular fluid can be further distinguished as **plasma** (the fluid portion of circulating blood) and interstitial fluid (Figure 11-2 ■). (**Interstitial** relates to spaces within a structure, such as the spaces within a tissue or an organ.)

Before discussing how this fluid moves within the child's body, it is necessary to review certain terms. Fluids consist of liquids and solids. A **solute** is a substance that is dissolved in a solution or fluid. The liquid in which a substance or solute is dissolved is called a **solvent**. A **solution** is formed when one or more solutes are dissolved in a solvent.

The solution of fluids and electrolytes constantly moves across the cell membrane to maintain the work of oxygenation, metabolism, excretion, and other body processes. This movement is accomplished by four methods: osmosis, diffusion, filtration, and active transport (Figure 11-3 ■).

Osmosis is the movement of fluid, the solvent, across the cell membrane from an area of lesser solute concentration to an area of greater solute concentration. Osmosis causes the concentration of solutes on both sides of the cell membrane to become equal.

Through the process of **diffusion**, solutes move across the cell membrane from an area of higher concentration to an area of lower concentration.

Filtration is a process by which solvents and solutes are pushed across a cell membrane from an area of higher pressure to an area of lower pressure. This pressure is called *hydrostatic pressure* or *capillary blood pressure*.

The movement of solutes across the cell membrane by means of metabolic activity and carrier cells is called **active transport**. Active transport uses energy to carry a solute from an area of lower concentration into an area of higher concentration. For example, normally, sodium is most abundant outside the cell and potassium is most abundant inside the cell. To maintain balance of these electrolytes, the sodium-potassium pump assists in the process. The pump works by employing carrier or transport cells to assist movement across the cell membrane.

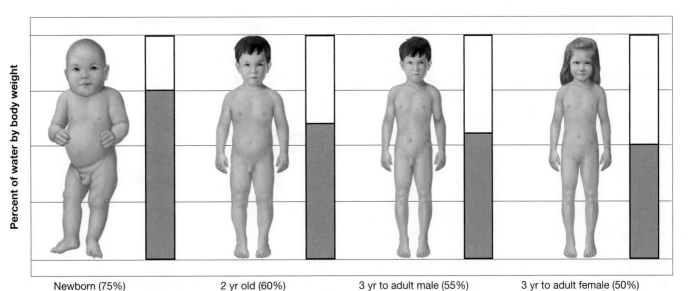

| Percent of water by body weight | | | |
| Newborn (75%) | 2 yr old (60%) | 3 yr to adult male (55%) | 3 yr to adult female (50%) |

Figure 11-1. ■ Percentage of water by body weight changes dramatically from 75% in infants to about 50% to 55% in adults. The greater percentage of water in infants makes them highly susceptible to fluid imbalance.

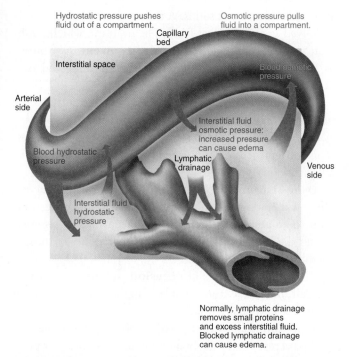

Normally, lymphatic drainage removes small proteins and excess interstitial fluid. Blocked lymphatic drainage can cause edema.

Figure 11-2. ■ When fluid is inside the body's arteries, veins, and capillaries (*vasculature*), it is plasma. When fluid moves across the *space* from circulatory structures to cells, it is interstitial fluid. Once it moves into cell structures, it is called intracellular fluid.

The movement of fluids and electrolytes assists the body in maintaining homeostasis. Homeostasis is also affected by fluid intake, hormonal regulation, and fluid output.

Fluid intake is primarily regulated through the thirst mechanism. For individuals to have adequate intake, they must be both alert and capable of pursuing fluids to drink. Therefore, infants, small children, and ill children are at great risk for inadequate fluid intake.

A variety of hormones assists the process of homeostasis. Antidiuretic hormone (ADH) makes the kidneys more permeable to water. Aldosterone assists in the regulation of sodium and potassium. Renin increases the perfusion of the kidneys and controls sodium levels. The body must also get rid of excess fluid and electrolytes by controlling fluid output. Fluid is lost from the body through the kidneys, skin, lungs, and GI tract.

ELECTROLYTES

Electrolytes are solutes within the body fluid; they may also be called minerals or salts. An electrolyte is dissolved in a solvent and is broken down into ions. These ions carry an electrical charge (hence the name). Electrolytes are measured in milliequivalents per liter (mEq/L). Milliequivalents represent the number of grams of the electrolyte dissolved in a liter of plasma.

Cations are positively charged electrolytes. Potassium (K^+), sodium (Na^+), and calcium (Ca^+) are common cations. Sodium is the body's most abundant electrolyte. It controls the balance of the body's water. It is regulated mainly through dietary intake and aldosterone. Potassium is found mostly in the intracellular space. Its main function is to control muscle contractions. Potassium is regulated by dietary intake and renal excretion. Calcium is stored in the bones, plasma, and body cells. The chief functions of calcium are to maintain bones and teeth and to assist in blood clotting. Calcium is mainly regulated by protein albumin.

Anions are negatively charged electrolytes. Chloride (Cl^-), bicarbonate (HCO_3^-) and sulfate (SO_4^{2-}) are common anions. Chloride is found in the extracellular fluid. It functions in conjunction with sodium and is regulated by dietary intake and the kidneys. Bicarbonate is found in the extracellular and intracellular fluid. Its primary function is to maintain acid-base balance. Bicarbonate is regulated by the kidneys. Acid-base balance is discussed later in the chapter.

Brief Assessment Review

In the child who is ill, the assessment of fluid balance is essential. Vomiting and diarrhea lead quickly to fluid and electrolyte loss (see Figure 11-1) and could lead to hypovolemic shock (see Chapter 14 ⟳). Measuring output might be difficult because the child may not be able to follow directions of vomiting into a basin or collecting stool in the proper receptacle. Weighing dry diapers, writing the weight on the outside, and then weighing them again when wet is the most accurate method of determining urinary output in infants (1 g = 1 mL). The moisture of mucous membranes, skin turgor, and level of consciousness can also be helpful in evaluating fluid loss. Intake, output, urine specific gravity, and daily weight are usually monitored in hospitalized children.

> **clinical ALERT**
>
> Daily weights are the best way to monitor fluid balance. Because the client's family may give fluids or even empty urine without informing the nurse, intake and output records may be inaccurate.

Table 11-1 ■ provides information about assessing fluid and electrolyte status in infants and children. Procedure 11-1 ■ reviews intake and output measurement.

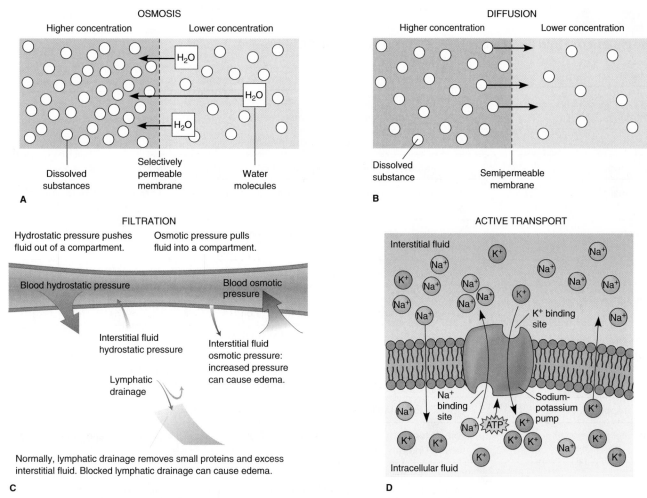

Figure 11-3. ■ (**A**) Osmosis. Water moves across a selective permeable membrane into an area of higher solute concentration and out of the area of lower solute concentration. (**B**) Diffusion. Molecules move across a semipermeable membrane from an area of higher solute concentration to an area of lower solute concentration. (**C**) Filtration is the process by which water and solutes move across capillary membranes driven by fluid pressure. The pumping action of the heart and gravity push water and solutes into the interstitial space. Note that water is returned into the vascular space by osmosis. (**D**) Active transport. The movement of sodium and potassium ions across cell membranes against their concentration gradients.

FLUID AND ELECTROLYTE DISORDERS

Recall that homeostasis is maintained when the child's intake and output are balanced. In states of illness, body fluids and the electrolytes contained within them may become unbalanced. Both fluid loss (e.g., through diarrhea, vomiting, or burns) and fluid gain (e.g., from IV fluid overload or cardiac and kidney disease) can create these imbalances in fluids and electrolytes.

Deficient Fluid Volume (Dehydration)

Dehydration is a condition of deficient fluid volume in the intravascular and interstitial fluid compartments.

Dehydration is often accompanied by imbalances in sodium. This disease process can be classified as isotonic, hypotonic, or hypertonic.

■ The most common type of dehydration in children is **isotonic dehydration**. This is a loss of fluid and sodium in equal proportions (as from vomiting). Sodium levels are normal, and most of the fluid lost is from the extracellular compartment.

■ **Hypotonic dehydration** is fluid and sodium loss in which relatively more sodium than fluid is lost (as in renal disease). Less salt than normal remains in the body. As sodium levels fall below normal range, fluid shifts into the intracellular space from the extracellular space.

TABLE 11-1

Assessment of Fluid and Electrolyte Status in Infants and Children

HISTORY	
Chronic diseases	Ask about cancer, diabetes, ulcerative colitis, or anorexia.
Past trauma	Ask about burns, head injuries, or massive trauma with hemorrhage.
Past surgeries	Ask about surgeries, especially those involving the GI tract, respiratory system, or kidneys.
Medications	Ask about medications that might affect F&E status such as diuretics or steroids.
Nutritional status	Ask about type of diet, typical fluid intake, increase or decrease in child's thirst, or recent weight gain or loss.
Elimination	Ask if the child has experienced oliguria, anuria, nocturia, polyuria, diuresis, diarrhea, or constipation.
Exercise/activity	Ask about the typical activity level of the child.
Neurologic status	Ask about any headaches, numbness, disorientation, muscle weakness or cramping, tremors, confusion, memory impairment, lethargy, or blurred vision.
PHYSICAL	
Weight	Weight is the most accurate physical assessment of F&E status. Children are usually weighed on admission to the health care facility and then daily. Generally 1 g of weight loss is equal to 1 mL of fluid loss. Observe for edema and ascites to indicate fluid gain.
General appearance	Observe for irritability, lethargy, unusual cry, or twitching.
Head	Palpate fontanels on the infant. A depressed fontanel is indicative of fluid loss, and a bulging fontanel indicates fluid gain.
Eyes	Observe for the presence of tears. Remember that tears are not present until 4 months of age. Lack of tears and sunken eyes indicate fluid loss. Periorbital edema indicates fluid gain.
Throat and mouth	Fluid loss is indicated by a dry mouth, decreased salivation, cracked lips with fissures, and furrows on the tongue. Fluid gain may be marked by increased mucus production, and edema of the tongue may leave impressions of the teeth on the child's tongue.
Cardiovascular	Observe jugular vein. A flat vein may indicate fluid loss, whereas a distended vein indicates fluid gain. A weak pulse rate greater than 160 in infants and greater than 120 in children may be related to fluid loss. The blood pressure may also be decreased in severe fluid loss. A full and bounding pulse and increased blood pressure are associated with fluid gain. A third heart sound may also be heard with fluid gain. ECG changes occur with potassium and acid-base imbalances.
Gastrointestinal/urinary	Observe the abdomen. It may be sunken in fluid loss, distended in malnutrition, and fluid-filled with ascites. Auscultate bowel sounds. In early fluid loss, there will be hyperactive bowel sounds. In later fluid loss, the sounds may be hypoactive. Describe and measure stools, vomitus, and urinary output.
Respiratory	Observe the respiratory rate and effort. Fluid gain and acid-base imbalances may cause a change in rate and effort. Auscultate the lung sounds. Moist sounds may be heard in fluid gain.
Neurologic	Assess muscle tone. Tone is likely to be increased with hypocalcemia and decreased with hypokalemia and hypercalcemia. Assess DTRs. In hypocalcemia, they are increased, and in hypercalcemia, they are decreased or absent.
Integumentary	Assess the skin's appearance. In fluid loss, it may be pale, gray, or mottled. In fluid gain, it may be red or shiny. Assess skin temperature. Skin temperature is typically decreased in fluid loss and increased in fluid gain. Assess the degree of pitting edema, if present. This is a sign of fluid gain. Assess skin turgor. Poor skin turgor is indicative of fluid loss.

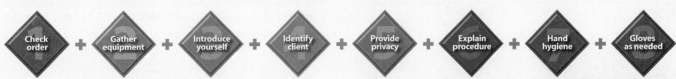
Purpose

■ To contribute to the assessment of a child's fluid and electrolyte balance

Equipment

■ Chart form
■ Specimen pan
■ Measuring cup

Check order ✛ **Gather equipment** ✛ **Introduce yourself** ✛ **Identify client** ✛ **Provide privacy** ✛ **Explain procedure** ✛ **Hand hygiene** ✛ **Gloves as needed**

Interventions and Rationales

1. Perform preparatory steps (see icon bar above).

2. Instruct parent and child to measure and record all intake and output (Figure 11-4 ■).

3. Carefully measure all oral intake such as gelatin, ice chips, ice cream, soup, juice, and water. Include fluids obtained through feeding tubes. Intake also includes IV fluids and medications, tube feedings, and blood products. Fluid requirements for children are calculated by weight (see Chapter 8 ⚭). Fluid deficit or overload can easily be identified by calculating daily intake. Children weighing 2.2 to 22 pounds (1–10 kg) should receive 100 mL/kg of fluid per day. Children weighing 22 to 44 pounds (10–20 kg) should receive 1,000 mL plus 50 mL/kg over 10 kg per day. Children weighing more than 44 pounds (20 kg) should receive 1,500 mL plus 20 mL/kg over 20 kg per day.

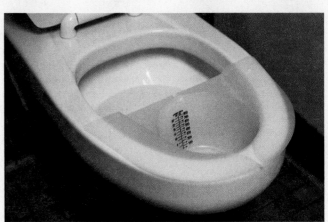

Figure 11-5. ■ A urine collection device can be placed in the toilet for children who are out of diapers.

4. Carefully measure all output, including urine (Figure 11-5 ■), diarrhea, vomitus, gastric suction, and drainage from wounds or tubes. For children in diapers, weigh diapers. One gram equals 1 mL of urine. *Fluid deficit or overload can be identified by calculating daily output. Urine output for infants and toddlers is more than 2 to 3 mL/kg/hour; for preschoolers and younger school-age children, it is more than 1 to 2 mL/kg/hour; and for older school-age children and adolescents, it is more than 0.5 mL/kg/hour.*

5. Total the intake and output for the entire shift and record on the chart form in the child's permanent record. Comparing the daily intake and output record can identify trends related to fluid and electrolyte imbalances.

SAMPLE DOCUMENTATION

(date) 1500 (Note: I&O portion of documentation only) 10-year-old boy 3 days postsurgery for appendicitis. Consumed 50% of breakfast tray, 100 mL apple juice, and 25 mL whole milk. Voided 55 mL clear, yellow urine. M. Manning, LPN

	CLIENT LABEL		
	Intake and Output Record		
INTAKE	0600-1800	1800-0600	TOTAL
Oral			
Tube feeding			
IV (primary)			
IV Meds			
TPN			
Blood			
TOTAL			24-Hour Total
OUTPUT	0600-1800	1800-0600	TOTAL
Urine			
Emesis			
G.I. Suction			
Stool			
TOTAL			24-Hour Total

Figure 11-4. ■ The intake-output chart is an important tool for monitoring fluid status.

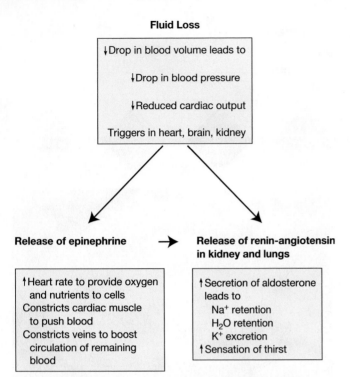

Fluid Loss

↓Drop in blood volume leads to

↓Drop in blood pressure

↓Reduced cardiac output

Triggers in heart, brain, kidney

Release of epinephrine → **Release of renin-angiotensin in kidney and lungs**

↑Heart rate to provide oxygen and nutrients to cells
Constricts cardiac muscle to push blood
Constricts veins to boost circulation of remaining blood

↑Secretion of aldosterone leads to
  Na⁺ retention
  H₂O retention
  K⁺ excretion
↑Sensation of thirst

Figure 11-6. ■ The body's response to fluid loss involves several body systems.

■ **Hypertonic dehydration** is fluid and sodium loss in which relatively more fluid than sodium is lost (as in diabetes). An excess of salt remains in the body. Fluid shifts from the intracellular space into the intravascular space.

As fluid is lost within the child's body, there is a loss of circulating fluid volume, which lowers cardiac output and blood pressure. The body tries to compensate for lack of fluid (Figure 11-6 ■). As the blood pressure lowers, triggers in the heart, kidneys, and brain increase cardiac output and sodium and water retention. These triggers also release epinephrine, which increases the heart rate, cardiac contractility, and venous constriction, increasing the circulating rate of the remaining blood volume.

Blood volume is increased through the release of renin-angiotensin (which causes the kidneys to decrease urine production). Sensors also stimulate the thirst mechanism and water retention. However, these compensatory mechanisms will fail if the dehydration is not treated promptly.

Close to 10% of pediatric hospitalizations can be attributed to some type of dehydration (Figure 11-7 ■). Isotonic dehydration is caused by vomiting and diarrhea; it can also occur during periods of food and fluid restriction, such as before and after surgery. Hypotonic dehydration is caused by gastroenteritis, burns, renal diseases, nasogastric suctioning, and inappropriate IV fluid replacement without

electrolytes. (See Chapter 21 ⊙⊙ for more discussion on burns in children.) Hypertonic dehydration is caused by diabetes or IV fluid replacement containing high concentrations of electrolytes. All forms of dehydration require attention. Some cultures have periods of fasting that may conflict with rehydration needs (Box 11-1 ■). In most cases, medical conditions exempt a person from following strict fasts.

Manifestations

Dehydration is classified by the percentage of body weight lost. Symptoms increase in severity as weight loss increases (Table 11-2 ■). In general, the child's pulse becomes rapid and may feel thready, the blood pressure drops, there is decreased urinary output and increased urine specific gravity, mucous membranes are dry, there is a lack of tears, skin turgor is poor, and an infant's fontanel is sunken. Table 11-3 ■ provides typical laboratory values for urine specific gravity and other common indicators of fluid or electrolyte imbalance.

clinical ALERT

The nurse must be aware of impending signs of shock, including a mottled, cyanotic appearance; dropping blood pressure; behavior from expressionless to restless; increasing respiratory rate with shallow breaths; and increasing blood urea nitrogen (BUN) levels.

Diagnosis

A careful history of the symptoms leading up to dehydration is essential in making a diagnosis. The nurse can also assist in gathering physical data related to dehydration. Weight loss is the most accurate physical assessment used to determine dehydration and the degree of dehydration. The weight of a pediatric client should be assessed on admission to the health care facility and then daily thereafter. Procedure 11-2 ■ describes how to calculate weight loss. See Procedure 8-2 ⊙⊙ for more about obtaining weights.

Laboratory data are also used in the diagnosis of dehydration. Loss of fluid causes concentration of the solutes within the plasma, so hemoglobin, hematocrit, glucose, BUN, creatinine, and protein levels are elevated in dehydration. The urine specific gravity is also found to be elevated.

Treatment

Treatment of dehydration is based on the degree of dehydration. Fluid and electrolyte replacement is essential. The underlying cause must also be treated. Fluid replacement can occur orally or intravenously.

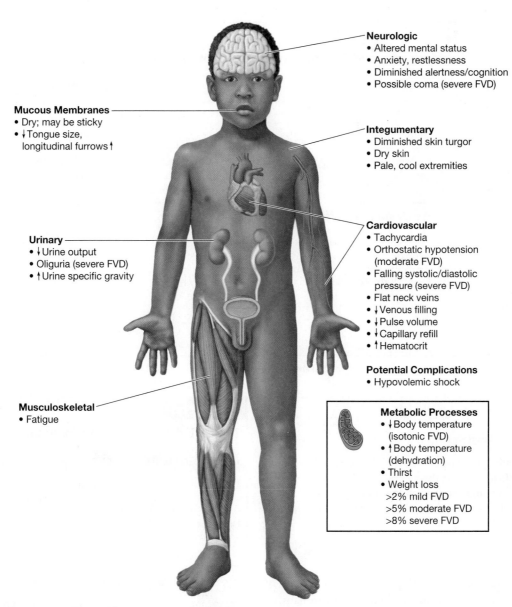

Neurologic
- Altered mental status
- Anxiety, restlessness
- Diminished alertness/cognition
- Possible coma (severe FVD)

Mucous Membranes
- Dry; may be sticky
- ↓Tongue size, longitudinal furrows↑

Integumentary
- Diminished skin turgor
- Dry skin
- Pale, cool extremities

Urinary
- ↓Urine output
- Oliguria (severe FVD)
- ↑Urine specific gravity

Cardiovascular
- Tachycardia
- Orthostatic hypotension (moderate FVD)
- Falling systolic/diastolic pressure (severe FVD)
- Flat neck veins
- ↓Venous filling
- ↓Pulse volume
- ↓Capillary refill
- ↑Hematocrit

Potential Complications
- Hypovolemic shock

Musculoskeletal
- Fatigue

Metabolic Processes
- ↓Body temperature (isotonic FVD)
- ↑Body temperature (dehydration)
- Thirst
- Weight loss
  >2% mild FVD
  >5% moderate FVD
  >8% severe FVD

Figure 11-7. ■ Multisystem effects of fluid volume deficit (FVD). Dehydration is a common cause of hospitalization in children.

TABLE 11-2

Manifestations of Mild, Moderate, and Severe Dehydration

CLINICAL ASSESSMENT	MILD	MODERATE	SEVERE
Percent of body weight lost	Up to 5% (40–50 mL/kg)	6–9% (60–90 mL/kg)	10% or more (100+ mL/kg)
Level of consciousness	Alert, restless, thirsty	Irritable or lethargic (infants and very young children); thirsty, restless (older children and adolescents)	Lethargic to comatose (infants and young children); often conscious, apprehensive (older children and adolescents)
Blood pressure	Normal	Normal or low; postural hypotension (older children and adolescents)	Low to undetectable
Pulse	Normal	Rapid	Rapid, weak to palpable

(continued)

TABLE 11-2

Manifestations of Mild, Moderate, and Severe Dehydration (continued)

CLINICAL ASSESSMENT	MILD	MODERATE	SEVERE
Skin turgor	Normal	Poor	Very poor
Mucous membranes	Moist	Dry	Parched
Urine	May appear normal	Decreased output (less than 1 mL/kg/hour), dark color; increased specific gravity	Very decreased or absent output
Thirst	Slightly increased	Moderately increased	Greatly increased unless lethargic
Fontanel	Normal	Sunken	Sunken
Extremities	Warm; normal capillary refill	Delayed capillary refill (greater than 2 seconds)	Cool, discolored; delayed capillary refill (greater than 3–4 seconds)
Respirations	Normal	Normal or rapid	Changing rate and pattern

Source: Ball, J. W., & Bindler, R. C. (2003). *Pediatric nursing: Caring for children* (3rd ed.). Upper Saddle River, NJ: Prentice Hall, p. 314, Table 10-3.

BOX 11-1 CULTURAL PULSE POINTS

Voluntary Fluid Restrictions

Muslim families require fasting or restriction of food and beverage from sunrise to sunset in the holy month of Ramadan. When a child requires oral rehydration, this tradition may become flexible. However, the devout Muslim family may have some concerns about disregarding this fast.

TABLE 11-3

Typical Laboratory Results for Infants and Children

COMPONENT TESTED	NORMAL LABORATORY VALUES
Hematocrit	Newborn: 44–65%; 1 to 3 years old: 29–40%; 4 to 10 years old: 31–43%
Urine specific gravity	Newborn: 1.001–1.020 mEq/L; Child: 1.005–1.030 mEq/L; Adolescent: 1.010–1.035 mEq/L
Blood urea nitrogen	Infant: 5–15 mg/dL; Child: 5–20 mg/dL
Potassium	Infant: 3.6–5.8 mEq/L; Child: 3.5–5.5 mEq/L; Adolescent 3.5–5.0 mEq/L
Sodium	Infant: 134–150 mEq/L; Child and Adolescent: 135–145 mEq/L
Calcium	Newborn: 3.7–7.0 mEq/L or 7.4–14.0 mg/dL; Infant: 5.0–6.0 mEq/L or 10–12 mg/dL; Child: 4.5–5.8 mEq/L or 9–11.5 mg/dL; Adolescent: 8.5–10 md/dL
Blood gases pH PaCO$_2$ HCO$_3^-$	Child: 7.36–7.44; Adolescent 7.35–7.45 Child and Adolescent 35–45 mm Hg Child and Adolescent 22–26 mEq/L

Note: Lab values may vary. Consult the laboratory at your health care agency.

ORAL FLUID REPLACEMENT. Teach parents the importance of maintaining oral hydration in children. On warm days, children may lose enough fluid through the skin and respiration to become dehydrated. Because of limited communication skills, they may have difficulty knowing they are thirsty or requesting a drink of water. Parents should develop a habit of offering water hourly, especially on hot days.

If it has been determined the child is dehydrated, fluid replacement must be started. Oral rehydration is ideal because it is the most natural and least invasive. Box 11-2 ■ highlights important information about fluid requirements and oral rehydration amounts by different weights in children.

The nurse and parents will need to be creative in administering oral fluids. Children often prefer sweetened flavored solutions such as Popsicles®, gelatin, decarbonated cola, or ginger ale. However, these can make diarrhea worse because of the osmotic effect of the sugar. When used, they should be diluted by 50%. Commercially prepared oral replacement solutions are preferred because they contain necessary electrolytes and less sugar. Some choices are listed in Box 11-3 ■. If the child's condition worsens or does not improve after 4 hours of oral fluid replacement, the doctor should be consulted.

| PROCEDURE 11-2 | **Calculating Weight Loss** |

Purpose

- To contribute to the assessment of a child's fluid and electrolyte imbalance, particularly fluid loss

Equipment

- Calibrated scale
- Documentation of child's previous weight

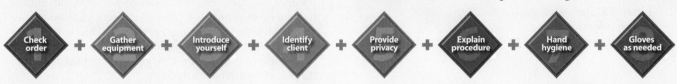

Interventions and Rationales

1. Perform preparatory steps (see icon bar above).
2. Review documentation of the child's previous weight.
3. Weigh the child on a calibrated scale in the same manner as the child was weighed previously (e.g., without shoes or with clothes; before or after meals; and using the same scale if available). *Changing these variables can give a false reading about changes in weight.*
4. Subtract the child's current weight from the previous weight.
5. Divide this value by the child's previous weight to obtain the percentage of weight loss. For example:

    Previous weight: 25 lb

    Current weight: 20 lb

$25 - 20 = 5$

Weight loss: 5 lb

$5/25 = 0.20 = 20\%$

Percent weight loss: 20%

SAMPLE DOCUMENTATION

(date) 0800   5-year-old male child. Admission weight 40 lb. Current weight, day 5 of hospitalization, 38 lb. Percent weight loss = 5%. W. Smartt, LVN

BOX 11-2

Fluid Requirements in Children and Oral Rehydration

Fluid Requirements

- Fluid requirements for children are calculated by weight (see Chapter 8).
- Children weighing 2.2 to 22 pounds (1–10 kg) should receive 100 mL/kg of fluid daily.
- Children weighing 22 to 44 pounds (10–20 kg) should receive 1,000 mL plus 50 mL/kg over 10 kg per day.
- Children weighing more than 44 pounds (20 kg) should receive 1,500 mL plus 20 mL/kg over 20 kg per day.

Oral Rehydration Amounts

- Fluids are given by mouth in small amounts frequently, for example, 1 to 2 tsp (5–10 mL) every 10 to 15 minutes. Continue giving oral fluids even if the child

vomits because some of the fluid might be absorbed.

- For mild dehydration, the child should be given almost 1 fluid ounce per pound (50 mL/kg) of body weight every 4 hours, plus the amount of fluid lost by vomiting and/or diarrhea during the same time.
- For moderate dehydration, the child should be given about 2 fluid ounces per pound (100 mL/kg) of body weight every 4 hours plus the amount lost through emesis and/or stool.
- For severe dehydration, the child is hospitalized, and fluids are given intravenously.

BOX 11-3 NUTRITION THERAPY

Commercial Rehydration Agents

Oral Agents

Pedialyte, Rehydralyte, Infalyte, Oral Maintenance Solution—for mild to moderate dehydration

Intravenous Agents

Normal saline—isotonic solution for restoring water and sodium

Lactated Ringer's—isotonic solution for burns, bleeding, and prolonged diarrhea

D_5W—isotonic solution for fluid loss and hypernatremia

BOX 11-4 LIFE SPAN CONSIDERATIONS

Overcoming Fear of IV Insertion in Toddlers

The initiation of intravenous therapy can cause fear and anxiety in toddlers. To help children understand that this therapy will help and not hurt them, provide a straw and a glass of water. Have the child take a drink. Ask where the water went when he or she took a drink. Explain that when the body needs a special type of drink, you need to put a tiny straw in the arm to bring the drink into the body. Enlist the parents to assist with distraction during the procedure. Parents can use toys, video games, music, or television to focus the child's attention. Another nurse should assist in keeping the child still during the procedure. With proper preparation, the child's anxiety can be reduced and the procedure can be successful.

INTRAVENOUS FLUID REPLACEMENT. When severe dehydration has occurred, the child should be hospitalized and IV fluid administered. Because children have small veins, inserting an IV needle can be a challenge. Younger children especially can be traumatized by IV insertion. Box 11-4 ▪ provides some suggestions for communicating with younger children about IV insertion. Figure 11-8 ▪ shows alternative pediatric IV sites. In some areas, the initiation of IV therapy is not an LPN/LVN function. However, assisting with the monitoring of the infusion might be required. The nurse must know and follow the state's nurse practice act and facility policy.

The needle is protected to prevent infiltration and the need to change sites. Padded limb boards and limb restraints may be needed to protect the child and prevent the needle from becoming dislodged (see Figure 8-43 ⚭). An IV infusion control device is used to prevent too rapid administration of fluids. This device should be locked to prevent accidental adjustment of the rate of infusion. Usually the rate is most rapid for the first few hours and then the rate is decreased. Careful frequent monitoring of the rate, site, and reaction to the therapy is essential. See Procedure 8-38 ⚭ for more information.

Excess Fluid Volume (Hypervolemia)

Fluid volume excess (FVE) occurs when there is retention of fluid and, in some cases, sodium in the extracellular compartment. It may also be called **hypervolemia**. FVE may arise due to cardiac disorders such as congestive heart failure and renal disorders. The affected child may also be taking glucocorticoids. FVE may also be caused by an overload of IV fluids, particularly those containing sodium (Figure 11-9 ▪). Low protein intake and high sodium intake might also cause FVE.

Manifestations

Symptoms of FVE include acute weight gain and edema. Edema is usually generalized in infants and *dependent* (occurring in lower legs, feet, or other areas affected by gravity) in children. The child's vital signs change. The pulse becomes fast and bounding. The blood pressure and respiratory rate increase. The child may also become

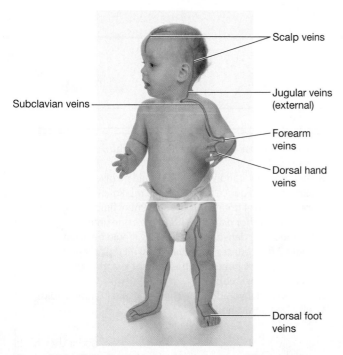

Scalp veins

Jugular veins (external)

Subclavian veins

Forearm veins

Dorsal hand veins

Dorsal foot veins

Figure 11-8. ▪ Pediatric access sites are more difficult to use because of the small size of the veins.

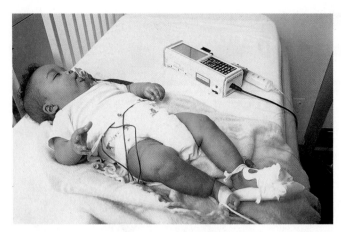

Figure 11-9. ■ If isotonic fluid containing sodium is given too rapidly or in too large an amount, an extracellular fluid volume excess will develop. It is important to monitor fluid intake, excretion, and retention in infants and children.

dyspneic. On auscultation to the chest, crackles are heard. Urine output may also increase.

Diagnosis

Diagnosis of FVE is usually made by symptom recognition, especially weight gain. The following lab results may also be associated with FVE:

- Decreased hematocrit (HCT)
- Decreased urine specific gravity
- Decreased BUN.

The lab values are due to hemodilution. Fluid may be seen in the lungs on x-ray.

Treatment

Medical treatment of hypervolemia is primarily focused on treating the cause of the condition. Other treatments may include sodium and fluid restriction, as well as diuretic administration to promote fluid loss. In severe cases, hemodialysis may be required.

Nursing Considerations

Accurate measure of daily weight and careful documentation of the child's intake and output are important nursing interventions. The nurse must carefully explain and monitor fluid and sodium restrictions. Foods containing sodium must be discussed with the parent and child. Edematous tissue is fragile; therefore, careful nursing attention should be given to promoting skin integrity. If the child is dyspneic, the nurse can promote breathing by elevating the head of the bed (HOB) to 30 degrees, loosening restrictive clothing, and administering oxygen as ordered.

clinical ALERT

Hypervolemia can progress to pulmonary edema. The nurse needs to be alert and must quickly recognize symptoms of pulmonary edema. These include restlessness, tachypnea, labored breathing, a full and bounding pulse or a weak and thready pulse, possible crackles on lung auscultation, and profuse diaphoresis. This condition is considered to be a medical emergency. The nurse must position the child to facilitate breathing and contact the physician promptly. Narcotics, diuretics, and bronchodilators may be ordered. Careful attention must be given to avoid complicating the child's condition with an overload of IV fluid. (See more on listening to the heart in Chapter 8, Procedure 8-2, and Chapter 13. See more on lung conditions in Chapter 12 ⚭.)

Sodium Imbalance

Sodium is found in high levels in extracellular fluid and in lower levels in intracellular fluid. Each cell is equipped with a sodium-potassium pump (see Figure 11-3D) that maintains sodium concentrations. Otherwise, the laws of diffusion would cause movement of the sodium outside the cell into the area of lower concentration (inside the cell).

HYPONATREMIA

Hyponatremia is a state of sodium deficit related to the body's water. It is caused by excessive water gain or excessive sodium loss. Excessive water intake can occur in:

- IV fluid overload, especially with hypotonic solutions
- Children with congestive heart failure
- Overuse of tap-water enemas
- Oral ingestion of excessive tap water; infants are particularly at risk for hyponatremia if parents are diluting formula incorrectly and because their thirst mechanism is not developed fully.

Excessive sodium loss can occur in diarrhea, vomiting, cystic fibrosis, burns, and renal disease.

Manifestations

Hyponatremia is manifested as headaches, lethargy, confusion, muscle weakness, and decreased deep tendon reflexes. In severe cases the child may develop seizures, and lethargy may progress to coma.

Diagnosis

Lab values related to hyponatremia are sodium levels below normal limits for the age group, decreased urine specific gravity, and serum osmolality greater than 280 mOsm/kg.

Treatment

Mild hyponatremia is treated by fluid restriction, oral sodium supplements, isotonic IV solutions, and a diet high in sodium. More severe cases require a hypertonic IV solution, diuretics, and admission to the intensive care unit.

PROCEDURE 11-3 Assisting with Fluid Restriction

Purpose

- To assist children who have excesses in fluid volume to limit oral intake

Equipment

- Measuring cups

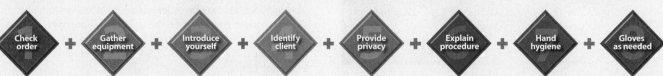

Interventions and Rationales

1. Perform preparatory steps (see icon bar above).
2. Explain the rationale for the restriction to the child and the parent. *Compliance can be increased when a connection can be made between the restriction and the restoration of health.*
3. State clearly the amount of fluid, if any, permissible in a 24-hour period. Post signs in the child's room to alert other health care personnel.
4. Inform the child and parent that ice chips, gelatin, ice cream, and broth are considered to be fluid intake.
5. Develop a plan that will allow the child to have fluids throughout the day. Consult the child and parent when devising this plan. Be sure to include oral intake required to swallow medications and brush the teeth. *Children are typically more active between 7:00 a.m. and 3:00 p.m., so more oral intake is needed during these hours.*
6. Monitor oral hygiene carefully. *Limited fluid intake or the restriction of fluid intake dries the mucous membranes and puts the child at risk for cracking and drying of the lips and mouth.*
7. Provide distraction activities. *A child who is not busy may focus on the desire for oral intake. Distraction activities such as group games, videos, or special toys may assist the child in managing fluid restrictions.*

8. Record fluid intake. *Documenting the oral intake improves patient compliance and assists health care personnel in appropriately managing oral intake.*

SAMPLE DOCUMENTATION

(date) 0700   Fluid restriction of 1,000 mL ordered. Discussed fluid restriction with child and parent. Plan of care developed: 240 mL breakfast, 100 mL midmorning snack, 240 mL lunch, 100 mL afternoon snack, 20 mL medication administration, 240 mL dinner, 20 mL medication administration, 40 mL bedtime snack. Signs posted above bed and on client's door.
L. Lowman, LPN

Nursing Considerations

Children with hyponatremia are at risk for injury due to muscle weakness and possible seizure activity. The nurse must provide a safe environment and watch carefully for seizures. Parents and children need to be taught about fluid restriction (Procedure 11-3 ■). Monitoring and documentation of vital signs, intake and output, and lab values are important interventions for the child with hyponatremia.

HYPERNATREMIA

Hypernatremia is a state of sodium excess related to the body's water. The thirst mechanism is the body's best line of defense against hypernatremia. Infants or children who cannot react to thirst are vulnerable.

Hypernatremia can be caused by excessive administration of a hypertonic IV solution. Excessive water losses from diarrhea, burns, and pulmonary infections also cause hypernatremia.

Manifestations

Symptoms of hypernatremia are most commonly thirst and neurologic symptoms. Restlessness, confusion, stupor, seizures, and coma may occur. The child may also have dry mucous membranes, a low-grade fever, oliguria, and flushed skin.

Diagnosis

Lab values include serum sodium levels greater than expected for the age group and increased or decreased urine specific gravity, depending on the cause.

Treatment

Medical management of hypernatremia includes oral and IV rehydration. This must occur gradually to avoid a rapid shifting of water into the brain cells, causing cerebral edema. The child may be placed on a low-sodium diet, and diuretics may be administered.

Nursing Considerations

Assist the child and the parents with oral rehydration by providing a variety of fluids and encouraging them to set a schedule for oral intake. The nurse can assist the child in making appropriate low-sodium diet choices. Oral hygiene and moisturizer for the child's mouth should be provided frequently because of dry mucous membranes. The nurse should observe closely for symptoms of fluid overload. Seizure precautions and other safety measures are necessary when the child's neurologic status is compromised.

Potassium Imbalance

HYPOKALEMIA

Hypokalemia occurs when there is a decrease in serum potassium levels to below normal range. Potassium loss can be caused by increased excretion, decreased intake, a shift into the cells from the extracellular fluid, and loss of potassium by vomiting or nasogastric suctioning. Hypokalemia is also related to inappropriate use of diuretics, diarrhea, alkalosis, anorexia nervosa, bulimia, and hypomagnesemia. Children who have ingested large amounts of black licorice may be at risk for hypokalemia because the candy increases renal excretion of potassium.

Manifestations

Clinical manifestations of hypokalemia include weakness, fatigue, intestinal distention, polyuria, and cardiac irregularities (Figure 11-10 ■). Serum potassium levels will be decreased according to the child's age (see Table 11-3).

Diagnosis

Diagnosis of hypokalemia is made by reviewing symptoms and laboratory values of potassium.

Treatment

Medical management of hypokalemia is focused on treating the causative factor. Potassium is replaced orally or intravenously. Prompt management of hypokalemia will avoid life-threatening complications.

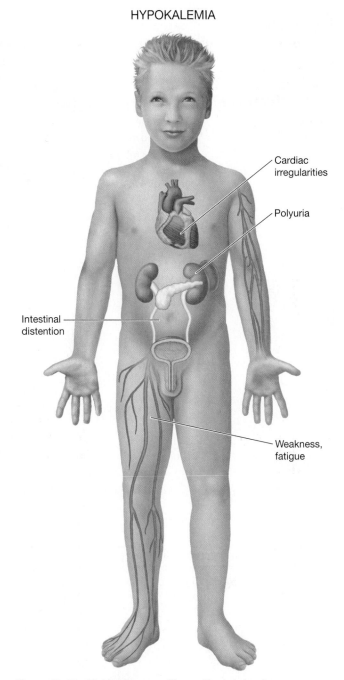

HYPOKALEMIA

Cardiac irregularities

Polyuria

Intestinal distention

Weakness, fatigue

Figure 11-10. ■ Multisystem effects of hypokalemia.

Nursing Considerations

Priority nursing interventions will include replacing potassium, as ordered, either orally or intravenously. Table 11-4 ■ provides more information about potassium supplementation. Children and their parents will also need to be taught about increasing potassium in the diet. The nurse teaches about foods containing potassium and ways to incorporate them into the diet (Box 11-5 ■).

Because potassium imbalances have the potential to affect cardiac and respiratory status, the nurse must vigilantly monitor the child's pulse and respiratory rate and

TABLE 11-4				
Pharmacology: Drugs for Replacing or Removing Potassium				
DRUG (GENERIC AND COMMON BRAND NAME)	**USUAL ROUTE/DOSE**	**CLASSIFICATION AND PURPOSE**	**SELECTED SIDE EFFECTS**	**DO NOT GIVE IF**
Potassium chloride (Klor)	PO: 1–3 mEq/kg/day in divided doses IV: up to 3 mEq/kg/d at less than 0.02 mEq/kg/minute	Potassium supplement used to treat hypokalemia due to vomiting, diarrhea, diuresis	Nausea, vomiting, ECG changes	Urine output is not within normal limits for age group. PO: dilute in water or juice; instruct child not to crush or chew. IV: Never give IV push. Dilute carefully before administering. Mix well. Any signs of blood vessel irritation occur. Stop infusion immediately with recognition of symptoms.
Sodium polystyrene sulfonate (Kayexalate)	PO 1 g/kg every 6 hours PR 1 g/kg every 2–6 hours	Sulfonic cation-exchange resin that removes potassium from body by exchange of sodium ion for potassium, especially in large intestine; resin is excreted	May cause gastric upset, sodium retention, hypocalcemia, hypokalemia, hypomagnesemia	Child shows clinical signs of hypokalemia Child has hypersensitivity to the drug Client cannot tolerate even a small increase in sodium load (e.g., congestive heart failure)

BOX 11-5   NUTRITION THERAPY

Foods High in Potassium

- Apricots
- Bananas
- Cantaloupe
- Carrots
- Dates
- Fish
- Meat
- Milk and milk products
- Oranges
- Peas
- Potatoes
- Raisins
- Spinach
- Tomatoes

rhythm. If electrocardiogram (ECG) monitoring is ordered, it must be observed closely as well.

The nurse must also keep strict intake and output records. Imbalances should be reported promptly. The effects of hypokalemia may cause the child to be at risk for injury. Safety measures should be implemented.

HYPERKALEMIA

Hyperkalemia occurs when there is an increase above normal range in serum potassium levels. Hyperkalemia is associated with renal dysfunction and failure, burns, sickle cell anemia, blood transfusions, prematurity, severe hypovolemia, lead poisoning, and acidosis. It can also be the result of an excessive IV infusion of potassium supplementation.

Manifestations

Clinical manifestations for hyperkalemia include anxiety, hypotension, dysrrhythmias, diarrhea, weakness, and cardiac arrhythmias progressing to cardiac arrest.

Diagnosis

Serum potassium levels will be increased according to the child's age (see Table 11-1). Diagnosis of hyperkalemia is made by reviewing symptoms and laboratory values of potassium.

Treatment

Medical management for hyperkalemia includes restricting intake of potassium. Kayexalate may be given to promote excretion of potassium. Peritoneal dialysis may also be necessary. IV calcium gluconate may be given to decrease cardiac effects. Insulin and glucose or sodium bicarbonate may be ordered to promote shifting of potassium into the cells.

Nursing Considerations

When caring for a child with hyperkalemia, the nurse will closely monitor serum potassium values and report imbalances promptly. Because potassium imbalances have the potential to affect cardiac and respiratory status, the nurse must vigilantly monitor the child's pulse and respiratory rate and rhythm. If ECG monitoring is ordered, it must be closely observed as well.

Kayexalate causes bowel excretion of potassium. Frequent hygiene must become a priority nursing action. This will facilitate the child's comfort and protect skin integrity.

Calcium Imbalance

HYPOCALCEMIA

Hypocalcemia is characterized by decreased serum calcium levels below normal levels. The condition may be caused by poor dietary intake of calcium accompanied by lack of vitamin D intake, lack of exposure to sunlight, surgical removal of the parathyroid, acute pancreatitis, and steatorrhea. The child who receives multiple blood transfusions is at risk for hypocalcemia. This is because citrate, which is a preservative in the blood, competes for calcium-binding sites; it causes calcium to be flushed through the body without being metabolized. Medications associated with hypocalcemia include overuse of antacids and laxatives, anticonvulsants, antineoplastics, and

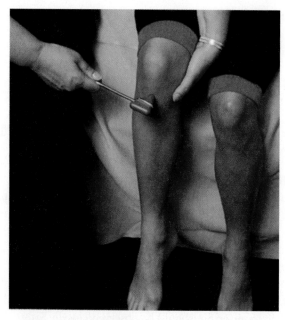

Figure 11-11. ■ The child with hypocalcemia may exhibit increased deep tendon reflexes.

phosphate-containing preparations. Hypocalcemia is also seen in the premature newborn. The exact cause is unknown but may be related to periods of asphyxia and resulting calcitonin levels increasing. Table 11-5 ■ provides a comparison of the causes of hypo- and hypercalcemia.

Manifestations

Clinical manifestations of hypocalcemia include numbness and tingling in the fingers and around the mouth, muscle cramps, pathologic fractures, and increased deep tendon reflexes (DTRs) (Figure 11-11 ■). The newborn with hypocalcemia may develop congestive heart failure.

TABLE 11-5		
Causes of Hypocalcemia and Hypercalcemia		
RELATED FACTOR	**HYPOCALCEMIA**	**HYPERCALCEMIA**
Vitamin D	Lack of dietary calcium and vitamin D	Overdose
Endocrine imbalance	Hypoparathyroidism	Hyperparathyroidism
Disease or disorder	Malabsorption Chronic renal insufficiency Chronic diarrhea Alkalosis	Bone tumors and other cancers
Medications/drugs	Laxative abuse	Thiazide diuretics
Medical procedure	Rapid infusion of plasma expanders Large blood transfusion (citrated blood)	—
Congenital basis	—	Familial hypercalcemia

Diagnosis

Serum calcium levels will be decreased for the child's age (see Table 11-1).

Treatment

Medical management of hypocalcemia includes administering calcium supplementation orally or intravenously. Vitamin D supplementation may also be prescribed. The child should also have a diet high in calcium.

Nursing Considerations

The nurse should slowly administer calcium gluconate diluted in D_5W. Rapid IV infusion may cause dizziness, hypotension, and cardiac arrhythmias. Monitor the child's IV site carefully for infiltration, which can cause tissue sloughing and necrosis. In an effort to decrease GI upset, the nurse should give PO calcium at least 1 hour after meals or administer it with milk. Vital signs, including cardiac monitoring, should be observed closely. Safety measures and seizure precautions are important to implement.

HYPERCALCEMIA

Hypercalcemia is a condition characterized by an increase in serum calcium above normal levels. The condition may be caused by hyperparathyroidism, prolonged immobilization, leukemia, bone tumors, and intake of excessive calcium, including total parenteral nutrition with excessive calcium content.

Manifestations

Clinical manifestations of hypercalcemia include decreased muscle tone, nausea, vomiting, weakness, decreased level of consciousness (LOC), renal calculi, cardiac arrhythmias, and possible cardiac arrest.

Diagnosis

Serum calcium levels will be increased according to the child's age (see Table 11-1).

Treatment

Medical management of hypercalcemia includes hydration to encourage excretion of calcium through diuresis. Diuretics may also be administered. Glucocorticoids may be used to decrease intestinal absorption of calcium and bone resorption. Dialysis may be necessary to facilitate removal of calcium.

Nursing Considerations

The nurse caring for a child with hypercalcemia should promote adequate fluid intake to keep urine dilute and to prevent constipation. It may be necessary to strain urine for calculi. The child with hypercalcemia is at risk for falls due to weakness. The nurse should ambulate the child with care and promote safety measures.

NURSING CARE
PRIORITIES IN NURSING CARE

When caring for a child with fluid and electrolyte imbalances, priority must be given to monitoring daily weight, intake and output, and lab values. Even slight variations in these objective findings could be significant in children. The nurse will need to report variations immediately to the health care provider in order for the child to receive prompt care. Communicating on an age-appropriate level with increased compliance (Table 11-6 ■).

TABLE 11-6				
Communicating Across the Life Span: Child with Hypovolemia				
	TODDLER	**PRESCHOOLER**	**SCHOOL-AGE CHILD**	**ADOLESCENT**
Nurse	To the parent, "What types of beverages does your child like? It is important to strongly encourage the child to drink adequate amounts of fluid."	To the child, "Would you like a juice box or a sport drink? I'm going to bring you something else to drink after you watch this cartoon."	To the child, "The diarrhea has caused your body to lose important fluid. If you will drink a lot this will replace the lost fluid. What can I bring you to drink?"	To the teenager, "You will need to drink fluids to replace those lost when you have diarrhea. Water or a sport drink every hour will protect your body."
Client	"I like juice."	"I'm so thirsty."	"I'll try to drink enough water and lemonade."	"I'd really rather have colas, but I guess that's too many colas in one day."

ASSESSING

The nurse needs to obtain adequate baseline vital signs, weight, and physical assessment data. These findings are then compared to data obtained throughout the course of the illness. Closely monitor changes in skin turgor, edema, moisture in mucous membranes, and lung sounds. Review the child's hematocrit, hemoglobin, urine specific gravity, BUN, creatinine, and electrolyte studies. Once treatment has begun, an improvement in these values should be demonstrated.

DIAGNOSING, PLANNING, AND IMPLEMENTING

Nursing diagnoses for fluid and electrolyte imbalances might include:

- Deficient **F**luid Volume related to excessive GI loss
- Excess **F**luid Volume related to excessive accumulation of fluid
- Imbalanced **N**utrition: Less than Body Requirements related to inadequate intake
- Impaired **S**kin Integrity related to irritation caused by diarrhea

Some outcomes for fluid and electrolyte imbalances are as follows. The child will:

- Exhibit symptoms of hydration to include moist mucous membranes, proper skin turgor, and vital signs WNL.
- Demonstrate symptoms of fluid balance to include lack of edema, vital signs and electrolyte values WNL.
- Maintain caloric and fluid intake, appropriate for weight and age.
- Maintain intact skin.

The nurse's role in providing support to these clients would include the following nursing interventions:

- Administer oral rehydration as ordered. *Oral fluids replace fluid losses but must be given slowly, in small amounts, to children with vomiting and diarrhea.*
- Assist with IV rehydration as ordered (see Procedure 8-22 ⊙⊙). *IV rehydration allows for more rapid fluid replacement when the child is severely dehydrated.*
- Monitor IV infusion closely. *Fluid overload could occur with rapid infusion of IV fluids.*
- Teach parents how to recognize signs and symptoms of fluid loss. *Timely recognition of symptoms will facilitate treatment.*
- Teach parents the appropriate method of oral rehydration (see Box 11-2). *Parents who recognize early symptoms of fluid loss can initiate rehydration early and possibly avoid severe imbalances.*
- Administer diuretics as ordered and monitor effectiveness. *Diuretics assist in removing excess fluid.*

- Assist the child and the parents in restricting fluids, if ordered. *Compliance will be improved if the child assists in planning for fluid restriction.*
- Ensure that the child changes position every 2 hours. *Edematous skin tears easily. Position changes will prevent skin breakdown.*
- Advance diet slowly, as ordered. *Food needs to be reintroduced slowly to avoid GI distress. Initial foods should be low in fiber and bland.*
- Encourage breastfeeding mothers to resume feedings. *Breast milk reduces the severity of the imbalance.*
- In infants with diarrhea, change the diaper frequently. *The diarrhea stool may contain excessive acid and irritate the skin.*
- Use a mild soap and water to cleanse the perineal area with each diaper change. *Soaps with high alcohol content and fragrances or commercial baby wipes may further irritate the skin.*
- Apply protective ointment as ordered. *Ointments can provide a moisture barrier to protect the skin.*

EVALUATING

Expected outcomes for a client with fluid and electrolyte include return of adequate hydration, weight gain or weight loss, and intact skin. The nurse can accurately evaluate these outcomes by monitoring vital signs, intake and output, lab values, and symptoms related to the imbalances. Documentation should include response to client teaching, tolerance to rehydration and diet changes, physical findings related to the imbalance, daily intake and output, daily weight, and lab values. Lack of response to treatment and worsening of symptoms must be reported to the charge nurse or physician promptly.

NURSING PROCESS CARE PLAN
Client with Diarrhea

Wesley is a 3-month-old infant who is formula fed. He is typically a pleasant child who has regular bowel habits. His big brother, Mark, has been home from school with a stomach virus this week. Today, after his morning bottle, Wesley has had several loose stools and is irritable when awake. His mother calls the pediatrician's office for advice.

Assessment.   The nurse should gather the following data during the phone call:

- Changes in diet by obtaining a 24-hour diet history
- Onset of diarrhea
- Color, consistency, frequency, amount, and odor of stools
- The presence of mucus in the stools
- Associated symptoms such as vomiting, fever, and lethargy.

When the child is seen in the pediatrician's office, gather the following data:

- Current weight
- Vital signs
- Skin turgor and texture
- Presence of skin breakdown in diaper area
- Bowel sounds
- Abdominal distension (by measuring abdominal circumference).

Nursing Diagnosis. The following important nursing diagnosis (among others) is established for this client:

- Deficient **F**luid Volume related to active fluid loss

Expected Outcomes

- The child will have balanced intake and output in the next 24 hours.
- The child will have adequate hydration, as evidenced by moist mucous membranes, good skin turgor, lab values, and vital signs within normal limits.

Planning and Implementation

- Obtain daily weight. *This provides important data for determining fluid status.*
- Maintain strict record of intake and output during each shift. *This provides important data for determining fluid status.*
- Document and review vital signs as ordered. Report abnormal values promptly. *Abnormal values may signal complications.*
- Review serum electrolytes, urine specific gravity, BUN, creatinine, and hematocrit lab values during each shift. Report abnormal values promptly. *Abnormal values must be addressed, because imbalances can be life threatening.*

- Carefully administer oral and IV fluids, as ordered. *Fluid balance can be affected by intravenous and oral fluid intake. Even slight variations from the ordered amount could compromise the child's health.*
- Provide frequent perineal hygiene. *Diarrhea could lead to impaired skin integrity.*
- Provide frequent oral hygiene. *Frequent oral care provides comfort and helps to lessen dryness of the mouth and mucous membranes.*
- Instruct parent in recognition of symptoms of fluid volume deficit and management techniques (see Box 11-2). *Client teaching is important for parents, both for follow-up care and for handling future situations appropriately.*

Evaluation. The child's intake and output are balanced. Return of hydration is evident in mucous membranes, skin turgor, lab values, and vital signs. The child's bowel and bladder habits return to normal.

Critical Thinking in the Nursing Process

1. A dangerous risk of diarrhea in a child is hypovolemic shock. How would the nurse recognize hypovolemic shock?
2. Wesley's mother asks if the formula caused her son's diarrhea. She wants to know if she should change formulas. What is the most appropriate nursing response?
3. Wesley's mother wonders if his brother gave him the stomach virus. She does not understand how this could have happened because they do not share eating utensils. What does she need to be taught about the spread of infectious diarrhea?

Note: Discussion of Critical Thinking questions appears in Appendix I.

ACID-BASE DISORDERS

Principles Related to Acid-Base Disorders

The principle of homeostasis, or balance, also applies to the balance of hydrogen ion concentration within the body. The concentration has 1 part carbonic acid (H_2CO_3) to 20 parts bicarbonate (HCO_3^-) (Figure 11-12 ■). Homeostasis of the hydrogen ion is measured by determining the pH of the blood. Normal blood pH for a child is 7.36 to 7.44. The condition of **acidosis** develops when there is an increase of hydrogen ion concentration. In acidosis, the body's pH will be less than 7.36. The condition of **alkalosis** develops when there is a decrease of hydrogen ion concentration. In alkalosis, the body's pH will be greater than 7.44.

When pH levels become abnormal, certain body mechanisms are initiated in an effort to correct the abnormal value

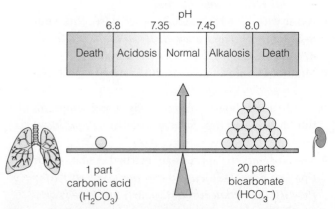

Figure 11-12. ■ The normal ratio of bicarbonate to carbonic acid is 20:1. As long as this ratio is maintained, the pH remains within the normal range of 7.35 to 7.45.

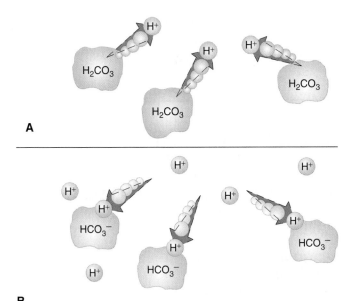

B

Figure 11-13. ■ Buffer response to acid-base. (**A**) The way in which buffers respond to an excess of base. If the blood has too much base, the acid portion of a buffer pair (e.g., H_2CO_3 of the bicarbonate buffer system) releases hydrogen ions (H^+) to help return the pH to normal. (**B**) The way in which buffers respond to an excess of acid. If the blood has too much acid, the base portion of a buffer pair (e.g., HCO_3^- of the bicarbonate buffer system) takes up hydrogen ions (H^+) to help return the pH to normal.

and restore the child's acid-base balance. There are three body mechanisms that compensate for abnormal pH levels: the buffer system, the respiratory system, and the renal system.

BUFFER SYSTEM

The buffer system is activated within seconds of detecting the abnormal value. The buffer system uses various chemicals such as bicarbonate, phosphate, hemoglobin, and protein to compensate for imbalances. Chemical reactions either rid the body of excess hydrogen ion or seek to conserve hydrogen ion when there is a hydrogen deficit (Figure 11-13 ■).

RESPIRATORY SYSTEM

The respiratory system is activated next, usually within minutes of a detectable imbalance. Normal respiration involves breathing in oxygen and breathing out carbon dioxide (CO_2) and water. CO_2 is continuously formed in the body. It moves out of the cells and into the interstitial fluids, then into the intravascular fluid. It is transported through the venous system to the lungs and is exhaled from the body.

If CO_2 becomes excessive, the CO_2 combines with body water and forms an acid. This chemical reaction causes a decrease in the body's pH. The body recognizes the imbalance and stimulates the respiratory system to increase the rate and depth of respirations to "blow off" excess CO_2.

If CO_2 is deficient, there is less than normal CO_2 to mix with water and form the acid the body needs. In this case, the

body's pH increases. The body recognizes the imbalance and decreases the rate and depth of respirations, conserving CO_2.

RENAL SYSTEM

The final compensation method to occur takes place in the renal system. It may take several days for this method to be initiated. When a person is healthy, the kidneys excrete more hydrogen ion and conserve bicarbonate (hydroxide). A normal, healthy person's urine has a pH of 6.

However, when there is too much hydrogen ion in the blood, the body will increase urinary output. When this occurs, there is more hydrogen ion in the urine than normal, making the urine pH less than 6. When there is too little hydrogen ion in the blood, the body will decrease urinary output. In this case, there is less hydrogen ion in the urine than normal, making the urine pH increased, or greater than 6.

ARTERIAL BLOOD GAS ANALYSIS

Arterial blood gas (ABG) analysis is an essential part of the data used to assess acid-base imbalances. ABG actually determines the functioning of the respiratory system. The nurse needs to understand the analysis process and be able to detect imbalances so they can be reported promptly. Table 11-3 lists normal values related to arterial blood gases.

ABG specimens may be obtained by an RN, lab technician, or respiratory technician. They are usually drawn from an arterial site such as the radial, brachial, or femoral artery. A heparinized syringe is used to avoid clotting of the specimen. Care must be taken not to allow air to enter the syringe. If air in the environment mixed with the blood specimen, it would alter the gas content of the blood. To reduce metabolism of the cells, the syringe containing the specimen is submerged in crushed ice and is taken to the lab immediately.

To analyze ABG results accurately, memorize the following principles:

- pH measures the hydrogen ion concentration of the specimen.
- $PaCO_2$ measures the partial pressure of the CO_2 in arterial blood. This is an indication of the effectiveness of ventilation.
- HCO_3^- measures the metabolic content of the arterial blood.
- The pH and $PaCO_2$ values move in opposite directions when the client has a respiratory condition. For example, pH 7.33 and $PaCO_2$ 51 indicates respiratory acidosis.
- The pH and HCO_2 values move in the same direction when the client has a metabolic condition. For example, pH 7.51 and HCO_3^- 28 indicates metabolic alkalosis. Box 11-6 ■ provides steps for reviewing ABG lab results.

Practice in ABG Analysis

Here are five examples of ABG results. *After reading Box 11-6, test your knowledge by covering the answers with a book or paper and writing the condition after each set of data.*

BOX 11-6	NURSING CARE CHECKLIST

Reviewing ABG Results

Follow these steps when reviewing ABG results:

☑ Review the pH to determine acidosis or alkalosis. pH less than 7.36 indicates acidosis; pH greater than 7.44 indicates alkalosis.

☑ Review the $PaCO_2$. Is it normal? Remember the principle: The pH and $PaCO_2$ values move in opposite directions when the client has a respiratory condition. For example, a respiratory condition is indicated when the pH is increased and the $PaCO_2$ is decreased or when the pH is decreased and the $PaCO_2$ is increased.

☑ Review the HCO_3^-. Is it normal? Remember the principle: The pH and HCO_3^- values move in the same direction when the client has a metabolic condition. For example, a metabolic condition is indicated when the pH and HCO_3^- are both increased or when pH and the HCO_3^- are both decreased.

☑ If all three values are abnormal, the body is compensating for the imbalance.

1. pH 7.34, $PaCO_2$ 50, HCO_3^- 22 _____
2. pH 7.33, $PaCO_2$ 44, HCO_3^- 20 _____
3. pH 7.46, $PaCO_2$ 45, HCO_3^- 30 _____
4. pH 7.47, $PaCO_2$ 33, HCO_3^- 25 _____
5. pH 7.33, $PaCO_2$ 50, HCO_3^- 30 _____

Answers:

1. respiratory acidosis
2. metabolic acidosis
3. metabolic alkalosis
4. respiratory alkalosis
5. respiratory acidosis with compensation

Respiratory Acidosis

Respiratory acidosis is an accumulation of CO_2 caused by states of hypoventilation, altered perfusion, or inadequate respiratory diffusion. In children, respiratory acidosis can be caused by airway obstruction resulting in CO_2 retention. As CO_2 builds, the pH decreases. The body seeks to compensate for this imbalance by increasing the rate and depth of respiration. The kidneys also conserve bicarbonate in an effort to raise the body's pH.

Respiratory acidosis is associated with diseases that impair the child's ability to breathe normally. These diseases include severe pneumonia, pneumothorax, cystic fibrosis, and croup (see Chapter 12 ⚭). Central nervous system (CNS) injuries also compromise the child's ability to ventilate properly. These injuries include brain tumors, head injuries, and spinal cord injuries. Respiratory acidosis can also occur with the use of anesthetics, sedatives, and narcotics that impair the respiratory effort.

Manifestations

Acidosis, a lowering of the body's pH, results in CNS depression characterized by disorientation, lethargy, and headaches. CNS depression can also progress to unconsciousness. Cardiac symptoms of respiratory acidosis include tachycardia, hypotension, and ventricular fibrillation. The child may have muscle weakness or convulsions, depending on the cause of the imbalance. Respirations are rapid and shallow.

Diagnosis

ABG findings, along with clinical manifestations, assist in the diagnosis of this imbalance. Serum pH is decreased, PCO_2 is increased, and the bicarbonate is normal unless compensation is occurring, at which time the bicarbonate increases. During compensation, the urine pH is decreased.

Treatment

Medical management of respiratory acidosis involves improving ventilatory status. The cause of the imbalance must be corrected. All avenues should be explored to determine the cause (see Health Promotion Issue on pages 302 and 303). Treatment often includes administration of bronchodilators, oxygen, and antibiotics; chest physiotherapy; mechanical ventilation; and removal of foreign objects that are obstructing the airway.

Nursing Considerations

Nursing care for the child with respiratory acidosis is focused on restoring adequate ventilation. A simple nursing measure is to raise the head of the bed and to avoid positioning that would allow chest compression or slumping to the side (Figure 11-14 ■). Emergency methods may be necessary to remove objects obstructing the airway. See Chapter 6 ⚭ for more information about preventing airway obstruction. The child may require temporary ventilatory support. See Chapter 12 ⚭ for more information on nursing care related to ventilators.

Safety is also a consideration for children with respiratory acidosis. Environmental hazards need to be assessed and removed if present. Sedation should be avoided to promote safety and to avoid further depressing the CNS. Parents will need reassurance and support.

Respiratory Alkalosis

Respiratory alkalosis, commonly known as hyperventilation, is a condition characterized by a low level of CO_2 in the blood.

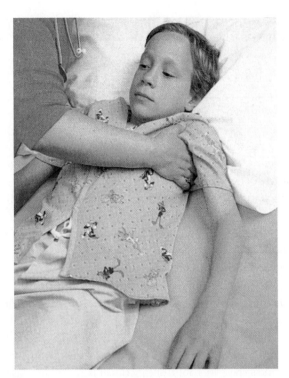

Figure 11-14. ■ Positioning to facilitate chest expansion. Positioning the child to avoid chest compression or slumping to the side will help correct respiratory acidosis.

Lack of CO_2 causes the serum pH to increase. In children, the most common cause of respiratory alkalosis is anxiety, fear, or panic. These emotional states cause the child to breathe rapidly and deeply. Other causes of respiratory alkalosis include pain, salicylate poisoning, altitude sickness, meningitis (see Chapter 15 ⬭), septicemia, and mechanical overventilation (see Chapter 12 ⬭).

Manifestations
The earliest symptom of this imbalance is tingling of the fingers and toes with a rapid, deep respiratory rate. Because the CNS is stimulated in alkalosis, the child may become light-headed, confused, anxious, and unable to concentrate. Other clinical manifestations include tachycardia, dysrhythmias, tetany, numbness, and hyperreflexia.

Diagnosis
ABG values show an increased serum pH, decreased PCO_2, bicarbonate within normal limits without compensation, and a decreased bicarbonate when compensation is occurring.

Treatment
Medical treatment seeks to correct the cause of respiratory alkalosis and restore CO_2 levels to within normal limits. Oxygen therapy is ordered for acute hypoxemia. Sedatives and antianxiety agents are used for children expressing anxiety, fear, pain, or panic.

Nursing Considerations
The simplest corrective action for early respiratory alkalosis is to encourage rebreathing of the child's own expiratory CO_2 by asking the child to breathe into a paper bag or cupped hands. Ensure that proper ventilation is promoted and mechanical ventilation is functioning properly.

The nurse also instructs the child in anxiety-reducing techniques and attends to the emotional needs of the child. Pharmacologic and nonpharmacologic pain relief methods are indicated for children experiencing pain. See the Nursing Care Plan Chart on page 304.

Metabolic Acidosis

Metabolic acidosis is a condition involving an excess of acids in the body. It results from the process of metabolism or a loss of bicarbonate through urine or gastrointestinal (GI) fluids. When the body produces an abundance of ketone bodies, metabolic acidosis may result.

Metabolic acidosis, called **ketoacidosis**, occurs when glucose storage is depleted and fat storage must be used for energy needs.

Manifestations
Metabolic acidosis may also occur as a result of starvation, anorexia nervosa, bulimia, severe diarrhea, intestinal malabsorption, drug toxicity, draining GI fistulas, diabetes, and renal failure. Children who ingest aspirin or toxic chemicals such as antifreeze may develop metabolic acidosis. The child may manifest symptoms of hyperventilation. **Kussmaul respiration** (rapid and deep respiration) may be present. The CNS is depressed, and the child may exhibit general malaise that progresses to unconsciousness. Hypotension, ventricular fibrillation, a dull headache, muscle weakness, nausea, vomiting, and abdominal pain may also occur.

Diagnosis
Diagnosis is accomplished by observing for symptoms and evaluating ABG values. Serum pH levels and bicarbonate will be decreased. The PCO_2 will be within normal limits if uncompensated and decreased if compensation is occurring. Urine pH levels will be decreased if compensation is occurring.

Treatment
Medical treatment seeks to correct the cause of metabolic acidosis. Insulin will be administered to correct ketoacidosis. Severe metabolic acidosis will be treated with IV sodium bicarbonate. For the renal client or child with an overdose, dialysis may be required. Antidiarrheal drugs may be used to treat diarrhea.

HEALTH PROMOTION ISSUE

SELF-ASPHYXIATION AS A GAME

The LPN/LVN works for the local school system and frequently visits several middle schools with an RN to provide health screenings, administer medications, and provide wellness information to students. One week a month, the nurses have lunch in each school in an effort to get to know the students better. This lunchtime visit also provides an opportunity for the students to learn to trust the nurses.

Recently, the nurses overheard a group of eighth-grade students planning a gasp party. The students appeared to be familiar with the nature of this type of party and only interested in obtaining information about the party particulars, such as time, date, and location.

When the crowd began to disperse for class, the LPN approached a female student whom she had previously befriended. The LPN asked the student for more information about the nature of a gasp party. The nurse was careful not to appear overly concerned and anxious. The student, who was not involved in the planning of this party, was willing to give the nurse information because she, too, was concerned about the health risks of this activity.

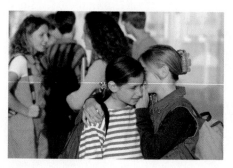

The LPN and the RN met with representatives from the school to discuss what might be done to protect the students from this dangerous activity. This group's first action item was to discover more information about this game.

DISCUSSION

In alarming numbers, preteen and early teens are engaging in an asphyxiation game that momentarily alters consciousness and causes a 10- to 20-second "high" or "rush." The game can be played in groups or alone. When the game is played in groups, a child's chest or neck is compressed to arrest the blood flow, and therefore, the oxygen flow, to the brain. The resulting hypoxia induces feelings of light-headedness, numbness, or tingling. There is a distinct possibility of loss of consciousness during this time. Children report feelings of euphoria, timelessness, and peace during this stage. Next, the pressure to the chest or neck is released, causing the blood to course quickly through the carotid arteries on its way to the brain, returning consciousness. This provides a "rush" sensation.

When the "choking game" is played alone, the child loses consciousness and is likely to be unable to loosen the constriction around his or her own neck. Hypoxia quickly proceeds to anoxia. Death can result in just a few minutes.

The game is believed to be addictive, and there have been reports of children playing the game for many hours in a row. During these marathon sessions, a child may actually lose consciousness several times.

The game is known by names other than the choking game. Some of the most common names are gasp, the American Dream game, space monkey, black out, pass out, space cowboy, rising sun, airplaning, funky chicken, flat liner, tingling and suffocation roulette, the fainting game, ghost, and the something dreaming game.

The choking game is most popular among middle school children ages 9 to 14. These children are usually popular in school and in their communities and are seemingly well adjusted. Their families state that they are close and maintain habits of functional families, such as eating meals together, taking vacations together, and keeping regular schedules. These children rarely cause trouble at home or school and are found to earn good grades.

It is difficult to gather exact figures on how many children are participating in this dangerous activity. Often, when the child is found dead, hanging from a rope or belt, the medical examiner determines the death a suicide instead of an accident due to the choking game.

Health risks associated with asphyxiation activities include injuries. They can be minor lacerations or sprained joints to more serious neck injuries causing permanent disability. Retinal damage has also been reported. The choking game may cause episodes of syncope. Ventricular arrhythmia can also be associated with the choking game. Brain damage and death, of course, are the most serious risks of the choking game.

PLANNING AND IMPLEMENTATION

The nurses and school staff developed a plan to raise awareness about this game. They also wanted to provide information to students, parents, and school officials about the health dangers associated with the choking game. First, they developed an informational pamphlet to be mailed to the homes of all middle school children. The pamphlet contained a detailed description of this game and the health risks associated with it. Warning signs and symptoms were also listed. These included:

- Linear abrasions or areas of ecchymosis on the neck
- Petechiae found on the face, eyelids, or conjunctiva
- Intermittent hoarseness when the child does not have a cold, sinus problems, or allergies
- Dog leashes, choke collars, bungee cords, ropes, belts, cords, or even wire clothes hangers draped in an unexplained manner over door frames or closet rods
- Frequent choice of high-necked shirts or turtlenecks, even in warmer months
- Frequent headaches
- A sudden increase in the amount of time spent alone in the child's bedroom

The pamphlet concluded with a plan for discussing these dangers with children. It was suggested that parents include the choking game in their discussion of other dangerous activities such as smoking, alcohol, drugs, and sexual activity. They were encouraged to ask the child to consider the consequences of the decision to play this game. Parents were advised to cite specific incidents in which children lost their lives to this activity. Parents were also encouraged to check the history and activity of a child's computer to determine if they are engaging in chat rooms where the game is discussed or visiting how-to websites related to the choking game. A contact number was given for more information and assistance.

The second intervention aimed at reducing the incidence of this game among middle school children was random health screening in the school setting for symptoms related to the choking game. Children would be given a questionnaire to determine their knowledge and involvement in the game. Children considered at risk would be referred to the school counselor.

The third intervention was a forum to discuss the issues with all school officials, including teachers, administrators, and support staff. Because this activity is often practiced on school grounds, school officials were encouraged to consider security cameras that would allow them to monitor for the activity.

School officials were also encouraged to be diligent in offering exciting alternatives to this type of risk-taking behavior. A variety of safe activities that appeal to a child's sense of adventure were encouraged.

SELF-REFLECTION

Consider the risk-taking activities you may have engaged in during your middle school and high school years. Did you have conversations with strangers who could have harmed you? Did you walk alone in wooded areas without someone knowing where you were? Did you drive recklessly? Were you in a car when your friend played "chicken" with oncoming traffic? Think carefully about what caused you to engage in these behaviors. What could have prevented your participation in these activities? How can you incorporate these findings into your own practice with children?

SUGGESTED RESOURCES

For the Nurse

Le, D., & Macnab, A. J. (2001). Self strangulation by hanging from cloth towel dispensers in Canadian schools. *Injury Prevention, V7*(3), 231–233.

Martin, A. (2006). The choking game: Important information for camp nurses. *Compasspoint, 16*(2), 22–23.

Waller, M., Hallfors, D., Halpern, C., Iritani, B., Ford, C., and Guo, G. (2006). Gender differences in associations between depressive symptoms and patterns of substance use and risky sexual behavior among a nationally representative sample of U.S. adolescents. *Archives of Women's Mental Health, 9*(3), 139–150.

For the Client

Shapiro, L. (2004). *The secret language of children: How to understand what your kids are really saying.* Naperville, IL: Sourcebooks. This book gives parents the tools to communicate more effectively with their children.

NURSING CARE PLAN CHART

Child with Respiratory Alkalosis

GOAL	INTERVENTION	RATIONALE	EXCEPTED OUTCOME
1. Ineffective Breathing Pattern, related to hyperventilation			
The child will demonstrate a respiratory rate and rhythm within normal limits.	Carefully document the child's respiratory effort	*Careful, complete documentation allows the nurse to evaluate respiratory status effectively.*	The child's respiratory rate is 18 bpm. Breaths are regular and even.
	Position the child for optimal chest expansion.	*Breathing is facilitated when the child's position allows for chest expansion.*	
	Encourage the child to take slow, deep breaths into a small paper bag placed over the child's mouth and nose.	*This method of breathing will aid in the correction of carbon dioxide levels.*	
The family will be able to recognize future symptoms of respiratory alkalosis and initiate prompt intervention.	Teach symptoms of respiratory alkalosis.	*Prompt recognition of physical conditions requires proper knowledge.*	The family recognizes symptoms of respiratory alkalosis and promptly initiates intervention.
	Teach the family to encourage the child to take slow, deep breaths into a small paper bag placed over the child's mouth and nose.	*This will correct carbon dioxide levels.*	
2. Anxiety related to situational crises			
The child will demonstrate the ability to manage anxiety.	Encourage the child to discuss anxious thoughts.	*Determining the child's thoughts allows the nurse to make an appropriate plan.*	The child demonstrates anxiety-reducing behaviors.
	Teach the child anxiety-reducing strategies including slow, deep breathing; reducing stimuli in the environment; and distraction techniques such as television, radio, or games.	*Anxiety can often be managed effectively by employing simple anxiety-reducing techniques.*	The family assists the child in identifying anxious behaviors. The family assists the child to develop skills to manage anxiety.
The family will assist the child in identifying symptoms of anxiety and to develop skills to manage anxiety.	Teach the parents to recognize symptoms of anxiety such as fidgeting, vague complaints of pain, and respiratory changes.	*Early recognition of symptoms of anxiety will assist the parent to manage the anxiety effectively.*	
	Encourage parents to provide a loving, constant presence in times of stress.	*A loving, constant presence can provide the child with a sense of security.*	

Nursing Considerations

The nurse closely monitors the child with metabolic acidosis for progressive respiratory, neurologic, and cardiac symptoms. Worsening symptoms must be reported promptly to the charge nurse and physician. Ventilation should be facilitated by proper positioning.

Oral hygiene should be provided for children with vomiting and rapid respirations. The child's lips also become dry because of rapid respiration. Lip balm should be applied as needed. Prompt attention is necessary to protect the skin from irritation due to diarrhea. The nurse may need to assist the child in conserving energy if muscle weakness and malaise are present.

Diabetic clients and their families need teaching on symptom recognition for ketoacidosis. They will also need instruction on management techniques for this condition.

Children who have overdosed, accidentally or purposefully, need to understand how to prevent this hazard. Referral to behavioral medicine units may be appropriate.

Metabolic Alkalosis

Metabolic alkalosis is a condition that results from a loss of metabolic acid or an excess of bicarbonate.

Loss of metabolic acids occurs due to vomiting, nasogastric suction, cystic fibrosis, inappropriate use of diuretics, and hypokalemia. Excess bicarbonate may occur:

- When the child ingests baking soda or an overdose of antacids
- Following blood transfusions with multiple units of blood
- In increased renal absorption

Manifestations
Clinical manifestations of metabolic alkalosis include abdominal distention, constipation, cardiac arrhythmias, polyuria, decreased rate and depth of respirations, tetany, seizures, weakness, confusion, lethargy, and coma.

Diagnosis
Lab work from a child with metabolic alkalosis reveals increased serum pH, increased HCO_3^-, normal PCO_2 when uncompensated, and increased PCO_2 when compensation is occurring.

Treatment
Medical management is focused on treating the causative factor. Treatment will include IV infusion with normal saline and administration of acetazolamide to facilitate renal excretion of bicarbonate.

Nursing Considerations
Nursing care for children with metabolic alkalosis includes assisting the child to breathe effectively and monitoring neurologic status closely. Measures must be implemented to keep safe the child who has an altered LOC.

Strict monitoring of intake and output for the child who is vomiting is essential to the nursing care plan. The child who is vomiting frequently also needs regular oral hygiene.

NURSING CARE
PRIORITIES IN NURSING CARE

Children experiencing an acid-base imbalance are at risk for ventilation and oxygenation difficulties. The nurse must be diligent in monitoring ventilation and oxygenation and in recognizing changes in these processes. The nurse should also prevent further compromise in these processes by positioning the child to facilitate ventilation, minimizing administration of narcotic pain relief, and keeping the airway free of obstruction through oral suctioning as necessary.

ASSESSING

In respiratory and metabolic acid-base imbalances, the nurse must give priority to assessing patency of the airway. Monitor respiratory rate, rhythm, and effort. Other vital signs, pulse and blood pressure, may also change in response to the imbalance and must be monitored closely. The child's neurologic status and cardiac function may indicate worsening of the condition. ABG values and pulse oximetry findings are assessed frequently.

DIAGNOSING, PLANNING, AND IMPLEMENTING

Nursing diagnoses for acid-base imbalances might include:

- Ineffective **B**reathing Pattern related to hyperventilation
- Impaired **G**as Exchange related to hypoventilation
- Risk for **I**njury related to central nervous system stimulation
- Disturbed **T**hought Processes related to central nervous system depression.

Some outcomes for acid-base imbalances might include that the child will:

- Demonstrate effective breathing pattern as evidenced by rate, rhythm, and effort of respirations within normal range.
- Demonstrate improved ventilation and oxygenation.
- Avoid injury until acid-base balance is restored.
- Regain usual thought process appropriate for age.

The nurse's role in providing support to these clients would include the following:

- Position the child to facilitate breathing. *Positions that promote lung expansion will improve breathing.*
- Encourage slow, deep breathing for respiratory acidosis. *Correcting hypoventilation is a priority goal.*
- Encourage rebreathing of CO_2 for respiratory alkalosis. *Respiratory alkalosis is marked by hyperventilation and CO_2 deficits.*
- Aspiration oral secretions as needed (prn). *Maintaining a patent airway might require assisting the child in removing oral secretions.*
- Administer humidified oxygen or carbon dioxide as ordered. *Oxygen administration prevents hypoxemia. Humidified oxygen assists in the thinning of secretions.*

Carbon dioxide replacement may be necessary in respiratory alkalosis.

- Administer IV solutions as ordered. *Corrects acidosis.*
- Administer sedation medications carefully. *In respiratory acidosis, sedation may be contraindicated because respiratory depression may occur. Sedation may reduce anxiety in respiratory alkalosis.*
- Create a safe environment for the child. Keep the bed in the lowest position. Keep the floor free of safety hazards. Assist the child to ambulate. *Muscle weakness and risk for seizure activity create a safety hazard for the child with an acid-base imbalance.*
- Encourage parents to monitor the child's muscle strength and neurologic status and to report noticeable changes. *Parents can often observe more subtle changes in the child's physical status. Early reporting of symptoms can lead to more effective treatment.*
- Provide brief and concise reorientation to reality. *Challenging the child's thinking would frustrate them. It is, however, important to present reality rather than agreeing with the child's distorted thinking.*
- Assure parents that distorted thinking is part of the acid-base imbalance. *This information relieves the parents' anxiety about the distorted thinking.*

EVALUATING

Expected outcomes for a client with acid-base imbalances include return of ABG values to normal limits, improved neurologic status, improved respiratory function, and improved cardiac function. Lack of response to treatment and worsening of symptoms must be reported to the charge nurse or physician promptly.

Note: The reference and resource listings for this and all chapters have been compiled at the back of the book.

Chapter Review

KEY TERMS by Topic

Use the audio glossary feature of either the CD-ROM or the Companion Website to hear the correct pronunciation of the following key terms.

Principles Related to Fluids and Electrolytes
homeostasis, plasma, interstitial, solute, solvent, solution, osmosis, diffusion, filtration, active transport, electrolytes, cations, anions

Deficient Fluid Volume
dehydration, isotonic dehydration, hypotonic dehydration, hypertonic dehydration

Excess Fluid Volume
hypervolemia

Sodium Imbalance
hyponatremia, hypernatremia

Potassium Imbalance
hypokalemia, hyperkalemia

Calcium Imbalance
hypocalcemia, hypercalcemia

Principles Related to Acid-Base Disorders
acidosis, alkalosis, respiratory acidosis, respiratory alkalosis, metabolic acidosis, ketoacidosis, Kussmaul respiration, metabolic alkalosis

KEY Points

- Children have a high percentage of water; therefore, fluid and electrolyte imbalances are much more dangerous in pediatric clients than in adults.
- Homeostasis is achieved by balance for fluid, electrolytes, acids, and bases.
- Careful measuring of intake and output is essential to detecting fluid and electrolyte imbalances.
- Obtaining accurate measurement of the child's weight can assist the nurse in correctly identifying imbalances in fluid and electrolytes.
- The treatment of dehydration requires rehydration. This may be accomplished with oral or IV fluids based on the degree of dehydration.
- Fluid restriction is a necessary treatment for some fluid and electrolyte imbalances. Younger children will have difficulty understanding why they cannot have oral fluids. The nurse must take care to explain the fluid restriction in terms the child can understand. It is also important when developing a plan for spacing the allotted fluid throughout the day to involve the child and his or her parents.
- Acidosis develops when there is an increase of hydrogen ion concentration. Alkalosis develops when there is a decrease of hydrogen ion concentration.
- Three body mechanisms that compensate for abnormal pH levels leading to acidosis or alkalosis are the buffer system, the respiratory system, and the renal system.
- The nurse must be able to analyze ABG results accurately by reviewing pH, CO_2, and HCO_3^- values.
- Children experiencing an acid-base imbalance are at risk for ventilation and oxygenation difficulties.

EXPLORE MediaLink

Additional interactive resources for this chapter can be found on the Companion Website at www.prenhall.com/adams.

Click on Chapter 11 and "Begin" to select the activities for this chapter.

For chapter-related NCLEX®-style questions and an audio glossary, access the accompanying CD-ROM in this book.

Animations:

Fluid balance

Acid–base balance

Evaluate deep tendon reflexes

FOR FURTHER Study

See Chapter 6 for more information about preventing airway obstruction.

For information about obtaining vital signs, taking weights, and providing IV medications, see Chapter 8.

For a discussion of meningitis, see Chapter 15.

For a discussion of mechanical ventilation, pneumonia, pneumothorax, cystic fibrosis, croup, and other respiratory disorders, see Chapter 12.

For more on hypovolemic shock, see Chapter 14.

See Chapter 21 for more discussion on burns in children.

Critical Thinking Care Map

Caring for a Client with Fluid Volume Excess
NCLEX-PN® Focus Area: Physiologic Adaptation

Case Study: Jayden, 3 days old, developed hyperbilirubinemia. The physician ordered placement of the newborn under phototherapy lights (bililights) and initiation of IV fluids to maintain adequate hydration. Following initiation of this therapy, the LPN noticed the IV rate infusing was greater than the rate ordered.

Nursing Diagnosis: Excess **F**luid volume related to intravenous overload

COLLECT DATA

Subjective

_____
_____
_____
_____
_____
_____

Objective

_____
_____
_____
_____
_____
_____

Would you report this? Yes/No
If yes, to: _____

Nursing Care

_____
_____
_____
_____
_____
_____
_____
_____
_____
_____
_____
_____

How would you document this? _____
_____
_____
_____
_____

Compare your documentation to the sample provided in Appendix I.

Data Collected
(use only those that apply)

- Flat fontanel
- Moist lung sounds
- Urine output 1 mL/kg/hour
- LPN states, "This rate is twice the rate ordered by the physician."
- Generalized edema
- Poor skin turgor
- Hemoglobin 30 g/dL
- Hematocrit 40%
- Urine specific gravity 1.000
- Sodium 133 mEq/L
- Pulse 110 bpm, bounding
- BUN 17 mg/dL

Nursing Interventions
(use only those that apply; list in priority order)

- Turn infant every 30 minutes.
- Monitor vital signs.
- Observe for edema of the extremities, face, and neck.
- Monitor and document intake and output.
- Weigh the infant daily and document.
- Hold feedings until approved by charge nurse.
- Monitor IV fluid rate.
- Observe closely for symptoms of pulmonary edema, including restlessness, tachypnea, labored breathing, a full and bounding or weak and thready pulse, possible crackles on lung auscultation, and profuse diaphoresis. Position the child to facilitate breathing, and notify the physician immediately if symptoms are present.
- Monitor lab values and report imbalances.
- Remove child from bililights until edema has resolved.

1 A nurse is caring for a 2-year-old with a diagnosis of fluid volume excess (FVE). The nurse knows that with FVE, certain clinical findings may be present. Which of the laboratory report findings reflects the diagnosis?

1. Urine specific gravity 1.019
2. BUN 15 mg/dL
3. Hematocrit 27%
4. Sodium 137

2 A 2-year-old client has had diarrhea for 1 week and now has hypernatremia. The nurse monitors the client for which of the following signs and symptoms of this disorder?

1. Thirst and neurologic symptoms
2. Anemia and other hematologic symptoms
3. Anorexia and other dietary symptoms
4. Constipation and other digestive symptoms

3 A nurse is assigned to a child with a diagnosis of hyperkalemia. The nurse prepares to care for the client and plans to do which of the following?

1. Monitor pulse, respiratory rate, and rhythm.
2. Monitor blood glucose levels every 3 to 4 hours.
3. Monitor for dependent edema every hour.
4. Monitor urine output hourly.

4 An infant is admitted with a diagnosis of hyponatremia. The nurse knows to monitor the client for _____ _____, a common sign of a worsening condition with this diagnosis. (Hint: Two words)

5 A pediatric client with hypercalcemia has just been admitted to the hospital. The child is weak and vomiting. Which of the following orders written by the physician should the nurse caring for this client complete first?

1. Strain all urine.
2. Monitor for decreased LOC.
3. Monitor for weakness.
4. Administer diuretics as ordered.

6 The nurse has just finished giving instructions to the parents of a 3-year-old client with dehydration. The nurse realizes that the parents need more instruction about intake and output when they say:

1. "We don't have to worry about noting if Susie vomits."
2. "We will weigh Susie's diapers."
3. "We will record all fluids Susie takes."
4. "We know we have to record if Susie has diarrhea and estimate the amount."

7 A pediatric client has just been admitted with a diagnosis of dehydration. The nurse anticipates all but one of the following written orders by the physician:

1. Obtain daily weight.
2. Maintain strict intake and output.
3. Take vital signs as ordered.
4. Provide fluids as wanted.

8 A 4-year-old pediatric client has suspected respiratory alkalosis. When reviewing the laboratory report, the nurse knows which of the following is most likely indicative of this diagnosis?

1. pH 7.40
2. PCO_2 25 mm Hg
3. Na^+ 140
4. K^+ 4.0

9 The nurse assesses a child and suspects the child is dehydrated. The nurse's suspicions are confirmed when she observes the following:

1. Bounding, strong pulse
2. Increased blood pressure
3. Weak, thready pulse
4. Edematous tongue

10 Calculate the following percentage of weight loss. The infant's birth weight was 7 lb 12 oz. At 3 days after birth, the infant weighs 7 lb 8 oz. Weight loss is _____%.

Answers for NCLEX-PN® Review and Critical Thinking questions appear in Appendix I.

Chapter 12

Care of the Child with Respiratory Disorders

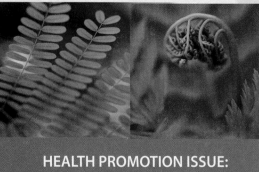

HEALTH PROMOTION ISSUE:
Tonsillectomy

NURSING CARE PLAN CHART:
Respiratory Syncytial Virus

NURSING PROCESS CARE PLAN:
Client with Asthma

CRITICAL THINKING CARE MAP:
Caring for a Client with
Respiratory Infection

BRIEF Outline

Anatomy and Physiology
Process of Respiration
Brief Assessment Review
UPPER RESPIRATORY DISORDERS
Epistaxis
Upper Respiratory Infections
Foreign Body Obstructed Airway

LOWER RESPIRATORY DISORDERS
Respiratory Disorders Associated with the Newborn and Infant
Congenital Respiratory Disorders
Lower Respiratory Infections
Additional Respiratory Disorders
Nursing Care

LEARNING Outcomes

After completing this chapter, you will be able to:
1. Define key terms.
2. Discuss the anatomy and physiology of the pediatric respiratory system.
3. Describe respiratory disorders including upper respiratory infections, respiratory distress, bronchopulmonary dysplasia, meconium aspiration, tracheoesophageal fistula, cystic fibrosis, asthma, and lower respiratory infections.
4. Explain appropriate nursing interventions for children with respiratory disorders.
5. Discuss clinical manifestations, diagnostic procedures, medical management, and nursing interventions related to respiratory trauma.

Disorders of the respiratory system include congenital malformations, infections, and diseases resulting from chromosomal abnormalities or unknown causes. Respiratory conditions may be acute or chronic. Often they have life-threatening implications and create great trauma and anxiety in the lives of pediatric clients and their families.

Anatomy and Physiology

Prenatally, the respiratory system begins as lung buds during the 6th week of development and is formed by the 23rd week, but is not capable of maintaining gas exchange outside the uterus. By week 20 to 23 the primitive lungs begin to produce surfactant. **Surfactant** is a substance that decreases the surface tension of fluid inside the alveoli, allowing the lungs to expand. By the 24th week, the lungs are capable of maintaining gas exchange outside the uterus. Therefore, the age of **viability** (the ability to live outside the uterus) is 24 weeks. An infant born at this time would most likely require intensive nursing care, including ventilation support. Surfactant production matures by the 35th week, making the prognosis more favorable.

The respiratory system is divided into the upper respiratory system and the lower respiratory system. The upper respiratory system contains the nose, nasal sinuses, pharynx, and larynx. The lower respiratory system contains the trachea, bronchial tree, and alveoli inside the lungs. The right lung is divided into three lobes, and the left lung is divided into two lobes. The entire respiratory system is lined with a continuous mucous membrane that produces approximately 125 mL of mucus daily. The underlying epithelial cells of the lower respiratory system contain cilia, which are hairlike structure extending outward from the cell membrane. The cilia continuously move the mucus toward the pharynx. Figures 12-1 ■ and 12-2 ■ show the differences in upper respiratory structures between a child and an adult.

NOSE AND SINUSES
Air enters the nares or nostrils and flows through the nasal cavities. Protruding into the nasal cavity from the sides are three shelflike structures called **conchae**. These structures, covered with mucous membrane, increase the surface area for warming and humidifying the air and trapping foreign particles. The four pairs of nasal sinuses open into the nasal

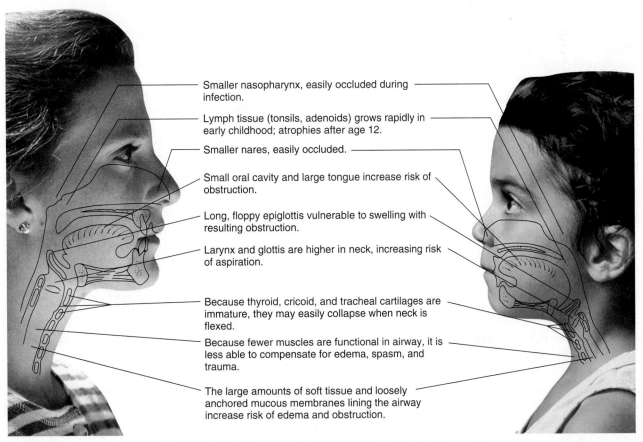

Smaller nasopharynx, easily occluded during infection.

Lymph tissue (tonsils, adenoids) grows rapidly in early childhood; atrophies after age 12.

Smaller nares, easily occluded.

Small oral cavity and large tongue increase risk of obstruction.

Long, floppy epiglottis vulnerable to swelling with resulting obstruction.

Larynx and glottis are higher in neck, increasing risk of aspiration.

Because thyroid, cricoid, and tracheal cartilages are immature, they may easily collapse when neck is flexed.

Because fewer muscles are functional in airway, it is less able to compensate for edema, spasm, and trauma.

The large amounts of soft tissue and loosely anchored mucous membranes lining the airway increase risk of edema and obstruction.

Figure 12-1. ■ The child's airway is clearly smaller and less developed than an adult's. Because of this, serious consequences may occur in the child with an upper respiratory tract infection, allergic reaction, or malpositioning of the head and neck during sleep. Swallowed objects pose a serious danger to the child.

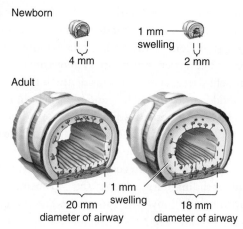

Figure 12-2. ■ The diameter of an infant's airway is approximately 4 mm; the adult's airway is 20 mm. An inflammation process that narrows the adult airway to 18 mm could easily narrow the infant's airway to 2 mm (see upper section of illustration).

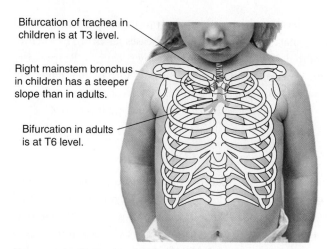

Figure 12-3. ■ Trachea position. In children, the trachea is shorter, and the angle of the right bronchus at *bifurcation* (place where it splits in two) is more acute than in the adult. When you are resuscitating or suctioning, you must allow for the differences.

cavity. The frontal, sphenoidal, ethmoidal, and maxillary sinuses lighten the weight of the head, as well as warm and humidify the air. The openings of the sinuses into the nasal cavity are small and easily blocked by swelling of the mucous membrane. Development of the nose begins in puberty along with the secondary sex characteristics. The lacrimal (tear) sacs also open into the nasal cavity.

PHARYNX

The pharynx or throat is made up of the nasal pharynx at the top, oral pharynx behind the mouth, and laryngopharynx above the larynx. The pharynx is simply a connection between the nasal cavity and the larynx and esophagus. Both air and food pass through this structure. The eustachian (auditory) canals from the middle ear open into the nasal pharynx. In infants, the eustachian tube is practically horizontal (see Figure 15-30B); by age 12, it tilts diagonally down into the nasopharynx and so is less likely to promote middle ear infection. Because of the differences in angle of the eustachian tube, the pinna of a child younger than 3 years is pulled down and back to straighten the ear canal for visualization or medication administration, whereas the pinna of an older person is pulled up and back (see Figure 8-2).

TONSILS

Masses of lymphatic tissue or tonsils are embedded in the wall of the pharynx. The pharyngeal tonsils (adenoids) are located in the nasal pharynx. The palatine tonsils are located on each side of the oral pharynx, and the lingual tonsils are located between the back of the tongue and the epiglottis. The tonsils begin to atrophy in midadolescence, so tonsillectomy and adenoidectomy are rarely performed after age 15. The epiglottis is a cartilage "door" that covers the larynx during swallowing in order to prevent food from entering the airway.

LARYNX

Besides a passageway for air to enter the lungs, the larynx contains the vocal cords. The larynx is surrounded by cartilage for protection. Muscles attached to the vocal cords control the pitch of the voice.

TRACHEA

The trachea or windpipe extends from the larynx to the bronchi in the chest (Figure 12-3 ■). The trachea is held open by C-shaped rings of cartilage.

BRONCHI AND LUNGS

The remainder of the respiratory tree is made up of branches of the trachea called bronchi and smaller bronchioles. Each bronchiole ends in an air sac or **alveoli**. Each alveolus is surrounded by capillaries through which gas exchange takes place.

The lungs are situated in the chest cavity with the base of the lungs at the level of the diaphragm. The left lung has two lobes, whereas the right has three. Respiration in children up to 6 years is achieved by movement of the diaphragm, abdomen, and intercostal muscles. After this time, the child breathes mainly with assistance from the muscles of the thoracic cage.

Process of Respiration

In utero, the placenta provides necessary gas exchange to the fetal lungs and tissues. At birth, the newborn must make a physiologic adaptation to extrauterine life. Changes in intrathoracic pressure occur as the newborn enters the world. In addition, exposure to new sensations of noise, temperature, and light assists the newborn to take his first gasp of air. As pulmonary blood flow increases, the foramen ovale and ductus arteriosus closes to complete the newborn's efforts to maintain respiratory effort. See Chapter 13 for further information.

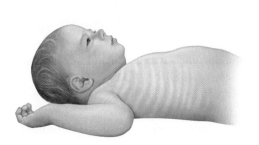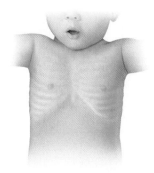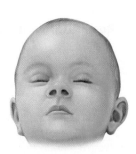

Figure 12-4. ■ Severe retraction. Marked retraction of posterior rib cage (*left*), marked retraction of anterior rib cage (*center*), and marked nasal flaring (*right*).

The mechanism of breathing is a complex process of changing pressure. Inside the aorta and carotid arteries (the major blood vessels leaving the left side of the heart) are specialized cells or chemoreceptors. When the carbon dioxide level in the blood rises, the chemoreceptors sense the elevation and send a message to the brain. The brain responds by stimulating a contraction of the **diaphragm** (the large muscle dividing the chest and abdominal cavities) and **intercostal muscles** (the muscles between the ribs). The contraction of these muscles causes the ribs to move outward and the diaphragm to flatten. The result is an increase in the size of the chest cavity, creating a vacuum that draws air into the body. The pressure of oxygen inside the alveoli is greater than that in the blood, allowing oxygen to move into the capillaries. The carbon dioxide level in the blood is greater than that in the alveoli, allowing carbon dioxide to move into the alveoli. The diaphragm and intercostal muscles relax, moving the ribs and diaphragm back to a resting state and pushing air out of the lungs. This cycle repeats 20 to 40 times a minute in the child.

Up to approximately 6 months of age, the infant is a nose breather. The newborn has an irregular breathing pattern, which gradually becomes regular over the first 3 to 4 months. Breathing pattern in the newborn is predominantly diaphragmatic, with the chest rising with the abdominal movements. Respirations are usually irregular with brief periods of apnea. If there are no color or heart rate changes, these brief apneic episodes are considered normal.

The normal breathing pattern (**eupnea**) is regular in rate and depth. The child with congestion may open the mouth to breathe. **Hypoventilation** refers to slow, shallow respirations that can indicate a central nervous system function depressed by drugs or other disorders. **Hyperventilation** refers to deep rapid respirations that occur from exercise, disorders that increase metabolism, or psychological stress. **Dyspnea** is difficulty breathing as evidenced by retractions or upward movement of the rib cage by contracting the neck muscles (Figure 12-4 ■). If dyspnea is relieved by sitting or standing, it is called **orthopnea**. If the breathing stops for a brief period, it is called **apnea**. Alternating hyperventilation and apnea is termed **Cheyne-Stokes respiration** (CSR). CSR is an ominous sign of declining condition in critical disorders such as congestive heart failure or neurologic disorders. Abnormal breathing patterns may be accompanied by **circumoral cyanosis** (bluish discoloration of the skin around the mouth). The child could have a productive or nonproductive cough. Whenever a child has a respiratory disorder, the nurse should monitor the oxygen saturation level.

The nurse should listen to all lung fields with the stethoscope. Lung sounds should be clear. **Crackles** (fine, dry sounds, formerly called rales), **rhonchi** (coarse, wet sounds), and wheezing are common sounds in the child with respiratory disorders. These sounds result when airways are partially obstructed by mucus or bronchial muscle spasms. Differentiating expiratory wheezes from inspiratory wheezes can be difficult because of the normally rapid respiratory rate. Occasionally, the child develops **stridor** (a high-pitched inspiratory crowing sound caused by severely narrowed airways).

clinical ALERT

When a child develops stridor, prompt medical attention is needed to prevent total airway obstruction. While awaiting medical assistance, continue to observe the child's respiratory effort. If the child becomes quiet, total occlusion of the airway may have occurred. CPR should be initiated.

Brief Assessment Review
HISTORY

■ Inquire about symptoms of respiratory conditions such as cough, fever, shortness of breath, dyspnea, sore throat, and fatigue.

■ Determine the course of the current illness.

■ Determine the child's history of colds, respiratory infections, and respiratory disorders.

TABLE 12-1

Normal Respiratory Rate by Age

AGE	RESTING RESPIRATORY RATE
Newborn	30–50 breaths/minute
1 year	20–40 breaths/minute
3 years	20–30 breaths/minute
6 years and older	16–22 breaths/minute

- Inquire about known allergies.
- Determine whether the child is exposed to second-hand smoke.
- Review the child's immunization status.

PHYSICAL

Because the child may not be able to tell you subjective information, observation of respiratory patterns and skin color is critical. The child should be quiet in order to allow accurate assessment of breathing rate, depth, regularity, and lung sounds.

To assess respiratory rate and breathing patterns accurately, the child must be in a position with the chest exposed so the nurse can watch the chest rise and fall. Table 12-1 ■ identifies the normal respiratory rate by age. The child's respiratory rate gradually slows, and by age 6 it approximates that of the adult.

- Assess and document the depth and rate of respirations and characteristics of the child's respiratory effort and/or cough. Note both the quality (clear, moist) and the strength of the cough.
- Observe for signs of respiratory distress (tachypnea, nasal flaring, retractions, inspiratory stridor). In the infant, listen for grunting with respirations.
- Observe rise and fall of chest and abdomen (simultaneous movement is normal; paradoxical movement is abnormal).
- Auscultate the lungs, anterior and posterior, for adventitious sounds.
- Observe the child's skin and nailbed color. Respiratory distress progresses from pallor to mottled skin to cyanosis, with central cyanosis signaling the worst condition. Crying may increase or decrease changes.
- Monitor oxygen saturation.
- Note level of consciousness, behavior, and restlessness or irritability. Hypoxia may cause changes in the child.
- Inspect for level of hydration, which can be affected by respiratory status.

UPPER RESPIRATORY DISORDERS

Epistaxis

Epistaxis or nosebleed is common in school-age children. The anterior nares, rich in blood vessels, are the usual source of bleeding. Blood vessels can be irritated by trauma, including nose picking, foreign bodies, and low humidity resulting in drying of the mucous membranes. The posterior septum can also be a source of nosebleeds. Posterior nosebleeds have a variety of causes that may include systemic conditions such as bleeding disorders, leukemia, and hypertension. Other causes could be allergies, forceful blowing of the nose, and infection. The mucous membrane may also be irritated by drug use, either prescribed or illicit.

Manifestations

Bleeding may occur from the anterior or posterior septum. Most nosebleeds coming from the anterior septum stop in 10 minutes with treatment. Posterior nosebleeds are usually more difficult to stop and may need medical attention.

clinical ALERT

If a nosebleed does not stop within 10 minutes or occurs frequently without identifiable cause, the child needs medical attention.

Diagnosis

Diagnosis is made by observation of obvious blood draining from the nares or down the throat and from a history of the child's condition and events that may have caused epistaxis. The physician may also examine the nasal mucosa.

Treatment

First aid treatment of nosebleeds includes applying direct firm pressure to the bleeding naris where the nose attaches to the maxillary bone. By pushing the outer side of the naris against the nasal septum, blood supply is slowed and clot formation can begin. The child should hold the head slightly forward to prevent blood from going down the throat and into the stomach, which can cause nausea and vomiting. A cold cloth applied to the forehead and back of the neck can slow circulation to the nose and aid in clot formation. Once the nosebleed stops, the child should not blow the nose for several hours to prevent a second nosebleed.

Upper Respiratory Infections

Upper respiratory infections in young children are common. Infections stimulate the immune system to develop antibodies that will protect the young child in later life. However, if the immune system is immature or is overwhelmed by multiple infections or other disorders, the life of the child may be in danger. Upper respiratory system infections include bacterial and viral infections of the nasal and oral pharynx, tonsils, middle ear, and epiglottis.

NASOPHARYNGITIS

The most common infection in children, **nasopharyngitis,** also called **rhinitis**, **coryza,** or the "common cold," is inflammation of the nasal mucosa often caused by a viral infection (e.g., rhinovirus, coronavirus) or bacteria (especially group A *Streptococcus*).

Manifestations

The classic symptoms include erythema and edema of the nasal and pharyngeal mucosa. Clear nasal discharge either through the nares or down the pharynx is common. Tonsils may be enlarged and vesicles may appear on the soft palate and the pharynx. Fever and irritability or general discomfort may occur. If the discharge becomes yellow or greenish, a bacterial infection should be suspected. Mouth breathing leads to drying of the mucous membranes, further irritation, and pain.

Diagnosis

Diagnosis is based on symptoms, nasal swabs, or throat culture.

Treatment

Nasopharyngitis usually resolves within 10 days. Parents may assist the child by providing humidified air when the child is sleeping. Saline nose drops can be administered every 3 to 4 hours and may be helpful to infants when given just prior to feeding. Older children may use drops or sprays. Decongestants or antihistamines may be prescribed. Parents should be taught to use over-the-counter medicines only if approved for use in children and only in the dosage recommended for the child's age and weight. They should not give children aspirin because of its association with Reye's syndrome. See Chapters 10 and 15 ⌾ for more on Reye's syndrome.

The child with nasopharyngitis becomes asymptomatic when the condition resolves. If the infection persists or recurs frequently, the child should be evaluated by the primary care provider. Antibiotics, decongestants, and antihistamines may be prescribed. Persistent or recurring respiratory infections could indicate an unresolved bacterial infection or a more serious condition, such as leukemia or diabetes mellitus. Herbal remedies are sometimes employed to assist with symptoms (Box 12-1 ■). Teach parents to review home remedies with the care provider to ensure safety.

TONSILLITIS

Tonsillitis, inflammation of the palatine tonsils, commonly spreads from the nasopharynx through the drainage of lymphatic fluid. Tonsillitis may be caused by a virus or bacteria, and the condition tends to recur.

BOX 12-1	COMPLEMENTARY THERAPIES

Herbal Agents Used for Respiratory Disorders

Herbal remedies may be used to achieve balance in the body. Common herbs used to prevent or treat respiratory disorders are:

- Eucalyptus—Clears stuffy nose and congested sinuses when the water is boiled and the steam breathed. Parental supervision is required. Care must be taken to prevent injury from hot water.
- Garlic—Treats cough and may have some antibiotic effect when eaten raw.
- Mullein—Soothes and relaxes airway and relieves cough when mixed with water and taken orally.
- Echinacea—Boosts the immune system to help prevent infection.

Manifestations

The inflammation causes the tonsils to enlarge, resulting in pain, difficulty swallowing (**dysphagia**), and a risk for airway obstruction (Figure 12-5 ■). Frequently, the swelling of the mucous membrane narrows or closes the eustachian tubes, trapping fluid in the middle ear. Microorganisms can be trapped in the middle ear as well, resulting in otitis media (see Chapter 15 ⌾).

clinical ALERT

Any child presenting with an upper respiratory infection should be evaluated for otitis media. Any child presenting with otitis media should be evaluated for an upper respiratory infection. These infections often occur simultaneously.

Diagnosis

When a child presents with a sore throat and swelling and redness of the tonsils, a culture is needed to determine the causative agent. The tympanic membranes

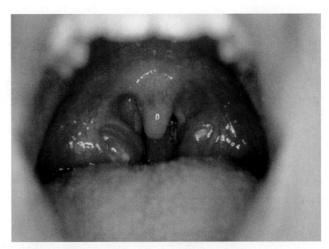

Figure 12-5. ■ Infected tonsils can swell and obstruct the airway. (Custom Medical Stock Photo Inc.)

are visualized and assessed for redness and fluid in the middle ear.

Treatment

When tonsillitis is caused by a virus, treatment is symptomatic until the infection resolves. Acetaminophen eases throat pain and reduces fever. Cold, nonacidic liquids such as water and sports drinks or frozen Popsicles® can soothe the throat and help prevent dehydration. A home humidifier can aid breathing during sleep. Teach parents to make a mild saltwater solution by dissolving 1/4 tsp of common salt in 8 oz warm water. Parents may need to show the child how to gargle with this solution in order to wash and soothe the swollen tissue in the throat.

When tonsillitis is caused by bacteria, antibiotics are generally prescribed. Because some bacteria, such as beta-hemolytic *Streptococcus*, can cause more serious infections (e.g., rheumatic fever), it is important to encourage parents to obtain treatment in a timely manner.

If a child has frequent recurrent episodes of bacterial tonsillitis, consideration may be given to surgical removal of the tonsils (**tonsillectomy**). The Health Promotion Issue below discusses this topic.

HEALTH PROMOTION ISSUE

Tonsillectomy

Parents worry about their children's tonsils, either because the tonsils are large, making swallowing difficult and causing snoring, or because of frequent episodes of tonsillitis. Ear, nose, and throat specialists are reluctant to surgically remove the tonsils. When should tonsils be removed?

DISCUSSION

The tonsils, lymphatic tissue found in the posterior oral pharynx, function to drain the lymph from the nose and sinuses. The nasal passages are the first line of entry for airborne bacteria and viruses. The lymph from the nose may contain these bacteria or viruses. Once the lymph enters the tonsil tissue, the microorganisms are destroyed by white blood cells. At times, the number of microorganisms entering the nose or multiplying within the lymph is greater than the white blood cells can destroy. When this occurs, the tonsils become swollen, red, and painful. If tonsillitis is the result of a virus, the infection will usually resolve spontaneously in 10 days to 2 weeks. If tonsillitis is from a bacterial infection, the child may need antibiotics to help stop the infection. This is especially likely when the causative organism is beta hemolytic streptococcus, which can invade and damage heart tissue.

Two common indications for tonsillectomy are chronic tonsillitis, having continuous symptoms for more than 3 months, or recurrent tonsillitis, having at least five episodes of tonsillitis in a year. However, the American Academy of Otolaryngology recommends that children have tonsillectomy if they have three or more episodes of tonsillitis in a year. In contrast, a study by Jack L. Paradise, MD (2002), reported that the modest benefit of a tonsillectomy in children who are moderately affected with sore throats (seven per year) does not seem to justify the risks, morbidity, or cost.

Sometimes the tonsils and adenoids become so enlarged that they cause obstructive sleep apnea (OSA). Children with OSA snore and have labored breathing, observed apnea, restlessness, excessive daytime sleepiness, and learning or behavior problems. Once the diagnosis of OSA is made, the child usually has both the tonsils and the adenoids removed.

Children with large tonsils can also have difficulty swallowing, resulting in feeding problems, failure to thrive, mouth breathing, and speech problems. As the child ages, the tonsils usually get smaller. If it is believed that the child will not outgrow the enlarged tonsils in a reasonable amount of time, or if the child is losing weight, a tonsillectomy may be performed.

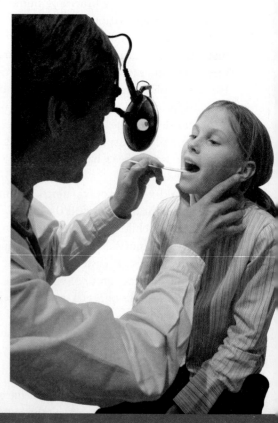

Nursing Considerations

When a tonsillectomy is planned, the nurse must provide preoperative teaching for the child and parents. The age and development of the child will influence the method of presenting information to the child. (See Chapters 6 and 7 ⊙⊙ for information about communicating with children.) Generally, routine preoperative care will be needed. This includes NPO for at least 4 hours, assessing the mouth for loose teeth, initiating an IV line, and giving sedation as ordered.

Postoperatively, the child's throat will be sore and the child may not want to swallow. Cold fluids such as Popsicles® may help relieve discomfort and increase fluids. Milk products are generally not given because they increase mucus production. Red fluids are also avoided so secretions do not appear to be blood. Liquid analgesics may be ordered.

The primary complication of a tonsillectomy is bleeding in the first 24 hours and again when the scab (**eschar**) sloughs off around day 10. Excessive swallowing may indicate blood is draining down the back of the throat. The nurse must use a flashlight to look into the child's oral pharynx to assess for bleeding.

The child may be discharged from the hospital within 24 hours after surgery. Parents should be taught to keep

---

The nurse collects data regarding the number of sore throats the child has had over time. It is important to obtain a throat culture to document the cause of the illness and to provide the correct medical treatment. Sore throat from postnasal drip does not count as an episode of tonsillitis unless the tonsils have pus on them. It is important for the nurse to question the child and parent regarding a current cold or sinus drainage. The severity of the symptoms should also be determined. If symptoms are so severe that the child misses a week of school with each episode of tonsillitis, a tonsillectomy may be warranted.

When a child presents with behavioral or attention problems, questions regarding sleep habits, snoring, and restlessness should be addressed. If the child is not growing at an acceptable rate or states dysphagia, the nurse should look in the throat to assess the size of the tonsils.

PLANNING AND IMPLEMENTATION

Parents need information about the child's specific disorder. If the child has recurrent or chronic tonsillitis, it is important for the nurse to teach the parents methods of preventing infection. Instruction must include hand washing, diet, adequate sleep, and avoiding infected persons. The nurse should answer questions about possible surgery, preoperative and postoperative care, and administration of antibiotics (including their side effects).

Even though the tonsils offer an important line of defense for the body, there are times when tonsillectomy is a necessary procedure. Continuous or recurrent tonsillitis can lead to more serious heart conditions and must be treated promptly. Sleep apnea is also a serious condition, and the parents should not wait for the child to outgrow the tonsil problems.

SELF-REFLECTION

Think of one time when you were out of breath from running or swimming. You may recall leaning forward over your knees (orthopneic position) and inhaling forcefully as you tried to "catch your breath." Gradually, your breathing returned to normal and your body relaxed. Knowing that in tonsillitis the child may experience restricted breathing, think of measures you can use to assist the child. Review both pharmacologic and nonpharmacologic measures.

SUGGESTED RESOURCES

For the Nurse

Marcus, C. L., Chapman, D., Ward, S. D., & McColley, S. A. (2002). Clinical practice guideline: Diagnosis and management of childhood obstructive sleep apnea syndrome. *Pediatrics, 109*(4), 704–712.

Paradise, J. L. (2002). Tonsillectomy and adenotonsillectomy for recurrent throat infection in moderately affected children. *Pediatrics, 110*(1), 7–15.

Ray, R. M., & Bower, C. M. (2005). Pediatric obstructive sleep apnea: the year in review. *Current Opinion in Otolaryngology & Head and Neck Surgery, 13*(6), 360–365.

Temple, R. H., & Timms, M. S. (2001). Pediatric coblation tonsillectomy. *International Journal of Pediatric Otorhinolaryngology 61,* 195–198.

For the Client

Gordon, M. (2000). *Let's talk about when you have to have your tonsils out.* New York: Power Kids Press.

Hatkoff, C., Hatkoff, J., & Mets, M. (2004). *Goodbye tonsils.* London: Puffin Books.

the child quiet for a few days, offer soft foods, and increase fluid intake. Bleeding will continue to be a concern until healing is complete in 7 to 14 days. Teach parents to contact the doctor immediately if bleeding is noticed. Any trauma to the back of the throat will increase the risk of bleeding. For this reason, drinking straws should be avoided and the child should be supervised while brushing the teeth. During the healing process, the dark scab will turn white and eventually slough off. Most commonly, the child will swallow the scab without noticing. Until healing is complete, the child's breath may have a strong foul odor. Gargling with mouthwash or saltwater is not recommended because of the increased risk of trauma that could cause bleeding. The odor will subside once healing is complete.

EPIGLOTTITIS

Epiglottitis is inflammation of the epiglottis caused by a bacterial infection of the pharynx and soft tissue of the larynx. As the epiglottis swells with inflammation, complete respiratory obstruction is possible. Therefore, epiglottitis is a potentially life-threatening condition.

Manifestations

Typically, the child develops a sudden high fever (higher than 102 °F or 39 °C), a sore throat, muffled or hoarse voice (**dysphonia**), and difficulty swallowing (dysphagia). As swelling progresses, respiratory distress and inspiratory stridor begin. Because of dysphagia, the child does not swallow saliva, resulting in drooling. Orthopnea is common. Anxiety is almost always present when the child has difficulty breathing.

clinical ALERT

The child might insist on sitting upright, leaning forward with the chin thrust forward, mouth open, and tongue protruding. This is called the **tripod position** (see Figure 12-13). The child should be allowed to maintain this position because it helps keep the epiglottis from obstructing the airway.

Diagnosis

Diagnosis is based on symptoms. Visual inspection is contraindicated because of the danger of triggering laryngospasm and airway obstruction in the child. A lateral x-ray view of the neck may be taken. Culture is postponed until an endotracheal tube or tracheostomy is in place.

Treatment

Medical treatment includes the insertion of an endotracheal tube in order to maintain the airway (see Procedure

8-28 🔗 for assisting in airway insertion). IV antibiotics are given to treat the infection. Acetaminophen or ibuprofen may be used to reduce the fever and discomfort. The child with epiglottitis is often cared for in the intensive care unit (ICU).

Nursing Considerations

Nursing care consists of managing the airway, administering prescribed medications, maintaining hydration, and providing emotional support for the child and family. Crying should be avoided as it stimulates the airway, increases oxygen consumption, causes the respiratory system to work harder, and could cause laryngospasm, which would totally occlude the airway. Provide a calm, quiet environment and a confident manner. Avoid any painful or frightening procedure until after the airway is secured. At times, light sedation may be needed.

clinical ALERT

Because of the life-threatening nature of epiglottitis, infants and toddlers who cannot ask for help must not be left alone during the acute phase of epiglottitis.

Difficulty swallowing, breathing, and speaking are frightening to the child and parents. The unfamiliar environment of the hospital creates additional stress. The nurse can reassure the child and family by remaining calm, explaining the various pieces of equipment, and providing care in a professional manner. Remaining in the room, or leaving for only a brief time, reassures the child and family that their needs will be met. Keep parents informed, and reassure them that any loss of voice is temporary. Most children show rapid response to treatment of cool mist, fluids, and antibiotics. The endotracheal tube can usually be removed in 24 to 36 hours. Home care involves completing the antibiotics as ordered. Parents need instruction in medication administration and potential side effects of the specific medication.

Foreign Body Obstructed Airway

The airway can become obstructed when the child puts a foreign body such as a small object, toy, or food in the mouth. Infants and young children must be observed closely while eating and be taught not to put small objects in the mouth. Table 12-2 ■ provides ways of communicating this teaching to children and parents. Even with

TABLE 12-2

Communicating Across the Life Span: Teaching Related to the Hazards of Choking

	TODDLER	PRESCHOOLER	SCHOOL-AGE CHILD	ADOLESCENT
Nurse	To the Parent: The small diameter of the airways makes obstruction more likely (see Figure 12-2). For example, the size of the child's trachea is about the diameter of the little finger. Small toys or bits of food such as raisins and hard candy can block the airway with serious consequences.	To the Parent: Preschoolers can choke easily. They should be taught not to put small items in their mouths.	To the child: Food should be eaten at the table and chewed and swallowed carefully before any activity. It is dangerous to run or play games when eating. You could get food caught in your throat and not be able to breathe.	To the adolescent: Choking can be a very dangerous thing. You are old enough to learn the signs of choking and what to do about it. Let me demonstrate the Heimlich maneuver for you.
Client/Parent	It will be important that I monitor mealtime, the types of foods my child eats, and his play time, so that he doesn't put small things in his mouth.	At Christmas time I need to buy large candy canes rather than small peppermint candies. I will need to tell my child that he should say "No" to any small candy offered to him.	I guess I'll have to quit eating my granola bar as I walk to school every morning.	I think I could save somebody's life if I see them choking in the cafeteria at school.

appropriate care, foreign body obstruction of the airway can occur. In this emergency situation, the care provider must immediately open the airway. To determine if the airway is obstructed, observe the child's facial expression, ask the child if he or she can talk, and observe for respirations. If the object can be seen in the back of the throat, try to remove it with a finger sweep, taking care not to push it deeper into the airway. If the object cannot be removed, the Heimlich maneuver (Figure 12-6 ■) is the recommended procedure to clear an obstructed airway safely. The size of the child will determine the position and procedure used.

NEWBORN

Newborn resuscitation requires special training and certification plus review courses to ensure that the nurse is using

up-to-date methods and is following the most current guidelines. The American Academy of Pediatrics offers the Neonatal Resuscitation Program (NRP) and the American Heart Association offers the Pediatric Advanced Life Support (PALS) program.

CONSCIOUS INFANT

To perform the Heimlich maneuver on an infant, the prone position is used with the baby's head lower than the trunk (see Figure 12-6). Support the head and neck with one hand, with the torso on the forearm. Use the heel of the other hand to give five forceful back blows between the shoulder blades. If the object is not dislodged after the back blows, the free hand is placed over the back of the neck, sandwiching the infant between the hands. The infant is turned over, maintaining the head-down position. Two to three fingers are placed just below the nipple line at the center of the chest. Five chest thrusts are given at a rate of one every 3 to 5 seconds. This procedure is repeated until the airway is cleared. Abdominal thrusts are not used on infants because of the risk of damaging the internal organs.

Cardiopulmonary resuscitation (CPR) (Figure 12-7 ■) may be needed once the airway is open. (CPR training is not reviewed in detail in this text. Nurses often obtain training for CPR through the American Heart Association,

clinical ALERT

In the health care setting, emergency care to infants and children related to respiratory or cardiac resuscitation should only be provided by a member of the health care team who has been trained and certified in these efforts. Organ and musculoskeletal damage may occur when improper techniques are applied during the Heimlich maneuver or cardiopulmonary resuscitation.

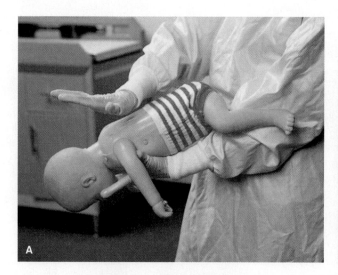

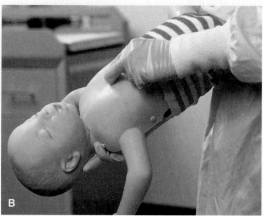

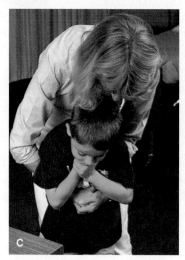

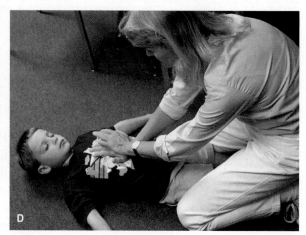

Figure 12-6. ■ Clearing a foreign object. (**A**) Back blows. (**B**) Chest thrusts on infant. (**C**) Standing thrusts (Heimlich maneuver) must be done more gently in a child than in an adult. (**D**) Chest thrusts on an unconscious child.

the American Red Cross, or their employing agency. Nurses may be expected or required to maintain current certification throughout their practice.)

CONSCIOUS CHILD

The Heimlich maneuver is performed on a child the same as on an adult. However, the smaller the child, the more gently the abdominal thrusts are given. If the child is sitting or standing, grasp the child from the back with both arms wrapped around the child's abdomen. With one hand made into a fist, place the thumb side against the child's abdomen, slightly above the umbilicus and well below the xiphoid process of the sternum (see Figure 12-6C). The fist is grasped with the other hand and pressed into the child's abdomen with a quick upward thrust.

Abdominal thrusts are repeated until the object is expelled or the child becomes unconscious.

UNCONSCIOUS CHILD

The unconscious child is positioned supine. Kneeling at the child's feet (standing at the feet if the child is on a table), place the heel of one hand on the child's abdomen, at the midline, slightly above the umbilicus, and well below the xiphoid process of the sternum (see Figure 12-6D). With the other hand on top of the first, press into the child's abdomen with a quick upward thrust. Repeat until the object is dislodged from the airway. Sometimes, the object is expelled into the mouth and can be removed with a finger sweep, taking care not to push the object back into the airway. CPR may be needed once the airway is opened.

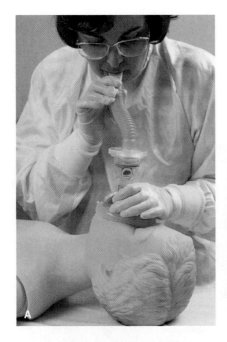
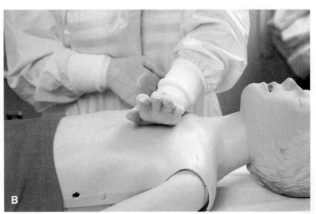
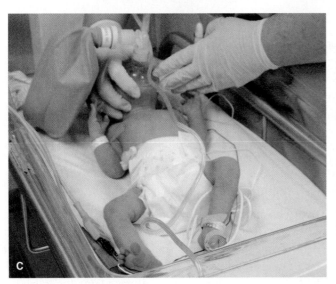
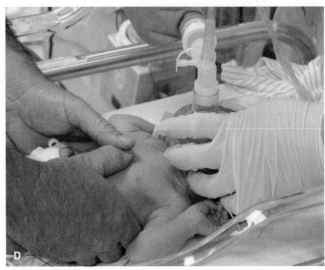

Figure 12-7. ■ CPR. (**A**) Mouth-to-mouth resuscitation using a mask with a one-way valve. (**B**) Hand position for chest compressions with a child. (**C**) Demonstration of resuscitation of a newborn with bag and mask (Ambu-bag). Note that the mask covers the nose and the mouth and the head is in a neutral, "sniff" position. The resuscitating bag is placed to the side of the baby so that chest movement can be seen. (**D**) Chest compression can be done with two fingers of one hand or using the pads of both thumbs. In either case, the sternum is compressed at a rate of 90 beats per minute.

LOWER RESPIRATORY DISORDERS

Respiratory Disorders Associated with the Newborn and Infant

NEONATAL RESPIRATORY DISTRESS SYNDROME

Neonatal respiratory distress syndrome (RDS) is a condition commonly seen in premature infants. RDS is defined as an inadequate production of surfactant. Surfactant is a mixture of phospholipids and apoproteins that attach to the internal surface of the alveoli, reducing the surface tension and improving the lungs' ability to remain inflated during exhalation. Without adequate amounts of surfactant, the alveoli collapse (Figure 12-8 ■), and the infant must work hard to reinflate the alveoli with each breath.

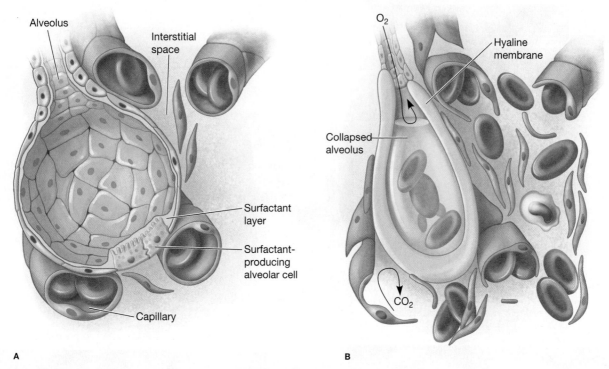

Figure 12-8. ■ Respiratory distress syndrome (RDS). When the newborn lung is lacking in surfactant, alveoli can collapse. (**A**) Healthy alveolus. (**B**) Collapsed alveolus.

Manifestations

The infant will exhibit signs of respiratory distress, including respirations greater than 60, retractions (see Figure 12-4), nasal flaring, and audible grunting. Lung sounds will be greatly decreased. Within a few minutes, symptoms can worsen.

Diagnosis and Treatment

Diagnosis, based on clinical symptoms, must be made rapidly in order to save the infant's life. Treatment includes oxygen administration and assisted mechanical ventilation (see Procedures 13-25 to 13-28 ⊙). Synthetic surfactant, given within 24 hours, may be helpful in treating **atelectasis** (an airless state of the lung).

Nursing Considerations

Infants with RDS will be cared for in the ICU. Infants will be placed in a warmer to maintain body temperature and reduce metabolic demands. Oxygen use in premature infants must be monitored closely as it can lead to bronchopulmonary dysplasia (discussed later) or blindness (called *retinopathy of prematurity*). Thorough assessment of intravenous fluid intake can prevent pulmonary edema.

Besides providing intensive care, the nurse must support the parents. The nurse may need to call clergy or family to be with the parents. Teaching about treatment can help alleviate the parents' fear of losing their child. Parents will need to learn CPR and oxygen administration. They may also need to learn how to use an apnea monitor or other equipment at home. Referral to a support group may be useful.

BRONCHOPULMONARY DYSPLASIA (BPD)

Bronchopulmonary dysplasia (BPD) is a chronic lung disease that affects infants with RDS, congenital heart defects, meconium aspiration, or other conditions that result in assisted mechanical ventilation. Most infants with BPD have been on a mechanical ventilator for at least 3 days. The immature lung becomes damaged from the high ventilator pressure and oxygen toxicity, resulting in pulmonary inflammation, cellular damage, and death of tissue.

Manifestations

The infant with BPD has persistent signs of respiratory failure due to bronchial edema and fibrosis of the lung tissue. There may be wheezing, crackles, retractions, nasal flaring, and grunting. Normal activities, such as feeding, place additional work on the respiratory system and may result in failure to thrive.

Diagnosis and Treatment

Diagnosis is based on chest x-rays. Medical management involves ventilation with progressive weaning from mechanical assistance, oxygen administration, nutrition, and antiinflammatory medication. A tracheostomy is indicated for long-term mechanical ventilation. Long-term complications include asthma and recurrent pulmonary infections. Some infants require a gastrostomy tube for feeding in order to obtain adequate caloric intake to support growth.

Nursing Considerations

Nursing care focuses on promoting respiratory function and preparing the family for home care. The infant with BPD can become acutely ill with respiratory complications at any time, and parents must be alert for early symptoms. Parents must be taught to administer feedings, oxygen, and medication. They must also learn to manage the required equipment. (See Figure 7-16 and respiratory Procedures 8-25 through 8-28 in Chapter 8 ⬀.) At home the infant may continue mechanical ventilation, oxygen, and medication. Parents who are fearful of assuming responsibility for their baby may require home nursing assistance. Referrals for respiratory supplies, medications, financial support, and follow-up care should be planned and coordinated before discharge.

SUDDEN INFANT DEATH SYNDROME

Sudden infant death syndrome (SIDS) is the sudden, unexplained death of an infant younger than 1 year. SIDS most often strikes infants between 2 and 4 months of age and is more common in males. Other factors common in SIDS include Native American or African American descent, low birth weight, and multiple births (twins or triplets). SIDS is the leading cause of death of infants between 1 month and 1 year of age. Box 12-2 ■ identifies risk factors associated with SIDS.

Manifestations

When SIDS strikes, the infant is typically found not breathing, and emergency medical help is summoned. The infant is usually in a normal state of nutrition and hydration. In more than 50% of infants, blood-tinged frothy fluids are present in and around the mouth and nose. The diapers are filled with urine and stool. The infant may be clutching a blanket. There is no audible outcry at the time of death. Skin is a white, ashen color, not the expected cyanotic blue found with respiratory distress. An autopsy will need to be performed to identify the cause of death.

Prevention and Treatment

SIDS remains unpredictable. The main preventive measure is to place infants on their backs to sleep. If a child is found in respiratory arrest, CPR must be initiated immediately and emergency medical services called. Parents of children at risk should be taught CPR methods.

BOX 12-2	ASSESSMENT

Risk Factors for SIDS

Infant
- Prematurity
- Low birth weight
- Twin or triplet birth
- Race (in decreasing order of frequency): most common in Native American infants, followed by African American, Hispanic, White, and Asian infants
- Gender: more common in males than females
- Age: most common in infants between 2 and 4 months of age
- Time of year: more prevalent in winter months
- Exposure to passive smoke
- History of cyanosis, respiratory distress, irritability, and poor feeding in the nursery
- Sleeping prone

Maternal and Familial
- Maternal age younger than 20 years
- History of smoking and illicit drug use (increases incidence 10 times)
- Anemia
- Multiple pregnancies, with short intervals between births
- History of sibling with SIDS (increases incidence four to five times)
- Low socioeconomic status; crowding
- Poor prenatal care, low birth weight gain

Nursing Considerations

The impact of SIDS on the family is one of extreme shock followed by extreme outrage. Family members commonly experience guilt, either self-blaming or projecting blame onto other family members or caregivers (e.g., a babysitter). Older children may fear SIDS will happen to them as well. Siblings may also believe that the infant died because of bad thoughts or desires they had toward their brother or sister.

The nurse has an important role in both supporting the family and educating the public. Recall that by 2 months infants are able to reposition their head to breathe. Ordinary mattresses and bedding are incapable of causing hypoxia to the point of suffocation. This knowledge can be used to help family members understand that the death was not their fault.

Although the need for support of parents and siblings is obvious, grandparents will need additional support. Grandparents will be experiencing grief at the loss of their grandchild, but also extreme hurt at watching their own children suffer. Family members should be allowed to hold the infant, and receive handprints, footprints, and a lock of hair. Provide the family with information about local support groups.

MECONIUM ASPIRATION

The passage of **meconium** (sterile substance present in the intestine of the fetus) by the fetus is a common occurrence in response to hypoxia or stress during the pregnancy. During birth, the newborn can inhale the amniotic fluid containing meconium (**meconium aspiration**). Severe meconium aspiration increases the possibility that the newborn will develop persistent pulmonary hypertension, pneumothorax, and pneumonia.

Congenital Respiratory Disorders

Tracheoesophageal fistula (TEF), a connection between the trachea and the esophagus, is the most common congenital anomaly affecting the respiratory system. TEF is associated with **esophageal atresia** (EA), in which the esophagus ends in a blind pouch instead of connecting to the stomach. EA and TEF are potentially life-threatening defects (see Figure 17-4 ⬤⬤). They may be found separately but are most commonly found together. When the newborn ingests breast milk or formula, the food will enter the trachea through the fistula, resulting in respiratory distress, aspiration, and possibly pneumonia. The infant with EA and TEF presents with copious amounts of thin mucus shortly after birth. The secretions clear with suctioning, but they soon reappear. If a TEF only is present, the stomach may become trapped with air and distended. If the defects are not identified prior to feeding, the infant will regurgitate the feeding, or the feeding will be aspirated into the lungs.

In the absence of other anomalies, surgical repair is usually completed in the first few days of life. If other anomalies are present, gastrostomy feedings may be necessary until the infant is stabilized. These disorders are discussed in further detail in Chapter 17 ⬤⬤, Care of the Child with Gastrointestinal Disorders.

CYSTIC FIBROSIS

Cystic fibrosis (CF) is an inherited autosomal recessive disorder of the exocrine glands affecting predominantly White children. In CF, there is defective chloride-ion and water transport across the cell membranes of mucus-secreting cells. This defect causes production of thick, tenacious mucus that obstructs organs with mucous ducts such as the pancreas and the lungs. Electrolytes are lost through sweat, saliva, and mucous secretions. The disease affects primarily the respiratory and gastrointestinal systems, but it has some effect on the integumentary, musculoskeletal and reproductive systems as well (Figure 12-9 ■). The life expectancy is 30 years.

CYSTIC FIBROSIS

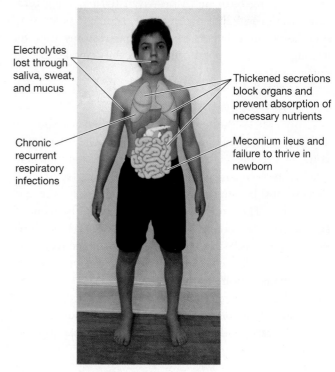

Electrolytes lost through saliva, sweat, and mucus

Chronic recurrent respiratory infections

Thickened secretions block organs and prevent absorption of necessary nutrients

Meconium ileus and failure to thrive in newborn

Figure 12-9. ■ Multisystem effects of cystic fibrosis.

Manifestations

In the newborn, presenting symptoms may be meconium ileus (a small bowel obstruction), failure to thrive, or chronic recurrent respiratory infections. The child's stools typically appear fatty or greasy (**steatorrhea**), frothy, float, and have a foul smell. The child may also be constipated. The child will have a chronic moist, productive cough with thick, sticky mucus and frequent respiratory infections. Despite a ravenous appetite, children will have trouble gaining weight. There may be clubbing of fingers related to a reduction in oxygen reaching the tissues.

Diagnosis

Diagnosis is made by a positive sweat test (Figure 12-10 ■). Table 12-3 ■ describes this test. Diagnosis may be made before 1 year of age, but children with a mild form of the disease may not be diagnosed until adolescence. CF is not generally terminal until adulthood.

Treatment

Medical treatment is aimed at maintaining maximum respiratory function and nutrition for as long as possible. Postural drainage or chest physiotherapy, also called bronchial hygiene therapy, is ordered to help the child eliminate respiratory secretions. Procedure 12-1 ■

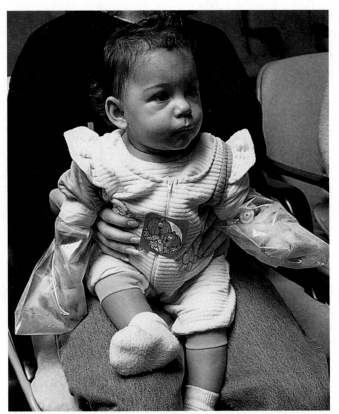

Figure 12-10. ■ Sweat test. The parent may hold and reassure the infant or small child being evaluated for cystic fibrosis with the sweat test. Sweat will be collected from the skin under the plastic wrappings for evaluation of sodium and chloride content. Note that sweat tests performed on infants younger than 4 weeks of age may not provide accurate results.

provides information on performing chest physiotherapy. Aggressive treatment of respiratory infections or allergies is required.

Pancreatic enzymes; vitamins A, D, E, and K; and a diet high in carbohydrates and protein are prescribed to manage the gastrointestinal complications of CF. On hot days, the child may need extra fluids and salt.

Nursing Considerations

When assessing a child with CF, pay close attention to respiratory function. Thick mucus can obstruct the bronchi, resulting in hypoxia and infection. The priority nursing intervention must be to open and maintain a patent airway (see Respiratory Procedures section in Chapter 8 ⬮). Children with CF are frequently admitted to the hospital with an acute respiratory infection. Respiratory therapy several times a day and antibiotics will be ordered to help clear the airways. Parents will need to be taught how to provide postural drainage with percussion. Procedure 12-1 provides steps for how to perform percussion.

Children with CF are growth retarded even with a ravenous appetite. The thick mucus blocks the production of pancreatic enzymes, resulting in an inability to digest nutrients. Fat-soluble vitamins are poorly absorbed. Digestive problems can be eased with special medication and diet modification. Pancreatic enzymes should be given with each meal and each large snack. The goal of care is to achieve near-normal stools and maintain adequate weight gain.

CF is a chronic, long-term illness that is ultimately fatal. With adequate treatment and prevention of complications, some children live into adulthood. However, the stress on the child, family members, and community resources is great. The child needs to be encouraged to participate in activities consistent with his or her level of development and physical endurance in order to maintain as "normal" a life as possible. Parents will need emotional support as they work daily to keep their child healthy.

CF takes a financial toll on the family resources as well. The nurse should provide referral to support groups and other resources to assist families.

MediaLink Cystic Fibrosis Research and Treatment

TABLE 12-3				
Sweat Test for Cystic Fibrosis				
TEST	**PURPOSE**	**METHOD OF SPECIMEN COLLECTION**	**NORMAL FINDINGS**	**ABNORMAL FINDINGS**
Sweat test (pilocarpine iontophoresis)	To analyze sodium and chloride content	Two electrodes covered with special gel are placed on child's forearms. A small electric current is passed through electrode for 5 minutes. Some tingling may be noted. Electrodes are removed, and sweat collector is applied to same area. Sweat is collected for 30 to 45 minutes. Sweat collector is sent to laboratory for analysis.	Sodium: 10–30 mEq/L; Chloride: 10–35 mEq/L	Chloride: 50–60 mEq/L is suspicious More than 60 mEq/L with other signs is diagnostic

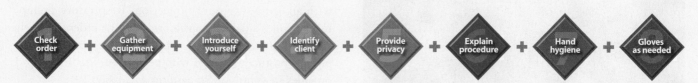

PROCEDURE 12-1 Postural Drainage with Percussion (Chest Physiotherapy)

Purpose

■ To clear the airway of thick mucus

Equipment

■ Bed or table
■ Pillows
■ Hand towel

Check order ✚ Gather equipment ✚ Introduce yourself ✚ Identify client ✚ Provide privacy ✚ Explain procedure ✚ Hand hygiene ✚ Gloves as needed

Interventions and Rationales

1. Perform preparatory steps (see icon bar above).

2. Position the child on one side, usually with the head lower than the hips. (The various positions for chest

physiotherapy are shown in Figure 12-11 ■.) The upper arm should be positioned over the head or across the anterior chest, exposing the lateral chest. Pillows may be

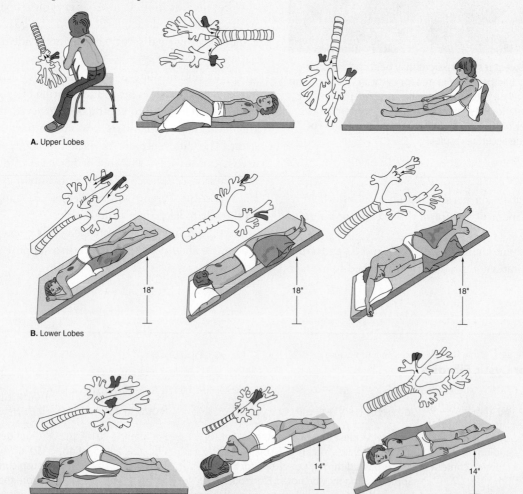

A. Upper Lobes

B. Lower Lobes

C. Lower Lobes (continued)

Right Middle Lobe

Left Upper Lobe

Figure 12-11. ■ Positions for postural drainage of different parts of the lung. The area of the lung to be drained is illustrated directly above the client's position.

used to support the child in position. *Positioning with the head down utilizes gravity to facilitate movement of mucus from small bronchioles to the larger bronchi.*

3. Place folded towel over the chest. *The towel protects the skin from trauma.*

4. With cupped hands (Figure 12-12 ■), gently clap on the lateral chest for 3 to 5 minutes. Turn the child to the abdomen to expose the back. Clap on the back over each lobe of the lung for 3 to 5 minutes each. Turn the child

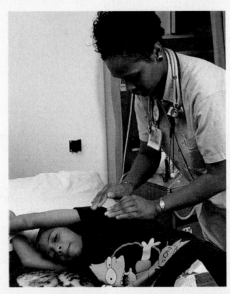

Figure 12-12. ■ The cupped-hand position is used to clap against the chest well over the segment to be drained. This creates a vibration that helps dislodge secretions. Various body positions are used, depending on the location of the obstruction. See Figure 12-11 for positions.

to the opposite side and continue clapping over each lung field. *Clapping on the chest with cupped hands causes vibration inside the lung, moving mucus to larger airways.*

5. Sit the child up and have him or her deep breathe and cough. *Coughing helps expel mucus.*

6. With the child in a sitting position, clap over the upper chest to clear the right and left upper lobes. *The upper lobes are anterior to the main bronchus; therefore, the child must be sitting for gravity to pull the mucus toward the large airway.*

7. A mechanical vibrator can be purchased to provide percussion instead of clapping with the hands. The child's position will be the same. *Mechanical vibrators can be used with postural drainage to move mucus out of small airways.*

SAMPLE DOCUMENTATION

(date) 0730   Respirations labored, accessory muscles used with inspiration. Lung sounds diminished in right middle and lower lobes. Postural drainage with percussion to all lung fields performed by mother. Productive cough of a moderate amount of thick white mucus. Lung sounds clear bilaterally. Respirations less labored.
_____L. Hines, LPN

Lower Respiratory Infections

Infections of the lower respiratory system include viral and bacterial infections of the bronchi and alveoli. The symptoms and nursing care of lower respiratory infections are similar. Medical treatment is specific to the causative organism.

BRONCHIOLITIS

Bronchiolitis is an infection and inflammation of the smaller airways or **bronchioles**. A buildup of mucus and swollen mucous membranes results in wheezing from partial obstruction. The most common causative organism is the **respiratory syncytial virus** (RSV).

RSV occurs in epidemics from October to March. This virus is easily transmitted and most children have been infected by age 3. RSV is transmitted through direct or close contact with respiratory secretions of infected individuals. The virus invades the cells of the bronchial mucosa, causing the cells to rupture. Cell debris irritates the airway, causing an increase in secretions that obstruct the bronchioles.

Manifestations

When the airways are partially obstructed, wheezing and crackles can be heard on auscultation. As the blockage continues, breath sounds diminish, causing impaired gas exchange and eventually leading to respiratory failure.

Symptoms of RSV begin with nasal stuffiness and fever, but within a few days they progress to frequent, deep cough; rapid, labored breathing; and respiratory distress, including retraction and nasal flaring. Parents report that the child appears sicker, refuses to eat and is less playful. Labored lung sounds may diminish as airflow to the lungs decreases. The child may also be dehydrated.

Diagnosis

Diagnosis is made by history, culturing nasopharyngeal secretions (e.g., with enzyme-linked immunosorbent assay [ELISA]), and chest x-ray.

Treatment

Depending on the degree of symptoms, the child with RSV may be hospitalized for treatment. The physician will order IV fluids, humidified oxygen, and medications to open the airways, decrease inflammation, thin the secretions, and lower the temperature. The respiratory therapist will be a valuable resource in maintaining a patent airway and administering breathing treatments.

Nursing Considerations

When hospitalized, the child with RSV requires special precautions to prevent transmission of the organism to others. These precautions would include a private room and the use of gowns and gloves (some facilities also require masks) when in the child's room. (See Procedure 8-26, Administering Oxygen to Children ⚭.) The Nursing Care Plan Chart below discusses nursing care for this infection.

Nursing Care Plan Chart

Respiratory Syncytial Virus

GOAL	INTERVENTION	RATIONALE	EXPECTED OUTCOME
1. Ineffective Airway Clearance related to inflammation of the bronchioles			
The child's airway will be clear within 48 hours	Monitor vital signs every hour.	*The child's condition can change rapidly and therefore must be closely monitored*	The child will be able to breathe at a rate and depth considered within normal limits (see Table 12-1).
	Monitor oxygen saturation continuously. See Procedure 8-29 ⚭.	*Continuous monitoring of oxygen saturation will alert the nurse if the child's condition deteriorates.*	Oxygen saturation will be at 95%.
	Administer oxygen as ordered. See Procedure 8-28 ⚭.	*Oxygen is administered to maintain oxygen saturation above 95%.*	
	Anticipate worsening respiratory distress by monitoring breath sounds, respiratory effort, and level of consciousness.	*Anticipating a worsening of the child's condition allows the nurse time to prepare for airway maintenance.*	
	Reposition every ½ hour.	*Frequent position changes facilitate drainage of respiratory mucus*	
	Administer IV fluids via appropriate equipment.	*IV fluids are administered by infusion pump to prevent accidental fluid overload*	
	Administer medications with careful attention to dosage.	*Pediatric dosage is individualized based on body weight. If dosage is not calculated carefully, overdosage or underdosage could occur. To maintain medication blood level in a therapeutic range, medications must be administered on time*	
The family will be able to execute an effective plan of care for the child at home.	Teach the family to recognize changes in respiratory status.	*Prompt recognition of symptoms will facilitate treatment*	The family effectively manages the child's respiratory needs at home.
	Demonstrate and observe a return demonstration of postural drainage techniques.	*Learning is enhanced when procedures are demonstrated and correct learning can be documented by return demonstration*	

CROUP

Croup is a term used to represent a group of respiratory illnesses that results from inflammation and swelling of the larynx, trachea, and large bronchi (Figure 12-13 ■). The causative agent can be either viral or bacterial. Although laryngotracheobronchitis is the most common, epiglottitis (discussed previously) and bacterial tracheitis are the most serious because of possible airway obstruction. Laryngotracheitis is caused by viral agents while epiglottitis and bacterial tracheitis are caused by bacterial agents. See Chapter 10 ⬮ for discussion of infectious diseases such as pertussis (whooping cough).

Manifestations

When a child has croup, **inspiratory stridor** (a high-pitched, musical sound caused by narrowing of the airway) will be present. A barking, seal-like cough and hoarseness are also present. The infant or child may have been ill for several days before the airway became partially obstructed and caused symptoms. Others may be healthy and develop severe symptoms in a matter of a few hours. Fever may or may not be present. The child may refuse to swallow saliva because of severe throat pain and swelling, resulting in drooling. The child may sit leaning forward (see Figure 12-13) in the tripod position.

Diagnosis

Diagnosis is based on clinical findings. An x-ray may be taken to rule out foreign body obstruction. Pulse oximetry is used to detect hypoxemia.

Treatment

The goal of treatment is to reduce the swelling and open the airways. Cool mist administered by mask or tent (see Figure 8-33 and Procedures 8-25 to 8-28 ⬮) may be ordered. If a bacterial infection is present, appropriate antibiotic therapy will be prescribed. Endotracheal intubation may be needed to keep the airway open. Medications to reduce airway swelling may be ordered.

Nursing Considerations

As with other respiratory conditions, the child should be observed closely for airway patency, oxygen saturation, and retractions. It is important to deliver cool mist to the child in a quiet environment. The child should not be left alone because very young children may not be able to summon help. Crying can induce laryngospasm and therefore should be avoided. Avoid probing the throat, including obtaining throat cultures, to prevent laryngospasm and complete obstruction.

Most children show rapid improvement once cool mist, oxygen, antibiotics, and fluids are started. The endotracheal tube, if used, can usually be removed in 24 to 36 hours. Discharge teaching includes the continued use of cool mist and administration of prescribed antibiotics, including side effects.

PNEUMONIA

Pneumonia is inflammation or infection of the bronchioles and alveoli in the lung or lungs (Figure 12-14 ■). The most common causative organism in infants and young children

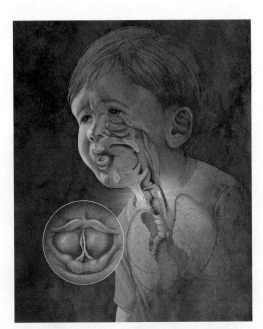

Figure 12-13. ■ In croup, the epiglottis swells and occludes the airway (*see inset*). The trachea swells against the cricoid cartilage, causing airway restriction. (Phototake NYC)

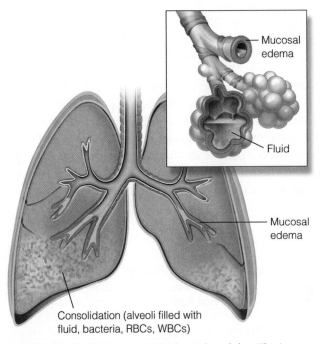

Figure 12-14. ■ Pneumonia in the lower lung lobes. The *inset* shows the buildup of fluid in the alveoli.

is viral; however, there are many causative agents. In premature infants and older children, the causative agent is more commonly bacterial (*Pneumococcus*). Whether viral or bacterial in origin, the pathophysiology of pneumonia is the same. The infecting organism causes inflammation and swelling of the mucous membranes. Macrophages move to the area and engulf the organisms by phagocytosis. Thick mucus, dead cells and other debris accumulate in the alveoli and small air passages where they block gas exchange. If the mucus remains in the small airways, it can cause **consolidation** (creating a solid or firm, inelastic lung) and become more difficult to remove.

Manifestations

The child with pnuemonia will develop a fever, malaise, and a cough. On auscultation, breath sounds may be diminished or absent in consolidated areas and wheezing may be heard. Respirations will be rapid (**tachypnea**) and labored. The child will be tired and want to sleep, but may be unable to rest because of dyspnea.

Diagnosis

Sputum cultures and chest x-rays are used to diagnose pneumonia.

Treatment

Medical treatment depends on the causative organism and includes antibiotics, oral and intravenous fluids, cough suppressants, and antipyretics. If diagnosed early, the child may be treated at home. The hospitalized child will require oxygen (see Procedures 8-25 to 8-28 ⬮), chest physiotherapy, and IV fluids. Most children recover in a short period of time.

The culture of the sick child can influence the way the family chooses to treat respiratory and other diseases. Box 12-3 ■ describes one cultural view of pneumonia.

Nursing Considerations

Like other respiratory disorders, the priority of care is to maintain the airway and provide symptom relief for pain and fever. The child requires constant attention. Parents need support because seeing their child in respiratory distress is frightening. The nurse provides teaching as appropriate for the situation and age of the child.

BOX 12-3	CULTURAL PULSE POINTS

Pneumonia as a "Cold" Disease

Various cultures, especially some Asian cultures, believe that physical disorders result from a hot or cold imbalance in the body fluids. Pneumonia is a disorder that is considered a "cold" disease and should be treated with "hot" fluids (e.g., hot tea). Other respiratory disorders are also considered "cold" in nature.

TUBERCULOSIS

Tuberculosis (TB) is an infection of the respiratory system by the acid-fast bacillus *Mycobacterium tuberculosis*. Individuals with TB may be immunocompromised with disorders such as HIV/AIDS, leukemia, or other disorders affecting the white blood cells. When a child develops TB, it is most commonly due to close association with a TB-infected adult. If left untreated, the disease leads to lung damage and central nervous system involvement. Tuberculosis meningitis, coma, and death are also complications.

The organism enters the body by droplets from an infected individual. Once inside the lungs, the organism rapidly divides and spreads throughout the body via the lymphatic and circulatory systems. Granulomas develop around the site of primary exposure. The granulomas contain and destroy the bacteria, eventually scarring the lung tissue. Pockets of infection may survive the immune response and lie dormant for some time. A change in the body's internal environment can cause the disease to reactivate.

Manifestations

Exposure and infection may not result in the presence of symptoms. Symptoms of a persistent cough, weight loss, and fever can appear 1 to 6 months after exposure. The child may also have diminished breath sounds, wheezing, and crackles. In addition, active TB causes fatigue, anorexia, night sweats, and chills.

Diagnosis

Diagnosis is based on a combination of physical findings, positive purified protein derivative (PPD) skin tests (**Mantoux test**) (Figure 12-15 ■), x-rays, and laboratory isolation of *M. tuberculosis* in the sputum. In rare cases (Box 12-4 ■), the skin test may give a false-positive reading.

Treatment

Medical treatment typically includes the administration of isoniazid, rifampin, and pyrazinamide for 2 months, followed

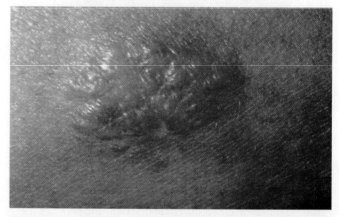

Figure 12-15. ■ Positive tuberculin skin test (Mantoux test), showing previous exposure to tuberculosis. (Custom Medical Stock Photo Inc.)

TABLE 12-4

Pharmacology: Drugs Used to Treat Tuberculosis

DRUG (GENERIC AND COMMON BRAND NAME)	USUAL ROUTE/DOSE	CLASSIFICATION	SELECTED SIDE EFFECTS	DON'T GIVE IF
Isoniazid (INH)	10–20 mg/kg/day; give 1 hour before meals	Antituberculosis agent	Peripheral neuropathy, GI upset, weakness	Low BP (give with caution); don't give if liver damage
Rifampin (Rifadin)	10–20 mg/kg/day in divided dose every 12 hours	Antituberculosis agent	Dizzy, GI upset, colitis	Children younger than 5 years (use not determined)
Pyrazinamide (Tebrazid)	20–40 mg/kg/day in divided dose every 12 hours	Antituberculosis agent	Hemolytic anemia, difficulty urinating	Severe liver damage

BOX 12-4   CULTURAL PULSE POINTS

Unusual Response to TB (Mantoux) Test
A false-positive tuberculin or Mantoux test can be expected from a child vaccinated in some countries, including the Philippines. This is due to the type of vaccine, bacille Calmette-Guerin, given to children of these countries. To diagnose tuberculosis in these children, chest x-rays and sputum cultures are necessary.

by 6 months of isoniazid or rifampin. Table 12-4 ■ describes drugs used in the treatment of TB. The PPD test will be permanently positive. Chest x-ray will be required to determine the elimination or recurrence of the disease.

Nursing Considerations

Nursing care is centered on family education. Drug resistance to TB has increased dramatically in recent years, so parents must be taught the importance of adhering closely to the medical regimen and completing treatment. Teaching should include preventing the spread of the infection to others and stressing the necessity of taking the prescribed medication. All people who have come in contact with the infected child need to be screened and treated as necessary.

If the child is hospitalized, standard precautions are sufficient unless there is extensive pulmonary infection. In this case, airborne precautions and use of a sealed particulate respirator for all patient contact is necessary. See Chapter 10 ⚭ for a discussion of the various types of precautions.

Additional Respiratory Disorders

ASTHMA

Asthma is a chronic inflammatory disorder of the tracheobronchial tree. A variety of triggers can cause asthma attacks, including allergens, smoke, medication, fumes, exercise, or

stress (Figure 12-16 ■). The stimulus that initiates the inflammatory process is specific to each individual. Before puberty, more boys have asthma, but by adulthood the disease is equally distributed between the genders.

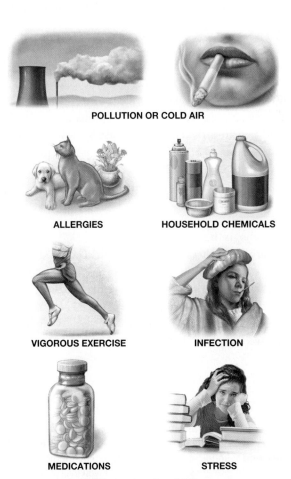

POLLUTION OR COLD AIR

ALLERGIES   HOUSEHOLD CHEMICALS

VIGOROUS EXERCISE   INFECTION

MEDICATIONS   STRESS

Figure 12-16. ■ Eliminating the child's exposure to potential asthma triggers requires significant lifestyle changes for the child and family, so be sensitive to the family's situation and needs. Culture sometimes plays a significant part in exposure to lifestyle triggers.

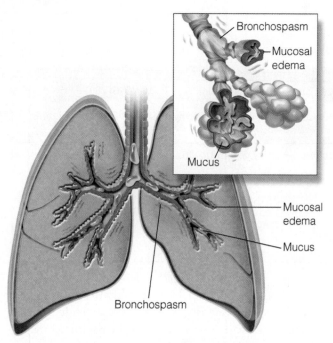

Figure 12-17. ■ When an asthma attack occurs, the bronchi constrict and spasm (*see inset*), and mucus obstructs the airway.

As the lining of the tracheobronchial tree becomes irritated by an allergen, fumes, or dust, the cells release histamine. Mucous membranes swell, mucus forms, and airway muscles contract (Figure 12-17 ■). Copious amounts of mucus block small airways, trapping air below the plug. Chronic irritation and swelling of mucous membranes cause damage to the cells lining the airway. The end result is scar tissue formation and hyperinflation of the alveoli.

Manifestations

The child who is having an "asthma attack" has fast, labored breathing with a productive cough. The child often wheezes on expiration. The child may complain of tightness in the chest and appear tired. There may be nasal flaring and intercostal retractions (see Figure 12-4). Young children may bob their heads to engage accessory muscles to breathe (see Figure 12-13).

clinical ALERT

A condition called *status asthmaticus* occurs when the child develops severe respiratory distress and bronchospasms that do not respond to medication. Without immediate medical attention, the child may die. Treatment may involve airway intubation and ventilator support. The child will be admitted to the ICU. The role of the LPN/LVN is to assist the RN in providing care. The nurse would also observe for signs of anxiety in the child and family.

BOX 12-5   ASSESSMENT

Child with Acute Asthma

The following provide important data for the assessment of a child with asthma:

■ Is the child able to talk, or does respiratory distress prevent speech?

■ Is the child wheezing?

■ What is the child's skin color and heart rate?

■ Is the child relaxed or fighting to breathe? Is the child crying?

■ Does the child hold on to parents, or is he or she lying calmly on the bed?

■ What is the family doing? Do they appear frightened? What is their tone of voice?

■ Do the parents ask appropriate questions?

Psychological reactions often intensify the symptoms of asthma. As the airway becomes blocked, the child becomes anxious and believes that he or she is suffocating. Severe anxiety intensifies the symptoms, and a vicious cycle ensues. Emotional stress may even trigger asthma attacks (Box 12-5 ■).

Diagnosis

Diagnosis of asthma is based on medical history, physical assessment, and pulmonary function tests. Peak expiratory flow rates (PEFRs) are used to determine the extent of damage. PEFR is the fastest speed at which air is exhaled. With asthma, airways collapse, trapping air in the alveoli and lowering the PEFR. Many allergens can be identified by skin tests.

Treatment

Asthma management involves avoiding triggers, regulating medications, family teaching, and ongoing follow-up. Drug management depends on the severity and frequency of the child's symptoms. Short-acting bronchodilators, inhaled corticosteroids, and long-acting oral antiasthmatics can be used alone or in combination. The newest class of drugs used to treat asthma is the leukotriene receptor antagonists. These drugs prevent the bronchoconstrictive and inflammatory action of leukotriene by blocking the receptor. Table 12-5 ■ lists common medications used in children with asthma.

Nursing Considerations

The child, with the help of the parents, may be able to avoid the specific allergens that trigger an asthma attack. Because exercise can bring on an acute asthma attack, the child should warm up well before exercising, avoid outdoor exercising in cold or dry air, and take prescribed medication 15 to 30 minutes before exercising.

TABLE 12-5

Pharmacology: Drugs Used to Treat Asthma

DRUG (GENERIC AND COMMON BRAND NAME)	USUAL ROUTE/DOSE	CLASSIFICATION	SELECTED SIDE EFFECTS	DON'T GIVE IF
Albuterol (Proventil, Ventolin)	PO: 2–6 years 0.1–0.2 mg/kg tid PO: 6–12 years 2 mg 3–4 times/day Inhaled: 6–12 years 1–2 inhalations every 4–6 hours	Beta-adrenergic agonist	Hypersensitivity, tremors, anxiety, blurred vision Call doctor if no relief	Epinephrine is being administered (possible additive effect)
Fluticasone (Flonase)	Inhaled: 1–2 inhalations bid	Antiinflammatory	Candidal infection of oral pharynx	Oral inhaler and nasal inhaler are not interchangeable
Prednisone (Solumedrol, etc.)	Acute asthma: PO: 1–2 mg/kg in divided doses Asthma: PO: 10–40 mg every other day, depending on age	Glucocorticoid	Edema, muscle weakness, hyperglycemia, growth suppression	Do not stop or alter dose without consulting primary care provider
Montelukast (Singulair)	PO: 4–5 mg daily in evening	Bronchodilator (respiratory smooth muscle relaxant), leukotriene receptor	Fever, headache, nasal congestion	Monitor periodic live tests
Theophylline (Theo-dur)	PO/IV 0.4–0.8 mg/kg/hour	Xanthine bronchodilator	Irritability, headache, tachycardia	Wait 4–6 hours after IV dose before starting PO Check IV incompatibility
Levalbuterol (Xopenex)	Inhaled 0.31 mg tid	Autonomic nervous system agent, bronchodilator (respiratory smooth muscle relaxant)	Allergic reactions, anxiety, headache, dizziness, increased blood glucose, tachycardia	Past allergic reaction, not recommended for children younger than 6 years

Parents need to be taught to administer medication by metered-dose inhaler and by continuous nebulizer (see Procedure 8-32 ⬮⬮). Older children can be taught to perform their own respiratory treatments.

PEFR monitoring devices can be used in the home or at school to monitor the child's condition and response to treatment, as well as to detect deteriorating lung function. Parents, children, and school personnel should receive instruction on the proper use of the PEFR equipment. The use of the PEFR allows the family greater control over the management of asthma and decreases the need for hospitalization by alerting parents to the need for adjustments to prescribed therapy.

Second-Hand Smoke

Research has confirmed that second-hand cigarette smoke contributes significantly to asthma and other chronic respiratory problems in children of all ages. This fact should be communicated to parents. If a parent is not ready to quit smoking, he or she may be willing to smoke outside, at least keeping the inside of the home free of smoke.

PNEUMOTHORAX

Pneumothorax, air in the chest cavity, can result from chest trauma or spontaneous rupturing of alveoli. When air enters the chest cavity, the normal negative pressure is lost and the lung cannot inflate (Figure 12-18 ⬛). Pressure from the intact lung can cause a shift of organs or **mediastinal shift** (Figure 12-18B) that compresses the great vessels, leading to shock. If bloody fluid is in the chest cavity, the disorder is called a **hemothorax.**

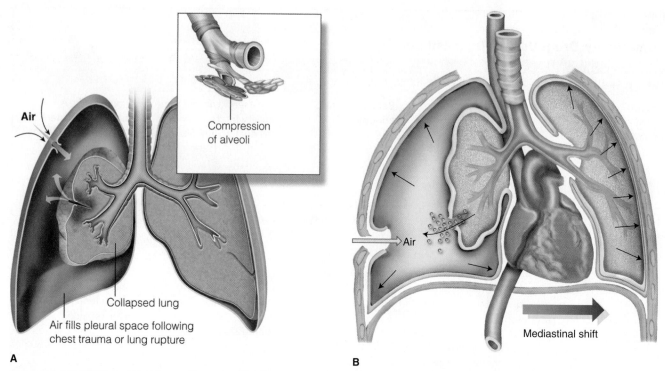

A

B

Figure 12-18. ■ (**A**) Pneumothorax. (**B**) Mediastinal shift caused by pneumothorax compresses the intact lung, further reducing the oxygen that can be provided to the body. Here compression of the great vessels occurs, leading to obstructive shock.

Manifestations

The child may complain of being unable to breathe. Because air is unable to enter the bronchi, lung sounds will be absent. Oxygen saturation will decrease.

Diagnosis

Clinical findings, coupled with history of chest injury or chronic lung disease, will usually result in further investigation with a chest x-ray.

Treatment

Immediate treatment is required to reinstate normal lung functioning and prevent shock. To reestablish the negative pressure in the chest cavity, the physician inserts a chest tube between two ribs and into the pleural space. If there is only air in the pleural space, the chest tube will generally be placed in the upper chest. If blood and fluid are in the pleural space (hemothorax), the chest tube will be placed low in the chest. The distal end of the chest tube is attached to an underwater seal (Pleur-evac®) and suction.

Nursing Considerations

The management of the underwater seal is the same for children as for adults. Prior to insertion of the chest tube, the nurse must set up the Pleur-evac® following the package directions (Figure 12-19 ■). The water seal chamber and the section chamber are filled with sterile water. The

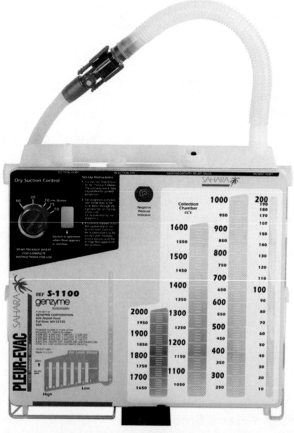

Figure 12-19. ■ Pleur-evac®. A disposable chest drainage system. (Courtesy of Teleflex Chemical.)

suction tube is connected to continuous wall suction. Once the physician has inserted the chest tube, it is attached to the client side of the Pleur-evac®. The suction is turned on to the prescribed level. The chest tube is sutured in place, and an occlusive dressing is applied. All tube connections are taped to prevent leaks. The tubes should be secured to the bed to establish straight drainage into the Pleur-evac®. The Pleur-evac® must be kept below the level of the chest tube. The nurse should observe the chest tube and Pleur-evac® frequently to maintain optimal function. The child's respiratory status should improve, and breath sounds should return in all lung fields. The chest tube can usually be removed in a few days.

Parents may be frightened to touch the child because of the chest tube. They should be reassured that the child can be touched, held, and played with as long as the chest tube is not pulled. Should an air leak occur, the chest tube should be clamped with large hemostats as close to the client as possible. The charge nurse and doctor should be notified immediately.

NURSING CARE

Priorities in Nursing Care
The priorities of nursing care for children with respiratory disorders are to maintain patent airway, prevent infection, promote healing, and prevent further respiratory damage. When planning and implementing care for the infant with severe respiratory disorders, the first priority is to establish and maintain an open airway. The nurse should ensure that artificial airways and suction equipment are available in case of airway obstruction.

ASSESSING

The infant or child with a respiratory disorder should be assessed for lung sounds bilaterally, oxygen saturation (see Figure 8-34 in Procedure 8-27 ⊙), elevated temperature, and stridor. If the throat is infected, the ears should be checked for signs of infection. Likewise, if the ears are infected, the throat should be assessed because of the communication between each through the eustachian tubes. Careful observation for signs of respiratory distress is critical. The airway of the infant is small and obstructs easily. The oxygen saturation should be monitored and reported to the supervising RN or physician if it falls below 90%. Many respiratory disorders affecting older children began in the younger years and continue into adolescence and adulthood. The older child should be assessed to determine whether he or she is ready to assume some responsibility for the daily management of his or her respiratory condition.

DIAGNOSING, PLANNING, AND IMPLEMENTING

The following nursing diagnoses are common among pediatric clients with respiratory disorders and their families:

- Ineffective **A**irway Clearance related to airway spasm or excessive mucus
- Risk for **I**nfection related to chronic disease
- Deficient **F**luid Volume related to inadequate fluid intake secondary to fatigue
- **F**ear and **A**nxiety related to difficulty breathing
- Deficient **K**nowledge related to lack of exposure to accurate information regarding respiratory condition

Some outcomes for pediatric clients with respiratory disorders might include that the child and/or their family will:

- Have an open airway
- Experience no evidence of respiratory infections
- Experience no evidence of fluid imbalance
- Appear calm and relaxed
- Verbalize understanding of respiratory disorder, medical treatment, and medication administration

The nurse's role in providing support to these clients would include the following:

- Take vital signs, including oxygen saturation measurements, at least every 2 hours in children with severe respiratory disorders. *The pediatric client condition may change rapidly, and the child may not be able to communicate this to the nurse.*
- Record intake and output if risk for deficient fluid volume exists. *The nurse must be alert for signs of dehydration, which can be life threatening.*
- Once the child is able to swallow, provide cool liquids. *Cool liquids can help decrease throat swelling, relieve discomfort, and maintain fluid balance.*
- Observe the child and the parents for signs of fear and anxiety. Remain with the child and family, and explain the need for the various pieces of equipment (Figure 12-20 ■). *Parents are fearful when the child is having difficulty breathing and has loss of voice. The hospital environment is frightening to the child and parents. The nurse's presence can be reassuring. Knowing about the equipment can reduce fear.*
- Explain all procedures to the parents and encourage their participation in care of the child to the extent possible. See developmental stages in Chapter 5 ⊙, and effects of hospitalization on children in Chapter 7 ⊙. *Infants and young children experience separation anxiety if the parents are not nearby.*
- Promote age-appropriate activities to the extent possible. *Children with chronic respiratory conditions still need to progress developmentally. Encouraging children to do all they can will promote self-esteem.*

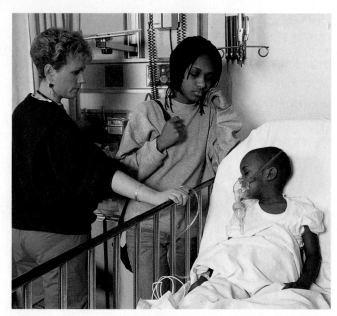

Figure 12-20. ■ Providing support to both the child and the parents is an important part of nursing care during acute episodes of asthma or other respiratory obstruction. This mother is exhausted after a sleepless night of caring for her son.

EVALUATING

Children with respiratory disorders are evaluated frequently for airway patency and oxygen saturation. An increase in urinary output indicates adequate fluid intake. Failure to complete ordered antibiotics can result in recurrence of the infection, so the importance of giving antibiotics as ordered must be emphasized with family members.

NURSING PROCESS CARE PLAN
Client with Asthma

Jimmy, a 7-year-old, is admitted to the pediatric unit with a diagnosis of acute asthma. His vital signs are T 98.4, P 112, R 36. He has high-pitched wheezing on expiration. The physician has ordered IV Solu-Medrol and breathing treatments.

Assessment

■ Wheezing respirations
■ Labored breathing
■ Clings to mother

Nursing Diagnosis

The following important nursing diagnosis (among others) is established for this client:

■ Ineffective **A**irway Clearance related to allergic response, inflamed bronchial tree.

Expected Outcomes

Expected outcomes for Jimmy are that:

■ Wheezing will resolve after administration of medication.
■ Respirations will return to within normal range.
■ Client will state that breathing is easier.
■ Parent and child will return demonstration of metered-dose inhaler for medication.

Planning and Implementation

■ Administer medication as ordered. *Medications relieve bronchial inflammation, decrease swelling, and open airways.*
■ Teach Jimmy and his parents how and when to use the handheld nebulizer. *Parent and child need instruction in technique and in proper use of the medication.*
■ Teach appropriate "play" techniques to extend expiratory time. *Increasing expiratory pressure and extending expiratory time improves breathing by keeping airways open, allowing air to leave the lungs.*
■ Supervise use of breathing equipment (e.g., inhalers, nebulizers, oxygen cannula/mask). *This ensures proper use of breathing equipment.*

Evaluation

Lung sounds will be clear, and breathing pattern will be within normal limits of 15 to 25 for a 7-year-old. Parents and child can verbalize and demonstrate use of breathing equipment.

Critical Thinking in the Nursing Process

1. What play activities could lengthen the exhalation time?
2. What questions should Jimmy and his parents be asked to help identify causative agents for the asthma attack?
3. What can the nurse do to help Jimmy express his feelings?

Note: Discussion of Critical Thinking questions appears in Appendix I.

Note: The reference and resource listings for this and all chapters have been compiled at the back of the book.

Chapter Review

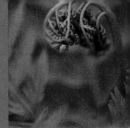

 KEY TERMS by Topic

Use the audio glossary feature of either the CD-ROM or the Companion Website to hear the correct pronunciation of the following key terms.

Anatomy and Physiology
surfactant, viability, conchae, alveoli

Process of Respiration
diaphragm, intercostal muscles, eupnea, hypoventilation, hyperventilation, dyspnea, orthopnea, apnea, Cheyne-Stokes respiration, circumoral cyanosis, crackles, rhonchi, stridor

Epistaxis
epistaxis

Upper Respiratory Infections
nasopharyngitis, rhinitis, coryza, tonsillitis, dysphagia, tonsillectomy, eschar, epiglottitis, dysphonia, tripod position

Respiratory Disorders Associated with the Newborn and Infant
neonatal respiratory distress syndrome, atelectasis, bronchopulmonary dysplasia, meconium, meconium aspiration

Congenital Respiratory Disorders
tracheoesophageal fistula, esophageal atresia, steatorrhea

Lower Respiratory Infections
bronchiolitis, bronchioles, respiratory syncytial virus, croup, inspiratory stridor, pneumonia, consolidation, tachypnea, tuberculosis, Mantoux test

Additional Respiratory Disorders
asthma, pneumothorax, mediastinal shift, hemothorax

KEY Points

- Respiratory disorders are potentially life threatening and must be monitored closely.

- Management of a patent airway is a priority nursing intervention for children with respiratory disorders.

- Upper respiratory infections can spread to the lower respiratory system.

- Viral infections should be treated with supportive care. Antibiotics should only be used for bacterial infections.

- Frequent swallowing after a tonsillectomy is the first sign of bleeding.

- Many respiratory disorders begin in early childhood and become chronic lifelong disorders.

- Pediatric clients can be taught to manage their chronic respiratory disorder.

- Management of asthma is focused on identifying and avoiding triggers, family education, medication administration, and follow-up care.

- Cystic fibrosis, an autosomal recessive trait, affects the child's respiratory and gastrointestinal systems. The life expectancy is 30 years.

- Health promotion activities, including immunizations, removing pollutants from the environment, and infection control measures, can help prevent or control pediatric respiratory disorders.

 EXPLORE Media Link

Additional interactive resources for this chapter can be found on the Companion Website at www.prenhall.com/adams.

Click on Chapter 12 and "Begin" to select the activities for this chapter.

For chapter-related NCLEX®-style questions and an audio glossary, access the accompanying CD-ROM in this book.

Animations:

Metered dose inhaler

Proper use of a metered dose inhaler (MDI)

Lung sounds

Asthma

Cystic fibrosis

FOR FURTHER Study

Review Chapter 5 for developmental levels of children as they relate to nursing care.

See Chapter 7 for information about communicating with children and effects of hospitalization by age and development.

See Respiratory Procedures section in Chapter 8 and Procedures 8-25 to 8-28.

Infectious diseases such as pertussis (whooping cough) are discussed in Chapter 10.

Reye's syndrome is discussed further in Chapters 10 and 15.

For additional information on otitis media, see Chapter 15.

Gastrointestinal disorders are discussed in Chapter 17.

Critical Thinking Care Map

Caring for a Client with Respiratory Infection
NCLEX-PN® Focus Area: Physiological Integrity

Case Study: Joseph, a 9-month-old infant, is admitted to the pediatric unit with a diagnosis of respiratory infection. He has a history of three episodes of bronchitis in the past 6 months. He has gained ½ lb since his last hospitalization 2 months ago. His mother states, "I don't know why he gets infections so easily."

Nursing Diagnosis: Ineffective **A**irway Clearance related to infectious process

COLLECT DATA

Subjective	Objective
_____	_____
_____	_____
_____	_____
_____	_____
_____	_____
_____	_____

Would you report this? Yes/No
If yes, to: _____

Nursing Care

_____

_____

_____

_____

_____

_____

_____

_____

_____

_____

How would you document this? _____

_____

_____

_____

Compare your documentation to the sample provided in Appendix I.

Data Collected
(use only those that apply)

- Lung sounds wheezy
- Crying
- T 103.2, P 148, R 40
- Reports not knowing cause of infection
- Nonproductive cough
- No eye contact
- Weight gain
- Labored breathing
- Withdrawn
- Circumoral cyanosis
- Jaundice
- Sleepy

Nursing Interventions
(use only those that apply; list in priority order)

- Note mother-infant interaction.
- Offer 1,000 mL clear liquids.
- Offer milk four times a day.
- Administer IV medication as ordered.
- Provide mist tent.
- Administer expectorant cough syrup.
- Provide droplet precautions.
- Provide contact precautions.
- Suction airway every 2 hours.

NCLEX-PN® Exam Preparation

TEST-TAKING TIP Look for the key terms in every question stem. A question that asks for an answer that is "most appropriate" may have more than one possible correct answer. The first step is to determine which answers might be correct. The second step is to determine which would be the FIRST nursing action.

1 An 18-month-old is in isolation for RSV. Which action by the nurse is most appropriate?
1. Wear sterile gloves when caring for the child.
2. Double-bag soiled diapers.
3. Have the child wear a mask when in the playroom.
4. Wear gown, mask, and gloves when feeding the child.

2 A 6-month-old child is receiving oxygen in a mist tent. Which of the following is an important consideration in caring for this young child?
1. Change bedding and clothing frequently.
2. Remove child from the tent if restlessness occurs.
3. Keep all objects outside the tent to prevent fire hazard.
4. Open the mist tent every hour to decrease the temperature inside the tent.

3 The day an 8-year-old is discharged after an acute asthma attack, her mother asks the nurse to recommend a pet for her child. The most appropriate pet for the child would be a:
1. Cat.
2. Fish.
3. Dog.
4. Parakeet.

4 A 7-year-old with cystic fibrosis is admitted with bronchial pneumonia. The physician orders postural drainage, primarily to:
1. Clear the lungs of mucus.
2. Dilate the bronchi.
3. Provide more room for lung expansion.
4. Remove bacteria from the lungs.

5 A toddler is being admitted to the pediatric unit with a diagnosis of epiglottitis. In planning care for this child, the nurse should:
1. Notify the respiratory therapist of the admission.
2. Have tracheostomy equipment available.
3. Make the child NPO.
4. Have antibiotics prepared when the child is admitted.

6 A 5-year-old had a tonsillectomy yesterday. The nurse would be least concerned by:
1. Halitosis.
2. Increased pulse.
3. Restlessness.
4. Crying.

7 The second day after a tonsillectomy, a child is receiving a full liquid diet. Which should be avoided?
1. Popsicles.
2. Jell-O.
3. Vanilla pudding.
4. Orange juice.

8 A 10-year-old is admitted with an acute episode of asthma after playing soccer. All of the following interventions are needed prior to discharge. Place these in order of priority.
1. Teach how to use prescribed inhalers.
2. Schedule follow-up appointment with primary care provider.
3. Stay with child to keep him calm.
4. Ask parents to identify triggers in the home environment.
5. Teach child the importance of warming up before playing soccer.

9 The nurse is teaching a mother how to administer 1 tsp of cough medicine to her 6-month-old child. The nurse should recommend which of the following?
1. Household measuring spoon
2. Silverware teaspoon
3. Plastic medicine cup
4. Plastic syringe (without needle) calibrated in milliliters

10 The doctor has ordered albuterol liquid 0.2 mg/kg for a 43-lb child. Albuterol is supplied in 2 mg/5 mL. How many milliliters will be administered to this child?

Answers for NCLEX-PN® Review and Critical Thinking questions appear in Appendix I.

Chapter 13

Care of the Child with Cardiovascular Disorders

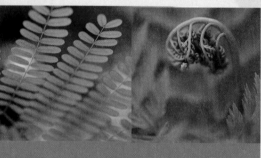

BRIEF Outline

LEARNING Outcomes

After completing this chapter, you will be able to:
1. Define key terms.
2. Discuss the anatomy and physiology of the pediatric cardiovascular system.
3. Describe cardiovascular disorders to include both congenital and acquired disorders.
4. Discuss clinical manifestations, diagnostic procedures, medical management, and nursing interventions related to cardiovascular disorders.
5. Explain appropriate nursing interventions for children with cardiovascular disorders.

Cardiovascular disorders in children can result from congenital heart anomalies or defects and acquired heart diseases. These disorders pose serious health threats. Connor (2002) estimates that one-third of children born with a congenital heart disease will die, with most of those deaths occurring in the first year of life. Because of the serious nature of cardiovascular disorders, the health care of these children may require frequent hospitalizations, including admissions to the intensive care unit. Nursing care for these children can be challenging. The LPN/LVN assists the physician and RN in providing safe, effective care to these children. Check the nurse practice act for your state and facility policy to determine whether specific interventions are within the scope of practice.

Anatomy and Physiology

To understand the pathology of heart defects, it is important to review the normal structure of the fetal heart (Figure 13-1A ■). Because fetal blood is oxygenated in the placenta, the lungs in the fetus need only enough blood to perfuse lung tissue. In the fetal heart, there are two structures to decrease the flow of blood to the fetal lungs. They are the foramen ovale and the ductus arteriosus. The foramen ovale connects the two atria, allowing blood to flow from the right atrium into the left atrium. The ductus arteriosus connects the blood flow from the pulmonary artery into the aortic arch.

At birth, with the infant's first breath, blood flow to the lungs must increase dramatically to allow full oxygenation.

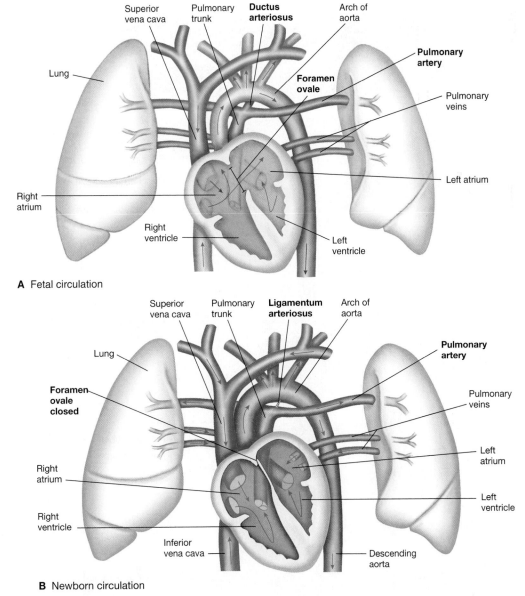

A Fetal circulation

B Newborn circulation

Figure 13-1. ■ **(A)** Fetal circulation. Notice the open ductus arteriosus above the heart and the flow of blood through the foramen ovale in the center of the heart. **(B)** Newborn circulation. Note that the ductus arteriosus has closed, showing two separate structures: the pulmonary arteries and the aortic arch.

Shortly after birth (usually within 24–48 hours), the foramen ovale and the ductus arteriosus structures normally close (see Figure 13-1B ■) (D'Amico & Barbarito, 2007). Now the right side of the heart pumps blood to the lungs for oxygenation, and the left side of the heart pumps oxygenated blood throughout the body. Figure 13-2 ■ illustrates the arteries and veins in the body. The pressure in the left side of the heart becomes higher than the pressure in the right side. An infant's heart muscle fibers are not developed fully, and the ventricles are not as compliant to **stroke volume** (the amount of blood forced out by the ventricles during a heart contraction). Therefore, the infant is very sensitive to

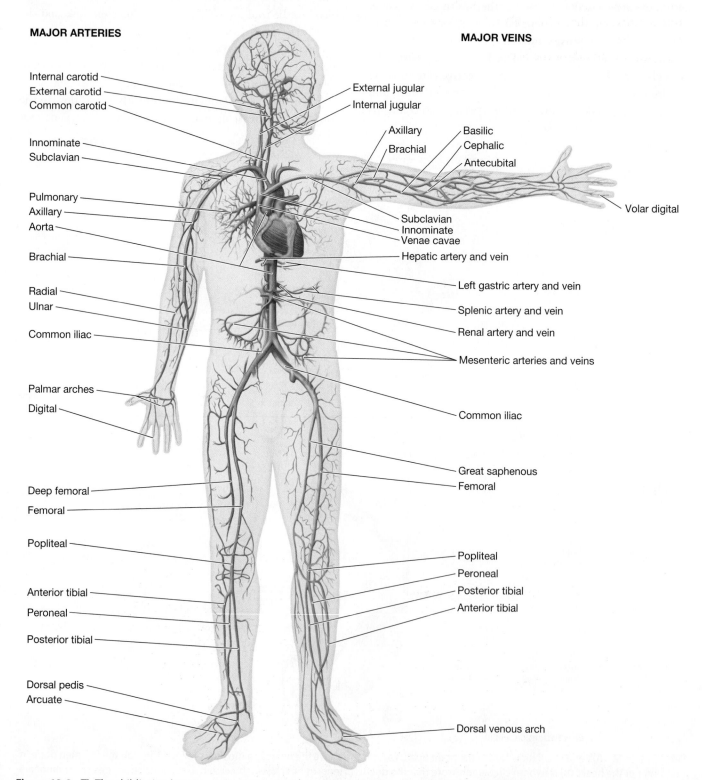

MAJOR ARTERIES

Internal carotid
External carotid
Common carotid

Innominate
Subclavian

Pulmonary
Axillary
Aorta

Brachial

Radial
Ulnar

Common iliac

Palmar arches
Digital

Deep femoral
Femoral

Popliteal

Anterior tibial
Peroneal

Posterior tibial

Dorsal pedis
Arcuate

MAJOR VEINS

External jugular
Internal jugular

Axillary
Brachial

Basilic
Cephalic
Antecubital

Volar digital

Subclavian
Innominate
Venae cavae

Hepatic artery and vein

Left gastric artery and vein

Splenic artery and vein

Renal artery and vein

Mesenteric arteries and veins

Common iliac

Great saphenous
Femoral

Popliteal
Peroneal
Posterior tibial
Anterior tibial

Dorsal venous arch

Figure 13-2. ■ The child's circulatory system. Major arteries are shown in red, and major veins are shown in blue.

volume and pressure overloads. **Cardiac output** is the total volume of blood forced out of the ventricles in 1 minute. Cardiac output is calculated by multiplying stroke volume with heart rate. Three things affect cardiac output. First is the **preload,** which is the volume of blood in the ventricles at the end of diastole. Second is the **afterload,** or the resistance against which the ventricles pump. Finally, the **contractility,** or the ability of the ventricles to stretch, affects cardiac output. Variations from these normal findings affect the health of the newborn and are discussed in this chapter.

Brief Assessment Review

HISTORY

- Inquire about a family history of cardiac disease.
- Ask the child or parent if there is any weakness or fatigue that develops on physical exertion.
- Inquire about symptoms of cyanosis, edema, dizziness, or poor weight gain.

PHYSICAL

To perform a brief focused assessment of the cardiovascular system, the nurse would:

- Observe the child's body posture. (e.g., squatting is often seen in a child with tetralogy of Fallot, hyperextension of the neck is seen with hypoxia).
- Observe for respiratory difficulty.
- Observe for edema, abdominal distention, or signs of dehydration.
- Inspect nail beds, sclera, and skin tone (Box 13-1 ■).
- Monitor body temperature, respiratory rate, and blood pressure (see Procedures 8-1, 8-3, and 8-4 ⚭).
- Palpate the peripheral, and auscultate the apical pulse (see Procedure 8-2 ⚭).
- Palpate for pitting edema if present.
- Auscultate heart and breath sounds (see Procedures 8-2 and 8-3 ⚭). Figure 13-3 ■ illustrates areas for auscultating the heart.
- Monitor arterial oxygen saturation as it is a key indicator of cardiac health. The normal amount of oxygen saturation

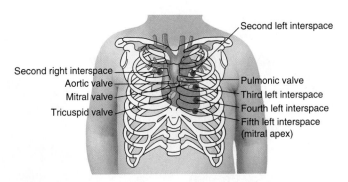

Figure 13-3. ■ Points for auscultating the heart.

TABLE 13-1	
Pediatric Lab Values for Oxygen Saturation	
Normal	95–98%
Mild hypoxemia	90–95%
Moderate hypoxemia	85–90%
Severe hypoxemia	85 or lower

in a child's blood is 95% to 98%. Table 13-1 ■ provides lab values for arterial oxygen saturation. Also see Procedure 8-29, Monitoring Oxygen Status ⚭ .

Congenital Heart Anomalies and Defects

Many congenital anomalies (e.g., patent ductus arteriosus, atrial septal defect, ventricular septal defect, coarctation of the aorta, tetralogy of Fallot, transposition of the great vessels) are identified at birth or within the first few weeks of life. It is important for the nurse to have an understanding of the pathology, symptoms, and related nursing care for these conditions. If the anomaly is life threatening, surgery is usually performed immediately to correct the defect. Other anomalies are not repaired until the child is stronger and better able to withstand the surgical procedure. Sometimes repair is performed in stages, and complete reconstruction may take months or years.

Congenital heart defects are more common when the child was exposed to rubella, alcohol, or drugs during intrauterine development. Other factors that increase the risk of congenital heart defects include other congenital or genetic defects, advanced maternal age, maternal disorders such as lupus and diabetes, and siblings or parents with congenital defects.

Congenital heart defects can be classified into four groups according to the way the defect affects circulation: defects with increased pulmonary blood flow, defects with

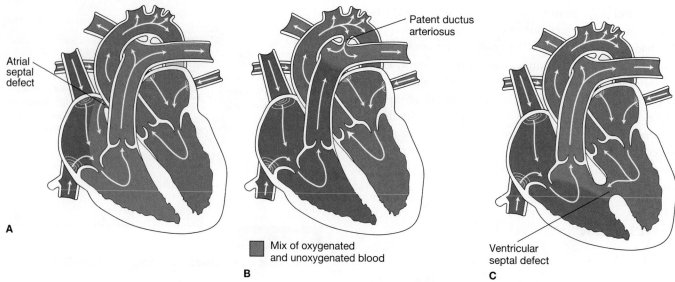

Figure 13-4. ■ **(A)** Atrial septal defect. Note that the defect is an opening between the right and the left sides of the heart. **(B)** Patent ductus arteriosus. Note that the connecting duct between the pulmonary artery and the aortic arch is still open. **(C)** Ventricular septal defect. Note the opening between the right and left ventricles.

decreased pulmonary blood flow, defects that obstruct systemic blood flow, and mixed defects.

DEFECTS WITH INCREASED PULMONARY BLOOD FLOW

Three heart defects that increase the blood flow to the pulmonary system are an atrial septal defect (ASD; Figure 13-4A ■), a patent (open) ductus arteriosus (PDA; Figure 13-4B), and a ventricular septal defect (VSD; Figure 13-4C).

Atrial Septal Defect

ASD describes the opening in the **septum** (wall) between the left and right atria that remains when the foramen ovale fails to close within a few hours after birth. Blood flows directly from the left atrium into the right atrium, increasing the amount of blood in the right side of the heart. Increased

pressure on the right side of the heart results in ventricular hypertrophy and increased pulmonary artery blood flow.

MANIFESTATIONS. The young child with ASD may be asymptomatic. Diagnosis may not occur until the preschool years, when symptoms of fatigue, delayed growth, and congestive heart failure occur. A soft systolic heart murmur may also be auscultated because of increased pulmonary artery blood flow.

DIAGNOSIS. An echocardiogram and chest x-rays are used to identify the defect. An ECG may be done but will not contribute much data unless the defect is large. Other tests that may be used include Doppler studies, cardiac catheterization, and an MRI of the chest. Table 13-2 ■ provides examples of how to discuss heart testing with children and with parents.

TABLE 13-2				
Communicating Across the Life Span: Preparing a Child for Cardiac Testing				
	TODDLER	**PRESCHOOLER**	**SCHOOL-AGE CHILD**	**ADOLESCENT**
Nurse	In preparation for an echocardiogram: "This medicine will make you very sleepy while we look at your heart. Your mommy will be right here."	In preparation for a chest radiograph: "While we take a picture of your heart, look at your daddy and take deep breaths with him."	In preparation for an electrocardiogram (ECG): "We want to really know how your heart is beating. These wires I've taped to your chest will tell us. The ECG will work better and faster if you hold very still. Why don't you shake everything right now to get the wiggles out and then pretend to be a wooden soldier."	In preparation for wearing a Holter monitor: "The monitor has to stay on for 24 hours. No showers, okay? It is important that you use this diary to record symptoms you experience, what activities you did, and when you slept during this 24-hour period."

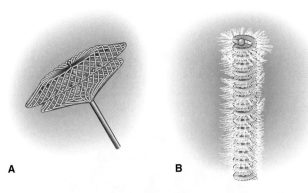

Figure 13-5. ■ **(A)** Septal occluder is used to close an atrial septal defect and less commonly to close a ventricular septal defect. **(B)** Coil used to close a patent ductus arteriosus. The coil of wire covered with tiny fibers occludes the ductus arteriosus when a thrombus forms in the mass of fabric and wire.

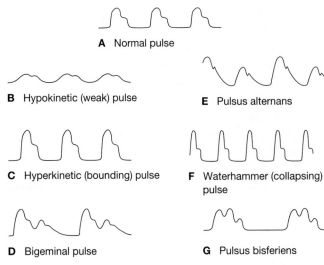

Figure 13-6. ■ Types of pulse patterns.

TREATMENT. The ASD can be closed surgically, requiring open heart surgery and the use of a heart-lung bypass machine during the procedure. Nonsurgically, the defect can be patched during cardiac catheterization using a septal occluder (Figure 13-5 ■). Antibiotics are given prior to either procedure to prevent **endocarditis**. Endocarditis is an inflammation of the endocardium and heart valves and may be caused by bacterial pathogens.

Patent (Open) Ductus Arteriosus

A patent ductus arteriosus (see Figure 13-4B) occurs when the ductus arteriosus fails to close. Closure is initiated with the first breath and normally occurs within 15 hours after birth, but it can take up to 3 months. In this defect, blood is pushed from the aorta to the pulmonary artery, resulting in an increase in blood flowing to the lungs. The increase in blood flowing to the lungs causes right ventricle hypertrophy and increased pressure in the pulmonary circulation.

MANIFESTATIONS. Clinical manifestations of a PDA include a full, bounding pulse; dyspnea; tachypnea; and delayed growth patterns. Figure 13-6 ■ illustrates a bounding pulse and selected other heart patterns. The infant with a PDA is at risk for respiratory infections and endocarditis due to increased pulmonary blood flow. The child is also at risk for congestive heart failure (CHF), **hepatomegaly** (enlargement of the liver), failure to grow, and intercostal retractions. A continuous systolic murmur can be auscultated, and a pulmonic thrill may be palpated at the left sternal border second to fourth intercostal space on a child with a PDA.

DIAGNOSIS. Auscultation of the characteristic heart murmur assists in confirming the diagnosis. A PDA can be positively diagnosed by chest x-ray, electrocardiogram (ECG), or echocardiogram.

TREATMENT. The symptomatic infant with a PDA is given indomethacin, or a nonsteroidal antiinflammatory that is also a prostaglandin inhibitor, intravenously to stimulate the closure of the ductus arteriosus. If unsuccessful, a surgical **ligation** (obstructing a vessel or duct using suture or wire ligature—see Figure 13-5) of the PDA may be necessary. In some children, closure may be accomplished nonsurgically via a transcatheter obstructive device. Fluid restriction is also important for these children to prevent cardiac overload.

Ventricular Septal Defect

A ventricular septal defect or VSD (Figure 13-4C) results from an abnormal opening in the septum between the ventricles. This allows blood to flow directly from the left ventricle to the right ventricle. The size of the VSD determines the degree of problems the child will have.

MANIFESTATIONS. Most children with a VSD are asymptomatic. If symptoms are present, the child may have dyspnea, tachypnea, delayed growth patterns, reduced fluid intake, or congestive heart failure (CHF). The child may have symptoms of pulmonary disease, such as pulmonary hypertension. A systolic murmur can be auscultated.

DIAGNOSIS. Auscultation of the systolic murmurs assists in confirming the diagnosis. A VSD can be diagnosed with a chest x-ray, ECG, or echocardiogram.

TREATMENT. Small VSDs may close spontaneously and not require medical intervention.

If surgical closure is required, it is done prior to age 2 years to prevent pulmonary artery hypertension. Pulmonary artery hypertension can lead to infectious endocarditis and cardiac failure. A **Rashkind procedure** (also known as balloon atrial septostomy) may be performed to relieve CHF until a more permanent surgical treatment can be accomplished. During the Rashkind procedure, an enlargement of the existing opening in the cardiac septum is made, allowing better mixing of oxygenated blood from the lungs with the systemic blood. Because the child will be at risk for endocarditis, prophylactic antibiotic administration prior to these procedures will be necessary.

DEFECTS WITH DECREASED PULMONARY BLOOD FLOW

Tetralogy of Fallot

When blood flow is decreased to the lungs, the amount of oxygen to all tissues decreases. Only one congenital heart defect that decreases blood flow to the lungs will be discussed here. Tetralogy of Fallot (TOF) is a combination of four defects: pulmonary stenosis, VSD, right ventricular hypertrophy, and an overriding aorta (Figure 13-7A ■). **Pulmonary stenosis** is a narrowing of the pulmonary valve. As the right ventricle tries to push blood through the tight pulmonary valve, the ventricular muscle enlarges and right ventricular hypertrophy occurs. As pressure in the right ventricle rises, blood is pushed through the VSD into the aorta, where it mixes with oxygenated blood from the left ventricle and is pumped throughout the body. The mixing of oxygenated and unoxygenated blood results in the common symptom of cyanosis.

MANIFESTATIONS. Clinical manifestations of TOF are determined by the severity of pulmonary stenosis. The infant may become cyanotic and hypoxic (Figures 13-7B and C). The older child may assume a knee-chest position to relieve lack of oxygen. Other symptoms include delayed growth, polycythemia, metabolic acidosis, exercise intolerance, and clubbing of the fingers. **Clubbing** is an enlargement of the end of the fingers, and in some cases the toes, and is associated with disorders causing cyanosis. A systolic murmur may be heard in the pulmonic area.

DIAGNOSIS. TOF can be diagnosed by chest x-ray, ECG, echocardiogram, or cardiac catheterization. The combined presence of pulmonary stenosis, VSD, right ventricular hypertrophy, and an overriding aorta denotes TOF.

TREATMENT. Surgical correction of the disorder is necessary prior to 6 months of age for the infant with severe symptoms. Otherwise, surgery can be delayed until the child is older than 6 months, typically 1 to 2 years.

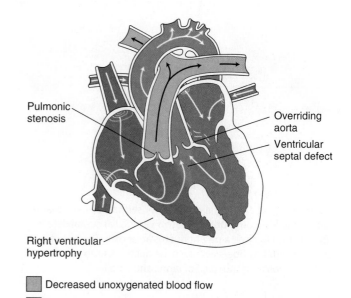

Pulmonic stenosis

Overriding aorta

Ventricular septal defect

Right ventricular hypertrophy

☐ Decreased unoxygenated blood flow

A ■ Mixed oxygenated and unoxygenated blood

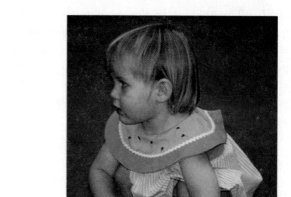

B

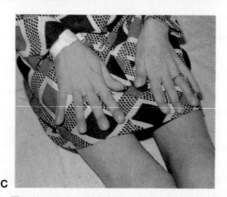

C

Figure 13-7. ■ (A) Tetralogy of Fallot involves four distinct problems: pulmonary stenosis, ventricular septal defect, right ventricular hypertrophy, and an overriding aorta. (B) A child with cyanotic heart defect squats (assumes a knee-chest position) to relieve cyanotic spells. (C) Clubbing of the fingers is one manifestation of a cyanotic defect in an older child.

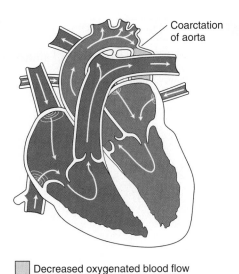

Decreased oxygenated blood flow

Figure 13-8. ■ Coarctation of the aorta. In most instances, the narrowing occurs in the aortic arch.

DEFECTS THAT OBSTRUCT SYSTEMIC BLOOD FLOW

Coarctation of the Aorta

Coarctation of the aorta (Figure 13-8 ■) is a *narrowing* of the aorta. The most common site of narrowing is in the arch of the aorta. The narrowed area restricts the flow of blood to the body. The left ventricle must work hard to force blood through the narrowed aorta. Over time, the obstruction leads to congestive heart failure. With coarctation of the aorta, blood pressure will usually be higher in the arms than in the legs.

MANIFESTATIONS. The degree of constriction dictates the severity of symptoms. Children with coarctation of the aorta may be asymptomatic, and their growth patterns may be unaffected. Or they may have CHF and altered blood pressure, with lower blood pressure and weak pulses in the legs due to reduced blood flow through the descending aorta; higher blood pressure in the arms, neck, and head; and strong, bounding brachial and radial pulses. Femoral pulses are weak or absent, and the older child may have weakness and pain in the legs following exercise.

DIAGNOSIS. Diagnosis of coarctation of the aorta can be made by ECG, chest x-ray, or MRI. Other tests that may be used are the echocardiogram and cardiac catheterization.

TREATMENT. Repair of the disorder is ideally performed in the first year of life. Balloon dilation, **angioplasty** (a mechanical widening of the aorta), or surgical resection relieves the symptoms. However, the coarctation may recur. The nurse must teach parents to observe closely for the return of signs and symptoms of coarctation of the aorta.

MIXED DEFECTS

Transposition of the Great Arteries

Mixed defects are those that affect both systemic and pulmonary circulation. When the positions of aorta and pulmonary artery are reversed (Figure 13-9 ■), the result is **transposition of the great arteries** (TGA). In this condition, unoxygenated blood enters the right side of the heart, travels through the right ventricle, moves out of the heart through the aorta, and flows back to the body. The oxygenated blood from the lungs enters the left side of the heart, travels through the left ventricles, moves out of the heart through the pulmonary artery, and flows back to the lungs. Unoxygenated blood becomes increasingly depleted of oxygen, while oxygenated blood is repeatedly exposed to oxygen. This condition is an immediate threat to the newborn's life.

MANIFESTATIONS AND DIAGNOSIS. TGA is characterized by cyanosis that may not improve with oxygen administration. The child may also have hypoxia, acidosis, CHF, tachypnea, and delayed growth. Parents may also report that the infant needs to rest frequently, particularly during feeding. A chest x-ray and echocardiogram are used for the diagnosis of TGA.

TREATMENT. Prompt treatment is necessary as survival without surgery is impossible. Prostaglandin E$_1$ is given to the newborn intravenously to maintain patency of the ductus arteriosus prior to surgical intervention. Surgical intervention, an arterial switch, can be performed before 1 week of life. **Balloon atrial septostomy** (Rashkind procedure described previously) may also be performed at 1 week to

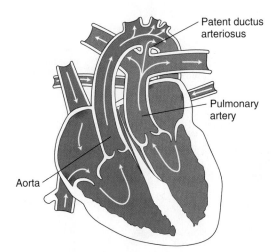

Figure 13-9. ■ Transposition of the great arteries. Note that the pulmonary artery and aorta are switched. Survival initially depends on the patent ductus arteriosus and foramen ovale. About 5% of children with congenital heart disease have this condition (Grifky, 1999).

3 months of age. Because the infant is at risk for endocarditis, prophylactic antibiotic administration prior to these procedures will be necessary.

Acquired Heart Diseases

CONGESTIVE HEART FAILURE

In CHF, a child has circulatory deficits that decrease cardiac output and can lead to cardiogenic shock (Figure 13-10 ■). CHF can result from congenital heart defects or acquired heart defects.

Manifestations

The symptoms of CHF can be grouped into three categories: cardiac, pulmonary, and metabolic. Cardiac symptoms include tachycardia, poor capillary refill, peripheral edema, fatigue, and restlessness. The child's heart may also be enlarged (called **cardiomegaly**) as the body attempts to maintain cardiac output. Pulmonary symptoms include dyspnea, tachypnea, cyanosis, feeding difficulties, and crackles and wheezing on auscultation. Metabolic symptoms are slow weight gain and perspiration. Box 13-2 ■ describes the differences in clinical manifestations related to age.

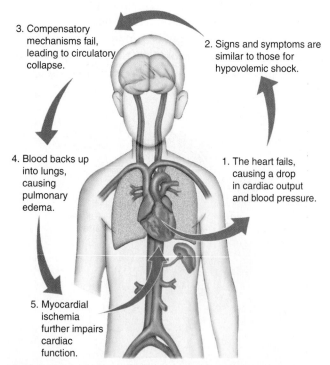

3. Compensatory mechanisms fail, leading to circulatory collapse.

2. Signs and symptoms are similar to those for hypovolemic shock.

4. Blood backs up into lungs, causing pulmonary edema.

1. The heart fails, causing a drop in cardiac output and blood pressure.

5. Myocardial ischemia further impairs cardiac function.

Figure 13-10. ■ Cardiogenic shock. When the heart fails, cardiac output and blood pressure decrease. Blood backs up into the lungs, causing pulmonary edema. Inadequate amounts of oxygen reach the myocardium, impairing the heart's pumping action. The result is cardiogenic shock.

| BOX 13-2 | LIFE SPAN CONSIDERATIONS |

Manifestations of Congestive Heart Failure by Age

Newborns and infants exhibit some different clinical manifestations of CHF than children or adolescents do.

Newborn/Infant
- Diaphoresis
- Cool extremities
- Restlessness
- Failure to thrive

Children and Adolescents
- Exercise intolerance
- Dyspnea
- Orthopnea
- Jugular vein distention
- Ascites

All Children
- Tachycardia
- Diminished pulses
- Wheezing/rales/rhonchi
- Poor weight gain
- Pallor
- Peripheral edema
- Diminished urine output
- Arrhythmias
- Hepatomegaly

Diagnosis

A diagnosis of CHF is based on the child or the parent's report symptoms. An x-ray of the heart can detect cardiomegaly or pulmonary edema. ECGs may be done to determine arrhythmias. Echocardiography can determine cardiac defects and changes in the heart.

Treatment

Children with CHF are treated with diuretics, potassium supplements, and **inotropic** (increases myocardial contractility) medications to increase the effectiveness of the heart. Heart transplantation may be required for children with end-stage cardiomyopathy. The nursing care for children with CHF is similar to that for children with other cardiac disorders. Priorities include a thorough assessment of the child's condition, promoting oxygenation, administering prescribed medications effectively, facilitating growth and development, and providing necessary teaching and support to the family.

SYSTEMIC HYPERTENSION

Elevated blood pressure in children is often secondary to kidney disease, coarctation of the aorta, hyperthyroidism, increased intracranial pressure (ICP), and side effects of certain medications. Hypertension may also be genetic or the

TABLE 13-3

Pharmacology: Antihypertensives

DRUG (GENERIC AND COMMON BRAND NAME)	USUAL ROUTE/DOSE	CLASSIFICATION AND PURPOSE	SELECTED SIDE EFFECTS	DON'T GIVE IF
Propranolol hydrochloride (Inderal)	Child: PO 1 mg/kg/day in two divided doses Neonate: PO 0.25 mg/kg every 6–8 hours	Beta-adrenergic antagonist for hypertension	Confusion, fatigue, drowsiness, bradycardia, paresthesia of the hands	Pulse is less than 60 bpm or systolic blood pressure is less than 90 mm Hg
Methyldopa (Aldomet)	Child: PO 10–65 mg/kg/day in two to four divided doses; IV 20–65 mg/kg/day in four divided doses	Central-acting hypertensive	Sedation, drowsiness, decreased mental acuity, sodium and water retention, nasal stuffiness	Child is receiving other drugs that decrease consciousness or if the child has decreased level of consciousness

result of family history and is called primary or essential hypertension.

Manifestations and Diagnosis

Severe hypertension can cause headaches, dizziness, and visual disturbances in children. A diagnosis of hypertension is made following three separate measurements of elevated blood pressure. Laboratory tests such as blood urea nitrogen (BUN), creatinine, blood glucose, electrolytes, complete blood count, urinalysis, and a lipid panel are also done. An echocardiogram is used to assess the degree of cardiac involvement.

Treatment

Clinical management of hypertension in children includes weight reduction for children who are overweight; a high-fiber diet low in calories, sodium, and fat; and regular exercise. Adolescents should be taught about the hazards of smoking and alcohol consumption. Antihypertensive medications are given to children with severe hypertension. Table 13-3 ■ describes drugs used to correct hypertension in children.

Nursing Considerations

Obtaining an accurate blood pressure measure is important. The appropriate size blood pressure cuff is essential. The child and family should be taught to take the blood pressure accurately. The blood pressure should be taken at different times during the day and after the child is at rest for at least 5 minutes (see Procedure 8-4).

The nurse can assist the child and family in making nutritional food choices that will help maintain a healthy blood pressure. The nurse should discuss specific foods appropriate for keeping the blood pressure low. The teaching plan should also include food choices at restaurants and fast-food restaurants. Box 13-3 ■ describes herbs and

vitamins that can be used as aids for the heart. However, herbs and vitamin supplements should be used with caution in children. Teach parents to review these with their care provider.

HYPERLIPIDEMIA

Hyperlipidemia is a condition characterized by increased total cholesterol, low-density lipoproteins, and triglycerides accompanied by decreased high-density lipoproteins. Children rarely exhibit symptoms of hyperlipidemia. Diagnosis is made by blood screening. See Table 13-4 ■ for expected laboratory values for cholesterol.

BOX 13-3   COMPLEMENTARY THERAPIES

Herbs and Vitamins for the Heart

In adults, several natural products have been said to promote heart health. These products are vitamin E supplementation, garlic, and the herb hawthorn. It is inappropriate to automatically assume that these same products are useful for children.

Herbal products are basically untested on children, and their production is unregulated in the United States. Parents who choose to give herbal products to their children should be advised to use products produced in developed countries to avoid contamination of lead, mercury, and steroids.

The National Institutes of Health (NIH) does report an apparent link between heart health and vitamin E supplementation. Parents of children should be taught about sources of vitamin E in foods. Foods containing vitamin E are almonds, sunflower seeds, peanut butter, spinach, broccoli, and kiwi. Physicians may recommend vitamin E supplementation for children with specific cardiac disorders. The following dosages of vitamin E are recommended by the NIH:

■ Ages 1–3: 9 IU/day
■ Ages 4–8: 10.5 IU/day
■ Ages 9–13: 16.5 IU/day
■ Ages 14 and older: 22.5 IU/day

TABLE 13-4

Laboratory Values for Cholesterol

TEST	NORMAL	BORDERLINE LEVELS	HIGH LEVELS
Total cholesterol	Less than 170 mg/dL	170–199 mg/dL	More than 200 mg/dL
Low-density lipoproteins	Less than 110 mg/dL	110–129 mg/dL	More than 130 mg/dL
Triglycerides	100 mg/dL	100–150 mg/dL	More than 150 mg/dL
High-density lipoproteins	More than 35 mg/dL	Less than 35 mg/dL	—

Children with hyperlipidemia should be encouraged to maintain a low-fat, low-cholesterol diet. They should implement a regular exercise plan. If these measures do not lower the lipid levels, cholesterol-lowering medication may be prescribed. See Health Promotion Issue on pages 352 and 353.

Nursing Considerations

The nurse should assist the child and family in making appropriate food choices (see Nutrition sections of Chapter 6 ⚭). Referral to a nutritionist may be necessary. Appropriate food choices for a low-fat, low-cholesterol diet include egg substitutes, chicken instead of red meats, and low-fat margarines and salad dressings.

Children with sedentary lifestyles are at greater risk for hyperlipidemia. The nurse can be instrumental in assisting the child and family with healthy lifestyle changes. Thirty minutes of aerobic activity, three to four times a week, is necessary to lower the child's lipid levels. The child should choose activities that are enjoyable.

KAWASAKI'S SYNDROME

Kawasaki's syndrome, an acute systemic inflammatory illness, is also known as mucocutaneous lymph node syndrome. Kawasaki's syndrome is more common in Asian children and male children (Taubert, 1994) but does affect other children as well. It is the most common cause of acquired heart disease in children, and it is increasing in incidence.

Manifestations

Three distinct phases of Kawasaki's syndrome can be identified. In the acute phase, the child is admitted to the hospital with fever, **conjunctival hyperemia** (an increased amount of blood in the conjunctiva), red throat, swollen hands and feet, rash, and enlarged cervical lymph nodes. The acute phase lasts for several weeks. As the child progresses from the acute to the subacute phase, the skin on the lips, hands and feet slough off or develop **fissures** (cracks or lines present on skin tissue) (Figure 13-11 ■). The child experiences joint pain. The heart is affected by thrombosis, large aneurysms of the coronary arteries, and myocardial infarction. The child gradually progresses through the convalescent phase with a decrease of inflammation. Most children fully recover, but damage to the heart is permanent and can lead to later complications.

Diagnosis

A diagnosis of Kawasaki's syndrome is made by evaluating the child's symptoms, and blood work such as erythrocyte sedimentation rate, platelet count, C-reactive protein level, and white blood cell count will be elevated. The child may have mild anemia, thrombocytosis, and hypoalbuminemia. An echocardiogram may also show vascular changes.

Treatment

Children with Kawasaki's syndrome will most likely be hospitalized during treatment. The child is given IV immunoglobulin and oral aspirin. High doses of these medications are given to prevent cardiac damage.

Nursing Considerations

In the acute phase, the child's temperature will need to be monitored every 4 hours. Large doses (80–100 mg/kg/day) of aspirin will be administered as ordered. Because of the antiplatelet action of aspirin, it is important to assess closely for bleeding. Monitor the conjunctiva, oral mucosa,

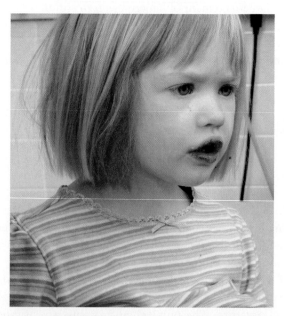

Figure 13-11. ■ This child has returned for one of her frequent follow-up visits to assess her cardiac status after treatment for Kawasaki's syndrome. Notice the lips that show the inflammation and cracking.

and skin every 8 hours for increasing edema, spreading of the red rash, and peeling of the skin. Assess the child for signs of dehydration and malnutrition. Auscultate the heart every 4 hours for abnormal sounds and rhythm.

Because Kawasaki's syndrome is very uncomfortable, all care should be provided as gently as possible. It is important to keep linens clean, dry, and free of wrinkles. Provide oral care using foam applicators to decrease trauma and bleeding of the gums. Bathe the child with cool water to decrease fever. A bed cradle may be needed to keep linens off the sensitive skin.

Fluid balance can be maintained by administering IV fluids. It may be difficult for the child to eat because of irritation of the oral mucosa. Soft foods of moderate temperature should be offered.

Activity is important to prevent complications of bed rest. However, periods of rest are also important to prevent cardiac complications. The child may be reluctant to move because of swollen, painful joints. Turn the child every 2 hours and provide passive and active range-of-motion (ROM) exercises to prevent skin breakdown and respiratory complications. Administer analgesics before activity to help keep the child comfortable.

All procedures should be explained to the child and family. Encourage parents to hold and rock the child to provide a sense of security. Teach them to provide care at home as well as the administration and possible side effects of medications. The Nursing Care Plan Chart below describes nursing care for this condition.

NURSING CARE PLAN CHART

The Child with Kawasaki's Syndrome

GOAL	INTERVENTION	RATIONALE	EXPECTED OUTCOME
1. Acute Pain related to inflammatory process			
The child will have relieved pain	Carefully protect the child's joints Offer the child warm baths Provide analgesics in a timely fashion	*Movement can increase pain and increase the risk of injury* *The application of warm water provides a nonpharmacologic method of pain relief.* *Pain is most effectively managed when analgesics are administered before pain becomes overly intense*	The child's pain is relieved by vital signs WNL, no expressions of pain, uninterrupted sleep patterns, appetite WNL
The family will recognize symptoms of pain and use methods of management within a timely fashion.	Teach the family how to administer pain medications after discharge; include frequency of administration, side effects, drug interactions, and precautions necessary Discuss with parents the importance of reporting promptly if pain is not relieved	*Adequate teaching will give parents the correct information to safely administer medications in the home setting* *Prompt reporting can minimize the amount of time the child suffers with unrelieved pain*	The family reports the child's pain to the nursing staff, implements nonpharmacologic pain measures such as adjusting the room environment and applying warm compresses.
2. Impaired Oral Mucous Membrane related to vasculitis of the oral cavity			
The child will demonstrate oral mucous membrane integrity	Provide lip balm Assist the child in choosing soft, bland, nonacidic foods and fluids Provide gentle mouth care with a soft toothbrush	*An oral protective paste or balm can restore the integrity of the oral mucosa* *These foods and fluids will not cause the child additional discomfort* *Oral hygiene must continue but should be accomplished without further trauma to the mouth*	Tissue of the oral cavity will be lesion free, moisture will be adequate, the child will be able to ingest foods and fluids without difficulty
The family will demonstrate effective oral care	Assist the family to identify substances that might irritate the oral mucosa and make different choices of food and fluids that will not irritate the child's mouth Encourage the parents to report any worsening of symptoms	*Explaining how certain substances, foods, and fluids irritate the oral mucosa will help the parents understand the importance of avoiding these. They can be instrumental in assisting their child to make choices of soft, bland, nonacidic foods and fluids* *Prompt reporting can minimize the amount of time the child suffers with an irritated oral mucosa*	The family assists in choosing appropriate food and fluids and provides lip balm and gentle mouth care to the child

HEALTH PROMOTION ISSUE

PROMOTING A HEALTHY HEART IN CHILDREN

Maria, a parent of a 7-year-old boy, Jason, asks the pediatrician's nurse what she can do to help her son avoid heart disease. Maria has been told by her family physician that there are many risk factors for heart disease in her family's history. Her son is 4 feet 2 inches tall and weighs 120 pounds. He enjoys reading, drawing, and playing educational video games. Maria and her husband smoke one pack of cigarettes per day. Their diet consists of mostly convenience foods.

DISCUSSION

Heart disease has been linked to being overweight, having a body mass index (BMI) greater than 95th percentile, high blood pressure, high cholesterol, diabetes, or cardiovascular disease before age 55 (for men) or 65 (for women). When a family member smokes, it also increases the child's risk.

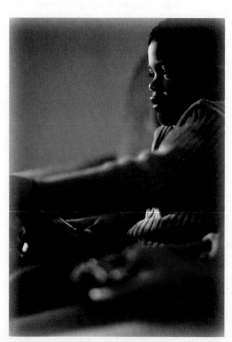

The BMI is determined by assessing gender, height, and weight. A score is then derived. If this score is less than or equal to the 5th percentile, the child is considered underweight. A BMI above 85th percentile to 95th percentile puts the child at risk for being overweight.

Hypertension can be defined as an average (based on two or more occasions) systolic and/or diastolic blood pressure that is at or over 95th percentile for gender, age, and height. To measure a child's blood pressure appropriately, the nurse uses auscultation and ensures that an appropriate size blood pressure cuff is used.

The American Heart Association suggests that children with a family history of high cholesterol or early heart disease have fasting lipids tested after age 2. Total cholesterol higher than 170 mg/dL is considered to be borderline. A level greater than 200 mg/dL is considered to be elevated. A low-density lipoprotein higher than 110 mg/dL is considered to be borderline, and a level more than 130 is considered to be elevated. A high-density lipoprotein of less than 35 mg/dL should be evaluated further, as should triglycerides that are higher than 150 mg/dL.

Prevention of cardiac disorders should include maintaining a healthy weight, remaining normotensive, keeping cholesterol levels within normal limits, preventing the development of diabetes, and avoiding smoking. There are many lifestyle considerations to assist in the prevention of heart disease. The nurse can be instrumental in assisting children and parents to develop ways to implement preventative measures.

PLANNING AND IMPLEMENTATION

Following a thorough assessment of Maria and her son's medical and social history, the nurse must develop a plan to address their needs. The LPN/LVN consults with the RN, a dietitian, and the pediatrician. Together, their plan will provide health maintenance and factors to help Maria's son prevent heart disease. Elements of the plan will also provide Maria and her husband with health benefits.

The nurse calculates Jason's BMI using a standardized chart. With a weight of 120 lb and height of 4 feet 2 inches, Jason's BMI is 33.8, which is above the 95th percentile. His ideal weight should be 61 lb. The nurse, dietitian, and pediatrician develop a plan for diet and exercise to help Jason manage his weight.

Jason, as a 7-year-old, needs about 2,000 cal/day. To lower his weight, fewer calories and increased energy expenditure are needed. The nurse and the dietitian decide to assess Jason's current diet by having him keep a 24-hour food and beverage journal with the assistance of his mother. Later, they will use this journal to help him maintain healthy habits.

The diet that the nurse and the dietitian design is low in sugar, fat content, and calories. They teach Jason the importance of healthy food choices and of eating three modest-size meals and two snacks daily. Beverages can constitute a high percentage of calories in a child's diet. Sodas and fruit juices should be avoided. Low-fat milk and water are better choices.

Jason needs to understand portion sizes to help him avoid overeating. He should be taught how to choose foods that fit into the food pyramid. Eating protein-rich foods at each meal and for each snack will keep Jason from being hungry.

The nurse spends time talking with Maria about food preparation. They discuss cooking methods such as baking, broiling, and grilling that can lower fat content and calories. They discuss buying fresh fruits and vegetables and preparing them for easy access. They discuss the fat and calorie content of favorite fast foods. Maria agrees that Jason will need to avoid fast-food meals in order to control his weight.

Jason does not have a regular pattern of exercise. Maria states that he enjoys sedentary activities such as reading, drawing, and video games. The nurse discusses a variety of activities with Jason to determine what type of activities he might enjoy. They discuss walking to the park or riding his bike several times a week. He also said he could take over the chore of walking the dog for his mother. They discuss rewarding himself with reading or drawing only after he has exercised. The nurse encourages Jason to do sit-ups and push-ups when watching television.

The nurse discusses with Maria and her husband about providing a good fitness example for Jason. The nurse

suggests exercising together as a family. They could take the stairs in public places instead of riding the elevator. They could park the car some distance from the store and walk briskly to their shopping destination. They could encourage Jason to get involved in a team sport such as soccer, which would give him the opportunity to exercise and build relationships with other active children.

The nurse also discusses with Maria and her husband the importance of keeping a positive attitude during the time they are changing their current habits of diet and exercise. They should not react heavy-handedly or punish Jason if he eats something unhealthy or does not exercise every day. Instead, if they remain complimentary and encouraging, Jason will be more likely to stick with the plan for diet and exercise.

The nurse explains to Maria and her husband that living in a smoking environment puts Jason in a higher risk category for heart disease. She also tells them that growing up in a household where smoking is the norm increases the chance that he will smoke as an adult. The nurse encourages Maria and her husband to join a smoking cessation class offered by a local hospital.

The nurse assists the pediatrician in assessing Jason's blood pressure, cholesterol, and blood glucose. At this time all values are normal, but the pediatrician

and the nurse plan to monitor this physical data on a regular basis. They also plan to schedule regular office visits to monitor Jason's weight. They will encourage Jason and his family to use the journal to record daily diet and beverage intake, as well as the type of exercise he does and the length of time spent in the activity. They will also encourage them to use the journal to record fears, struggles, thoughts, and feelings related to the weight management plan. Maria and her husband could also use the journal to record their successes and struggles with smoking cessation.

SELF-REFLECTION

Use the previous guidelines for heart disease risk factors to determine your personal risk. Do you know your cholesterol levels? What is your blood pressure? What is your blood glucose? Calculate your BMI. Are there changes that you need to make in order to decrease your own risk for heart disease? Develop a personal plan for improvement and discuss the plan with a trusted friend who will provide you with accountability.

SUGGESTED RESOURCES

For the Nurse

Kavey, R. E., Daniels, S. R., Lauer, R. M., Atkins, D. L., Hayman, L. L., & Taubert, K. (2003). American Heart Association guidelines for primary prevention of atherosclerotic cardiovascular disease beginning in childhood. *Circulation, 107*(11), 1562–1566.

National High Blood Pressure Working Group on High Blood Pressure in Children and Adolescents. (2004). The fourth report on the diagnosis, evaluation, and treatment of high blood pressure in children and adolescents. *Pediatrics, 114*(2), 555–576.

For the Client

Children's Heart Foundation (2004). *It's my heart.* Lincolnshire, IL: Author.

Jones, C., & Trujillo, E. (2005). *Eating for lower cholesterol: A balanced approach to heart health with recipes everyone will love.* New York: Marlowe and Company.

ACUTE RHEUMATIC FEVER

Acute rheumatic fever (ARF) is an inflammatory disorder that can follow a group A beta-hemolytic *Streptococcus* infection of the throat (pharyngitis, tonsillitis). ARF is more common in children between 6 and 15 years old. There has been a decrease in the number of cases of ARF due to the use of antibiotics in the treatment of beta-hemolytic strep infections. Although the exact pathology is unknown, it is believed that the group A beta-hemolytic *Streptococcus* triggers an autoimmune response that damages the heart, joints, central nervous system (CNS), and skin. ARF tends to recur, and with each recurrence, there is a threat of further damage to the heart.

Manifestations

Rheumatic fever most often occurs following a strep throat infection. The child could have had a mild sore throat that was relatively asymptomatic or a more severe respiratory illness. Within a few days to 6 weeks, the child presents with enlarged, painful, inflamed joints; a red rash; and a temperature of 100.4 °F (38 °C) or higher. The most commonly affected joints are the knees, elbows, and wrists. There may be increased heart rate, irregular rhythm, and abnormal sounds. Tachycardia, atrial fibrillation, murmurs, and friction rub may be caused by inflammation of the heart. Most commonly, it is the mitral and aortic valves that are permanently damaged by rheumatic fever. If the heart is involved, the child should be hospitalized during the acute phase of the illness.

Erythema marginatum, a red skin rash, rarely occurs with ARF. This transient rash is characterized by nonpruritic, red, macular lesions that blanch in the center. Frequently, the rash may be found on the chest, abdomen, buttocks, and proximal limbs. Although erythema marginatum is unpleasant, it does not cause permanent skin damage.

If the CNS is involved, the condition is known as *Sydenham chorea* (**St. Vitus's dance**). Changes in the CNS rarely occur until late in the disease process, possibly after other symptoms have subsided. The child experiences involuntary facial and upper extremity movements. There may be abnormal electroencephalogram (EEG) findings that gradually return to normal. **Chorea** (involuntary, spasmodic movements of the limbs and face) can last for a few weeks or as long as 2 years. Eventually the child returns to normal functioning.

Diagnosis

Diagnosis of ARF is based on clinical manifestations. Diagnostic laboratory findings will include presence of antistreptolysin O titer, the antistreptococcal antibody.

Treatment

The treatment of ARF includes the administration of antibiotics, antiinflammatories, and steroids for severe **carditis** (inflammation of the heart).

clinical ALERT

Polyarthritis of ARF responds to the antiinflammatory effects of aspirin. Parents should be instructed by the LVN/LPN to follow the physician's orders about medication administration and to recognize and report symptoms of Reye's syndrome. For more information on Reye's syndrome, see Chapter 10 ⚭.

Nursing Considerations

The assessment of the child must include a detailed assessment of these body systems. In the acute phase of rheumatic fever, the child is assessed every 4 hours for elevated temperature and heart function. Tepid baths or cool compresses may be provided to decrease temperature and provide comfort. IV fluids are monitored carefully because fluid overload could lead to CHF. Antibiotics and aspirin are prescribed. The nurse provides quiet activities to prevent the child from overtaxing the heart.

During the recovery phase, the child will be cared for at home. Parents need to be reassured that the rash, chorea, and arthritis will subside. The child will need to have limited activities but should be able to return to school and function normally. The child may remain on long-term antibiotic therapy.

clinical ALERT

It is important to tell future health care providers, including dentists and surgeons, of the history of rheumatic fever. Prophylactic antibiotics may be prescribed prior to invasive procedures.

Client teaching is important for long-term care after discharge (Box 13-4 ■). The child and parents should understand the need to prevent infection, treat sore throats, and monitor heart function.

Evaluation of heart function during and following ARF is a crucial part of care. The child and parents should be able to verbalize the need for follow-up evaluation. They should also be able to state the type and dosage of medications, the signs of infection, and the guidelines for seeking medical attention.

NURSING CARE

PRIORITIES IN NURSING CARE

When caring for children with cardiac disorders, priority should be given to several aspects of care. It is important to assess oxygen status and to promote oxygenation in these

---

BOX 13-4   CLIENT TEACHING

Discharge Teaching After Acute Rheumatic Fever

Activity limited to prevent heart damage: Plan quiet activities such as computer and board games and reading. As activities increase and the child returns to school, arrange periods of rest.

Medication: Long-term antibiotic therapy is necessary. It is important to take medication as prescribed to prevent heart damage.

Future health care: Tell future health care providers, including dentists and surgeons, of history of rheumatic fever. Prophylactic antibiotics may need to be given before procedures. Do not ignore future sore throats; the child may need increased antibiotics.

---

children (Figure 13-12 ■). The focus of care will be correct administration of oxygen therapy and positioning the child to facilitate breathing. Nursing care should also promote energy conservation in these children because they tire easily and have compromised circulation. Assessment of the child's respiratory and cardiac status, as well as fluid and electrolyte balance, is essential.

ASSESSING

Children with congenital and acquired heart defects exhibit signs and symptoms of CHF. These include, but are not limited to, altered vital signs, heart murmurs, cyanosis, respiratory distress, fluid retention, and activity intolerance. It is important for the nurse to monitor vital signs correctly, document them, and monitor for changes. See Procedures 8-1 to 8-4 ⚭. Some heart murmurs are loud and easily heard. Others are soft and can only be detected by a trained

practitioner. Murmurs are most easily heard with the bell of the stethoscope. Murmurs are graded according to the intensity of the sound from grade 1 to grade 6. A grade 1 murmur can barely be heard, whereas a grade 6 murmur is heard without a stethoscope.

Cyanosis can be either constant, generalized cyanosis or cyanosis around the mouth (**circumoral**). Circumoral cyanosis is seen only when the child is active, nursing, or crying. Clubbing is an advanced sign of cyanosis. To determine clubbing, ask the child to place index fingers of the right and left hand together with nails facing one another. When clubbing is not present, a diamond-shaped opening forms at the base of the nails. When clubbing is present, fingertips do not touch and there is less than a 160-degree angle created between the skin and the nail base.

The child should be observed for respiratory distress. Signs of respiratory distress include tachypnea, orthopnea, grunting, flaring nostrils, and chest retractions (see Figure 12-4). Fluid retention may be evidenced by bulging fontanels, fewer than six wet diapers per day, moist lung sounds, and generalized tissue edema. Restlessness, crying, and lethargy can be signs of intracranial edema. Young children may display activity intolerance by increased respiratory effort, resting frequently, or squatting while at play.

DIAGNOSING, PLANNING, AND IMPLEMENTING

Prior to surgical intervention, the following diagnoses may be applicable:

- **A**ctivity Intolerance related to impaired circulation
- Risk for **I**nfection related to inadequate defense mechanisms

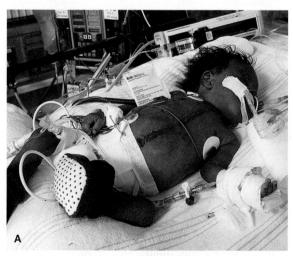

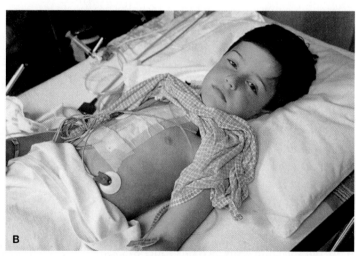

Figure 13-12. ■ **(A)** This child is continuously monitored for congestive heart failure. **(B)** Surgery is performed with this type of defect to prevent pulmonary vascular obstructive disease.

- Imbalanced **N**utrition: More than Body Requirements related to excess intake of sodium- and/or fat-containing foods
- Impaired **S**kin Integrity related to hyperthermia or peripheral edema
- Risk for Imbalanced **F**luid Volume related to impaired circulation.

Nursing diagnoses for children who have had surgery for heart defects might include:

- Ineffective **B**reathing Pattern related to pulmonary edema, increased work of breathing, or poor respiratory effort
- Decreased **C**ardiac Output related to mechanical defects
- Acute **P**ain related to operative site.

Goals for the child include:

- Tolerance of activity will be achieved by balancing rest and activity
- Freedom from signs and symptoms of infection
- Improved diet based on prescribed regime
- Skin will be lesion free
- Fluid and electrolyte balance will be maintained
- Breathing will improve and the need for oxygen will be reduced
- Parents report child appears more comfortable
- Child is able to take food orally

Nursing interventions are supportive measures for the child and family:

- Group activities and alternate them with periods of rest to promote energy conservation. *It is important to conserve the child's energy, balancing rest and activity.*
- Encourage a balanced diet with adequate iron, protein, and vitamins. Diet should be low in sodium and fat. Supplements may be needed. *Adequate nutrients are needed to produce red blood cells, maintain tissue integrity, and maintain fluid balance.*
- Establish a routine of skin care to include assessing on a daily basis, changing positions frequently, keeping diaper area clean, changing bed linens frequently, and providing mouth care prn. *These measures will prevent skin breakdown and improve tissue perfusion that is currently compromised.*
- Instruct child and parents in the importance of hand hygiene, especially after toileting, before meals, and after interacting with other children. *Prevention of transfer of harmful bacteria is essential to preventing infection.*
- Encourage maintenance of all immunizations. *Immunizations will prevent a majority of serious childhood diseases.*
- Closely monitor the child's intake and output. See Procedure 11-1 ⚭. *Intake and output is an essential measure of the child's fluid and electrolyte status.*
- Weigh the child daily. See Procedure 8-8 ⚭. *Subtle changes in weight can assist in the diagnosis of fluid and electrolyte imbalances.*

- Monitor lab values such as urine-specific gravity, BUN, and electrolytes. Report abnormal findings. *Slight changes in these values indicate fluid and electrolyte imbalances. These imbalances may not be tolerated by the child with a cardiovascular disorder and must be addressed promptly.*
- Position the child to assist respiration. *Upright positions allow for adequate inspiration and expiration.*
- Encourage the use of slow, deep abdominal breathing during times of respiratory distress. *Slow, deep abdominal breathing can ensure adequate oxygen exchange and reduce anxiety.*
- Monitor oxygen saturation. Report abnormal findings. See Table 13-1. Also see Procedure 8-29, Monitoring Oxygen Status ⚭. *Oxygen saturation provides data about the child's ability to utilize available oxygen.*
- Older children and adolescents need to be taught that smoking increasingly compromises respiratory health. *The nurse explains the risks of smoking in an effort to deter this behavior.*
- Explain oxygen therapy and the necessity of it to the child and parents. See Procedure 8-28 ⚭. *This teaching should assist compliance.*
- Administer prescribed medications and treatments in a timely manner. Monitor continually until the child is stable. Observe closely for side effects. See Procedures 8-31 through 8-40 ⚭. *This may be the primary role of the RN. LPNs/LVNs assist or administer medications as state regulations and facility policy allow.*
- Provide emotional support to the family. *Parents and family will be anxious and concerned about the child's health. This may interfere with learning about the condition.*
- Reinforce teaching about the child's condition. For example, if an infant becomes cyanotic, the parent can place the infant supine and bend the knees to bring the child to a knee-chest position. *Reinforcement of teaching can be useful. The knee-chest position increases vascular resistance in the lower extremities.*
- Help the child hospitalized with a cardiac condition to feel some sense of control. *Examples of measures that can increase a child's sense of control are allowing the child to have input regarding the day's schedule (i.e., when to bathe), or giving the child a choice of acceptable food items.*

EVALUATING

Children with cardiac defects should be evaluated frequently for fluid balance, signs of infection, and side effects of medication. The nurse will monitor to be sure the child stabilizes over a few hours to days postoperatively. Oxygen will gradually be reduced. The child will be comfortable and able to take oral nutrients. Parents should be able to verbalize and demonstrate needed home care prior to discharge. Encourage follow-up appointments to evaluate health status, including normal growth and development patterns. Because many cardiac defects can be long term and life-threatening, therapeutic communication is valuable in evaluating the infant's and family's emotional status.

NURSING PROCESS CARE PLAN
Child with Hypertension

Branson, age 13, has been recently diagnosed with hypertension. Branson's mother asks the pediatric nurse how to help Branson lower his blood pressure. She knows he needs to lose weight and reduce the stress in his life. She is also concerned about the antihistamines that Branson takes daily for his environmental allergies. She states, "The physician said that his allergy medicine might make his blood pressure worse."

Assessment.   The client has a height of 5 feet, 4 inches, and weighs 175 lb. Vital signs are T 97.8, P 100, R 18, BP 140/90. Branson states, "I'm always concerned about my grades. It's very important to me to make all As. I want to be able to get into an Ivy League college." Client says he does not have many friends, and other students only make fun of him anyway. Denies any hobbies, sports activities, or other interests.

Nursing Diagnosis.   The following important nursing diagnoses (among others) are established for this client:

- **A**nxiety related to threat to role status
- Imbalanced **N**utrition: More Than Body Requirements related to lack of basic nutritional knowledge and lack of physical exercise

Expected Outcomes.   The expected outcomes for the plan of care might include the following:

- Demonstrates anxiety-relieving strategies
- Lists foods to assist in maintaining appropriate intake of calories, fats, and other nutrients
- Participates in a regular exercise program

Planning and Implementation.   The following interventions are planned and implemented for Branson:

- Encourage verbalization of anxious thoughts related to academic success. *Verbalization of thoughts allows the nurse to understand the child's anxiety level and plan appropriate interventions.*
- Provide teaching on creating a calm environment. *A calm environment contributes to lowering the child's anxiety level.*
- Discourage the use of caffeine or other stimulants. *Stimulants can contribute to the child's anxiety level.*
- Teach anxiety-reducing techniques such as breathing patterns, relaxation methods, meditation, and massage.

These measures utilize the gate control theory to block unpleasant sensations.
- Design, along with Branson, a regular schedule for assessing body weight. *Encouraging the child's participation in planning will increase his compliance with the plan of care.*
- Obtain an accurate record of food intake. *Documenting food intake will allow for evaluation of the plan of care.*
- Obtain an accurate record of daily physical activity. *Documenting level of activity will allow for evaluation of the plan of care.*
- Provide teaching on appropriate daily intake of calories and nutrients. *Knowledge will allow the child to make educated food choices.*
- Suggest appropriate food choices. *Providing examples of food choices will assist the child in making good food decisions.*
- Assist Branson in developing an exercise regimen. *Providing suggestions of how to accomplish the required level of activity will improve compliance with the plan of care.*

Evaluation.   At the follow-up visit, the nurse inquires as to whether Branson is experiencing less stress. He states that he is really enjoying his regular physical activity at the gym. This time gives him an opportunity to get his mind off his studies. He is walking on the track and lifting weights with his trainer four times a week after school. He has also made a new friend at the gym who has similar interests. He and his new friend sometimes spend time at the book store together.

The nurse asks Branson about his diet. He states that he is learning to like fruits and vegetables. He has replaced meals of pizza and soda with sandwiches of meat, cheese, and lettuce and bottles of water. He also states that his desire for sweets is diminishing, and he is excited to have lost 5 pounds already.

Critical Thinking in the Nursing Process

1. Excessive sodium in the diet may contribute to hypertension. Provide suggestions for Branson to reduce the sodium in his diet.
2. Design a plan for teaching Branson to monitor his blood pressure.
3. How can Branson manage his allergies and reduce his intake of antihistamines?

Note: Discussion of Critical Thinking questions appears in Appendix I.

Note: The reference and resource listings for this and all chapters have been compiled at the back of the book.

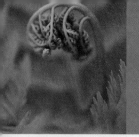

Chapter Review

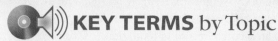 **KEY TERMS** by Topic

Use the audio glossary feature of either the CD-ROM or the Companion Website to hear the correct pronunciation of the following key terms.

Anatomy and Physiology
stroke volume, cardiac output, preload, afterload, contractility

Congenital Heart Anomalies and Defects
septum, endocarditis, hepatomegaly, ligation, Rashkind procedure, pulmonary stenosis, clubbing, coarctation, angioplasty, transposition of the great arteries, balloon atrial septostomy

Acquired Heart Diseases
cardiomegaly, inotropic, hyperlipidemia, conjunctival hyperemia, fissures, erythema marginatum, St. Vitus's dance, chorea, carditis, circumoral

KEY Points

- An infant's heart muscle fibers are not developed fully, and the ventricles are not as compliant to stroke volume. Therefore, the infant is very sensitive to volume and pressure overloads.

- Volume and pressure overloads cause CHF in infants.

- CHF is characterized in children according to the type of heart defect. Symptoms of left-sided heart defects are cyanosis, dyspnea, respiratory crackles, orthopnea, tachycardia, fatigue, and restlessness. Right-sided heart defects are characterized by distended neck veins, tachycardia, liver enlargement, weight gain, and edema.

- Congenital heart defects may arise when the fetus is exposed to infections, alcohol, or drugs in utero.

- Congenital heart defects can be classified into four groups according to the way the defect affects circulation: defects with increased pulmonary blood flow, defects with decreased pulmonary blood flow, defects that obstruct systemic blood flow, and mixed defects.

- Elevated blood pressure in children is often secondary to kidney disease, coarctation of the aorta, hyperthyroidism, increased ICP, and side effects of certain medications.

- Obtaining an accurate blood pressure measure in children with cardiovascular disorders is important. The appropriate size blood pressure cuff is essential.

- Nursing care for children with cardiac disorders should include assessing oxygen status, promoting oxygenation, and energy conservation. Assessment should also include fluid and electrolyte balance.

- Because rheumatic fever most often occurs following a strep throat infection, the nurse must educate parents on the symptoms and encourage them to report these symptoms.

- Polyarthritis of ARF responds to the antiinflammatory effects of aspirin. Parents should administer aspirin only under the supervision of the physician and be instructed to report symptoms of Reye's syndrome.

 EXPLORE MediaLink

Additional interactive resources for this chapter can be found on the Companion Website at www.prenhall.com/adams.

Click on Chapter 13 and "Begin" to select the activities for this chapter.

For chapter-related NCLEX®-style questions and an audio glossary, access the accompanying CD-ROM in this book.

Animations:
The heart
Heart sounds
Chambers of the human heart
Dysrhythmia
Capillary pressure
Congenital heart defects

FOR FURTHER Study

Nutrition is discussed by age group in Chapter 6.
Pediatric procedures are found in Chapter 8.
For more information on Reye's syndrome, see Chapter 10.
Figure 12-4 illustrates some manifestations of respiratory distress.

Caring for a Client with Acute Rheumatic Fever

NCLEX-PN® Focus Area: Physiologic Integrity

Case Study: Mrs. Ness called the pediatrician's office and reported that her 10-year-old daughter, Emma, has symptoms of a red rash; a temperature of 101 °F; and sore, painful wrists and elbows. On reviewing the client's chart, the LPN notes that Emma had a positive strep culture 3 weeks ago and received a prescription for penicillin.

Nursing Diagnosis: Acute Pain related to joint inflammation

COLLECT DATA

Subjective	Objective
_____	_____
_____	_____
_____	_____
_____	_____
_____	_____
_____	_____

Would you report this? Yes/No

If yes, to: _____

Nursing Care

_____
_____
_____
_____
_____
_____
_____
_____

How would you document this? _____

_____
_____
_____
_____
_____

Compare your documentation to the sample provided in Appendix I.

Data Collected
(use only those that apply)

- Winces when wrist and elbow are moved
- "I'm just not hungry. Nothing tastes good."
- Reports joint pain to be a 6 on a scale of 10
- Vital signs: T 101.1°F, P 110, R 12, BP 110/60
- Takes Tylenol every 4 to 6 hours for joint pain
- "Rash doesn't itch."
- "The medication caused diarrhea, so we didn't finish the prescription."
- Denies sore throat
- Reports resolution of diarrhea since discontinuing medication
- Right wrist enlarged
- Diffuse macular lesions noted on chest and abdomen
- Throat without erythema

Nursing Interventions
(use only those that apply; list in priority order)

- Teach the child and parent to properly clean skin and prevent moisture.
- Develop a plan to reevaluate the child's pain.
- Monitor the child's hydration level and encourage additional oral intake.
- Note the size, color, and any exudate related to the child's rash.
- Teach the child and parent the proper administration of prescribed pharmacologic agents to include route, dosage, side effects, reportable symptoms, and drug interactions.
- Use cooling measures to lower body temperature.
- Teach the child and parent nonpharmacologic methods of pain relief such as gentle joint massage, ROM exercises, application of heat, control of environmental factors (lighting, noise, room temperature), and relaxation techniques.
- Thoroughly assess the child's pain. Include location, characteristics, onset/duration, frequency, quality, intensity, precipitating factors, and relief methods.

NCLEX-PN® Exam Preparation

TEST-TAKING TIP Use logic and memory to help you answer a question. For example, a congenital heart problem might affect the upper body differently than the lower body. Use this information to help you pinpoint the correct answer..

1 The nurse is caring for a child with congestive heart failure and has just finished teaching the parents about diuretics and why they are given. The nurse realizes more teaching is needed when the father states:

1. "The diuretic should be given at the same time each day."
2. "The diuretic helps take away the fluid."
3. "If my child throws up the diuretic, I can give him another right away."
4. "I realize my child has to be monitored closely while on the diuretics."

2 A child has been diagnosed with Kawasaki's syndrome. The father is asking about the disease, and the nurse explains that Kawasaki's syndrome is:

1. A circulatory deficit with decreased cardiac output.
2. A mixed cardiac defect that affects both the systemic and the pulmonic circulations.
3. An inflammatory disorder caused by group A beta-hemolytic *Streptococcus* infection.
4. A systemic, acute inflammatory disease also known as mucocutaneous lymph node syndrome.

3 The nurse is caring for a child with Kawasaki's syndrome. The child is in the subacute phase of the disease. Which manifestations would the nurse expect to observe? Select all that apply.

1. Swollen hands and feet
2. Sloughing of the skin of the lips, hands, and feet
3. Conjunctival hyperemia
4. Pain in the joints
5. Enlarged cervical lymph nodes

4 The nurse has assumed care of a child with suspected rheumatic fever. The lab reports have just come back. The nurse reviews them. Which lab report would be helpful in confirmation of this diagnosis?

1. Antistreptolysin O titer
2. Erythrocyte sedimentation rate
3. Glucose tolerance test
4. Red blood count

5 The nurse is monitoring the intake and output of an infant with congestive heart failure. Which of the following indicators alerts the nurse that the child is accumulating fluid?

1. Sunken fontanel
2. Bradycardia
3. Crackles heard on auscultation
4. Capillary refill of 2 seconds

6 A nurse is caring for an infant with a diagnosis of tetralogy of Fallot (TOF). The nurse knows that there are four defects associated with TOF. They are:

1. Left ventricular hypertrophy, arterial septal defect, aortic stenosis, and overriding aorta.
2. Right ventricular hypertrophy, pulmonary stenosis, arterial septal defect, and overriding pulmonary artery.
3. Right ventricular hypertrophy, pulmonary stenosis, ventricular septal defect, and overriding aorta.
4. Left ventricular hypertrophy, pulmonary stenosis, arterial septal defect, and overriding aorta.

7 The nurse is caring for a child with a diagnosis of coarctation of the aorta who has congestive heart failure. Which of the following symptoms is also related to this diagnosis?

1. Weak, thready pulses in the right arm and bounding pulses in the lower extremities.
2. Strong, bounding pulse in the left arm and thready pulses in the lower extremities.
3. Strong, bounding pulses in the arms, thready and weak pulse in the right femoral artery.
4. Strong, bounding pulse in both arms, thready and weak pulses in the legs.

8 The mother of a child with a diagnosis of transposition of the great arteries asks what kind of medication the nurse is giving the child. The nurse tells the mother that the child is receiving prostaglandin E_1. The mother asks why this medication is necessary. The nurse replies that the medication:

1. Maintains adequate cardiac output and oxygen saturation.
2. Prevents endocarditis.
3. Is given prophylactically to prevent infection before surgery.
4. Prevents the progression of central nervous system involvement.

9 The nurse is caring for a child with Kawasaki's syndrome and reviews the medication orders expecting to find orders for:

1. Aspirin and immune globulin.
2. Cephalosporin and furosemide.
3. Glucagon and phenobarbital.
4. Digoxin and cisplatin.

10 A nurse is caring for a 15-year-old child with hyperlipidemia and is implementing a teaching plan for this child. Select all the interventions the nurse would anticipate for this client.

1. Low-fat, low-cholesterol diet
2. Pain medication
3. Regular exercise plan
4. Consultation with a dietitian
5. Anticoagulants
6. Cholesterol-lowering medications

Answers for NCLEX-PN® Review and Critical Thinking questions appear in Appendix I.

Chapter 14

Care of the Child with Hematologic or Lymphatic Disorders

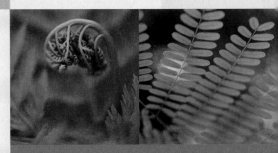

BRIEF Outline

Anatomy and Physiology
Brief Assessment Review
Bleeding Disorders
Anemias
Thalassemia

Cancers of Hematologic or Lymphatic Systems
Hematopoietic Stem Cell Transplantation (Bone Marrow Transplant)
Nursing Care

LEARNING Outcomes

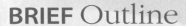

After completing this chapter, you will be able to:

1. Define key terms.
2. Describe the anatomy and physiology associated with the hematologic system.
3. Describe the anatomy and physiology associated with the lymphatic system.
4. Discuss the clinical manifestation of disorders of the hematologic and lymphatic systems.
5. Discuss the medical management of disorders of the hematologic and lymphatic systems.
6. Discuss nursing considerations related to disorders of the hematologic and lymphatic systems.

HEALTH PROMOTION ISSUE:
Dealing with Side Effects of Chemotherapy

NURSING CARE PLAN CHART:
The Child Undergoing Chemotherapy

NURSING PROCESS CARE PLAN:
Client with Sickle Cell Anemia

CRITICAL THINKING CARE MAP:
Client with Hodgkin's Lymphoma

Disorders of blood and lymph in children range from life altering, such as those causing chronic fatigue, to life threatening, such as Hodgkin's lymphoma. They may be inherited (e.g., sickle cell disease) or not (e.g., leukemia). Because blood and lymph support all body organs and systems, these disorders can have profound effects. Care of children with blood and lymph disorders will entail emotional support and teaching, as well as physical care.

Anatomy and Physiology

Hematology is the study of blood and blood-forming tissues. It includes the study of the bone marrow, blood, spleen, and lymph system. Knowledge of hematology is important to client care because it assists the nurse in determining the body's ability to deliver oxygen and other important nutrients to the body.

Blood cells are produced in the bone marrow by a process called **hematopoiesis.** The function of blood includes transportation of oxygen and other nutrients to the body; regulation of fluids, electrolytes, and acid-bases; and protection of the body through clotting and infection control.

Blood is composed of plasma and a variety of blood cells (Figure 14-1 ■). **Plasma** is mainly water. It also includes proteins such as albumin, globulin, and fibrinogen. Plasma contains small amounts of waste products, ions, gases, and nutrients. The three types of blood cells are erythrocytes, leukocytes, and thrombocytes. **Erythrocytes** are also called red blood cells (RBCs). RBCs carry oxygen and carbon dioxide to the body's tissues and regulate the body's acid-base balance. These RBCs are pliable and able to change their shape so they can be transported in the narrow passages of the capillary. RBCs are produced by a process called **erythropoiesis** and destroyed by a process called **hemolysis.**

Leukocytes are also called white blood cells (WBCs). WBCs are involved in infection control for the child. There are two types of WBCs: the *granulocyte* and the *agranulocyte.* When a harmful bacteria, virus, or atypical cell is noted by the WBC, the granulocyte can destroy it. The agranulocyte provides the body's immune response by assisting in the development of antibodies. A common agranulocyte is the *lymphocyte.* (Disorders of the immune system are discussed in Chapter 22 ⊙⊙.)

The **thrombocytes,** also called platelets, assist the body's clotting mechanism. These cells are important in minimizing blood loss when a child is involved in an injury. Following an injury, vasoconstriction occurs to decrease bleeding from the site. After vasoconstriction, platelets begin the process of clumping or **agglutination.** Platelets also activate clotting factors so coagulation can occur. Examples of clotting factors are fibrin and thrombin.

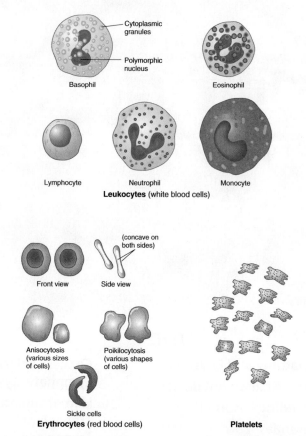

Figure 14-1. ■ Types of blood cells: *leukocytes* (white blood cells) at top, *erythrocytes* (red blood cells) at bottom left, *platelets* (also called *thrombocytes*) at bottom right.

The body has a mechanism in place so excessive clotting does not occur, compromising circulation. Anticoagulants are agents that keep blood from clotting or dissolve fibrin when it forms.

The liver, spleen, and lymphatic system are also parts of the hematologic system. The liver produces the coagulants. The spleen produces RBCs during fetal development; filters RBCs and their by-products; and stores lymphocytes, monocytes, and platelets.

The lymphatic system (Figure 14-2 ■) transports fluid and filters the fluid between the interstitial spaces and the intravascular system. The lymphatic system is also important in the body's immune response. This system consists of lymph, lymphatic capillaries, ducts, and lymph nodes. When the body is fighting infection, more granulocytes are produced. Debris from destruction of bacteria or viruses is carried away by lymph. An acute infection causes swelling of the lymph nodes as the body works rapidly to destroy and remove infection. For this reason, lymph nodes are important in physical assessment.

Lymph capillaries and ducts form a circulation system that drains lymph and fluid from tissues. Lymph contains leukocytes. The lymph flows through lymph nodes, which act as filters. The body has both deep (impalpable) and superficial (palpable) lymph nodes. There are two collecting

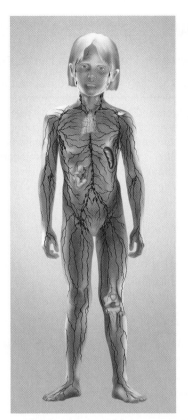

Figure 14-2. ■ Lymph system in the child. (Phototake NYC)

ducts for lymph fluid, the right lymphatic duct and the thoracic duct. The right lymphatic duct drains the upper body, and the thoracic duct drains the lower body. Eventually, all lymph is returned to the intravascular system. (Disorders of the cardiovascular system are discussed in Chapter 13 ⬭.)

Brief Assessment Review

HISTORY

- Inquire about the child's activity level. Has the child had weakness or fatigue?
- Is the child experiencing acute or chronic pain?
- Has there been a recent illness or infection? Any fever? Any weight loss?
- Has the child been in contact with anyone with an illness or infection?
- Does the child bruise easily? Any bleeding, especially uncontrolled bleeding? Nosebleeds?
- Does the child have wounds that do not heal properly?
- Inquire about the family history related to cancer, anemia, and other blood and lymph disorders.
- Is the child with chronic conditions experiencing low self-esteem, anxiety, body image alterations, symptoms of depression, social isolation, difficulty with relationships, or difficulties performing activities of daily living?

PHYSICAL

- Observe posturing to facilitate breathing.
- Observe for bruising, noting location, size, and color.
- Note skin color, including the color of the sclera and mucous membranes.
- Note shape of nails and capillary refill.
- Review lab work, noting especially complete blood count values.
- Compare height and weight to growth charts.
- Palpate for lymph nodes (Figure 14-3 ■), noting size, mobility, consistency, tenderness, and temperature.

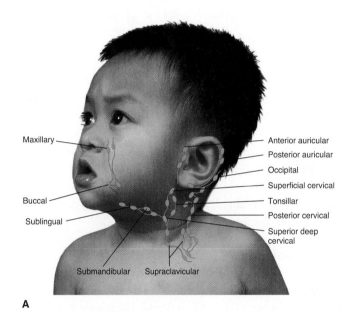

A

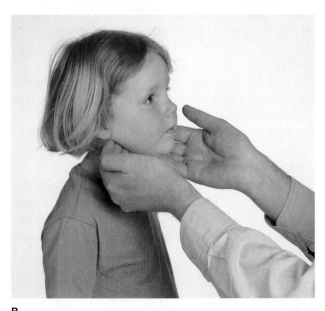

B

Figure 14-3. ■ **(A)** The lymph nodes in the neck are often palpated to determine the presence of infection. **(B)** Care provider assessing the lymph nodes in a young client. (B. Dorling Kindersley Media Library)

Bleeding Disorders

Bleeding disorders are the result of a decreased amount of blood clotting factors or a decreased number of platelets. Often there are few symptoms until after 6 months of age, because of the limited mobility of the child. Once the infant becomes more mobile, excessive bruising may be evident. It is important to evaluate the infant to differentiate bleeding disorders from child abuse. More information on recognizing child abuse can be found in Chapter 16 and Box 20-7 ⬤.

HEMOPHILIA

Hemophilia (types A and B) is a rare hereditary X-linked recessive disorder causing a deficiency in a specific blood clotting factor. The disorder almost exclusively affects males.

Manifestations

The hallmark symptom is bleeding into soft tissue and joints or prolonged bleeding during invasive procedures such as dental procedures, surgery, or trauma. Parents may first notice symptoms of joint pain, tenderness, and edema caused by bleeding into the joint. Impaired wound healing (Hoffman, Harger, & Lenkowski, 2006), bruising, epistaxis, and hematuria may also be noted. For more information on the nursing care related to epistaxis, see Chapter 12 ⬤.

Diagnosis

Diagnosis of hemophilia is made based on history, physical examination, and laboratory tests. Laboratory tests reveal decreased factor VIII or IX and prolonged activated partial thromboplastin time. Usually, prothrombin time, thrombin time, fibrinogen, and platelet counts are within normal limits.

Treatment

When major hemorrhages occur, treatment of hemophilia includes intravenous transfusion of the missing clotting factor. In mild cases desmopressin acetate or DDAVP (a synthetic drug that increases factor VIII activity) is effective. Aminocaproic acid has an unlabeled use of stopping bleeding related to dental procedures (Ball & Bindler, 2006). Gene therapy provides a promising future for a child with hemophilia to clot more effectively, have reduced symptoms, or even begin producing clotting factor. Researchers are seeking to develop a method to insert better functioning factor VIII or factor IX genes into the cells of people with hemophilia (National Hemophilia Foundation [n.d.]).

Nursing Considerations

Parents and children should be taught safety measures to prevent injury (Box 14-1 ▪). They should be taught to avoid medications that alter blood clotting, such as those

---

BOX 14-1 | LIFE SPAN CONSIDERATIONS

Safe Exercise for Children with Hemophilia

The child with hemophilia must choose appropriate activities in order to prevent injury that might cause bleeding. For toddlers, head, elbow, and knee protection may be necessary when the child plays simple games such as skipping, jumping rope, and playing hide and seek. School-age children and adolescents can obtain necessary exercise on stationary equipment such as a treadmill or bicycle. Swimming is an appropriate activity for any age group.

---

containing aspirin. Encourage parents to have the child wear a bracelet identifying the child as a hemophiliac, because this helps medical personnel to provide necessary care in case of bleeding.

---

clinical ALERT

Children with bleeding disorders should avoid the following activities to prevent excessive bleeding.

- Rectal temperatures
- Rectal suppositories
- Frequent blood pressure monitoring
- Unnecessary invasive procedures such as intramuscular or subcutaneous injections and venipunctures
- Medications containing aspirin
- Contact sports
- Body piercings and tattoos

IDIOPATHIC THROMBOCYTOPENIA

Idiopathic thrombocytopenic purpura (ITP) is a bleeding disorder of unknown cause that leads to a decrease in the number of platelets. Thrombocytopenia is more common in children between the ages of 2 and 5 years. Frequently, the child has had a recent viral infection such as chickenpox, varicella zoster, or rubella.

Manifestations

Symptoms include **purpura** (a rash in which blood cells leak into the skin, as shown in Figure 14-4 ▪), **petechiae** (pinpoint microhemorrhages under the skin), hematuria, blood in the stool, nosebleeds, and **ecchymosis** (hemorrhage into the skin that is larger than petechiae). The disorder may spontaneously go into permanent remission. **Remission** is defined as lack of evidence of any clinical symptoms of a disorder.

Diagnosis

Diagnosis of ITP is made through reviewing the child's history and physical findings. Laboratory data include a decreased platelet count, decreased antiplatelet antibodies, presence of antinuclear antibodies, and positive direct Coombs' test.

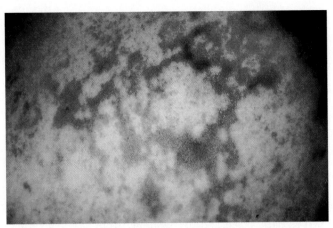

Figure 14-4. ■ Nonpalpable purpura with bleeding into the tissue below the skin. (Courtesy of the Department of Hematology/Oncology, Children's Medical Center, Washington, DC.)

Treatment

Corticosteroid therapy is indicated for platelet counts less than 50,000 mm³/dL. For platelet counts less than 20,000 mm³/dL, IV immune globulin is administered. Platelet replacement may be required if the child is experiencing hemorrhage. If the disorder continues long term, a splenectomy may be performed with some success in controlling the disorder.

Nursing Considerations

Nursing care would include controlling bleeding (Box 14-2 ■) and teaching the child and family measures to decrease risk of bleeding (Clinical Alert, page 364). Parents should also be aware of the signs and symptoms of occult (hidden) bleeding, such as tarry stool (**melena**). Occult blood may also be present with tumors of the GI tract, ulcers, or inflammatory bowel disease.

Anemias

Anemia is a decrease in the number of RBCs, a decrease in hemoglobin, or both. Anemia can be caused by blood loss, a destruction of RBCs, or a decrease in production of RBCs. Three types of anemia that affect children—iron-deficiency anemia, sickle cell anemia, and thalassemia—are discussed.

IRON-DEFICIENCY ANEMIA

Iron-deficiency anemia is a condition that results when the demand for stored iron is greater than what the body can supply. The number of RBCs may be normal, but the hemoglobin level is low, resulting in decreased oxygen-carrying capacity. The cause of iron-deficiency anemia in infants can be blood loss, but more commonly it is due to poor intake of iron and iron-rich foods after 6 months of age. Infants have adequate iron stores from birth to 4 to 6 months. In children and adolescents, iron-deficiency anemia may develop during periods of rapid physical growth.

BOX 14-2   NURSING CARE CHECKLIST

First Aid for Bleeding

☑ Obtain assistance from another health care worker.

☑ Apply personal protective equipment.

☑ Apply direct pressure with sterile gauze to the site of bleeding for at least 15 minutes.

☑ If gauze becomes soaked, do not remove. Add additional gauze.

☑ Raise the site of bleeding above the heart while applying pressure.

☑ Apply ice packs to promote vasoconstriction.

☑ If bleeding has not slowed after 15 minutes of the above measures, apply additional pressure to the pulse site above the wound.

☑ Monitor vital signs closely.

☑ If the child does not have venous access, initiate access to administer IV fluid or blood replacement as ordered.

☑ Offer emotional support to the child and his or her family.

Manifestations

The child with iron-deficiency anemia will appear pale, tired, and irritable (Figure 14-5 ■). If undiagnosed or untreated for a long period of time, the child can display tachycardia, muscle weakness, systolic heart murmur, and growth retardation and can be mentally delayed. Over time, the nail beds become deformed.

clinical ALERT

Anemia may be associated with **pica**, a craving to eat substances that are not food. A child who is seen eating dirt, clay, chalk, glue, ice, starch, hair, or other nonfood substances should be assessed to determine whether anemia is the cause. Teach parents to recognize and report these symptoms promptly.

Diagnosis

Diagnosis of iron-deficiency anemia is made by history, physical examination, and laboratory tests. Hemoglobin, hematocrit, reticulocyte counts, serum ferritin, and serum iron concentration will be decreased while RBC count and total iron-binding capacity are increased. See Table 14-1 ■ for classifications of iron-deficiency anemia.

Treatment

Treatment for iron-deficiency anemia includes administration of oral supplemental iron preparations (Table 14-2 ■). Dietary counseling is also important to ensure adequate dietary intake of iron. For instance, children are more apt to eat raisins and enriched cereals or breads than green, leafy vegetables. Reevaluation of laboratory findings is necessary

ANEMIA

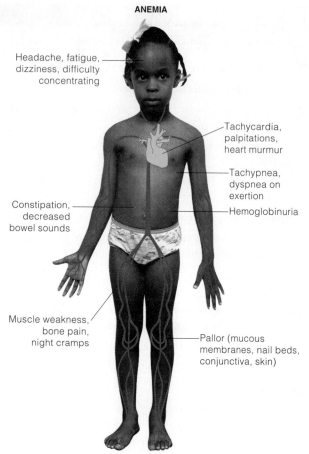

Headache, fatigue, dizziness, difficulty concentrating

Tachycardia, palpitations, heart murmur

Tachypnea, dyspnea on exertion

Constipation, decreased bowel sounds

Hemoglobinuria

Muscle weakness, bone pain, night cramps

Pallor (mucous membranes, nail beds, conjunctiva, skin)

Figure 14-5. ■ Multisystem effects of anemia.

after 2 months of treatment. If findings are satisfactory, iron supplementation is decreased and laboratory tests are repeated in 6 months to determine whether dietary intake is sufficient.

TABLE 14-1

Hemoglobin Levels in Anemia

ANEMIA CLASSIFICATION	HEMOGLOBIN LEVEL
Mild	9.5–11 g/dL
Moderate	8–9.4 g/dL
Severe	Less than 8 g/dL

Nursing Considerations

Parents should be taught to provide a diet high in iron, such as dark green and deep yellow fruits and vegetables, dried fruits such as raisins, red meats, fish, poultry, and whole grains. Box 14-3 ■ lists foods that can help in absorption of iron. Infants who are formula fed should be given formulas containing iron. When solid food is introduced, iron-fortified cereals are encouraged.

Because young children have difficulty swallowing pills, liquid iron preparation may be ordered. Liquid preparations

BOX 14-3	COMPLEMENTARY THERAPIES

Foods to Increase Absorption of Iron

Vitamin C–containing foods can increase the absorption of iron when ingested at the same time. The nurse can give the child and parent several examples of meals that will facilitate absorption of iron:

- Hamburger with tomato slice
- Chicken and broccoli casserole
- Spinach salad with orange slices
- Whole-grain cereal (dry) sprinkled over fresh strawberries
- Baked fish with a glass of pure fruit juice fortified with vitamin C

TABLE 14-2

Pharmacology: Drugs for Iron Deficiencies

DRUG (GENERIC AND COMMON BRAND NAME)	USUAL ROUTE/ DOSE	CLASSIFICATION AND PURPOSE	SELECTED SIDE EFFECTS	DON'T GIVE IF
Ferrous sulfate (Feosol)	For deficiency: less than 6 years old, 75–225 mg/day PO; 6–12 years old, 600 mg/day PO	Iron preparation	Nausea; heartburn; constipation; black, tarry stools	Crushed; within 1 hour of bedtime; undiluted
Ferrous fumarate (Feostat)	For deficiency: 3 mg/kg three times a day PO For supplementation: 3 mg/day once daily PO For the infant: 1–15 mg/kg/day PO	Iron preparation	As above	As above
Ferrous gluconate (Fergon)	For deficiency: 100–300 mg/day PO For supplementation: 100–300 mg/day PO	Iron preparation	As above	As above

should be diluted and given through a straw or placed on the back of the tongue to prevent staining of the teeth. Liquid iron preparation may not be compatible with milk or juice. Iron preparations may turn the stool black, cause constipation, and create an unpleasant aftertaste. Adequate fluids, a high-fiber diet, and exercise will help the child avoid constipation.

clinical ALERT

Iron overdose is possible, and parents should be taught to recognize the symptoms. These symptoms include abdominal pain, vomiting, blood diarrhea, shortness of breath, and shock. Immediate recognition and prompt reporting of these symptoms is essential. The child will need immediate treatment.

Hemoglobin S and Red Blood Cell Sickling

Sickle cell anemia is caused by an inherited autosomal recessive defect in Hb synthesis. Sickle cell hemoglobin (HbS) differs from normal hemoglobin only in the substitution of the amino acid valine for glutamine in both beta chains of the hemoglobin molecule.

When HbS is oxygenated, it has the same globular shape as normal hemoglobin. However, when HbS off-loads oxygen, it becomes insoluble in intracellular fluid and crystallizes into rodlike structures. Clusters of rods form polymers (long chains) that bend the erythrocyte into the characteristic crescent shape of the sickle cell.

SICKLE CELL ANEMIA

Sickle cell anemia is a hereditary disorder affecting the formation of hemoglobin. Normal hemoglobin (Hgb) is replaced by hemoglobin S (Hgb S) that causes the RBC to form an "S" or "C" shape (Figure 14-6 ■). This changing of the RBC shape is called **sickling.** The abnormally shaped RBCs cannot travel normally through the capillaries, resulting in decreased blood flow and decreased oxygen-carrying capacity.

Sickle cell anemia is a recessive trait affecting primarily African Americans, but it has been found in other races as well, such as those of India and the Mediterranean countries. Approximately 1 in 12 African Americans carries the recessive gene, but most do not exhibit symptoms of sickle

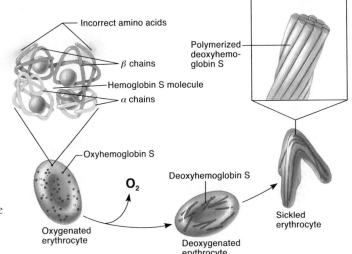

The Sickle Cell Disease Process

Sickle cell disease is characterized by episodes of acute painful crises. Sickling crises are triggered by conditions causing high tissue oxygen demands or that affect cellular pH. As the crisis begins, sickled erythrocytes adhere to capillary walls and to each other, obstructing blood flow and causing cellular hypoxia. The crisis accelerates as tissue hypoxia and acidic metabolic waste products cause further sickling and cell damage.

Sickle cell crises cause microinfarcts in joints and organs, and repeated crises slowly destroy organs and tissues. The spleen and kidneys are especially prone to sickling damage.

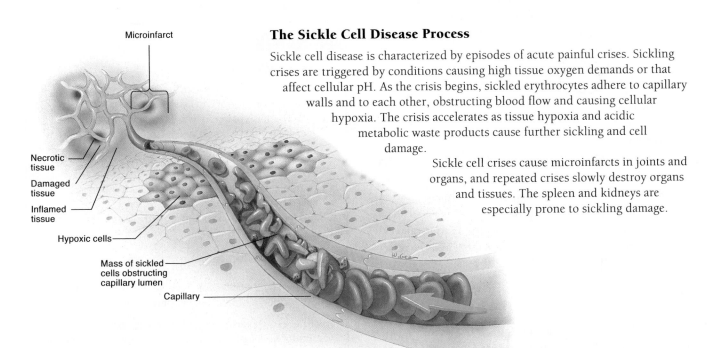

Figure 14-6. ■ Pathophysiology of sickle cell anemia and sickle cell crisis. Obstruction of capillaries causes acute pain.

cell anemia. If both parents carry the recessive gene, there is a 25% chance that each child will have sickle cell anemia. Such parents should be counseled about the possibility of having a child with sickle cell anemia.

Manifestations

The infant with sickle cell anemia will be asymptomatic until approximately 4 to 6 months of age because sickling is inhibited by fetal hemoglobin. Not all RBCs will be misshapen, and the infant will be healthy much of the time. For the child, during periods of stress, such as rapid growth, or illness more sickle-shaped cells will be released into the circulation. Sickle cells have a short life span, living 10 to 20 days instead of the usual 120 days of normal RBCs. The difficulties associated with sickle cell anemia are a combination of sickle cells obstructing circulation (**vasoocclusion**) and anemia from not enough normal RBCs and hemoglobin. They result in pathologic changes to body systems and structures (Table 14-3 ■).

Children with sickle cell anemia experience symptoms characterized as a sickle cell crisis (see Figure 14-6). The **sickle cell crisis** is an acute episode of severe symptoms. The crisis may be brought on by fever, dehydration, altitude, vomiting, emotional distress, fatigue, alcohol consumption, pregnancy, or excessive physical activity.

During a sickle cell crisis, the child will experience severe pain, localized to the area of the vasoocclusion. For example, an obstruction in the spleen would cause severe left upper quadrant pain. If occlusions occur close to the dermis, discoloration, pallor, and coolness of the skin would be present. Nausea, fever, swelling and pain in the joints (**arthralgia**), vomiting, anorexia, and diarrhea may also be present.

The three most common types of sickle cell crisis (Box 14-4 ■) are:

- Vasoocclusive (or thrombotic) crisis
- Splenic sequestration
- Aplastic crisis

Diagnosis

Diagnosis of sickle cell anemia can be made for infants through a blood test called hemoglobin electrophoresis. For children older than 6 months, another blood test, a Sickledex test, is used for screening purposes. If the Sickledex is positive, a hemoglobin electrophoresis can verify the diagnosis. The Hgb will be decreased, and the reticulocyte count will be increased.

Treatment

If given early in crisis, a blood transfusion can relieve the anemia and make the sickled blood less thick or viscous. Whole blood, packed RBCs, fresh frozen plasma, cryoprecipitate, clotting factors, or albumin may be prescribed. Parenteral

TABLE 14-3

Effects of Sickle Cell Anemia on Body Structures and Systems

ORGAN AFFECTED	PATHOLOGIC CHANGES
Brain	Stroke (cerebrovascular accident), headache, aphasia, convulsions, visual disturbances
Bones	Infections and bone degeneration resulting from chronic ischemia (osteoporosis, osteomyelitis, spinal deformities, aseptic necrosis of the femoral head)
Eyes	Diminished vision from retinal detachment, retinopathy
Extremities	Vasoocclusion and chronic ischemia leading to peripheral neuropathy, weakness, arthralgia
Kidneys	Ischemia leading to enuresis, hematuria, inability to concentrate urine
Liver	Impaired blood flow leads to enlargement and scarring (hepatomegaly, cirrhosis)
Penis	Obstruction of microcirculation and engorgement of penis (priapism)
Skin	Decreased peripheral circulation (leg ulcers)
Spleen	Infarct in spleen leads to fibrosis (nonfunctioning spleen, increased number of infections) Crisis involving spleen can be life threatening within hours

BOX 14-4

Types of Sickle Cell Crisis

Vasoocclusive (Thrombotic) Crisis
- Most common type of crisis; painful
- Caused by stasis of blood with clumping of cells in the microcirculation, ischemia, and infarction
- Signs include fever, pain, and tissue engorgement

Splenic Sequestration
- Life-threatening crisis; death can occur within hours
- Caused by pooling of blood in the spleen
- Signs include profound anemia, hypovolemia, and shock

Aplastic Crisis
- Diminished production and increased destruction of red blood cells
- Triggered by viral infection or depletion of folic acid
- Signs include profound anemia and pallor

Source: London, M., Ladewig, P., Ball, J., & Bindler, R. (2007). *Maternal and child nursing care*, 2nd ed. Upper Saddle River, NJ: Pearson Education. Table 49-5, p. 1497.

analgesics are administered routinely to control pain. Continuous IV infusion of fluid is common during crisis to correct dehydration. Oxygen therapy may also be implemented. Because the child with sickle cell anemia has a decreased ability to fight infection, prophylactic antibiotic administration is given. Pain management is also a priority in the treatment of the child with a sickle cell crisis.

clinical ALERT

The child who requires frequent blood transfusions is at risk for **hemosiderosis** (iron overload, the buildup of iron in tissues and organs). Therefore, an iron-chelating agent such as deferoxamine is also given, which binds to iron so it can be excreted by the kidneys. Vitamin C may also be used to promote iron excretion.

Nursing Considerations

The child should be observed closely for signs of anemia, including pallor, fatigue, lethargy, and irritability. If the child is under physical stress, mild cyanosis may be present. The nurse should encourage a diet high in calories and protein with adequate fluid intake. Because children who are chronically ill are at greater risk for infection, and infection can stimulate crisis, it is essential to prevent infection. Immunizations, including the pneumococcal vaccine, should be kept up to date. The child should avoid contact with infected persons. Frequent hand washing is a must. Prophylactic antibiotic administration may be prescribed.

Administration of blood products is often the role of the registered nurse, who starts the infusion and documents that the blood to be infused matches the child's blood type. The LPN/LVN should follow state regulations and facility policies regarding administration of blood. In many states, LPNs/LVNs may administer blood products once they are IV certified. LPNs/LVNs may monitor the infusion and the client and obtain vital signs frequently. The LPN/LVN should also be aware of the clinical manifestations of blood transfusion reaction (Box 14-5 ■) and stop the transfusion at the first indication of this potential complication.

Assisting the child with sickle cell anemia in pain management is a priority nursing task. Pain should be managed before it becomes overwhelming to the child. A combination of nonpharmacologic and pharmacologic techniques should be used. Nonpharmacologic techniques include positioning, breathing and relaxation techniques, distraction, massage, and warm baths. The nurse should ensure the routine administration of pharmacologic pain relief methods in addition to the nonpharmacologic methods.

Knowledge about the disease helps ensure compliance with preventative measures and treatment. Family members should be encouraged to share their feelings. Because sickle cell anemia is a chronic, life-threatening, genetic

BOX 14-5	ASSESSMENT

Blood Transfusion Reaction

- Urticaria
- Respiratory distress
- Fever
- Chills
- Headache
- Chest or back pain
- Hypotension
- Nausea
- Productive cough
- Distended neck veins

Note: In some states, LPNs/LVNs may administer blood products once they are IV certified. Be sure to observe state policy.

disease, a lot of additional stress will be placed on the family unit. Family members need help coping with guilt, fear, and depression. Support groups may be available to assist and support families of sickle cell children.

Thalassemia

Thalassemia is an inherited disorder caused by abnormal hemoglobin synthesis. Thalassemias are classified as either *beta* or *alpha*. Both beta and alpha thalassemias are defects in the production of hemoglobin. Beta thalassemia is the most commonly occurring type. In beta thalassemia, the RBCs are fragile and can be easily destroyed. Beta thalassemia is an autosomal recessive disorder, so if both parents are carriers, each child has a 25% chance of having the condition. Children of Mediterranean descent and those from the Middle East, Asia, or Africa are more likely to have these conditions (Box 14-6 ■).

Manifestations

The by-product of hemolysis is **hemosiderin,** which can be deposited in the skin of the child, creating a tanned appearance. As anemia progresses, the child can have pathologic

BOX 14-6	CULTURAL PULSE POINTS

Genetic Risk for Thalassemia

Health officials in Greece have developed extensive public service campaigns to advise citizens of their potential genetic risk for thalassemia. Prenatal screening programs have been successful in reducing the incidence of the disease. Therapeutic abortion rates are also high among women who discover the trait in the fetus they are carrying. Thalassemia is a risk for all women of Mediterranean descent.

fractures and skeletal deformities. Pallor, lethargy, activity intolerance, headache, and bone pain are also clinical manifestations. The liver and spleen may also become enlarged.

The symptoms of alpha thalassemia are similar to those of beta thalassemia. They are, however, typically milder unless a significant number of the child's genes are affected. In alpha thalassemia, a fetus may develop **hydrops fetalis** (a fetal condition of accumulation of fluid within two or more fetal compartments) and congestive heart failure.

Diagnosis

Thalassemia can be detected by genetic testing in pregnancy. History, symptoms, and physical examination assist in the formation of a diagnosis in the infant or child. Laboratory tests include hemoglobin electrophoresis, complete blood count (CBC), chest x-ray, and magnetic resonance imaging (MRI) of the liver.

Treatment

Medical management of thalassemia is supportive and not curative. The child may be given blood transfusions every 2 to 4 weeks to address symptoms related to anemia. An iron-chelating agent (e.g., deferoxamide) is given to prevent iron overload (*hemosiderosis*). If the spleen is enlarged, a splenectomy may be considered.

Nursing care for the child with thalassemia is similar to that in other forms of anemia and includes strategies to minimize infection, help the child conserve energy, and teach the parent and child about the disease and treatment.

Cancers of Hematologic or Lymphatic Systems

HODGKIN'S LYMPHOMA

Hodgkin's lymphoma (Figure 14-7 ■) is a rare, malignant disorder of the lymphoid system. Together with non-Hodgkin's lymphoma, it is the third most common form of childhood cancer in the United States (Ries et al., 1999). In children younger than 14 years, Hodgkin's disease is rare. The incidence of the disease increases with age and is especially high in 15-year-old males. With early diagnosis and treatment of Hodgkin's lymphoma, the long-term prognosis is favorable (80–90% survival rate).

Manifestations

The symptoms of Hodgkin's disease include nontender, firm, enlarged lymph nodes, usually in the cervical and supraclavicular area. Occasionally, the mediastinal lymph nodes are involved, resulting in respiratory distress from pressure against the trachea. Some adolescents experience fever, night sweats, and weight loss.

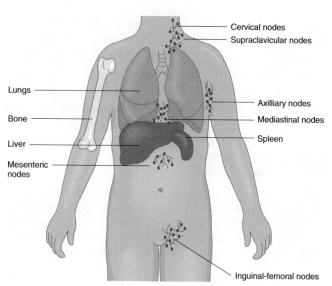

Figure 14-7. ■ Hodgkin's disease. Lymph nodes and organs affected in Hodgkin's disease in children.

Research indicates a relationship between herpes virus, cytomegalovirus, and Epstein-Barr virus and Hodgkin's disease. Hodgkin's disease has been reported in families, suggesting a genetic factor as well.

Diagnosis

The erythrocyte sedimentation rate and leukocyte counts may be elevated in children with Hodgkin's disease. Diagnosis is made by lymph node biopsy. Once the diagnosis is made, further tests must be made to determine the extent to which the disease has spread throughout the body. This process, called **staging,** classifies the extent of the spread of cancer into four main stages with substages. Box 14-7 ■

BOX 14-7

Staging of Hodgkin's Lymphoma

- Stage I: The disease is confined to a single lymph node area.
- Stage IE: The disease progresses from the single lymph node area to adjacent regions.
- Stage II: The disease is in two or more lymph node areas on one side of the diaphragm.
- Stage IIE: The disease extends to adjacent regions of at least one of the affected nodes.
- Stage III: The disease is in lymph node areas on both sides of the diaphragm.
- Stage IIIE: The disease extends into adjacent areas or organs.
- Stage IIISE: The disease extends into adjacent areas or organs and/or into the spleen.
- Stage IV: The disease has spread from the lymphatic system to one or more other organs, such as the bone marrow or liver. Lymph nodes associated with these organs may or may not be affected.

TABLE 14-4

Combination Antineoplastic Agents Used to Treat Hodgkin's Lymphoma

COMBINATION	DRUGS INCLUDED
ABVD	**A**driamycin, **b**leomycin, **v**inblastine, **d**acarbazine
MOPP	**M**echlorethamine, vincristine (**O**ncovin), **p**rocarbazine, **p**rednisone
BCVPP	**B**armustine (Bi**C**NU), **c**yclophosphamide, **v**inblastine, **p**rocarbazine, **p**rednisone

shows the staging system for Hodgkin's lymphoma. These stages assist the physician to order treatment related to the location of the disease. Other tests to assist the diagnosis include computed tomography (CT) or MRI scans, lymphangiogram, blood counts, bone marrow biopsy, and staging laparotomy.

Treatment

Treatment usually consists of a combination of four or five antineoplastic agents or chemotherapeutic agents. Table 14-4 ■ lists the antineoplastic agents commonly used to treat Hodgkin's lymphoma. There are several reasons for using a combination of antineoplastic agents. First, there is less chance that the cancer cells can develop a resistance to one of the drugs. Second, drug combinations allow the health care provider to select drugs with different patterns of toxicity; this helps to prevent damage to other body organs. Third, by using drugs that affect cells at different stages of their growth cycle, a higher numbers of malignant cells can be destroyed in a shorter period of time. Side effects of antineoplastic drugs include bone marrow depression, nausea, vomiting, **stomatitis** (inflammation of the mucous lining of the mouth), and hair loss. Many antineoplastic drugs are excreted unchanged in the urine.

Low-dose radiation may be added to the treatment plan.

Nursing Considerations

The side effects of antineoplastic drugs, coupled with the disease process and radiation treatments, may make the child feel tired, sick, and embarrassed by the change in appearance. The adolescent, who felt invincible prior to developing Hodgkin's disease, may suddenly be confronted with his or her own mortality. Because exposure to infection must be avoided when WBCs are low, the child may need to decrease contact with his or her friends, remain home from school, and limit social interaction. The child's lack of contact with the peer group could lead to feelings of isolation, depression, and anger. Table 14-5 ■ provides some ways of discussing the diagnosis of cancer with children and their parents.

Antineoplastic agents are typically given intravenously. In most cases, these drugs are administered by an RN with certification or additional training beyond his or her original degree. This training is usually offered by the clinical facility. The LPN/LVN caring for the client would need to work closely with the RN. Clients must be assessed for signs of infection, open lesions, and bleeding. Their mental health status should be evaluated, and emotional support provided. Precautions must be taken to prevent the care provider from being contaminated by body fluids containing the antineoplastic drugs.

NON-HODGKIN'S LYMPHOMA

Non-Hodgkin's lymphoma (NHL) is a type of lymphoma with a rapid onset and widespread involvement. It presents in children from infancy to adolescence. The greatest incidence of occurrence is in children between ages 7 and 11. The true cause of non-Hodgkin's lymphoma is not known, but T-cell abnormalities have been isolated. Children with

TABLE 14-5

Communicating Across the Life Span: Talking with Children About a Cancer Diagnosis

SPEAKER	TODDLER	PRESCHOOLER	SCHOOL-AGE CHILD	ADOLESCENT
Parent with assistance from the nurse	"We are going to a special doctor's office, next to the hospital to get some special medicine, in a shot. It will help you get better."	"I know you feel tired today. It's because there are some cells in your body that don't need to be there. You are getting this medicine to get rid of those cells."	"The cancer cells are making you tired. It's going to be important to rest every day. This should keep you from being so tired."	"Fatigue is something you'll have to live with right now. I know it's important to be with your friends, so you'll have to try and eat good food and rest every day."
Client	"I don't like to get shots."	"I want to feel better so I can play soccer."	"I guess I could take a nap when I get home from school."	"It's not fair. I'm tired of having cancer. I don't even feel like eating most days."

immunodeficiencies have a higher incidence of the disease. Depending on the extent of the disease at diagnosis, 80% of children have a 5-year survival.

Manifestations

The child with NHL usually presents with a sudden onset of pain and inflammation located at the site of enlarged lymph nodes or tumors. Depending on the site of the tumor, the child may have dyspnea, jaw pain, abdominal pain, nausea, or vomiting. Fever, weight loss, and night sweats also occur, though less commonly than in Hodgkin's disease.

Diagnosis

A thorough history of the child's health can assist the physician in ruling out a diagnosis of NHL. Blood work will include CBC, renal and liver function studies, electrolytes, uric acid, and LDH. Chest x-rays, CT scans, and MRIs can locate the areas of involvement. Once these areas are identified, tissue biopsy of the location will confirm the diagnosis. The extent of the disease is designated by a staging system. NHL has four stages and progresses from stage I (with a single tumor and no lymph nodes involved) to stage IV (with numerous tumors, CNS involvement, and bone marrow metastases).

Treatment

Chemotherapy is tailored according to the stage of the disease. Radiation or surgery may be necessary to relieve pressure on vital organs. Stem cell transplantation is also an option for the child with recurrent disease.

LEUKEMIA

Leukemia is cancer of the blood-forming organs. It is characterized by an increase of abnormal WBCs. Several different types of leukemia are differentiated by the rate of disease progression and the specific cells affected. Chronic leukemia, although common in adults, is rare in children. The exact cause of leukemia is unknown, yet some researchers theorize that exposure to viruses before or after birth can predispose a child to leukemia. Two types of acute leukemia, acute lymphoblastic leukemia and acute myeloid leukemia, are common in children and are discussed here.

Acute Lymphoblastic Leukemia

Acute lymphoblastic leukemia (ALL) is the overproduction of immature lymphocytes. ALL, the most common leukemia of childhood, has the highest incidence in White boys who are 3 to 4 years of age (Figure 14-8 ■).

Normally, lymphocytes are formed from stem cells in the bone marrow and migrate to lymphatic tissue where they

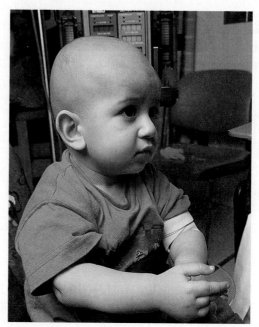

Figure 14-8. ■ Acute lymphoblastic leukemia is the most common type of leukemia in children and the most common cancer affecting children younger than 5 years.

become mature functioning cells. In ALL, the lymphocytes divide rapidly but fail to mature. Lymphoblasts (immature lymph cells) have no normal function. As lymphoblast numbers rise, fewer and fewer normal lymph cells are produced, and the high numbers of lymphoblasts crowd out normal WBCs, RBCs, and platelets.

Acute Myelogenous Leukemia

Acute myelogenous leukemia (AML) occurs when cancer cells develop in the bone marrow (*myeloid tissue*). AML is a less common form of leukemia in children. In AML, cancer cells replace normal bone marrow, and immature WBCs, RBCs, and platelets are found circulating throughout the body. Because in both ALL and AML bone marrow is replaced by blast cells, the symptoms are very similar. Diagnosis, treatment, and nursing care are also similar.

MANIFESTATIONS. The child with leukemia presents with symptoms associated with a decreased number of normal blood cells. With a low WBC count, the child easily develops infections, most commonly respiratory infections. Low RBC count results in fatigue and other signs of anemia. With a low platelet count, bleeding gums and bruising are common.

DIAGNOSIS. Diagnosis is made by blood counts and bone marrow aspiration. Laboratory values reveal elevated leukocytes, decreased platelets, and decreased hemoglobin. The presence of abnormal lymphoblasts is seen in the bone marrow aspirate. The earlier a diagnosis is made and treatment

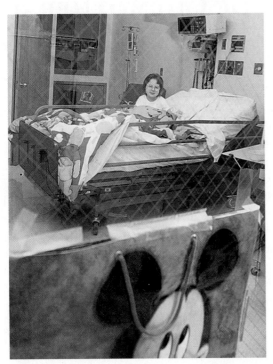

Figure 14-9. ■ Protective isolation. The child undergoing bone marrow transplantation is hospitalized in a special sterile unit while receiving chemotherapy before the transfusion. The child will remain in the unit for several weeks afterward until the new marrow produces enough cells to maintain health.

is begun, the better the prognosis. Left untreated, the life expectancy of a child with AML is several weeks to 6 months.

TREATMENT.   Treatment might include antibiotics, blood replacement, chemotherapy, and radiation. After remission is achieved, bone marrow transplant can be beneficial if a suitable donor is available. During treatment or after bone marrow transplantation, the child must be protected in as sterile an environment as possible, while the body rebuilds its defenses (Figure 14-9 ■). See Health Promotion Issue on pages 374 and 375.

Nursing Considerations

Assessment of bruising, bleeding, fever, and symptoms of infection during treatment should be done frequently. Chemotherapy is very damaging to the kidneys, so renal function must be monitored with specific gravity, intake and output, and daily weight. Chemotherapy and radiation can be harmful to the rapidly growing mucous membranes of the gastrointestinal system, resulting in nausea, vomiting, constipation, decreased sense of taste, lack of appetite, and sores in the mouth. Nutritional status and fluid balance should be assessed closely.

The child with leukemia needs periods of rest coupled with safe activities. During the acute phase of the illness,

the child may not have enough energy for a lot of physical activity, but quiet play can help maintain mobility as well as provide the child with a diversion from thoughts of cancer.

Having an acute life-threatening illness causes a lot of fear for the child and for the parents and family. Because of the rapid onset of symptoms of leukemia, the child appears well one day and extremely ill the next. Hospitalization, numerous invasive diagnostic procedures, and administration of toxic chemotherapy contribute to the fear and anxiety. The nurse is instrumental in providing support and teaching. The nurse also helps organize interdisciplinary resources to assist the client and family. Referral to family support groups may be made on request. More information about nursing care for the child undergoing chemotherapy is shown in the Nursing Care Plan Chart on page 376.

Hematopoietic Stem Cell Transplantation (Bone Marrow Transplant)

Hematopoietic stem cell transplantation (HSCT) is a medical procedure in which stem cells are transplanted into an individual diagnosed with certain hematologic and lymphatic system disorders, such as leukemia. The procedure may be referred to as a *bone marrow transplant*. Stem cells can be obtained from bone marrow, peripheral blood, and umbilical cord blood. When healthy, donor stem cells are transplanted, they migrate to the recipient's bone marrow and produce new blood cells in a matter of 2 to 4 weeks.

There are three types of donors for HSCT. The first is the **autologous donor** (person who donates for his or her own later use). These stem cells come from the child who has been diagnosed with a hematologic or lymphatic system disorder. Second is the **isogeneic donor** or **syngeneic donor.** In this type of donation, stem cells are harvested from an identical twin. Third is the **allogeneic donor,** in which stem cells are obtained from a relative, usually a sibling. The National Marrow Donor Program also provides stem cells when no match can be located within the child's family.

The process of HSCT is lengthy and requires the best medical and nursing care. Prior to the transplant, the ill child will undergo chemotherapy and possibly radiation in an effort to destroy blood cells and diseased bone marrow. The child will be hospitalized and placed in strict isolation in an effort to prevent infection while the child is in an immunocompromised state.

Compatible donors are identified by testing for the human leukocyte antigen (HLA). Donors are often given growth factors prior to harvesting to stimulate blood cell

DEALING WITH SIDE EFFECTS OF CHEMOTHERAPY

Nine-year-old Mandy recently completed her second chemotherapy treatment for leukemia. Her mother calls the physician's office and reports that Mandy had no side effects with the first treatment but has recently been fatigued to the point of not having enough energy to eat. Mandy and her mom have also noticed that Mandy's hair seems to be falling out. Mandy is particularly upset by this side effect. In fact, she is crying frequently and refusing to go out in public, including school.

Mandy's mom wonders if these side effects are normal and if other children experience them. She asks the nurse for advice on dealing with these issues. She is particularly interested in anything specific that will make Mandy feel more comfortable, increase her energy, and cause her to feel better about herself so she can continue her normal activities.

DISCUSSION

Fatigue is the most frequent symptom reported by cancer patients. This fatigue can feel quite different from general fatigue. It may also appear suddenly and may not be relieved by rest. This fatigue may last as long as the body is attempting to overcome the disorder. The child may see resolution of fatigue once her condition stabilizes.

Hair loss or *alopecia* is a common occurrence following chemotherapy. Alopecia can be thinning of the hair, loss of clumps of hair, or a complete loss of all hair, including hair on the head, face, arms and legs, underarms, and pubic area. The remaining hair may become dull and dry, making the child feel unattractive. When treatments are completed, the hair usually grows back. The new hair, however, may be a different color and a different texture.

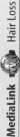

MediaLink Hair Loss

PLANNING AND IMPLEMENTATION

Fatigue

Encouraging rest for a child with fatigue due to chemotherapy is the most important nursing action. The nurse should make specific suggestions to assist Mandy and her mother in achieving an adequate amount of rest for Mandy. Carefully review Mandy's schedule. Prioritize essential activities. These priority activities should be accomplished when Mandy has the most energy. This is usually in the morning or immediately following a meal. Schedule rest breaks and naps between activities.

Physical activity can actually promote energy. Discuss activities that are desirable to Mandy. Begin with range-of-motion exercises performed in a seated position and progress to leisurely walks of short distance or exercise in a swimming pool. Encourage Mandy to participate in making a daily schedule to increase her sense of control over her life.

A healthy diet and adequate fluids are essential for combating fatigue. The nurse can teach Mandy that just as getting her chemotherapy treatment on a regular basis is essential for fighting the leukemia, getting adequate nutrition every day is equally important. The nurse can help Mandy view nutrition as part of her treatment.

Large meals can increase fatigue, so several small meals are more effective.

Meal preparation can be fatiguing, so proper meal planning, shopping, and preparing meals ahead of time conserves energy. Healthy, energy-producing snacks such as fruit juice, fruits, vegetables, soups, cheese, peanut butter, and nuts should be readily available.

The nurse should explain to Mandy that the fluids she drinks can also increase or decrease her fatigue. The best fluid to consume is water. Most clients enjoy water that is very chilled. Mandy can be encouraged to squeeze a slice of lemon, lime, or orange into her water for added flavor. Drinks containing caffeine and sugar only give temporary energy and eventually decrease the overall energy level. These types of drinks should be limited.

Several complementary therapies are available that may help Mandy focus her mind, body, and spirit. These therapies can reduce stress, lessen fatigue from chemotherapy, and enhance overall well-being. Examples of these therapies are biofeedback, visualization, massage, muscle tension and release, meditation and prayer, breathing techniques, yoga, music therapy, and pet therapy.

Biofeedback includes controlling heart rate, blood pressure, and muscle tension. A machine is used to sense signs of tension and provide a signal such as a sound or flashing a light. The machine also gives feedback when a relaxation response occurs.

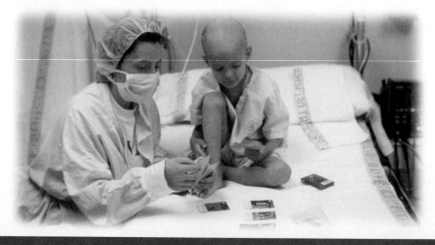

Visualization creates a mind picture. This mind picture can allow Mandy to turn her fearful thoughts and feelings into positive images. Visualization can reduce fear, promote positive thinking, and increase relaxation. Mandy can create mind pictures of herself as an energetic child or of her leukemia being rid from her body by the chemotherapy.

Many health care practitioners believe in the power of healing touch. Massage therapy involves touch and different methods of stroking and kneading the muscles of the body. The nurse can refer Mandy to a licensed massage therapist for massage therapy.

Mandy can learn several techniques for relieving tension at home between visits to the massage therapist. The nurse can teach these simple techniques. Mandy should find a comfortable, quiet environment. Taking slow, deep breaths will promote relaxation. Instructions for muscle tension and release are as follows: Breathe in through the nose, tensing the toes. Then breathe out through the mouth, releasing the tension and relaxing completely. Take several deep breaths, enjoying the relaxed state. Continue the process with all muscle groups, progressing from toe to head.

Meditation is a relaxation technique and state of mind allowing the client to focus his or her energy and thoughts. In meditation, the client can repeat a positive word or short phrase. For example, Mandy could repeat, "I have energy. My body is healing." The nurse should assess the family's spiritual beliefs. If prayer is a familiar practice, it should be encouraged. Prayer can provide strength, comfort, and inspiration throughout the cancer experience. The nurse may also want to refer Mandy to a pastor or priest.

The nurse can assist Mandy in becoming aware of her breathing. Paying attention to rate and depth of breathing can assist Mandy in recognizing stress and promoting states of relaxation. The following instructions can be used to teach breathing awareness: Ask the client to sit up straight, placing one hand, palm down, over the abdomen with the other hand on top; ask the client to breathe in and out normally, paying attention to how the abdomen rises and falls; and encourage the client to imagine a balloon in the abdomen, expanding during inspiration and collapsing during expiration. Mandy can be encouraged to slow her rate and rhythm of breathing when she detects stress in her life.

Yoga is described as a science of the inner world of the body and mind consciousness. It involves stretching, muscle tone, and relaxation. Yoga can be learned by taking a class, reading a book, or watching a DVD. The nurse can refer Mandy to available resources.

Music therapy can enhance physical comfort and reduce fatigue. Music is effective by activating the right brain and stimulating the autonomic nervous system. The nurse should encourage Mandy to decrease unpleasant noises by using earphones and turning off the television and radio, which can increase anxiety. If Mandy has an MP3 player, she can create a file of music to aid in relaxation. The nurse can assist Mandy in obtaining resources for relaxing music.

Pet therapy has been shown to improve the life span of clients, decrease blood pressure, and increase relaxation. Caring for a pet or just having a pet present is a source of comfort and provides a distraction or focus for clients. Interactions with pets allow clients to exercise their nurturing instinct and to feel safe and accepted unconditionally. The nurse can help Mandy and her family decide if a pet is appropriate for their lifestyle. Any pet—a dog, a cat, a bird, or a fish—could be beneficial for Mandy.

To assist Mandy, her mother, and the nurse in evaluating her fatigue level and the interventions implemented, Mandy should keep a journal of her diet, activity, and fatigue level. Mandy and her mom should review this daily and make adjustments as needed. Mandy should also bring this journal to her health care visits for review.

Alopecia

The nurse can help Mandy learn to care correctly for her hair and scalp during chemotherapy treatments. A mild shampoo, soft hair brush, and low heat during drying of the hair can help minimize hair loss. Using chemicals such as hair color, perms, or relaxing agents can irritate the scalp and increase the risk of hair loss. The nurse might suggest a shorter hairstyle. This would make hair loss easier to accept. Suggestions for preventing sun damage to the scalp include regular use of sunscreen and wearing a head covering such as a hat, cap, or scarf when outdoors.

When hair loss occurs, Mandy will need information about covering her head if she so chooses. Discuss alternative hairstyles or cuts that might make hair loss less traumatic. Children with shorter hair may be, but are not always, less upset with hair loss than those with much longer hair. Some children decide to purchase a wig prior to complete hair loss to obtain a more correct color and style match. A hairstylist can assist Mandy in styling her wig. The nurse can help Mandy's mom file for health insurance reimbursement, because the cost of a wig is typically covered when the client is receiving chemotherapy.

Anger and depression are common emotions expressed by clients who lose their hair. The nurse can assist Mandy and her mom in dealing with these emotions. The complementary therapies described here might be effective. Talking or journaling about the emotions may also prove to be helpful. The nurse may be able to put Mandy in contact with another young girl who has experienced hair loss during chemotherapy.

SELF-REFLECTION

What is your reaction when you see a child with alopecia? Shock? Horror? Pity? Sorrow? What unspoken messages are given to children when we compliment their hair? What messages are conveyed when we express approval only when their hair is well groomed and neat?

SUGGESTED RESOURCES

Leukemia and Lymphoma Society. The website provides information to health care professionals and the public on leukemia and lymphoma.

National Cancer Institute. The government website provides information to health care professionals and the public on various types of cancer.

NURSING CARE PLAN CHART

The Child Undergoing Chemotherapy

GOAL	INTERVENTION	RATIONALE	EXPECTED OUTCOME
1. <u>N</u>ausea related to side effects of chemotherapy			
The child will report relief from nausea			The child is able to ingest food and fluids without gastric distress.
	Apply cool, damp cloth to the child's forehead, neck, and wrists	*The application of cold to these sensitive areas improves nausea*	
	Reduce exposure to odor-producing substances and food	*Strong odors can elicit or accentuate nausea*	
	Administer antiemetics as prescribed	*These can help the child avoid and eliminate nausea*	
The family will be able to identify interventions that decrease nausea	Teach the family to avoid cooking in the child's presence	*Strong odors can elicit or accentuate nausea*	The family reports feeling confident that they can assist the child in managing nausea.
	Assist the child in restricting fluids 1 hours before and after meals	*Fluids on an empty stomach often accentuate nausea*	
2. Imbalanced <u>N</u>utrition: Less Than Body Requirements related to nausea and reduced caloric intake			
The child will report an adequate intake of nutritional foods with an improved energy level	Ascertain the types of food the child prefers	*The child is more likely to ingest foods that are preferred*	The child is able to eat the amount of calories prescribed on a daily basis. The child does not lose weight.
	Create an environment where meals can be enjoyed	*Odors, sights, and distractions can prevent the child from eating*	
	Consult with a dietitian as necessary	*The dietitian is trained to develop meal plans for special situations*	
The family will be able to provide the child with an acceptable diet	Teach the client and family about easily digestible foods such as broth, gelatin, and bananas	*When the child is nauseated and fatigued, these food will be easier to digest and assist them in avoiding nausea*	The family is able to plan and prepare meals that are pleasing to the child.
	Provide the family with information about when they should contact the physician	*The family needs to contact the physician if the child is lethargic, has dry mucous membranes, and is losing weight*	

growth. They must undergo a bone marrow aspiration in order to harvest the stem cells. Box 14-8 ■ provides more information on bone marrow aspiration. Harvested stem cells may be frozen until transplantation if necessary.

The healthy stem cells are transplanted to the ill child through an intravenous infusion. During the 2 to 4 weeks that the stem cells are reproducing, the child experiences **pancytopenia.** Pancytopenia is a state of decreased RBCs, WBCs, and platelets. During this time the child is at risk for infection, anemia, and bleeding.

Following the period of stem cell reproduction, the child is at risk for developing graft-versus-host disease. Even though tissue typing has been done, in some cases the

---

BOX 14-8

Bone Marrow Aspiration

Bone marrow aspiration is a painful procedure, so it is necessary to discuss the procedure with the child and the family. The child should be sedated for bone marrow aspiration. The child is positioned in either the prone or supine position. The aspiration site, usually the iliac crest or sternum, is prepped with Betadine. A needle with stylet is inserted through the skin into the bone. Once the stylet is removed, a 10-mL syringe is attached and bone marrow is aspirated. The child must remain on bed rest for 1 hour after the procedure. The nurse monitors vital signs, observes for signs of bleeding, and provides pain management.

child's body will have an immunologic (allergic) response to the donor cells. If symptoms of graft-versus-host disease occur within 100 days of the transplant, it is said to be an acute episode. In acute *graft-versus-host disease*, a pruritic rash begins on the extremities and progresses to the trunk. The child's skin may blister and feel as if it is burning. There may also be nausea, vomiting, diarrhea, and abdominal pain. Liver involvement may develop.

If symptoms of graft-versus-host disease occur more than 100 days after the transplant, it is said to be a chronic episode. The symptoms of chronic graft-versus-host disease include frequent infections that are not easily treated, thrombocytopenia, ulcers of the mouth, throat, and esophagus, and dry, irritated eyes. Both acute and chronic graft-versus-host disease is treated with immunosuppressant drugs such as prednisone, methotrexate, and cyclosporine.

NURSING CARE

PRIORITIES IN NURSING CARE

When caring for children with hematologic and lymphatic system disorders, priority nursing care includes improving tissue perfusion, infection prevention, injury prevention, improving nutritional status, adequate pain management, and improving activity intolerance. Administer iron replacement therapy as ordered. Encourage dietary intake of foods containing iron. Provide a safe environment for the child. Implement measures to prevent the spread of harmful bacteria. Provide pharmacologic and nonpharmacologic pain methods. Assist the child with activities of daily living (ADLs) and encourage periods of rest.

ASSESSING

To assess clients with these disorders adequately, the nurse should obtain a complete history, including past medical history and family history. Baseline physical data include weight, height, vital signs, inspection of the skin, nails, and mouth, and palpation of the lymph nodes.

DIAGNOSIS, PLANNING, AND IMPLEMENTING

Some common nursing diagnoses for children with these disorders include:

- Ineffective **T**issue Perfusion related to reduced hemoglobin content of the blood
- Risk for **I**nfection related to excessive white blood cell production
- Risk for **I**njury related to hematologic alterations

- Imbalanced **N**utrition: Less than Body Requirements related to inadequate dietary intake of iron
- Acute **P**ain related to hematologic alterations
- **A**ctivity Intolerance related to decreased oxygen supply

Outcomes for these children include:

- Tissue perfusion improves as evidenced by sensation, temperature, and color within normal limits.
- Child will be free of symptoms of infection.
- Child will avoid physical injury.
- Laboratory values will be within normal limits.
- Child will state that pain level is improved.
- Child will participate in ADLs without symptoms of fatigue.

For children with hematologic and lymphatic system disorders, the following interventions apply:

- Monitor fluid, electrolyte, and laboratory status. *Slight changes in these values could further compromise tissue perfusion.*
- Evaluate capillary refill, peripheral pulses, and edema. *Alteration in these findings may indicate compromised tissue perfusion.*
- Instruct the child and parents on the importance of hand washing. *Hand washing minimizes exposure to harmful bacteria.*
- Encourage the child and parents to avoid contact with individuals who are known to be ill. *This minimizes the child's exposure to harmful bacteria and viruses.*
- Assist the child with ambulation, prn. *Assistance with ambulation can prevent falls.*
- Remove environmental hazards. *Poor lighting, walkway obstructions, and stairways are examples of environmental hazards that may contribute to the risk for injury.*
- Assess diet for nutritional content. *Accurate evaluation of the child's diet gives the nurse data for developing a teaching plan specific to his or her client.*
- Develop a meal plan to increase the dietary intake of iron. *A specific plan will take into consideration a child's likes and dislikes and improve compliance.*
- Teach the use of nonpharmacologic methods of pain relief. *Nonpharmacologic methods of pain relief can supplement pharmacologic methods and assist in the reduction of pain.*
- Correctly administer pharmacologic pain relief methods. *The correct administration of pharmacologic agents for pain relief will be most effective.*
- Prioritize daily activities. *The child will have energy for important activities and not be tired by activities that are unnecessary.*
- Encourage frequent periods of rest. *Rest can restore the child's energy levels.*

EVALUATING

The nurse collects data for frequent assessment of the child with these disorders to determine effectiveness of treatment. The goal of treatment for children with hematologic disorders is a return to normal blood count levels. The child's energy level will return to normal, and they will be free of infection and hemorrhage. The child with lymphatic disorders will be free of infection and edema.

NURSING PROCESS CARE PLAN
Client with Sickle Cell Anemia

An 8-year-old girl was admitted yesterday to the facility in sickle cell crisis. Her family was vacationing when the crisis began, and they drove several hours back by car in order to admit their daughter to her "home" hospital. A blood transfusion and fluids have been administered. She is receiving oxygen at 2 liters per minute. The parents state that their son has a cold, but that they "were sure Yolanda did not have it" when they started their trip. When you enter the room, Yolanda is moaning. She cries when you say it is time to reposition her in bed. She states she does not want to have a position change because "it hurts too much to move."

Assessment. When caring for Yolanda, the following data should be collected:

- Status of pain: location, intensity, duration, alleviating factors
- Vital signs
- Intake and output
- Skin (pallor, cyanosis, tenting)
- Review of lab work

Nursing Diagnosis. The following important nursing diagnosis (among others) is established for this client:

- Acute **P**ain related to sickle cell crisis resulting from vasoocclusion in lower extremities

Expected Outcome. Client will state pain relief sufficient to allow movement, position changes, and range-of-motion exercises.

Planning and Implementation

- Administer pain medication promptly. *Pain of sickle cell is difficult for the child to manage and should be addressed before it becomes too severe.*
- Position the child carefully. *Careful positioning can prevent undue pain in joints and extremities.*
- Encourage the child and the family to notify the nurse if pain-relieving measures are not successful. *Management of the child's pain must include using alternative measures if the currently prescribed methods are not effective.*
- Ask the child and the family about nonpharmacologic pain relief measures that have been helpful in the past. Use these nonpharmacologic measures when providing care. *Nonpharmacologic measures complement pain medications.*

Evaluation. Yolanda reports that warm compresses prior to position changes reduce the discomfort and make movement easier.

Critical Thinking in the Nursing Process

1. What conditions may have led to the sickle cell crisis?
2. When performing physical interventions with this client, what concern will be most important?
3. What nonpharmacologic interventions can be used in this situation?

Note: Discussion of Critical Thinking questions appears in Appendix I.

Note: The reference and resource listings for this and all chapters have been compiled at the back of the book.

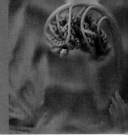

Chapter Review

 KEY TERMS by Topic

Use the audio glossary feature of either the CD-ROM or the Companion Website to hear the correct pronunciation of the following key terms.

Anatomy and Physiology
hematology, hematopoiesis, plasma, erythrocytes, erythropoiesis, hemolysis, leukocytes, thrombocytes, agglutination

Bleeding Disorders
hemophilia, idiopathic thrombocytopenic purpura, purpura, petechiae, ecchymosis, remission, melena

Anemias
anemia, iron-deficiency anemia, pica, sickle cell anemia, sickling, vaso-occlusion, sickle cell crisis, arthralgia, hemosiderosis

Thalassemia
hemosiderin, hydrops fetalis

Cancers of Hematologic or Lymphatic Systems
staging, stomatitis, leukemia, acute lymphoblastic leukemia, acute myelogenous leukemia

Hematopoietic Stem Cell Transplantation
autologous donor, isogeneic donor, syngeneic donor, allogeneic donor, pancytopenia

KEY Points

- The primary oxygen-carrying cell in the body is the erythrocyte or red blood cell.

- The primary cell in the body that helps prevent infections is the leukocyte or white blood cell.

- The primary cell in the body that assists with clotting is the thrombocyte or platelet.

- The priority nursing intervention when caring for a child with hemophilia is to prevent bleeding.

- Emergency measures are necessary to control bleeding of the child with hemophilia. These include applying pressure, elevating the site, applying ice, monitoring vital signs, and obtaining venous access.

- When caring for the child with iron-deficiency anemia, the nurse must teach the child and family about adequate dietary sources of iron.

- Liquid iron preparation causes staining of the teeth. The nurse can administer these preparations through a straw to prevent this complication.

- A common complication of iron supplementation is constipation. Fluids, exercise, and fiber are appropriate preventative measures for this complication.

- Children who suffer from sickle cell crises experience pain. The nurse must be vigilant in assisting the child to properly manage his or her pain.

- Common types of leukemia in children include acute lymphoblastic leukemia (ALL) and acute myelogenous leukemia (AML).

- Preventing infection in children with leukemia is a priority nursing intervention.

- Children, especially adolescents, must be assisted by the nurse in dealing with the side effects of antineoplastic drugs, which include bone marrow depression, nausea, vomiting, stomatitis, and hair loss.

 EXPLORE MediaLink

Additional interactive resources for this chapter can be found on the Companion Website at www.prenhall.com/adams.

Click on Chapter 14 and "Begin" to select the activities for this chapter.

For chapter-related NCLEX®-style questions and an audio glossary, access the accompanying CD-ROM in this book.

Animations:
Sickle cell anemia

Leukemia

Blood pressure

Hemodynamics

⊕ FOR FURTHER Study

For more information on nursing care related to epistaxis, see Chapter 12.

Disorders of the cardiovascular system are discussed in Chapter 13.

More information on child abuse can be found in Chapter 16.

Musculoskeletal signs of child abuse are described in Box 20-7.

Disorders of the immune system are discussed in Chapter 22.

Critical Thinking Care Map

Client with Hodgkin's Lymphoma
NCLEX-PN® Focus Area: Physiological Integrity: Reduction of Risk Potential

Case Study: Yolanda is a 15-year-old Black female recently diagnosed with Hodgkin's lymphoma. She has completed her first cycle of chemotherapy. She and her mother ask what they should expect over the next few weeks.

Nursing Diagnosis: Risk for Infection related to immunocompromised status following chemotherapy

COLLECT DATA

Subjective	Objective
_____	_____
_____	_____
_____	_____
_____	_____
_____	_____
_____	_____

Would you report this? Yes/No

If yes, to: _____

Nursing Care

_____
_____
_____
_____
_____
_____
_____

How would you document this? _____
_____
_____
_____
_____

Compare your documentation to the sample provided in Appendix I.

Data Collected
(use only those that apply)

- Current weight 110 lb
- Mother reports that Mandy's best friend has the flu
- Vital signs: T 99.0, P 59, R 12, BP 120/80
- States that she wants to see her friends as soon as possible and go to the movies
- Family history of breast cancer
- Height 5 ft, 4 in.
- WBC count 5,000 mm^3
- "The doctor said I could go about my normal life."

Nursing Interventions
(use only those that apply; list in priority order)

- Monitor white blood cell count.
- Encourage frequent mouth care regime.
- Teach client to monitor for symptoms of infection such as fever, redness, and cold symptoms.
- Teach good hand washing habits.
- Assess client's spiritual beliefs.
- Screen visitors for those that may be ill.
- Facilitate communication between client and his or her family.
- Avoid large crowds.
- Encourage well-balanced diet high in protein.

1 The nurse is caring for a pediatric client with sickle cell anemia. The parents ask the nurse about the causes of the disease. Which response by the nurse best describes the cause of this disease?

1. "It is caused by a recessive trait that primarily affects African Americans."
2. "It is caused by a demand for iron in the bloodstream."
3. "It is an inherited disorder caused by abnormal hemoglobin synthesis."
4. "It is a rare, malignant disorder of the lymphatic system."

2 The nurse is instructing the father of a child with sickle cell anemia about sickle cell crisis and causes. The father verbalizes understanding, but the nurse realizes more instruction is needed when the father identifies which of the following as a major contributor in a sickle cell crisis?

1. Iron deficiency
2. Fever
3. Stress
4. Vomiting

3 The nursing instructor is conducting a lecture about hematologic disorders in children and leads the discussion about the causes of thalassemia. The nurse tells the students that children who are at greatest risk for this blood disorder are those who are of:

1. German American heritage.
2. Australian descent.
3. Swedish descent.
4. Mediterranean descent.

4 The nurse knows that which of the following blood values indicate sickle cell disease?

1. High Hgb and low reticulocyte count
2. Low Hgb and low reticulocyte count
3. High Hgb and high reticulocyte count
4. Low Hgb and high reticulocyte count

5 A nurse is reading the health record of her client with Hodgkin's disease. Which of the following symptoms would the nurse expect to see in the record considering the diagnosis?

1. Tender, soft lymph nodes in the femoral area
2. Nontender, soft tumors in the abdominal area
3. Nontender, hard lymph nodes in the cervical area
4. Tender, soft tumors in the popliteal area

6 The nurse has just completed teaching the parents of a child who has started chemotherapy. The mother has been instructed about infection control during therapy. The nurse realizes the mother understands the teaching when she says:

1. "I will make sure to keep my child away from public places to prevent infection."

2. "It is all right for my child to go skiing as long as I give him vitamin C to prevent infection."
3. "The chemotherapy won't affect my son as long as he eats well."
4. "My son doesn't have to have blood tests until the chemotherapy has ended."

7 The nursing instructor asks a nursing student in the class to describe acute lymphoblastic leukemia (ALL). The instructor realizes the nursing student does not need further instruction in the disease when the student states:

1. "ALL occurs when cancer cells develop in the bone marrow."
2. "ALL is the overproduction of immature lymphocytes."
3. "ALL is a rare hereditary sex-linked disorder."
4. "ALL is a malignant disorder of the lymphatic system."

8 The nurse is reviewing the physician's orders for a child with hemophilia. Indicate the orders that the nurse might expect to see written in the child's chart.

1. Avoid rectal temperatures.
2. Avoid unnecessary invasive procedures.
3. Avoid salicylates.
4. Avoid carbonated beverages.
5. Avoid rectal suppositories.

9 A 5-year-old child is hospitalized with a suspected diagnosis of idiopathic thrombocytopenic purpura. The laboratory technician has just drawn the child's blood. Because of the suspected diagnosis, the nurse expects to see the following results on the child's lab report:

1. Increased platelet count, positive Coombs' test
2. Decreased platelet count, increased antiplatelet antibodies
3. Positive direct Coombs' test, absence of antinuclear antibodies
4. Decreased platelet count and antiplatelet antibodies

10 The nurse is discussing iron-deficiency anemia and knows the child with this disorder may crave substances that are not food. Select the following substances that children with this disorder may crave and eat:

1. Dirt
2. Hair
3. Olives
4. Starch
5. Bananas
6. Chalk
7. Glue

Answers for NCLEX-PN® Review and Critical Thinking questions appear in Appendix I.

Chapter 15

Care of the Child with Neurologic and Sensory Disorders

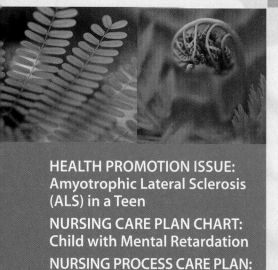

HEALTH PROMOTION ISSUE:
Amyotrophic Lateral Sclerosis
(ALS) in a Teen

NURSING CARE PLAN CHART:
Child with Mental Retardation

NURSING PROCESS CARE PLAN:
Child with Cerebral Palsy

CRITICAL THINKING CARE MAP:
Caring for a Client with
Meningitis

BRIEF Outline

LEARNING Outcomes

After completing this chapter, you will be able to:

1. Define key terms.
2. Discuss the anatomy and physiology of the pediatric neurologic system.
3. Describe common neurologic disorders as they relate to pediatric clients.
4. Explain appropriate nursing interventions for children with neurologic disorders.
5. Describe disorders of the eye and ear in children.
6. Explain appropriate nursing interventions for children with disorders of the eye and ear.

The child's neurologic system is not fully developed at birth. As the child ages, senses become more refined, control of muscles and bodily functions improves, and cognitive development occurs steadily. Disorders of the neurological system can cause this development to be hindered or arrested altogether. This chapter will discuss the disorders of the neurological system and the nursing care appropriate for children who are diagnosed with them.

Anatomy and Physiology

The nervous system can be divided into two parts: the central nervous system (CNS) and the peripheral nervous system (PNS). The CNS includes the brain and the spinal cord. The PNS includes the nerves, **ganglia** (groups of nerve cell bodies located in the PNS), and sensory receptors.

CENTRAL NERVOUS SYSTEM

Neurons are the nerve cells that transmit impulses from one part of the body to another. Each neuron contains three parts: the cell body, the axon, and the dendrite. The **axon** is a fiber carrying the impulse away from the **cell body** (the part of the cell that contains the nucleus and cytoplasm). The **dendrite** conducts the electrical impulses toward the cell body (Figure 15-1 ■). At birth, the infant has the same number of neurons as an adult, but the infant does not have the connecting axons and dendrites until later in childhood (Figure 15-2 ■).

At birth, the axons in a child's body are lacking **myelination** (development of the myelin sheath around the nerve fiber), and this allows for the presence of newborn reflexes. The **myelin sheath** is the lipoprotein covering of the axon. As the infant ages, myelination develops in a **cephalocaudal** (head to toe) direction. The process of myelination improves voluntary control of the muscles,

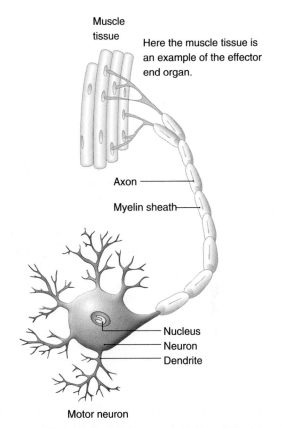

Figure 15-1. ■ Structures of the neuron. The dendrites bring information to the nucleus. The axon carries messages away from the nerve cell.

enabling the child to develop fine and gross motor skills and coordination.

Brain

Fetal development of the brain and spinal cord begins in the 3rd week of pregnancy. The nervous system is most vulnerable to harmful substances such as drugs, alcohol, cigarettes,

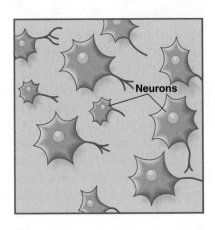
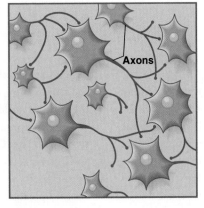
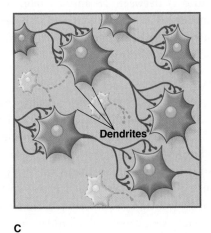

A   **B**   **C**

Figure 15-2. ■ The developing brain. (**A**) At birth, the infant's brain has a complete set of neurons but relatively few synaptic connections. (**B**) During the first year, the axons grow longer, the dendrites increase in number, and a surplus of new connections is formed. (**C**) Over the next few years, active connections are strengthened, while unused connections atrophy. (Reprinted from Kassin, S. [2001]. *Psychology* [3rd ed.]. Upper Saddle River, NJ: Prentice Hall.)

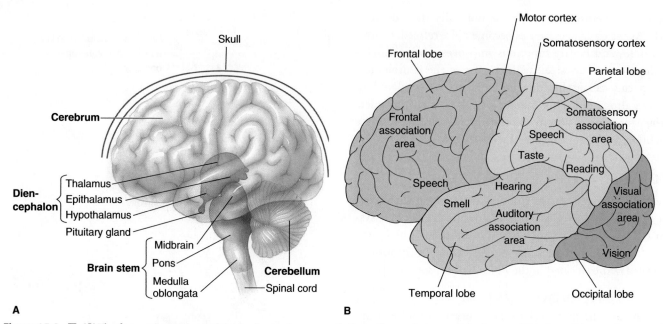

Figure 15-3. ■ (**A**) The four major regions of the brain: cerebrum, cerebellum, diencephalon, and brainstem. (**B**) Lobes of the cerebrum and functional areas of the cerebral cortex. The illustration shows what areas of the cerebrum are associated with what senses.

chemicals, and infection during the period of **organogenesis** (formation of organs, days 15 to 60 of pregnancy).

The developing brain is an intricate, delicate structure composed of many structures. There are four main regions of the brain: the cerebrum, the diencephalons, the brainstem, and the cerebellum (Figure 15-3 ■). It is important to understand the functions of each region.

At birth, the bony structure or **cranium** surrounding the brain is not fully fused, which allows for growth of the brain. Two sites of connective tissue joining the bones of the cranium are the anterior fontanel and the posterior fontanel (Figure 15-4 ■). The anterior fontanel closes when the child is between 18 and 24 months. The posterior fontanel closes around 2 months. The bones of the cranium are fully developed by age 12. Until then, risk of injury to the head and brain is greater.

Spinal Cord

The spinal cord is the structure extending from the brainstem to the lumbar region. It is surrounded and protected by the vertebrae. It supplies nerve impulses to the brain along the ascending and descending pathways. The ascending pathways transmit sensory impulses, and the descending pathways transmit motor impulses. Review Figure 15-5 ■ to understand the areas governed by each section of the spinal cord.

Physical sensation and stimulation are important to development. Children who are deprived of normal amounts of physical stimulation may develop broad developmental or emotional deficits (Box 15-1 ■). Likewise, overstimulation can have dramatic negative effects, especially

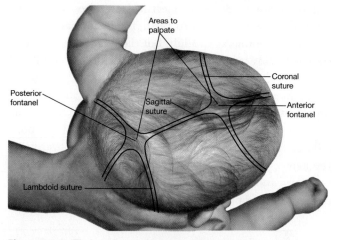

Figure 15-4. ■ Anterior and posterior fontanels.

in premature infants. Nursing care must take into account the importance of stimulation in the health and healing of infants and children (Box 15-2 ■).

Cerebrospinal fluid (CSF) transports nutrients and removes waste. CSF is the clear, colorless fluid that nourishes and cushions the brain and spinal cord. (See Figure 15-12 to note the circulation pattern of CSF.) CSF is formed in the choroid plexus and contains protein, vitamin C, glucose, and a few blood cells. In infancy, the child produces 100 mL of CSF/day. In adulthood, 500 mL are produced daily. CSF provides a cushion surrounding the brain and spinal cord and, therefore, protects these organs from trauma. The CSF also transports nutrients and removes waste.

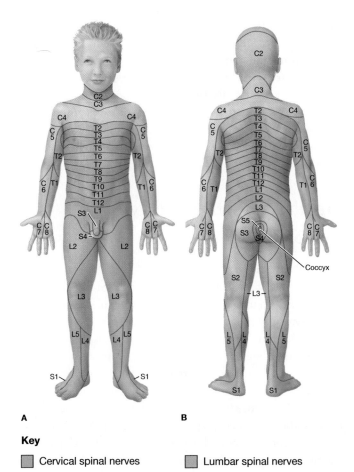

A   **B**

Key

☐ Cervical spinal nerves   ☐ Lumbar spinal nerves

☐ Thoracic spinal nerves   ☐ Sacral spinal nerves

Figure 15-5. ■ (**A**) Anterior dermatomes of the body. (**B**) Posterior dermatomes of the body.

Intracranial Pressure

Intracranial pressure (ICP) is defined as the force exerted within the cranial cavity by the brain, blood, and CSF. Normal pressure is 0 to 12 mm Hg. Until closure of the

---

BOX 15-1   CLIENT TEACHING

Importance of Emotional and Physical Care

Researchers (Wismer Fries, Ziegler, Kurian, Jacoris, & Pollack, 2005) studied 18 4-year-olds who had lived in Eastern European orphanages for an average of 16.6 months. These children were adopted into American families. After living with these families for an average of 34.6 months, the researchers studied hormone levels and compared them with 21 children of similar age who lived with biologic parents.

The hormone levels of oxytocin and arginine vasopressin were found to be lower in the children who had come from the orphanages. These hormones have been linked to the ability to form social bonds. This study raises the question of the long-term effects of neglect early in life. Nurses can use this study to develop teaching plans that encourage parents to provide both emotional and physical care to their children from birth.

BOX 15-2   COMPLEMENTARY THERAPIES

Music as an Aid in the NICU

Premature infants in the neonatal intensive care unit (NICU) are often bombarded with sounds, lights, and other excessive stimuli. These excessive stimuli can have negative effects on the improvement of the infant's condition. Simple positive changes in the environment of the NICU can have positive effects on the premature infant. One of these changes is using music therapy. Music therapy is defined as healing with music, voice, or sound. Several research studies have found music therapy to be effective in the NICU. Infants, after being exposed to calming music, were less likely to experience high arousal states, had shorter hospital stays, and weighed more than infants who were not exposed to music.

Olson (1998) provided six principles essential to the effective use of music therapy. (1) Music is a method of demonstrating caring. (2) Music has emotional and physical effects and can facilitate the healing process. (3) Music can bring a human approach to a clinical environment. (4) Music is a method of individualizing client care. (5) Tone, rhythm, pitch, and volume of music can create a peaceful environment. (6) Music of the child's religious faith provides spiritual care to the client.

---

fontanels, the infant can adapt more easily to ICP changes. The body compensates for increased ICP by shunting or diverting CSF and reducing cerebral blood flow. Early signs of increased ICP are headache, vomiting, level of consciousness changes, asymmetric pupils, and seizures. In the infant, a high-pitched cry, bulging fontanels, dilated scalp veins, and irritability may be noted. Later signs include significant changes in level of consciousness (LOC), respiratory distress, bradycardia, increased systolic blood pressure, fixed and dilated pupils, and death.

PERIPHERAL NERVOUS SYSTEM

The PNS consists of 31 pairs of spinal nerves, 12 pairs of cranial nerves, and somatic and autonomic reflexes. **Somatic reflexes** are those that control skeletal muscle contractions. **Autonomic reflexes** are those that control cardiac and smooth muscles and the glands.

Autonomic Nervous System

The autonomic nervous system (ANS) provides control of homeostasis within the body through the sympathetic nervous system and the parasympathetic nervous system. The **sympathetic nervous system** provides assistance to a person in a stressful or life-threatening situation (*right side* of Figure 15-6 ■). In response to frightening stimuli, the sympathetic nervous system causes physical changes that allow the person to respond quickly to danger (sometimes called "fight or flight" response). These changes include dilated pupils; diaphoresis; tachycardia;

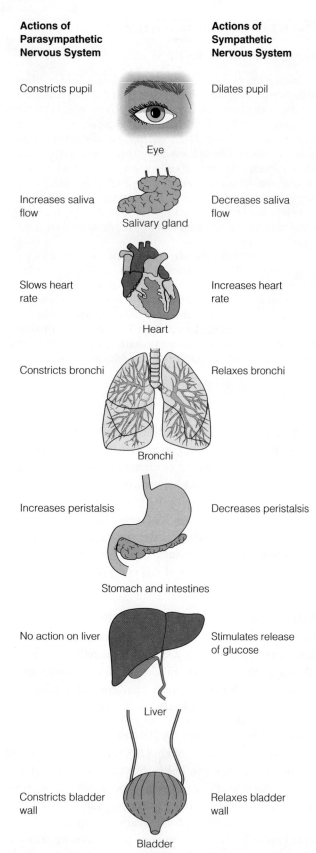

Actions of Parasympathetic Nervous System		Actions of Sympathetic Nervous System
Constricts pupil	Eye	Dilates pupil
Increases saliva flow	Salivary gland	Decreases saliva flow
Slows heart rate	Heart	Increases heart rate
Constricts bronchi	Bronchi	Relaxes bronchi
Increases peristalsis	Stomach and intestines	Decreases peristalsis
No action on liver	Liver	Stimulates release of glucose
Constricts bladder wall	Bladder	Relaxes bladder wall

Figure 15-6. ■ Autonomic nervous system and the organs it affects. (*Left side*) the actions of the parasympathetic nervous system. (*Right side*) the actions of the sympathetic nervous system.

dilation of bronchioles; decreased digestion; decreased urine output; and increased blood clotting, metabolic rate, and mental alertness.

The **parasympathetic nervous system** (*left side* of Figure 15-6) controls bodily processes in nonstressful situations. Clinical manifestations of parasympathetic nervous stimulation include constriction of pupils, decreased heart rate, constriction of bronchioles, and increased peristalsis.

Brief Assessment Review

HISTORY

All Children

Because neurologic disorders in children could be the result of incidents occurring during fetal development, obtaining a history of the pregnancy is an important aspect of assessment. The nurse should ask about drug use, infections, birth trauma, and complications in the immediate postpartum period. The Apgar score of the newborn may be the first screening tool used to determine neurological disorders. See Procedure 8-5 ⬀. The birth weight of the child could indicate prematurity or nutritional status. By assessing the mental status and reasoning ability of both parents, the nurse can gain information that will be useful in planning and implementing care for the child.

Infants

- Ask parents about tremors, unusual movements, irritability, and difficulties sucking or swallowing.
- Ask about intestinal cramps or colic.

Toddlers and Preschoolers

- Assess the child's ability to communicate, both verbally and nonverbally. Compare to the expected developmental level.
- Ask about headaches or seizure activity. Obtain as detailed a description as possible.
- Inquire about the child's behavior, including fears, concerns, aggressive behaviors, and attention span.

School-Age Children and Adolescents

The school-age child and adolescent may be reluctant to discuss some aspects of their behavior with parents present. The nurse should provide privacy and maintain confidentiality within legal requirements and facility policy.

- Ask about general mood or noticeable changes in behavior.
- Inquire about headaches, seizure activity, and alcohol or drug consumption.

PHYSICAL

Infants

- Measure head circumference. Compare the measurements with the normal range for the age of the child.
- Palpate the spine for intactness.

- Observe the infant's posture.
- Test the infant's reflexes and reaction to stimuli. See Procedure 8-13, Eliciting Newborn Reflexes ⚭.
- Assess level of consciousness; the Glasgow Coma Scale can be used. See Procedure 15-1 ■.

PROCEDURE 15-1 | # Glasgow Coma Scale

Purpose

- To provide a score related to level of consciousness
- To allow health care providers a benchmark assessment that will allow them to document either improvement or deterioration of the child's neurologic condition

Equipment

- Glasgow Coma Scale (Table 15-1 ■)

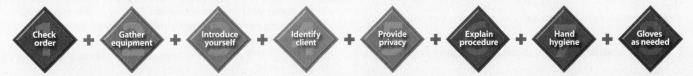

Interventions and Rationales

1. Perform preparatory steps (see icon bar above).
2. Use the Glasgow Coma Scale to assess the child with a neurologic injury or disorder. Assign a score, based on the criteria outlined, for eye opening, verbal response, and motor response.
3. A total score of 15 indicates adequate neurologic function. A total score of 3 indicates neurologic unresponsiveness.
4. Document results and report scores below 15 to the charge nurse.
5. Repeat the Glasgow Coma Scale as necessary.

SAMPLE DOCUMENTATION

(date) 1500   4-year-old-male admitted to pediatric intensive care following closed head injury due to 6-foot fall from tree as reported by father. Glasgow Coma Scale score 5. Score reported to charge nurse. _____
R. Roberts, LPN.

TABLE 15-1

Glasgow Coma Scale

FACULTY MEASURED	RESPONSE	SCORE
Eye opening	Spontaneous	4
	To verbal command	3
	To pain	2
	No response	1
Motor response	To verbal command	6
	To localized pain	5
	Flexes and withdraws	4
	Flexes abnormally	3
	Extends abnormally	2
	No response	1
Verbal response	Oriented, converses	5
	Disoriented, converses	4
	Uses inappropriate words	3
	Makes incomprehensible sounds	2
	No response	1

Note: 15 points = alert and oriented; 8 or less = comatose; totally unresponsive = 3.

Toddlers, Preschoolers, School-Age Children, and Adolescents

- Note general behavior, such as responsiveness and activity level. (See more about behavior and thought process disorders in Chapter 16 🔗.)
- Test balance, coordination, and accuracy related to motor skills.
- Assess sensations of touch, temperature, and pain.
- Assess deep tendon reflexes.
- Assess the child's short- and long-term memory.
- Observe for any signs of abuse. Suspected abuse should be reported to the charge nurse. (See legal information in Chapter 3 and discussion of abuse in Chapter 16 🔗.)

Pain

PHYSIOLOGY

Pain in children can be a result of ischemia, tissue pressure, injury, or tension created by air or fluid filling a body cavity. A pain impulse stimulates the nociceptor, causing *transduction* of pain sensation. The **nociceptors** are sensory receptors that detect and differentiate pain sensation. Following transduction, the pain impulse is transmitted along peripheral sensory nerves to the spinal cord and brain.

PERCEPTION

Pain perception occurs as the pain impulse reaches the brain. Depending on which sensory receptor is stimulated, the child may perceive dull, burning, sharp, localized, cutaneous, somatic, visceral, or chronic pain. The child may express the pain verbally or nonverbally. Verbal expressions of pain include crying, moaning, groaning, or screaming. Nonverbal expressions of pain include facial grimacing, posturing, splinting, restlessness, and sleep disturbances. Box 15-3 ■ provides one mnemonic for assessing pain. See the Pain Assessment section of Chapter 8 🔗 for more nursing information about assessing the child in pain.

PAIN THEORIES

The gate control theory (Figure 15-7 ■), developed by Melzack and Wall in 1965, is the most commonly used theory of pain and pain management. The gate control theory

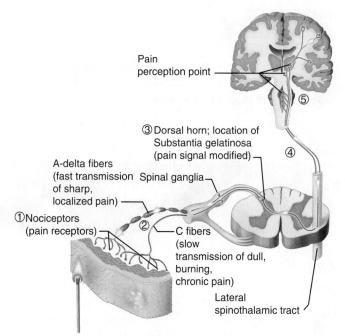

Figure 15-7. ■ In the gate control theory of pain, (1) nerve endings (*nociceptors*) transmit information about injury to the spinal cord via specialized nerve fibers. Biochemical mediators activate the nerve response or sensitize nerve endings. C fibers slowly transmit dull, burning, diffuse, or chronic pain. (2) A-delta fibers quickly transmit sharp, well-localized pain. (3) Depending on other stimuli, the pain signal may be modified at the dorsal horn of the spinal cord (*lower right*). (4) The pain signal is then transmitted to the brain, where perception occurs. (5) At the brain, emotional responses may increase or decrease the intensity of the pain perceived.

proposes that certain actions, if employed, can block pain transduction at the spinal cord before it reaches the brain. These behaviors include touch, distraction, and breathing and relaxation techniques. These are considered nonpharmacologic approaches to pain management.

PAIN MANAGEMENT

Treatment of Pain

The pharmacologic management of pain includes the use of narcotic and nonnarcotic medication. (Refer to Chapter 8 🔗 for discussion of pain as the "fifth vital sign" and for pain assessment, Procedure 8-6 🔗.) When possible, the oral route of administration is preferred for children. Careful dosage

---

BOX 15-3 ASSESSMENT

Pain in Children

Here is a quick way to remember how to assess for pain in children. Use the abbreviation PQRST:

- **P** Precipitating Factors—What caused the pain?
- **Q** Quality and Quantity—Describe the pain. Is it steady, or does it come and go?
- **R** Region, Radiation, and Related Symptoms—Describe the exact location of the pain. Does it radiate to other

parts of the body? What symptoms are associated with the pain?
- **S** Severity—Rate the pain as to its impact (e.g., Can you walk during the pain? Can you continue talking during the pain?).
- **T** Timing—What time of the day or night does the pain occur? Does it occur every day? Is it associated with other activities, such as breathing, lying down, or walking?

calculation is essential in preventing an overdose. If narcotics are used, monitoring the respiratory status is vital because narcotics can depress respiration. Narcotics are usually held if the respiratory is 12 or less. In cases of severe or prolonged pain, a PCA pump may be used (see Figure 7-11 ⚭).

Other nonpharmacologic nursing measures may be effective in the control of pain or enhance the use of pharmacologic methods. Distraction or involving the child in other activities and play can reduce anxiety and the awareness of pain. Massaging or rubbing the area of pain, or rocking and holding the child, provide a stimulus to compete with pain receptors and therefore decrease transmission of pain. The application of heat or cold may reduce swelling, inflammation, and muscle spasm causing the pain. Care must be taken to avoid damage to the skin with either heat or cold.

Pain can be associated with disorders of the neurologic system and also with conditions associated with the eye and ear. Neurologic disorders include congenital defects, infections, trauma, and disorders such as seizures, cerebral palsy, and fibromyalgia.

CONGENITAL NEUROLOGIC DEFECTS

Congenital neurologic defects can have a profound impact on quality of life. Defects vary from spina bifida to Down syndrome (discussed later in this chapter under Mental Retardation).

Spina Bifida

Spina bifida is an incomplete closure of the vertebra and **neural tube** (the fetal tissue that develops into the CNS). The cause of spina bifida is a genetic predisposition with a deficiency of the essential nutrient folic acid. If spina bifida exists, there is a high probability of other congenital defects, including clubfoot, hip defects, and hydrocephalus. The defect can be found anywhere along the spinal column and results in a variety of pathologies. Most commonly, the defect is located in the lumbosacral region. Defects affecting only the vertebrae may not be obvious until the toddler tries to walk.

In larger defects, meningocele or meningomyelocele may result. **Meningocele** is the herniation of the meninges through the vertebral defect. **Myelomeningocele** is a herniation of the spinal nerves and cord, as well as the meninges, through the vertebral defect (Figure 15-8 ■). The outer covering of the defect may be skin or the transparent, fragile meninges. If the spinal cord or spinal nerves are affected, there will be flaccid paralysis, bowel and bladder incontinence, and sensory deficits.

Diagnosis

During pregnancy, mothers can have an alpha-fetoprotein test between 16 and 20 weeks' gestation. This blood test can indicate the presence of neural tube defects. The diagnosis can be confirmed with high-resolution ultrasound prior to birth. After birth, further ultrasounds, x-rays, CT scans, and MRIs can determine the extent of the defect and the involvement of other organs such as the bowel and bladder, if present.

Treatment

Surgical correction to close the defect is completed as soon as possible. If hydrocephalus is present, a shunt may be placed at the same time. (Hydrocephalus is discussed later

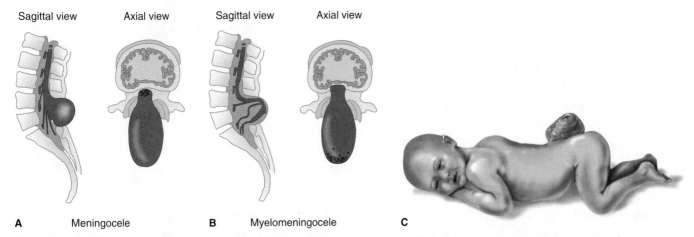

A   Meningocele   **B**   Myelomeningocele   **C**

Figure 15-8. ■ (A) Meningocele. A saclike protrusion through the bony defect in the spinal column containing meninges and cerebrospinal fluid. Sac may be transparent or membranous. **(B)** Myelomeningocele. Saclike herniation through the defect holding meninges, cerebrospinal fluid, and a portion of spinal cord or nerve root. Fluid leakage may occur because the lesion may be poorly covered. This defect is more common than the meningocele; 99% of children with this defect are disabled. **(C)** The infant with a myelomeningocele is placed prone or in a side-lying position, and the exposed sac is protected carefully and kept moist.

in this chapter.) Postoperatively, the infant is observed closely for signs of increased ICP, infection, bowel and bladder function, and movement of extremities. Prognosis is variable, depending on the location and severity of the defect.

Nursing Considerations

It is critical to protect the integrity of the sac until surgical correction can be completed. This is done by wearing sterile gloves and using sterile linens to cover the defect. The linens covering the sac are kept moist with saline. The infant must be positioned so as not to exert pressure on the meninges (see Figure 15-8C). A prone position is typically used. The nurse must monitor carefully for symptoms of infection. The infant should be kept warm. An isolette is appropriate to avoid placing heavy covers over the sac.

Emotional care and tactile stimulation are still vital for this infant. Encourage parents to hold their baby's hand and talk gently to him or her. For feeding, the baby may need to be placed on the parent's lap in a prone position with the head turned to one side. Parents will need assistance from the nurse to accomplish feeding because the baby cannot be held in typical feeding positions.

Postoperatively, the nurse will observe the child for signs of infection, changes in vital signs, and neurologic changes. Observe the skin closely to prevent breakdown from bony prominences of the pelvis as the child lies in the prone position. Change the child's position to side-lying or hold the child upright. Passive range-of-motion exercises are important to prevent contractures. The nurse should observe the infant for urinary and bowel retention because this disorder often causes sensory loss and loss of sphincter control. Older children and adolescents with spina bifida will be taught to perform clean intermittent catheterization to maintain urinary health if bladder defects are present.

Hydrocephalus

Hydrocephalus results from increased production, decreased absorption, or blockage of the flow of CSF. Blockage can be caused by a variety of pathologies, including infections, ventricular hemorrhages, tumors, cysts, or malformations (Figure 15-9 ■). Malformations include:

- *Chiari II malformation* (downward displacement of the cerebellum, brainstem, and fourth ventricle, along with herniation through the foramen magnum into the cervical spaces)
- Stenosis of the aqueduct of Sylvius, a recessive X-linked disorder
- *Dandy-Walker syndrome* (a disruption of fetal brain development in which the fourth ventricle enlarges into a cyst). Ventricles can be seen in Figure 15-12.

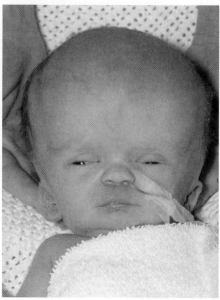

A

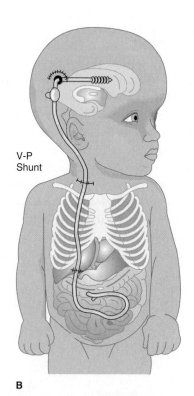

V-P
Shunt

B

Figure 15-9. ■ (A) Infant with hydrocephalus. **(B)** A ventriculoperitoneal shunt, which allows fluid to leave the cranial cavity and so reduces intracranial pressure, is usually placed at 3 to 4 months of age.

Manifestations

Sometimes hydrocephalus is obvious at birth, but more commonly it develops over time. The classic symptoms of hydrocephalus include the child's head circumference being greater than normal, with the forehead and top of